TEXTBOOK OF GYNECOLOGY

VOLUME 2:
DISORDERS, THERAPEUTICS, AND ADVANCES IN PELVIC HEALTH

Dr. Beatriz Lezama

ALLIED
HEALTH
PRESS

Textbook of Gynecology

Volume 2: Disorders, Therapeutics, and Advances in Pelvic Health

Author: **Dr. Beatriz Lezama**

Allied Health Press
4164 Lakeshore Road
Burlington ON L7L 1A4
Canada
www.alliedhealthpress.com
Email: orders@arclereducation.com

ISBN: 978-1-77956-848-9

ABOUT THE AUTHOR

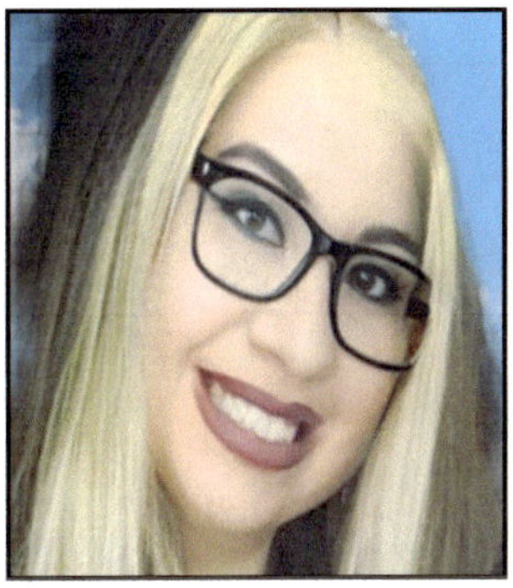

Dr. Beatriz Lezama is a pediatric specialist and fellow in neonatology, with a strong clinical foundation and a passion for early-life care. She holds certifications in general ultrasound, vascular Doppler, and maternal-fetal Doppler, enhancing her diagnostic and perinatal care skills. In addition to her clinical work, Dr. Lezama is an active health communicator and blog writer, with several health-focused articles published on LinkedIn. Her work bridges expert pediatric knowledge with accessible public education, promoting wellness and informed care for families and communities.

Brief Table of Contents

Getting Started with This Book

Chapter Openers

A list of Chapter Outline is presented providing a brief Introduction to what will be covered in the chapter.

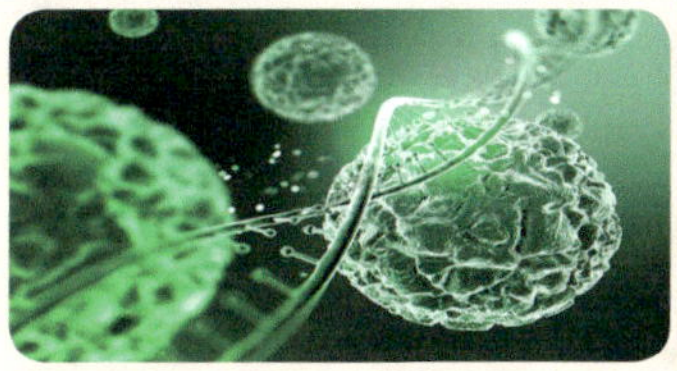

LEARNING OBJECTIVES

After studying this chapter, you will be able to:

1. Discuss the scientific method in biology;
2. Explain the cell theory;
3. Discuss the genetics and heredity;
4. Evolution and natural selection;
5. Focus on ecology and ecosystems;
6. Learn about human biology;
7. Evaluate the plant biology;
8. Explain the microbiology;
9. Focus on current trends in biology.

Introduction

Often referred to as the science of life, biology is a broad field of study aimed at comprehending the several kinds of life on Earth, from tiny creatures to sophisticated multicellular entities. Comprising several subfields, including molecular biology, ecology, and evolutionary biology, each of which advances our knowledge of living systems, this field clarifies the mechanisms controlling life events, including development, reproduction, and interaction with the surroundings, which is the central goal of biology. Moreover, biology fills in the void between the natural sciences and medicine by offering a necessary understanding of health, illness, and the interactions between organisms and their environments. Dealing with urgent global issues such as climate change, biodiversity loss, and new diseases depends on an awareness of these complex biological interactions, therefore highlighting the critical part biology plays in modern civilization. Fundamentally, biology explores and tests ideas about the living world using the scientific method. Through methodical observation and experimentation,

1.1. The Scientific Method in Biology

Learning Outcome

1. Describe the steps of the scientific method;
2. Focus on hypothesis formation;
3. Learn about experimental design.

Learning Outcomes

The beginning of each section of every chapter contains a set of Learning Outcomes that inform students of concepts they should understand. These outcomes help students understand what they should be able to do if they have mastered the material in that section.

Test Your Knowledge

Throughout each chapter, Test Your Knowledge cues you to note which topics have been covered and to self-test your understanding of the material presented.

Test Your Knowledge

1. Explain why correlation does not imply causation in scientific experiments.
2. How does the scientific method help reduce the influence of personal opinions in research?

Chapter Summary

The Summary Section appear at the end of each chapter and summarize main concepts covered throughout the chapter. These points provide key concepts in an engaging and meaningful way.

Summary

The investigation of biological principles highlights the importance of a comprehensive view of life by reflecting the intricate interactions that occur within living systems. The complexity of biology goes beyond individual species or systems, as this essay highlights; it also includes the interactions that mold ecosystems and affect biodiversity. Researchers can conduct in-depth analyses of metabolomic data using sophisticated technologies like MetaboAnalyst, which offer insights into the molecular mechanisms underlying these interactions. As demonstrated by the developments in MetaboAnalyst, for example, the integration of diverse omics data promotes a thorough understanding of metabolic pathways and helps identify important biological markers necessary for research on development and disease (Chong et al., 2018). Additionally, the phenomenon of ecological invasions is a key component of biological research and a vital field of study. The introduction of non-native species into unfamiliar habitats has significant ramifications and calls for multidisciplinary management strategies. Examining the origins and effects of these biological incursions, invasion science has become a crucial field that highlights the need to comprehend ecological dynamics and community interactions. As interest in biological invasions increases, new findings are emerging that put conventional ecological theories and practices to the test. The importance of incorporating various scientific viewpoints is shown by this developing discipline, which also highlights how invasive species shape ecosystems and advances our knowledge of ecological resilience (David et al., 2013). When taken as a whole, these discoveries from invasion science and metabolomics highlight the value of multidisciplinary biology research. Fostering cross-disciplinary collaboration and utilizing technological breakthroughs to improve our comprehension of intricate biological interactions are crucial as we look to the future of biological research. In addition to deepening our understanding of the complexities of life, this method lays the groundwork for tackling urgent environmental issues. Future studies can ensure the continued relevance of biology in a world that is constantly changing by acknowledging the interconnection of biological systems and opening the door to creative solutions that support sustainability and biodiversity conservation. We might imagine a thorough comprehension of life that serves both academia and society at large through ongoing investigation and integration of scientific knowledge.

Knowledge Assessment

The chapter includes material designed to review and reinforce each content. It includes Critical Thinking Questions to help test of your understanding of information presented in the chapter and Short answer Questions to review your understanding of the key concepts presented in the chapter.

Critical Thinking Questions

1. **Who is known as the "Father of Modern Biology"?**
   a. Aristotle
   b. Charles Darwin
   c. Gregor Mendel
   d. Louis Pasteur
2. **What is the basic unit of life?**
   a. Atom
   b. Molecule
   c. Cell
   d. Organism
3. **Which branch of biology studies the interaction of organisms with their environment?**
   a. Genetics
   b. Ecology
   c. Physiology
   d. Botany
4. **Which macromolecule is the main source of energy for living organisms?**
   a. Proteins
   b. Lipids
   c. Carbohydrates
   d. Nucleic acids
5. **DNA is primarily responsible for which function in living organisms?**
   a. Energy production
   b. Protein synthesis
   c. Storing genetic information
   d. Regulating body temperature

Short Answer Questions

1. What is biology, and why is it important to study biology?
2. What are the three main domains of life, and how are they different from one another?
3. Define homeostasis and give an example of how it works in living organisms.
4. What is the cell theory, and why is it fundamental to biology?
5. How do autotrophs and heterotrophs differ in the way they obtain energy?
6. What is the scientific method, and how is it applied in biological research?
7. Discuss how biology helps address global challenges such as climate change, disease, and food security.
8. Explain the levels of biological organization from the smallest unit to the largest. Provide examples at each level.
9. Describe the relationship between structure and function in biology, giving specific examples from cells or organs.
10. How has the discovery of genetics shaped our understanding of inheritance and variation among organisms?

Supplementary Materials

Key Terms: A list of key terms is given for quick reference

KEY TERMS FROM THIS CHAPTER

Annotation enrichment analysis	Biological structure	Cell
Cell theory	Cellular structure	Ecology
Ecosystems	Genetics	Human biology
Microbiology	Natural selection	Organism
Plant biology		

Further Resources: Recommendations for additional readings, websites, and multimedia resources.

References

1. Argelaguet, R., Velten, B., Arnol, D., Dietrich, S., Zenz, T., Marioni, J. C., Buettner, F., et al. (2018). Multi-omics factor analysis—A framework for unsupervised integration of multi-omics data sets. *Molecular Systems Biology, 14.* https://doi.org/10.15252/msb.20178124.
2. Bacher, S., Blackburn, T. M., Essl, F., & Genovesi, P. (2017). *Socio-Economic Impact Classification of Alien Taxa (SEICAT).* https://core.ac.uk/download/286567949.pdf (accessed on 8th March 2025).
3. Barnett, R., Brace, S., Cucchi, T., & Dobney, K. (2013). *Divergent Evolutionary Processes Associated with Colonization of Offshore Islands.* https://core.ac.uk/download/20664364.pdf (accessed on 8th March 2025).

Detailed Table of Contents

LIST OF FIGURES

non-viral systems, such as shRNA/siRNA/miRNA, DNA plasmids, lipid-based and polymeric NPs and CRISPR/Cas9 approaches. Of note, some of the above approaches, e.g., shRNA, were also delivered via lentiviral vectors

Figure 12.14. Main targeted gene therapy approaches for gynecological benign and malignant disorders. Strategies include (A) mutation compensation using adenoviral vectors to correct gene expression; (B) suicide gene therapy, such as HSV-TK, inducing cell death via toxic metabolites; (C) antiangiogenic gene therapy to inhibit tumor angiogenesis; (D) oncolytic virotherapy, where viruses replicate within and destroy cancer cells; and (E) immunopotentiation through delivery of cytokine genes to stimulate anti-tumor immunity

PREFACE

The issues of women's health move beyond the field of anatomy and physiology into a realm of complex clinical disease affecting fertility, structural integrity, and oncologic risk. Pathology as benign as uterine displacement and as malignant as neoplastic growth of genital tissues mandates a multifaceted approach that includes surgical skill, hormonal information, and psychosocial sensitivity. As the technologies improve—from complex imaging to targeted treatment and regenerative medicine—gynecologists must be well-versed in both old-fashioned surgical procedures and newer therapies. Such diverse conditions impact not only reproductive function but also overall quality of life, making the need for combined, evidence-based counsel even stronger.

Over the last several decades, our understanding of disorders such as endometriosis, pelvic organ prolapse, and infertility has been revolutionized by developments in pathogenesis and diagnosis. Practices of contraception have become more patient-specific and varied, with many options for long-term use available with favorable side-effect profiles. Similarly, management of sexually transmitted diseases and HIV infection in women requires coordination of prevention, antiretroviral therapy, and planning for reproduction. Trends in oncology toward immunotherapy and fertility-sparing surgery underscore the evolving nature of gynecologic cancer therapy. These advances reflect the dynamic interplay among basic science, clinical trials, and patient activism, illustrating how advancements in one area have implications for several dimensions of treatment.

Readers will find in *Textbook of Gynecology: Volume 2* a logical presentation of female pelvic disorders, reproductive function disorders, and systemic diseases with gynecologic implications. The content builds upon the foundational knowledge presented in Volume 1 to address both common and complex conditions encountered in practice. Emphasis is placed on pathophysiology, clinical presentation, diagnostic algorithms, and emerging treatments, including minimally invasive techniques, biologic therapies, and assisted reproductive technologies.

Chapter 1 outlines the classification, etiology, and treatment of uterine displacement, such as anteversion, retroversion, and prolapse. Chapter 2 addresses female infertility, discussing disorders of ovulation, tubal and uterine causes, and male factors, and introducing investigation and treatment protocols, including IVF and novel reproductive technologies.

Chapter 3 addresses the means of contraception, ranging from barrier devices and use of hormonal implants to intrauterine systems, with guidelines for counseling and follow-up. Chapter 4 addresses endometriosis and adenomyosis, outlining theories of causation, symptomatology, and the spectrum of medical and surgical management.

Chapter 5 details genital fistulae, including obstetric, traumatic, and iatrogenic etiologies, with surgical reconstruction and postoperative care. Chapter 6 addresses genital malignancy, from cervical and endometrial cancer to rare vulvar and vaginal neoplasms, with a focus on screening, staging, and multidisciplinary management algorithms. Chapter 7 addresses the pathogenesis and treatment of fibroids (leiomyoma), with a review of uterine-sparing procedures and uterine artery embolization.

Chapter 8 reviews sexually transmitted illnesses and HIV, including prevention, diagnosis, and antiretroviral therapy in reproductive health. Chapter 9 covers pelvic floor prolapse, with anterior, posterior, and apical defects, and covers options ranging from pessary use to laparoscopic repair.

Chapter 10 addresses the diagnosis and treatment of female genital tuberculosis with emphasis on its epidemiology in endemic regions. Chapter 11 addresses urinary incontinence and fistulas, combining urodynamic studies with surgery and non-surgical management.

Chapter 12, the final chapter, discusses radiotherapy, chemotherapy, immunotherapy, and gene therapy in gynecology, illustrating up-to-date protocols and new trends for benign and malignant conditions.

This text is aimed at gynecologists, urologists, oncologists, fellows in reproductive medicine, and trainees in women's health. It is also an authoritative guide for primary care physicians and allied health professionals involved in the continuum of care of women with pelvic and reproductive disorders. By giving both breadth and practical guidance, this text assists clinicians to deliver individualized, high-quality care for the full range of gynecologic practice.

DISPLACEMENT OF THE UTERUS

1

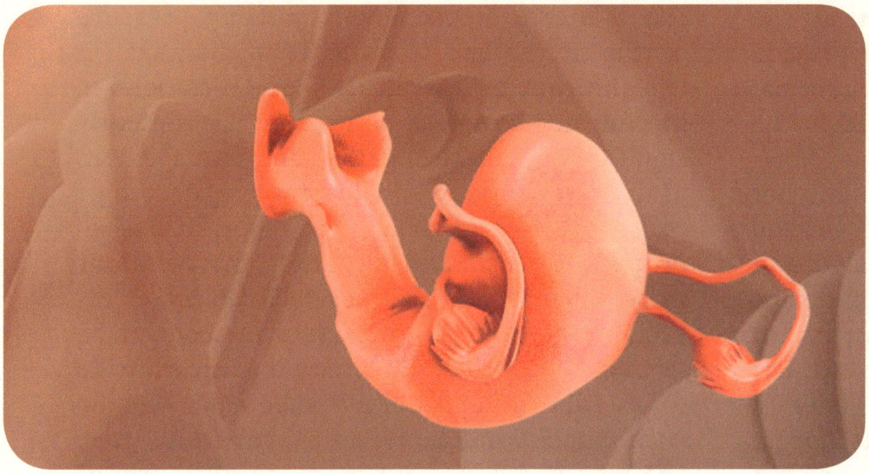

Introduction

The intricate anatomy and physiological processes of the uterus hold utmost significance in understanding conditions such as uterine displacement. This condition would signify the abnormal positioning of the uterus in the pelvic cavity, which could be due to various reasons such as anatomical variations, trauma, or post-surgical changes. In reproductive-aged females, uterine displacement may deeply affect not just sexual intercourse as well as menstruation mechanics but even overall reproductive health. The effect of such displacement underscores the necessity for thoroughgoing medical understanding because changes in uterine position may occur due to or may lead to clinical complications amenable to treatment. Thus, understanding uterine displacement provides insight not only into anatomical and physiological function but also lays the groundwork for an integrated comprehension of diagnostic and therapeutic management. Secondly, correct assessment of uterine displacement relies on advanced imaging modalities and strategies refined to register small changes in organ position

LEARNING OBJECTIVES

After studying this chapter, you will be able to:

1. Identify the anatomical structure and functions of the uterus.
2. Classify the various types of uterine displacement.
3. Explain the potential causes of uterine displacement.
4. Recognize the common symptoms associated with uterine displacement.
5. Describe the diagnostic methods used to assess uterine displacement.
6. Evaluate available treatment options for managing uterine displacement.

over the passage of time. Modalities such as ultrasound, MRI, and CT scans are important in imaging the uterus and surrounding organs in order for healthcare professionals to diagnose those conditions which may complicate pregnancy and affect women's overall health. Discussions on organ motion have featured center stage in the larger context of interventional imaging in the last few years, with these developments making treatment more precise. Advances in imaging modality, notably those that involve high-intensity focused ultrasound, demonstrate the ability of sophisticated technologies to provide noninvasive treatment of various abdominal and pelvic organ anomalies. As detailed in the literature, increased visualization not only allows for greater appreciation of displacement but also guides potential therapeutic intervention aimed at minimizing complications related to it (Celicanin et al., 2014). Associated with uterine displacement are the impacts on pregnant women, particularly as they pertain to surgical interventions. Pregnancy has long been a contraindication for certain operations due to concerns regarding maternal and fetal safety. However, the innovation in laparoscopic surgery and anesthesia has transformed such perceptions, rendering most operations feasible during pregnancy with safety. By thoroughly investigating these risks and benefits, practitioners can make informed decisions that precede the mother's and fetus's health outcomes. Conditions such as appendicitis and cholecystitis may necessitate surgery, highlighting the way in which the displaced uterus would affect surgical techniques and outcomes. Understanding the interactive dynamic of uterine displacement and surgical elements ultimately becomes a critical area of investigation in women's health, emphasizing the need for ongoing research and clinical vigilance (Godwin et al., 2015).

Definition of Uterine Displacement

The term uterine displacement is employed to signify the abnormal placement of the uterus in the pelvic cavity, an abnormality that can have serious reproductive consequences. The displacement can manifest in any of the forms, such as anteversion, retroversion, and lateral displacement, each with its own distinctive changes in the uterus's orientation. Anteversion implies forward angulation of the uterus, and retroversion implies backward angulation; both are susceptible to producing discomfort or pregnancy complications. Additionally, uterine fibroids or pelvic adhesions may cause lateral displacement, putting pressure on the uterus and altering its normal axis. It is significant to appreciate these variations in uterine displacement since they are similarly significant in the evaluation and management of infertility as well as other gynecologic conditions, highlighting the significance of proper diagnosis and treatment interventions in reproductive health services (Parry et al., 2019). The impact of uterine displacement on fertility cannot be overstressed, which attests to its role in reproductive medicine. Women with such conditions as retroverted uteri commonly present with infertility, perhaps due to disordered sperm transport or pelvic anatomy alteration impairing implantation. Furthermore, uterine displacement-related conditions, e.g., endometriosis or fibroids, have a tendency to propagate an inflammatory environment within the pelvis, also impairing fertility. One of the pillars of measuring uterine displacement is by imaging modalities, such as ultrasonography or hysteroscopy, by which health practitioners can identify structural abnormalities and quantify their effect on reproductive success. Office hysteroscopy, for instance, is referred to as the "gold standard" for intrauterine pathology diagnosis affecting implantation as well as pregnancy viability, indicating the importance of being aware of uterine positioning in fertility care (Kinsella et al., 2017). Management of uterine displacement is facilitated by a comprehensive approach, which may include surgery or conservative options. Hysteroscopic management is widely applied in the treatment of structural abnormalities that cause uterine displacement and subsequently improve reproductive outcomes. For example, hysteroscopic myomectomy in the removal of submucous fibroids has been reported to increase clinical pregnancy rates among affected women. Similarly, management of abnormalities such as intrauterine adhesions can greatly improve chances of conception and implantation success. However, treatment must be uniquely tailored to the patient based on the severity and extent of displacement, symptoms of the patient, and overall reproductive goals. Thus, there is a need for a multidisciplinary team with gynecologists, reproductive endocrinologists, and radiologists so that the maximal management regimens can be guaranteed and reproductive health outcomes in women with uterine displacement can be improved (Parry et al., 2019).

Importance of Understanding Uterine Displacement

Uterine displacement is significant in both healthcare practice and patient health. Uterine displacement can lead to severe health issues such as persistent pain as well as complications during pregnancy and childbirth. These issues might even necessitate the need for surgery or be linked with adverse fetal outcomes, thereby impacting not just the patient but the entire healthcare system as well. With careful analysis of causes, mechanisms, and implications of uterine displacement, medical practitioners are able to identify risk factors and implement effective management schemes to meet the unique requirements of individual patients. This information ensures an active approach in gynecology to enable early treatment and improved patient education to minimize the risks of uterine displacement and, therefore, enhance overall well-being. The social and economic consequences of uterine displacement are likewise significant, especially in low-resource environments. For example, maternal morbidity and mortality rates in Burkina Faso remain alarmingly high because of poor healthcare access and underlying vulnerabilities in women's health systems. The lives of women, as revealed through case studies, highlight how conditions such as uterine displacement can result in runaway health expenses, further entrenching existing societal inequities. These structural impediments can significantly limit women's resilience and capacity to cope with health conditions, thereby exacerbating a cycle of ill health and economic vulnerability. This context highlights the need to understand uterine displacement holistically, as raised awareness levels among clinicians can help promote greater advocacy for health reform and appropriate care support systems. Moreover, advancement in medical technology and research emphasizes the need to study uterine displacement both mechanically and biologically. Studies in allied disciplines such as fluid dynamics and reproductive biology are capable of bringing a breakthrough in uterine position and function mechanics. For instance, understanding the uterine environment and its interaction with reproductive physiology can reveal pivotal relationships between uterine displacement and fertility problems. Advanced knowledge in these fields can result in new treatment methods and prevention for victims. Thus, embracing a multi-disciplinary approach of the research of uterine displacement has the promise of producing holistic findings that not just address current health problems but also inform future research and clinical practice in obstetrics and gynecology.

1.1. Anatomy of the Uterus

Learning Outcome

1. Define the description of the normal position of the uterus
2. Describe the factors influencing uterine position
3. Identify the common variations in uterine anatomy

The structure of the uterus plays a crucial role in defining conditions related to its displacement. Physically, the uterus is a hollow muscular organ that is found within the pelvis, typically between the rectum and bladder. Its primary components include the fundus, body, and cervix, each with specific functions within the reproductive cycle. The uterine wall is made up of three layers: the endometrium (inward layer), the myometrium (middle muscular layer), and the perimetrium (covering outside). The complex architecture not only accommodates implantation and fetal development but also compensates for hormonal changes throughout the menstrual cycle. Uterine displacement—retroversion or anteversion—is regulated by a number of factors, including anatomical variations, pressure from adjacent organs, and fetal growth in pregnancy. Thus, intimate familiarity with uterine anatomy becomes essential in the diagnosis and cure of displacement effectively. Secondly, aberrations in uterine location can have significant clinical implications on physical well-being as well as on fertility. As an example, a retroverted uterus may not be able to engage during pregnancy and can lead to miscarriage or obstructed labor.

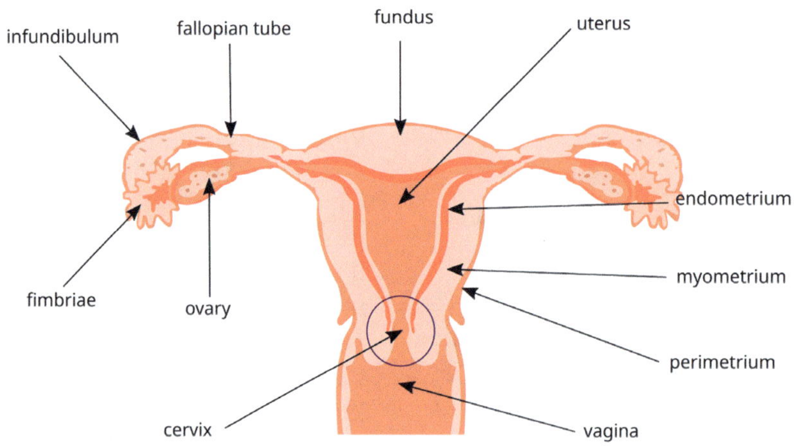

Figure 1.1. Uterus.

Source: https://prod-images-static.radiopaedia.org/images/69801917/ced5da2890b764ee2bffbe42be19c662c70da83bcb86d4d46cdf46574e3fb1ee_big_gallery.jpeg

In addition, the severity of displacement is often compounded by dysmenorrhea or dyspareunia and thus impacts quality of life. Causes of uterine displacement—heterogeneous as they are, from fibroids to pelvic inflammatory disease—highlight the significance of understanding anatomy as well as the functional interaction of the uterus with adjacent pelvic structures. Providers need to consider these anatomical considerations in diagnosing and treating patients with a displaced uterus, providing an individualized health-care strategy tailored to each patient's anatomical differences. Along with anatomy, new imaging technologies are also revolutionizing the assessment of uterine position and health. Techniques such as three-dimensional ultrasound provide accurate information on uterine shape and position, allowing for better assessments of displacement. Mentionable are digital health technologies, elaborated in the interorganizational records scoping review, which have the potential to improve decision-making procedures in clinical settings (Wiles et al., 2022). With healthcare embracing digitalization, the combination of increased imaging with a robust anatomical foundation will assist in more precise diagnostics (Lloyd et al., 2019). Last but not least, the integration of anatomical details and modern technology plays a significant role in developing effective treatment plans for individuals undergoing uterine displacement so that their overall health and reproductive health are optimized.

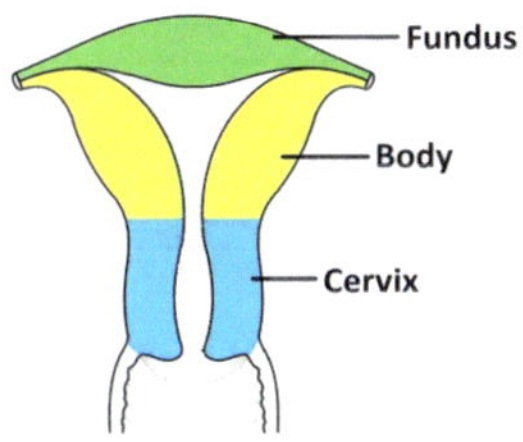

Figure 1.2. The three anatomical divisions of the uterus.

Source: https://teachmeanatomy.info/pelvis/female-reproductive-tract/uterus/

1.1.1. Description of the Normal Position of the Uterus

To know the typical position of the uterus is significant in knowing how its displacement is facilitated and how it could impact women's health. The uterus, which is typically located inside the pelvis, is located anterior to the rectum and posterior to the bladder. The uterus, when in a normal position, is also slightly forward tilted, also referred to as anteversion. This anatomical structure allows for the maximum support of the pelvic floor muscles and the surrounding ligaments, making it stable and functioning in various physiological changes, such as menstruation, pregnancy, and childbirth. Furthermore, regular uterine positioning is also influenced by conditions such as age, hormonal changes, and individual variations of the pelvic anatomy, which can additionally hinder clinical assessments and treatments concerning uterine positioning (Moustafa, 2014). Moreover, the uterus is normally described as pear-shaped so that it can support any increase in volume, particularly when one is pregnant. Supported by the round and broad ligaments, the upright position places the uterus in the center of the pelvis. Alteration of this position can lead to a variety of conditions, ranging from benign conditions like pelvic organ prolapse to severe consequences like miscarriage or infertility. The significance of identifying the normal position of the uterus also becomes apparent in cases where displacement has occurred, as it can compromise not only reproductive health but the overall health of an individual (Franco et al., 2017). An acute understanding of the normal anatomical position is important in facilitating clinicians to diagnose and manage uterine-related complications adequately (Franco et al., 2017).

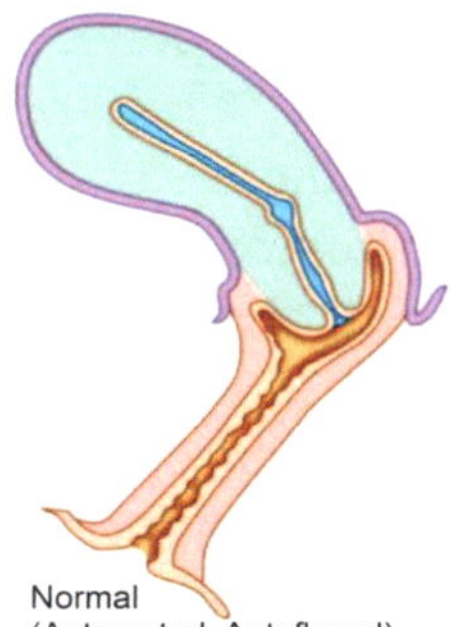

Figure 1.3. Normal uterus.

Source: https://oshimu.com/wp-content/uploads/2021/07/Gynaecology-DC-Dutta.pdf

Uterine displacement may be due to numerous reasons, including anatomical abnormalities, procedures, and lifestyle issues. These displacements have a long-range impact, which normally presents as long-standing pelvic pain, dysfunctional menstrual bleeding, and failure of the urinary tract. For instance, abnormalities like retroversion, where the uterus is tilted posteriorly instead of its normal anteverted position, may affect the bladder and surrounding structures, causing discomfort or other issues. Treatment of such displacements demands a proper understanding of the anatomy of the normal uterus. Use of specific interventions that restore the uterus to its proper position can greatly enhance not just the presented symptoms but the quality of life in the involved individuals as well. Ongoing research into the determinants of uterine position is imperative in optimizing treatment modalities for women with displacements (Moustafa, 2014).

1.1.2. Factors Influencing Uterine Position

The position of the uterus is influenced by a range of factors, which come together in complex ways to affect both its anatomical placement and overall functioning. The uterus is anatomically held in place by ligaments, connective tissue, and pelvic muscles, which become weakened or are altered under several factors. For instance, childbirth trauma, anatomical malformations, and previous operations are capable of initiating changes in uterine position, with resultant effects such as retroversion or prolapse. These changes not only impact female reproductive health but also general pelvic function. Accurate identification of these anatomical factors is crucial in the diagnosis and therapy of uterine displacement disorders, making extensive pelvic examination the cornerstone of clinical practice. Hormonal fluctuation and aging also play crucial roles in changing the uterine position. Reproductive hormones estrogen and progesterone play a role in the structural integrity of the pelvic support mechanism. With advancing age, particularly menopause, decreased levels of these hormones lead to weakening of the connective tissues and ligaments, leading to a shift in the position of the uterus. This loss of hormonal support, in addition to having effects on the displacement of the uterus, could also generate a variety of gynecological symptoms.

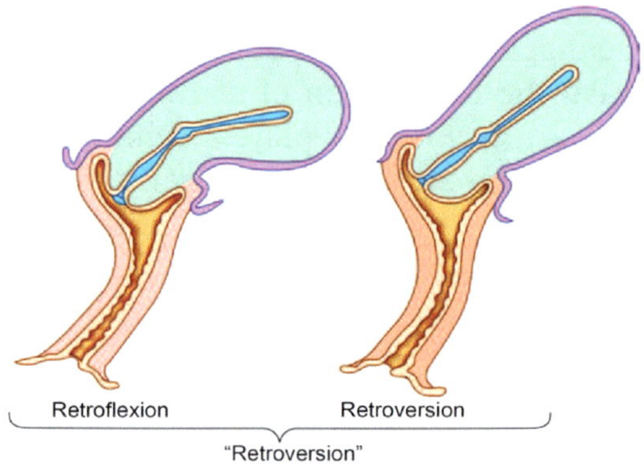

Figure 1.4. Retroverted uterus.

Source: https://oshimu.com/wp-content/uploads/2021/07/Gynaecology-DC-Dutta.pdf

In addition to this, lifestyle and obesity can further influence these age-related alterations in terms of adding additional stress to the pelvic floor, thereby making the clinical presentation of uterine displacement more complicated. Identification of these lifestyle and hormonal effects is important for the generation of evidence-based interventions to treat uterine displacement. Psychosocial factors, including lifestyle and occupational demands, can also indirectly affect uterine position. For example, the nature of work a woman undertakes, particularly in an occupation that involves heavy physical labor, may produce a cause of pelvic floor dysfunction, which subsequently can lead to a change in uterine position. Moreover, a stressful lifestyle can exacerbate symptoms such as muscle tension and contribute to causing pelvic pain syndromes, thus influencing uterine positioning. It is most crucial for healthcare providers to understand this psychosocial factor because it opens up the possibility of multimodal treatment approaches. Uterine positioning is determined not only physically but also psychosocially. Tackling both the physical and psychosocial determinants that impact uterine positioning may lead to more effective management interventions in the clinical setting. Compiling all these various influences—anatomical, hormonal, and psychosocial—medical workers can adopt a three-dimensional strategy toward the management of uterine displacement disorders.

1.1.3. Common Variations in Uterine Anatomy

The human uterus exhibits numerous anatomical variations, which have the potential to significantly influence reproductive well-being as well as the risk of uterine displacement. They range from variations in size, shape, and position and can be categorized into normal anatomical variants and pathologies. Variations such as bicornuate or septate uteri are the result of developmental anomalies during embryogenesis and lead to structural abnormalities that have the potential to influence implantation, gestation, and labor. Awareness of these anomalies is crucial because they put the patient at risk of developing complications like an increased likelihood of miscarriage and preterm labor. This emphasizes the importance of thorough clinical evaluation and imaging investigations to identify these anomalies in a timely manner so that management and intervention tactics can be offered based on the specific anatomical configuration of each patient. The function of the cervix is another significant uterine anatomy feature that is responsible for maintaining pregnancy and preventing complications. The integrity of the cervical canal's structure is vital, as otherwise, it can lead to a weak cervix that would not support the growing embryo properly, thus threatening miscarriage or preterm labor. In the assessment of common variation of uterine anatomy, the part played by the internal cervical os should be stressed in contributing to these findings. The mechanism by which cervical structural variation impacts physiological processes is complex and requires research; it is known that structural weakness can result from developmental abnormalities or underlying pathology. Through such associations, health care practitioners are in a position to utilize interventions to reinforce the internal os in vulnerable groups of individuals, basically eradicating the threat of preterm labor due to variation in uterine anatomy (Bonney et al., 2016).

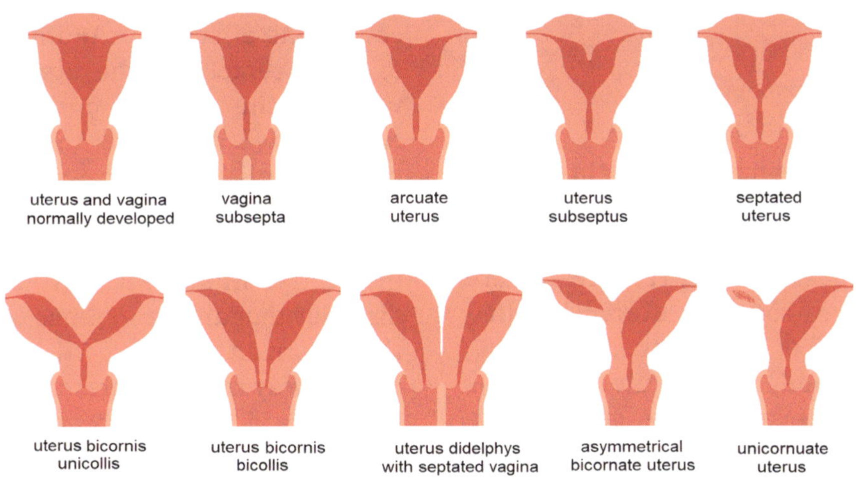

Figure 1.5. Malformations of the uterus.

Source: https://upload.wikimedia.org/wikipedia/commons/thumb/f/ff/Uterine_malformation.png/1200px-Uterine_malformation.png

In addition, new instruments and tools have emerged to assist in evaluating and treating conditions of uterine and cervical anatomy. For instance, the creation of measurement devices that establish the distance from the cervix to the rectum is valuable in treatment planning, particularly in the case of cervical cancer. These instruments enable clinicians to visualize and quantify anatomical relations that can affect surgical outcomes and radiation treatment planning (Fischell et al., 1981). Explicit familiarity with anatomical variations is not only required to manage existing conditions but also to direct preventative measures and optimize patient outcomes in reproductive health cases. With ongoing research, there is a hope that learning will be converted to individualized therapy interventions to address the intricate issues introduced by variability in uterine anatomy and therefore optimize the management of individuals thus affected and further enhance maternal-fetal medicine.

Test Your Knowledge

1. What is the normal anatomical position of the uterus in the female body?
2. Which factors can influence changes in the position of the uterus?

1.2. Types of Uterine Displacement

Learning Outcome

1. Define anteversion and retroversion
2. Explain the lateral displacement
3. Discuss the prolapse of the uterus

The uterine displacement can occur in various forms, impacting women's reproductive health. Among the various types that are typically encountered, retroversion and retroflexion are most common. A retroverted uterus is tilted backward toward the spine, and retroflexion occurs when the body of the uterus curves backward at the level of the cervix. The displacements have been explained by reasons such as congenital abnormalities, history of pelvic surgery, or the existence of fibroids. Many women may not exhibit any symptoms; however, in some cases, retroversion may lead to complications such as urinary incontinence or pelvic pain. Understanding these conditions is crucial because they can significantly impact a woman's quality of life, particularly when reproductive activities are involved. Ongoing research underscores the importance of determining uterine position in the diagnosis and treatment of accompanying medical conditions effectively. Another significant type of displacement of the uterus is anteversion, wherein the twisted position of the uterus turns forward toward the bladder. It is the usual condition of the uterus, but various pathological processes, such as endometriosis, can disrupt this position and lead to pain or infertility. Endometriosis is a multifaceted disorder that affects millions of women globally, characterized by the growth of endometrial-type tissue away from the uterine cavity and causing pelvic pain, infertility, and other sequelae (Smolarz et al., 2021). Notably, understanding the anatomical ramifications of anteversion can assist clinicians in a more precise diagnosis of patients with reproductive dysfunction. Management would vary from conservative measures to surgical intervention, as the severity and complications would determine. Therefore, a comprehensive understanding of the categories of uterine displacements is essential to individualize effective treatment techniques. In surgical procedures, the Large Uterus Classification System (LUCS) recognizes various kinds of uterine displacement that can influence the success of surgery. According to research, uteri are categorized based on vascular pedicle displacement, which affects the outcome of laparoscopic hysterectomy (Uccella et al., 2021). Type 1, without vascular displacement, should typically have lower operative times and rates of complications, while Types 2 and 3 are more strenuous. This form of classification is important since it can help clinicians define surgical risks according to each type and perhaps improve the quality of patient care during surgery. By extensive analysis of types of uterine displacement, clinicians can maximize patient counseling and planning for surgery and ultimately lead to improved postoperative results for women who undergo hysterectomies.

1.2.1. Anteversion and Retroversion

The words anteversion and retroversion become important to understand anatomical positioning and resultant complications secondary to uterine displacement. Anteversion means anterior bending of the organ, where the organ is bent forward at the junctional level between the cervix and body of the uterus. Retroversion means reverse inclination, such that the uterus inclines in the posterior direction. These are key positions for gynecological assessment because they can have a significant effect on menstrual, pregnancy-related, and overall reproductive symptomology. Uterine position can affect function within the pelvis and may be connected with pelvic pain or delivery complications. Understanding these differences enhances a clinician's capacity to reach a soundly informed decision regarding diagnosis and treatment in uterine displacement, emphasizing anatomy's relevance in gynecology. Uterine displacement complications can vary based on the direction of the uterus, emphasizing the importance of anteversion and retroversion in practice. For instance, a retroverted uterus might contribute to the difficulty of conducting certain gynecological interventions, and it might complicate surgical interventions such as hysterectomies or terminations. In some cases, a retroverted position might interfere with the success of interventions that are meant to address reproductive health issues, leading to what other practitioners have coined "situational challenges" when handling patients who come in with such displacements (Borgatta et al., 2009).

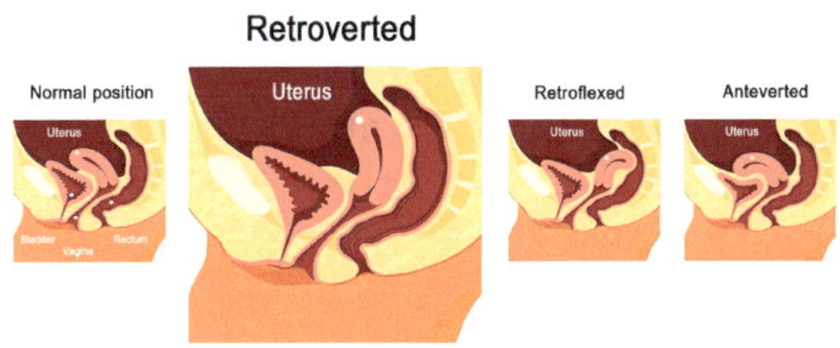

Figure 1.6. Retroverted uterus.

Source: https://fertilab.com/en/what-is-a-retroverted-uterus/

Conversely, while an anteverted uterus is generally regarded as normal anatomical positioning, it too may encounter challenges, like during childbearing, where atypical positioning can result in labor complications. Thus, awareness of these changes helps with preoperative planning and early intervention approaches. Awareness of anteversion and retroversion encompasses implications for the surgical process and outcome also. With progression in gynecologic surgery, the role of these positioning factors remains a priority in the creation of repair procedures, such as the Emmet procedure, which is used in the repair of lacerations of the cervix uteri (Goldspohn, 1896). Although the primary issue of this procedure is cervical trauma, it indirectly highlights the issue of uterine position in the operating room. Uterine unfavorable position is not only a complicating factor in the conduct of surgical procedures but also in the selection of the most appropriate method of intervention. An understanding of these anatomical terms, thus, enhances clinicians' capacity to manage the complexities of surgical gynecology and apply efficient approaches unique to the anatomy of patients as well as to reduce resulting complications due to uterine displacement.

1.2.2. Lateral Displacement

Lateral uterine displacement is a concept that frequently arises in the context of various physiological and pathological states of female reproductive well-being. This is a condition that can strongly manifest in early pregnancy, where the size and weight of the developing embryo result in lateral displacement of the uterus.

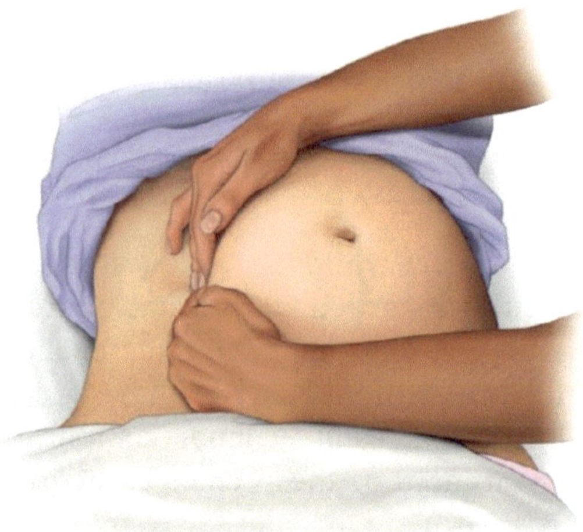

Figure 1.7. Left uterine displacement with 2-handed technique.

Source: https://www.researchgate.net/figure/Left-uterine-displacement-with-2-handed-technique-3_fig2_255976862

The positional changes that result from such displacement can have numerous clinical impacts, with complications that may confuse diagnostics as well as treatment protocols. As noted, lateral displacements are a common result in gynecological examination, which can lead to undue manipulations or surgical interventions that might not be the be-all and end-all of treating the root cause of results. Identification of normal uterine positioning parameters during pregnancy and other complications is crucial for practitioners to avoid misdiagnosis and to give appropriate care to patients suffering from these common physiological events (Crichton et al., 2018).

Furthermore, presentation of lateral displacement can be problematic diagnostically. The condition will probably be mistaken for more serious conditions, such as tumors or adnexal structural anomalies. For instance, lateral pelvic pain may be a manifestation of isolated fallopian tubal torsion, which, although uncommon, has associated symptoms that are overlapping with symptoms of uterine displacement. A thorough ultrasound will be capable of distinguishing between these conditions since excessive lateral uterine movement may be managed in a different manner than acute torsion or other pathology. In such instances, accurate diagnosis depends on meticulous clinical evaluation and adequate imaging, revealing the subtle interplay between uterine position and reproductive health (Padmalatha et al., 2012). In addressing cases of lateral displacement, clinicians are required to utilize an interdisciplinary practice by leveraging concepts in obstetrics and gynecology. Not only does the understanding of lateral displacement affect clinical interventions, but also patient education, allowing for the understanding of women's health issues more deeply. By appreciating the importance of lateral movements, healthcare providers can guide patients better throughout their reproductive lives, enhancing care and support. Additionally, because the clinical situation is dynamic with changes in imaging and surgical techniques, continued study of the pattern and implication of uterine displacement will be necessary to optimize outcomes for women who encounter these problems during their reproductive years (Crichton et al., 2018; Padmalatha et al., 2012).

1.2.3. Prolapse of the Uterus

Uterine prolapse is a severe reproductive disorder that occurs as a result of prolapse of the uterus into the vaginal canal due to weakened pelvic supportive structures. It often results from multiple causative factors, including childbirth, aging, and endogenous hormonal changes affecting the strength of the connective tissue. Female patients with a history of repeated pregnancies or those with a history of vaginal delivery are particularly vulnerable, since the strain on pelvic muscles and ligaments leads to progressive, more severe weakening. Lifestyle elements such as obesity and coughing also increase the risk of uterine prolapse. Identification of the above factors makes it possible to recognize high-risk populations and direct preventive interventions and management decisions in afflicted patients. Symptoms associated with uterine prolapse may have a significant effect on the quality of a woman's life, both physical and emotional. Symptoms range from a sensation of heaviness or pressure in the pelvic area, incontinence, and dyspareunia. These symptoms not only affect function in activities of daily life but also cause psychological manifestations like depression and anxiety.

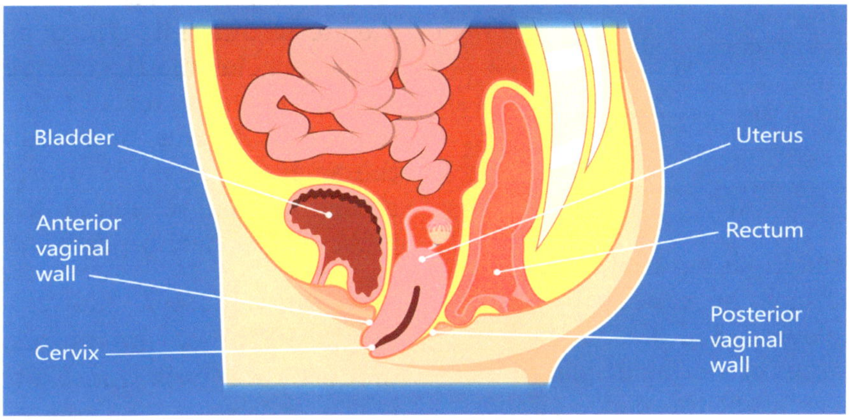

Figure 1.8. Uterine Prolapse.

Source: https://cdn.apollohospitals.com/health-library-prod/2021/09/Uterine-prolapse-scaled.jpg

Proper assessment of such symptoms is required to create an individualized treatment regimen. Doctors must talk closely to affected patients to understand their individual experiences and challenges due to this condition. This multi-faceted approach permits both physiological and psychological considerations in management, ultimately resulting in an overall healing process. Imaging modalities have become more valuable in both diagnosis and therapy of uterine prolapse with better visualization of the structures in the pelvis. Using ultrasound, especially 3D/4D multiplanar ultrasound, offers real-time assessment of the dynamics of the pelvic floor, enabling clinicians to visualize the way the uterus and surrounding tissue react to physical movements such as coughing or straining. This function is crucial in the diagnosis and prolapse severity stratification as well as the detection of concomitant risks such as delivery-associated avulsion injuries and hiatal overdistension. Data obtained through these imaging modalities not only benefit real-time clinical decision-making but also contribute to the comprehension of underlying pathophysiologic pathways. With ongoing research in urogynaecology, the use of combined contemporary imaging techniques will be the hallmark to drive both diagnostic and therapeutic performance in women presenting with uterine prolapse (Smolarz et al., 2021; Dietz, 2018).

Test Your Knowledge

1. How does an anteverted uterus differ from a retroverted uterus?
2. What are possible causes of lateral displacement of the uterus?

1.3. Causes of Uterine Displacement

Learning Outcome

1. Describe the congenital factors that affect the structure and function of the uterus
2. Examine acquired factors, including childbirth, that contribute to uterine changes or disorders
3. Analyze the role of hormonal influences on uterine health and function

Uterine displacement is a multi-factorial condition, and it may be caused by some anatomical, physiological, and lifestyle factors. One of the main causes of uterine displacement is structural weakening of the pelvic support tissues. The tissues include ligaments and connective tissue that assist in supporting the uterus's position in the pelvis. Factors such as childbirth, menopause, and age can lead to a progressive loosening or weakening of these supportive structures, resulting in conditions such as uterine prolapse. Besides, genetic connective tissue disease predisposes this event to happen, rendering women susceptible to uterine displacement. It is essential to recognize these causative factors since they signal the relevance of prevention as well as interventions in the susceptible groups. Aside from the structural causes, hormonal alterations play a significant role as well in uterine positioning. Conditions such as fibroids or endometriosis alter the shape and size of the uterine cavity and thus result in displacement. Hormones like estrogen and progesterone play critical roles in regulating the menstrual cycle and the overall health of the uterus. Hormonal imbalance may lead to abnormal tissue growth that can push the uterus out of its typical position, especially in cases of endometriosis or benign tumors. The contact between uterine stability and hormonal well-being is, thus, paramount in determining the overall cause of uterine displacement among women, reflecting the sophistication of reproductive health problems.

Lastly, lifestyle matters also affect the displacement of the uterus, particularly in modern life with inactivity becoming the standard. Women who do not engage in regular exercise are likely to experience muscular imbalance in the pelvic region, thereby weakening the supportive structures of the uterus. Prolonged lifting and coughing, which operate with pressure over the pelvic floor, exacerbate the situation. In addition, obesity has been found to have a correlation with higher intra-abdominal pressure, thereby influencing the pelvic organ positioning directly, such as that of the uterus. Modifying these lifestyle elements through lifestyle intervention and education may be an effective strategy towards preventing the risk of uterine displacement and improving the overall quality of life in affected women.

1.3.1. Congenital Factors

Understanding congenital factors is significant in the examination of uterine displacement, as these inborn factors can influence uterine functioning and position. Congenital abnormalities, which manifest during embryonic growth, can potentially lead to various forms of uterine malformations. These abnormalities range from minor deviations, such as an acquired tilt in the uterus, to more intricate forms, including duplication or agenesis of the uterus. A specific genetic link has been established; for instance, mutations in the NR6A1 gene have been related to both renal and uterine malformations, thereby demonstrating the connection between predispositions that are held at the genetic level and physical anatomy of reproductive structures.

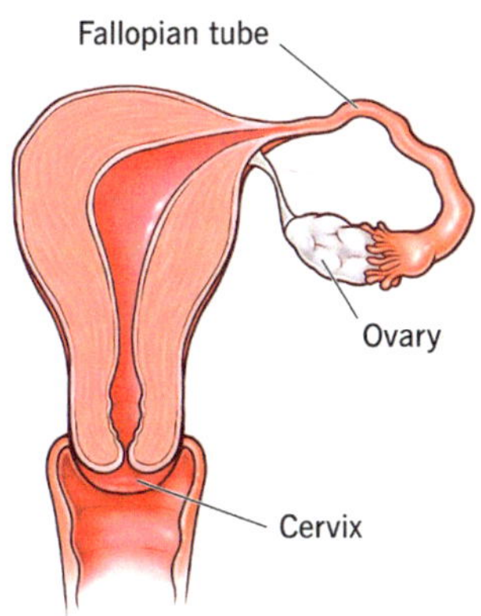

Figure 1.9. A unicornuate uterus is when you have half a uterus with only one working fallopian tube and ovary.

Source: https://my.clevelandclinic.org/health/diseases/23302-unicornuate-uterus

Such relations enable researchers to comprehend the manner in which developmental abnormalities result in such conditions as displacement of the uterus, and therefore the reason why genetic issues are important in reproductive health. The term congenital factors is broader than just anatomical; they can impact clinical results in patients with uterine displacement too. For example, women with existing congenital anomalies could be at higher risk during pregnancy because such abnormalities may have complicated events such as preterm labor or fetal malposition. Further, identification of congenital causes can help doctors create tailored preventive interventions and treatment protocols to address specific risks due to malformations of the uterus. With congenital uterine malformations, individualized patient care is critical, and comprehensive diagnostic workups become the norm.

By understanding the role of these congenital conditions, clinicians are more able to optimize their care and prevention of complications, ultimately improving outcomes of health in involved patients. Recent case reports illustrate the interaction between congenital factors and arising health complications and the importance of genetic conditions in the pathophysiology of uterine displacement. A notable example was the patient with hyperuтерин bleeding compounded by congenital thrombopathia, which highlights the unpredictable and severe nature of underlying congenital disorders. Concomitantly, even in the absence of familiar chronic disorders, congenital bleeding disorders compound uterine displacement problems and create considerable clinical issues. How these sexual health conditions interface with the remainder of the systemic abnormalities reminds practitioners of the complex interplay among congenital aspects in patient presentation. The ability to discern these associations not only enhances diagnostic accuracy but also guides overall-care strategies for women with uterine displacement and accompanying complications, in support of the dominant role of congenital drivers in reproductive health (Jacquinet et al., 2025; Pineda et al., 2025).

1.3.2. Acquired Factors, Including Childbirth

The uterine displacement process is significantly influenced by various acquired conditions, most notably childbirth. Vaginal delivery puts the pelvic supports under severe stress and strain, and hence, potential uterine displacement. This stress may alter the structural stability of the pelvic floor, leading to disorders such as pelvic organ prolapse. The forces of delivery in an acute fashion can elongate the levator ani muscle and associated connective tissueswell beyond their normal boundaries, initiating changes that predispose to subsequent uterine displacement. Because birth occurs so frequently in society, having knowledge of its influence on uterine position is essential to being able to adequately deal with women's health issues related to pelvic support tissue and their function regarding uterine displacement. Apart from childbirth, other acquired factors like age and parity also play considerable roles in uterine displacement. With increased age, the additive role of parity—i.e., successive births—contributes toward the diminution of the pelvic floor's supportive capacity. As a rule, the aging process leads to a loss of striated muscle fibers in significant supporting structures, thus compromising their function to maintain desirable pressure dynamics during normal activities. Studies reveal that with advancing age and increasing childbirth exposures, the probability of acquiring conditions associated with uterine displacement, i.e., urinary incontinence and prolapse of pelvic organs, also increases. These studies highlight the importance of preventive measures and targeted interventions in women undergoing these physiological changes, as an anticipatory strategy can decrease the chance of severe displacement and its effect on quality of life. In addition, biomechanics of childbirth categorically point to the need for more research on the interaction between uterine displacement factors and acquired factors. For instance, the co-operation of the levator ani muscles and connective tissues of the pelvis in supporting the uterus is a key issue. Notably, vaginal delivery subjects such structures to extreme tensile stresses, with possible damage or weakening and resultant displacement of the uterus. Recent research suggests that the individual strains encountered by the pudendal nerve and adjacent musculature during childbirth are key determinants for post-childbirth pelvic floor health. The pathomechanics of the same are a field that is still open to research; the studies will ultimately do justice to clinical methods of avoiding and treating uterine displacement appropriately (Parente et al., 2008; RE et al., 2007).

1.3.3. Hormonal Influences

The intricate interaction between hormonal effects and uterine displacement is pivotal in understanding many reproductive diseases, including endometriosis. Estrogen and progesterone, in particular, play an imperative role in regulating the menstrual cycle and maintaining the organizational structure of uterine tissue. Dysregulation of such hormonal levels will lead to pathological conditions, such as the formation of endometriosis lesions, where there is displacement of endometrium from the uterus. The presence of retrograde menstruation supports the theory that hormonal fluctuations contribute to the disease condition, as elevated levels of estrogen could lead to the growth of ectopic endometrial cells. Finally, the relationship between hormonal components and the position of the uterus anatomically is meant to emphasize the need for more study of treatment that attempts to bring hormonal balance back in a bid to offset the effect of such displacements (Smolarz et al., 2021).

Apart from progesterone and estrogen, other hormones, including those used in immune response pathways, have an important influence on uterine displacement as well. During pregnancy, for example, the body experiences dramatic changes in its hormone levels that necessitate a complex interaction of immune processes to support the developing fetus. The switch from Th1 to Th2 immunity is a reflection of this process, whereby the immune environment is altered by the presence of trophoblast antigens. This hormonal control also influences the position of the uterus, but not only its position, as it promotes implantation and fetal growth. But as soon as this hormonal state becomes dysregulated, it may lead to conditions like recurrent pregnancy loss or preeclampsia. Therefore, understanding the hormonal orchestration during pregnancy is crucial for performing implications based on uterine displacement and optimizing maternal and fetal health (Wang et al., 2020).

At last, the control exerted by hormones does not remain limited to certain menstrual phases or pregnancy. Syndromes such as polycystic ovary syndrome (PCOS) also depict how endocrine imbalance leads to uterine displacement. Elevations in androgen, which is a characteristic of PCOS, are known to lead to abnormal uterine positioning as well as morphological changes and impact fertility. In addition, the hormonal environment in PCOS is also one of the endocrine inflammatory syndromes that contribute to the exacerbation of uterine displacement. The interaction between the displacement of the uterus and the hormones explains the significance of hormonal regulation in maintaining reproductive health. By examining these complex interactions, researchers can design personalized therapies that aim to rebalance the hormonal levels and therefore treat the symptoms as well as the causes of uterine displacement disorders (Smolarz et al., 2021).

Test Your Knowledge

1. What are some common congenital factors that can affect the uterus or reproductive system?
2. How can childbirth lead to acquired changes in uterine position or structure?

1.4. Symptoms of Uterine Displacement

Learning Outcome

1. Define pain and discomfort
2. Explain the menstrual irregularities
3. Identify the impact on fertility

The signs of uterine displacement are often very heterogeneous in patients, making the clinical presentation complex and possibly even difficult to diagnose and treat. Many women may experience pelvic pain, which is a very nonspecific sign and may be confused with various other illnesses like ovarian cysts or endometriosis. This pain is aching or chronic and extends to the thighs or lower back, affecting a woman's quality of life and daily activities. To add, there are those who complain of changed menstrual patterns, like irregular menses or profuse menstrual flow, as the location of the uterus affects the hormonal regulation of menstruation. Therefore, there should be a consciousness of the mild signs of uterine displacement by clinicians so that they can put in place appropriate management strategies and alleviate pain for the patient. In some instances, an intrauterine device (IUD) results in worsened symptoms of uterine displacement. As seen in current literature, complications arising due to IUDs can encompass severe conditions such as device migration or perforation, which lead to extra symptoms and pain (Macheku et al., 2025). When an IUD is displaced, women can exhibit symptoms such as pelvic pain, heavy menstrual spotting, or abnormal discharge. Follow-up is made standard, as women might not show obvious symptoms after displacement and therefore require delays in interventions. The use of high-tech imaging like 3D ultrasound and computed tomography has been helpful in diagnosing IUD complications, enhancing the ability to assess the device placement and associated symptoms effectively (Li et al., 2024). Besides, psychological manifestations can also arise as a result of physical discomfort as a consequence of uterine displacement. Chronic pelvic pain and menstrual irregularities can lead to increased anxiety, stress, and poor quality of life that can force some women to seek psychological counseling or guidance. Physical and psychological interaction makes the case for a multidisciplinary approach to symptom management of uterine displacement more compelling. Clinicians are requested to remain cognizant not just of physical treatment modalities available but also of emotional support to which patients may be entitled. Both elements discussed ensure an integrative approach to care, leading ultimately to enhanced health benefits and quality of life in sufferers of the debilitating effects of uterine displacement.

1.4.1. Pain and Discomfort

The discomfort and aching of uterine displacement are multifaceted, influencing not only the health of women at the physical level but also their psychological and social lives. Pain, cramping, and dysmenorrhea are commonly felt with the imbalance of the uterus. They are not merely temporary inconveniences; they can greatly impact daily functioning and quality of life. The subtleties of this condition often require an interdisciplinary treatment regimen. For instance, the administration of various therapies, such as manual manipulation or drug therapy, can alleviate pain while addressing the concomitant displacement. Understanding the interplay between uterine positioning and symptom pattern is essential for practitioners to deliver effective treatment regimens that treat both the physical and psychosocial components of patient care. Particularly, the relationship between uterine displacement and specific menstrual complications shows the profound interconnectedness between anatomy and distress.

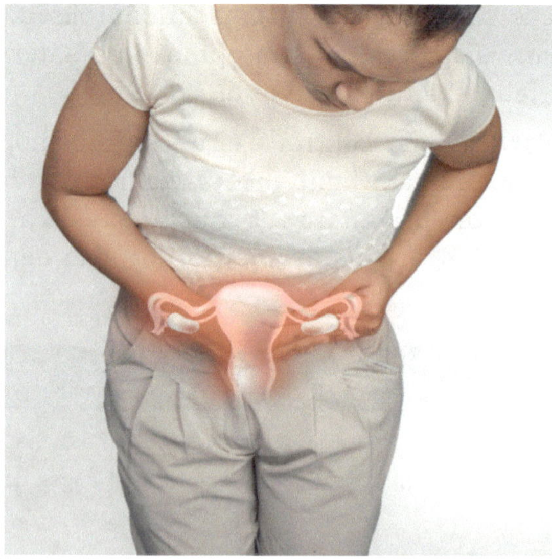

Source: https://i0.wp.com/drhyler.com/wp-content/uploads/2019/03/shutterstock_267973223.jpg?fit=1000%2C667&ssl=1

Disorders like Vataja Yoni Vyapad demonstrate the fine interplays between reproductive health and disabling symptoms connected with menstruation. This situation normally leads to severe distress, including severe dysmenorrhea and painful sensations in the vulval and vaginal regions. Treatment today is geared towards restoring balance in the body through oral drug therapy and local measures, including Sthanika Chikitsa. With such treatments, patients can find tremendous relief, some of which alleviates the pain associated with uterine displacement. Not only does this holistic technique treat physical pain, but it also promotes a new sense of well-being, emphasizing that a multifaceted approach is what is needed to effectively treat these conditions (Jana et al., 2025). Besides, recent findings in osteopathic gynecology add to the treatment benefit of an understanding of utero-pelvic mechanics in reducing pain arising from displacement. The osteopathic philosophies inform an integrated-person understanding of health, and anatomical relationships and their influence on function are emphasized. In combining traditional treatment protocols with osteopathic interventions, health professionals are able to provide a more effective pain management intervention. These interventions can alleviate pain by resolving the underlying mechanical tension that exacerbates the symptoms expressed with uterine displacement. While awareness in this field evolves, the potential for greater control of pain and discomfort with uterine displacement is clearer and contradicts current research to further mold and extend the treatment models (Woodall et al., 1902).

1.4.2. Menstrual Irregularities

Menstrual irregularities most often appear as deviations from the standard menstrual cycle, normally 21 to 35 days in duration and involving a four to seven-day period of flow. Irregularities can be attributed to several factors, including imbalance in hormones, anatomical differences, and extrinsic factors. With displacement of the uterus, the alteration in anatomy can result in irregular placement of reproductive organs, which can directly tamper with menstrual cycles. For instance, an abnormal uterine position can disrupt the normal shedding of the endometrial lining, resulting in abnormal patterns of bleeding, such as heavier or lighter menstrual periods, and the onset of intermenstrual bleeding. Discovery of this kind of abnormality is crucial to the understanding of the causes of discomfort or potential fertility problems, paving the way for appropriate medical action. Intrauterine device (IUD) placement, specifically nonhormonal IUDs, makes the process of interaction between menstrual abnormalities and uterine positioning more complicated. Studies indicate that IUD misplacement adds unexpected bleeding patterns, including extended duration of menstruation and spotting between cycles. Bleeding irregularities and assessment in relation to the correct placement of IUDs have gained importance in gynecological research. According to studies, the use of transvaginal ultrasonography and hysteroscopy is key in determining the exact position of such devices inside the uterine cavity, a procedure critical in the correction of the resulting menstrual disorders. Understanding the cytokine profile in these patients provides additional evidence of how the hormonal environment may change after insertion, thus providing better insight into the significant number of factors that influence menstrual health following invasive procedures (Watad et al., 2024).

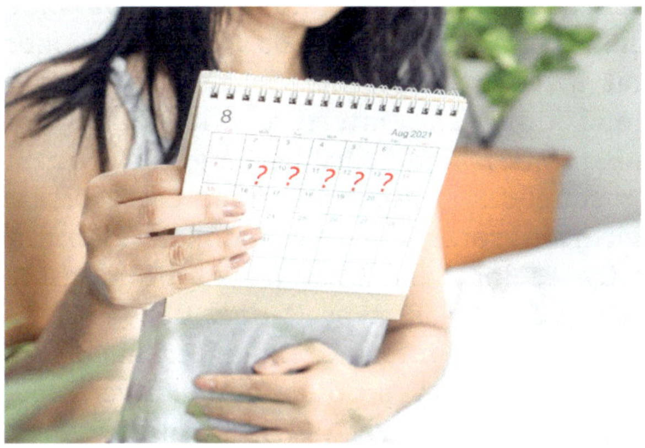

Source: https://charaklive.b-cdn.net/wp-content/uploads/2022/05/period-calender-1200x818.jpg

Furthermore, hormonal effects on menstrual irregularity may be compounded subsequent to bouts of illness or extensive surgical procedures. As a case in point, syndromes like Long COVID illustrate dramatic multi-system dysfunction, which may involve effects on the hormonal mechanisms that regulate reproductive activity. In accord with new reports, pre-existing disease and severity of any acute illness may make complicated not only the physiologic response but also the regularity of the menstrual cycle. To this effect, an understanding of how systemic conditions can affect menstrual health is fundamental in the provision of effective diagnosis and treatment. Given that the medical community is always observing and learning the impact of such conditions on menstrual cycles, it is essential to adopt a delicate strategy in developing tailored treatment plans that address both the symptoms and the underlying health conditions (Negruț et al., 2024).

1.4.3. Impact on Fertility

The relationship between uterine displacement and fertility is a multifaceted phenomenon that has raised substantial concern in reproductive medicine. One of the very important determinants of fertility complications is the presence of uterine leiomyomas, or more commonly, fibroids. Fibroids are benign tumors that distort the uterine cavity, alter uterine blood flow, and interfere with embryonic implantation, and hence become less probable for conception. Among various categories of uterine fibroids, the International Federation of Gynecology and Obstetrics type identifies a unique subclass type 3 ULs. Depending on their invasion into the endometrium, hybrid leiomyomas may produce cumulative effects that are particularly detrimental to women desiring to conceive. Because ongoing research is continuing to make progress in demystifying the complexities of such tumors, the understanding of their specific impacts on fertility remains a central point of concern in creating appropriate treatment protocols for the affected individuals (Chiantera et al., 2023).

Moreover, microbial and metabolic pregnancy conditions play an important role in fetal and maternal health, and hence any level of disruption, like uterine displacement, may lead to complications. For example, high-yielding dairy cows experience metabolic issues at the transition period, leading to conditions such as ketosis and generalized inflammation that adversely affect fertility. In a study assessing serum levels of lipoprotein, it was found that reproductive function during postpartum was greatly enhanced in cows with high levels of High Density Lipoprotein (HDL) before the dry period. Low HDL was correlated with increased chances of reproductive disorders, further supporting the contribution of metabolic health to fertility (Comin et al., 2017).

Transfer of these findings to human reproductive health underscores the importance of a holistic understanding of how physiological and metabolic contexts may influence uterine positioning and reproduction in general. The meaning of uterine displacement extends beyond anatomy, encompassing both biological and psychological influences on fertility. The stress produced by infertility, coupled with bodily pain due to displacement or the presence of fibroids, can result in increased levels of anxiety and depression among the sufferers. The psychological stress can also augment hormonal imbalances, which in turn may inhibit ovulation and reduce overall fertility levels.

With a focus on a comprehensive approach that takes into account the psychosocial nature of fertility, medical professionals can better address both the physiological and psychological implications for treating women with uterine displacement. As studies continue to advance, it is essential that both medical and psychotherapeutic treatments are integrated into treatment strategies in order to maximize fertility in women with such complex reproductive issues.

Test Your Knowledge

1. How can abnormal uterine positioning cause pain and discomfort?
2. What menstrual irregularities may be associated with uterine abnormalities?

1.5. Diagnosis of Uterine Displacement

Learning Outcome

1. Understand the physical examination techniques
2. Define imaging methods, such as ultrasound
3. Describe the role of patient history in diagnosis

Diagnosis of uterine displacement is an involved process requiring a good perception of both clinical presentation and modalities of diagnosis. History and physical examination are valuable in the initial management; patients commonly present with pelvic pain, abnormal uterine bleeding, or urinary symptoms, which are suggestive of displacement. Pelvic examination can perhaps provide evidence of uterine position, such as fornix tenderness or lateral displacement. Diagnostic imaging is also very important in making the diagnosis, with the most frequent first-line imaging being ultrasound. Transvaginal ultrasound can provide clear views of the uterus and the supporting structures and allow clinicians to identify any positional defects or structural abnormalities. When ultrasound imaging is non-diagnostic, other imaging modalities like MRI can be used for clearer visualization of pelvic anatomy and precise diagnosis of uterine displacement. The use of ultrasound in the diagnostic evaluation has changed the detection of uterine displacement. More specifically, by the use of transabdominal and transvaginal ultrasound, practitioners are able to assess the orientation of the uterus and detect any secondary pathologies, such as fibroids or endometriosis, that may be inducing displacement. The clinicians usually assess the bladder and rectum for abnormalities that not only indicate primary displacement but also make the patient's clinical picture more complicated. Besides, new knowledge about imaging technologies enables a better understanding of how the location of the uterus could affect surrounding structures. For example, comparative studies with 3D ultrasound have shown how changes in uterine position affect the anatomy and function of the pelvic floor. Such greater understanding can guide treatment and improve outcomes. Aside from imaging, more problematic clinical presentations, such as recurrent pregnancy loss and infertility, highlight the importance of the correct diagnosis of uterine displacement. An abnormally positioned uterus can prevent normal reproductive function, making natural conception impossible, and leading to adverse pregnancy outcomes. In the event of failure with conservative treatment, surgery may be indicated.

Therapy for uterine displacement varies with etiology and may vary from uterine suspension to total hysterectomy in the chronic form. Understanding the diagnosis and etiological factors of uterine displacement paves the way for customized management strategies and patient counseling. As reproductive health science continues to progress, the study of the effects of uterine displacement, particularly in relation to the establishment of surgical treatment and reproductive outcome, remains the most significant aspect of enhancing the quality of care for affected individuals.

1.5.1. Physical Examination Techniques

Uterine displacement has to be assessed using a systematic approach, beginning with an accurate history taking and observing the presenting complaint. A routine history of menstrual, pregnancy, and related pelvic pain is usually taken by clinicians. This is crucial in that it might throw some light on an underlying condition such as endometriosis or pelvic inflammatory disease—conditions known to have an impact on uterine position and overall gynecological health. This is followed by physical examination techniques that must include external and internal examinations. Abdominal examination may be employed to detect evidence of associated pathologies, while pelvic examination, performed with caution, offers a way to palpate the uterus and determine its mobility and size directly. These preliminary measures not only give needed information but also aid in rapport building for effective management of the patient. Following the initial assessment, practitioners usually employ more advanced imaging techniques to complement findings on physical examination. Of these, magnetic resonance imaging (MRI) and transvaginal ultrasound have become key to assessing uterine displacement, particularly when complicated by conditions like endometriosis that can complicate or mimic easy dislocations. MRI, given its increased resolution characteristics, provides a non-surgical alternative that outlines the uterine anatomy and the adjacent anatomical setting in a better manner. Such advanced modalities are crucial to gain an exhaustive evaluation because they provide visualization of pathologies that lead to displacement or mimic its symptoms.

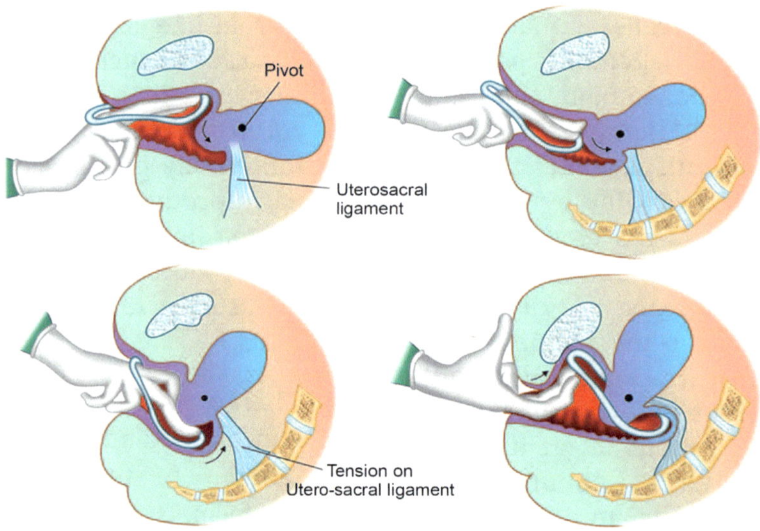

Figure 1.10. Methods of introduction of pessary to correct the position of a RV uterus.

Source: https://oshimu.com/wp-content/uploads/2021/07/Gynaecology-DC-Dutta.pdf

As suggested, two imaging modalities are applied in diagnosing endometriosis: ultrasound scan with endovaginal access and MRI, which is highly accurate in examining conditions of the uterus, including displacement (Anastasi et al., 2015). Integration of physical examination techniques and sensitive imaging enhances diagnostic performance, whereby healthcare providers can sufficiently prepare management for uterine displacement patients. After detection of probable causes, the treatment may vary extensively from conservative therapy in the form of physical therapy and lifestyle change to surgical intervention in complex presentations. Moreover, ongoing assessment by repeated examination and follow-up imaging is essential to determine the success of treatment and symptom progression. This cycle not only addresses current health problems but also prepares women for future pregnancy planning, in the event they opt for pregnancy. Thus, the incorporation of physical examination techniques into imaging procedures not only improves diagnostic information but also enables integrative treatment for women suffering from the displacement of the uterus (N/A, 1989).

1.5.2. Imaging Methods, Such As Ultrasound

Imaging methods, such as ultrasound, play a critical role in the assessment and management of uterine displacement. Ultrasound technology allows for the real-time visual assessment of the uterus and adjacent structures, allowing clinicians to identify abnormalities early. It is a non-invasive imaging procedure, which is valuable to identify the position of intrauterine devices (IUDs) in women, in addition to diagnosing disorders that can affect the location of the uterus. For instance, pre- and post-MRI pelvic ultrasounds in clinical trials have indicated that correctly placed Cu-IUDs are not affected in certain imaging conditions, in line with the reliability of such imaging techniques in device placement evaluation and displacement. The implications of these research studies are significant as they give evidence on patient safety and the effectiveness of various diagnostic approaches in managing uterine health, particularly for those patients undergoing treatment for conditions such as pelvic pain or abnormal uterine bleeding (Moy et al., 2024).

Furthermore, advancements in imaging technologies, including MRI and targeted ultrasound therapy, have broadened the scope of uterine health assessment. For instance, MRgFUS surgery has emerged as a promising option for the surgical resection of symptomatic uterine fibroids. The clinical value of the procedure has been compromised by surrounding anatomical structures, but recent technologies like bowel displacement have proved effective in breaching them.

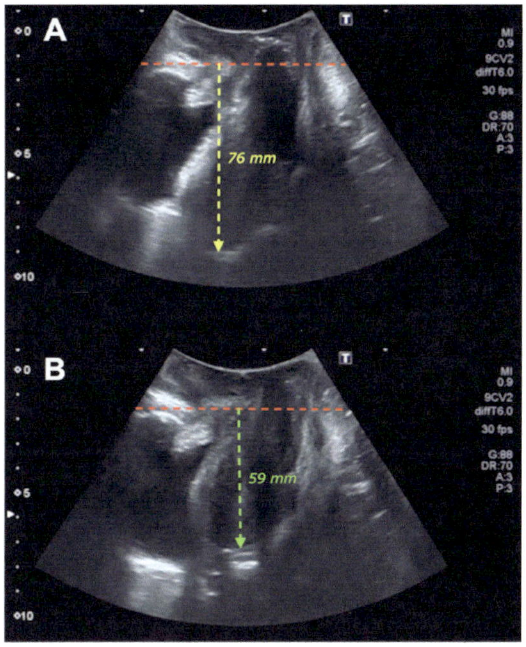

Figure 1.11. Ultrasound of uterine prolapse. Figure (A) shows the midsagittal plane of the pelvic floor at rest where the red line delimits the posteroinferior margin of the pubis and the yellow line the pubis–fundus distance at rest. Figure (B) shows the midsagittal plane of the pelvic floor in Valsalva where the red line establishes the posteroinferior margin of the pubis and the green line the pubis–fundus distance in Valsalva.

Source: https://www.mdpi.com/tomography/tomography-08-00144/article_deploy/html/images/tomography-08-00144-g001.png

Through strategic bladder and rectal filling, clinicians can create a straighter acoustic course for effective treatment, enhancing safety and rates of success during procedures. These advancements reflect advances in imaging technology sophistication and the central role it has in bettering surgical outcomes for uterine displacement and related conditions (Lai et al., 2022).

The integration of different imaging modalities, in this case, ultrasound and MRI, is fundamental in the comprehensive management of uterine displacement. Not only do they contribute to accurate diagnosis, but they also help in therapeutic intervention, hence optimizing patient care quality. Continually developing such imaging modalities and conducting research on alternative methods like bowel displacement enables healthcare providers to significantly enhance treatment outcomes. The collaboration between emerging imaging technologies and the practice setting is the most important, giving women effective, less invasive treatments for conditions created by uterine placement and displacement. With ongoing research, vigilance for patient safety and effectiveness of these imaging modalities as clinical decision guides is essential (Moy et al., 2024; Lai et al., 2022).

1.5.3. Role of Patient History in Diagnosis

In the diagnosis of uterine displacement, patient history can never be overemphasized since it has a vital role in revealing underlying pathology that may not be apparent through physical examination. Appropriate medical history enables health workers to assess the reproductive history of a patient, such as any past surgeries, obstetric history, and IUD use. For instance, IUD insertion can lead to displacement and perforation, and their detection is crucial early on. While conducting research at SGRRIM and HS, inappropriate IUD insertion was seen to lead to displacement and, therefore, strict follow-up and assessment of IUD insert patients with a history were required (Chaudhari et al., 2018). Understanding the patient's pre-existing diseases and treatments directs the diagnostic process such that a more individualized evaluation is achieved based on her own illness narrative. Further, some congenital abnormalities, such as Mullerian anomalies, can be key to the etiology of uterine asymmetry. A proper understanding of the patients reproductive history, including previous known congenital defects, can be useful in diagnosing conditions like a bicornuate uterus, which can influence uterine positioning and lead to displacement. Ultrasound scans of the pelvis remain an invaluable diagnostic tool in these cases, and they are found to be 99% sensitive in identifying such abnormalities (Gorman et al., 2023).

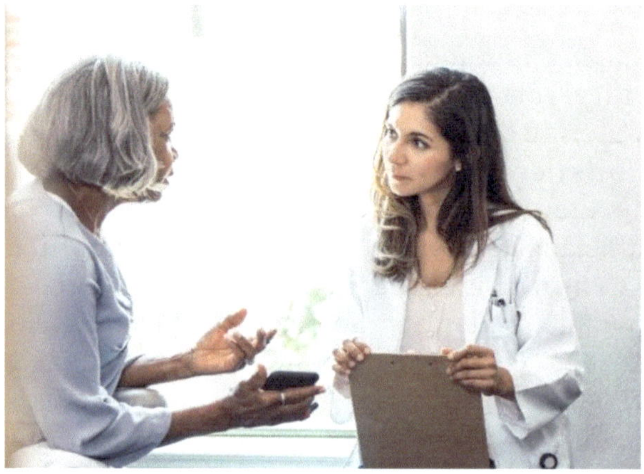

Source: https://i0.wp.com/medlrn.com/wp-content/uploads/2022/04/history-taking-tips-by-medlrn.jpg?resize=1000%2C500&ssl=1

Structural uterine anomalies have implications for future pregnancy and complicate the application of standard treatments for uterine displacement, underscoring the value of including patient history in clinical assessment. Through taking thorough histories, practitioners can more accurately predict complications associated with anatomical abnormalities and prior reproductive disease. Finally, patient history is not merely a data collection process; it provides a collaboration between the provider and patient that is essential to uterine displacement management success. Convincing patients to disclose their whole health histories, including psychological factors and lifestyle choices, can illuminate areas that can affect diagnosis and the resulting treatment plan. For instance, understanding the trends of a patient's menstruation cycle and symptoms that accompany them may be very useful in identifying the existence of displacement. Open communication may lead to more precise diagnosis in accordance with evidence that highlights the significance of accurate patient evaluation in obstetric practice (Chaudhari et al., 2018). In addition, since fetal effects are shaped by maternal health complexities, a holistic strategy taking both maternal background and the most recent physiological evaluation into perspective is vital for effectively managing the implications of uterine displacement.

Test Your Knowledge

1. What physical examination techniques are commonly used to assess uterine position and abnormalities?
2. How does ultrasound assist in diagnosing uterine anatomical variations?

1.6. Treatment Options

Learning Outcome

1. Discuss the non-surgical management strategies
2. Define surgical interventions
3. Explain the lifestyle modifications and physical therapy

With the treatment of uterine displacement, particularly uterine prolapse, on the agenda, there is a need for an appreciation of surgical procedures. Among the features championed is the use of abdominal surgery with a mesh, such as sacrocolpopexy and sacrohysteropexy. Literature indicates that the surgeries are effective in the management of women presenting with uterine or vaginal vault prolapse. Pertinent is the fact that a recent dissertation highlights that after one year of the surgery, there is no difference in outcome between abdominal and vaginal surgeries, offering the potential that both approaches can be good modalities for treatment. Also, new advancements in minimal invasive methods, specifically laparoscopic surgery, have been found to be successful with less blood loss and shorter hospital stays, emphasizing the advantages of modern surgical techniques in enhancing patient recovery and comfort (Oudheusden et al., 2023). In addition to the surgical methods, non-surgical management also forms an integral part of managing uterine displacement. Pelvic floor rehabilitation, for instance, is directed towards muscle strengthening of the pelvic floor and increased support to the uterus. Kegel exercises, for instance, are commonly prescribed to women as a conservative treatment to decrease symptoms of prolapse. Additionally, pessaries, objects inserted into the vagina to support the pelvic organs, also exist as a valuable non-surgical form of intervention. Pessaries may be fitted to meet the individual anatomical needs and can deliver relief from pain so that women may enjoy some degree of normality in their lives. The patients must be educated on how to use and care for pessaries correctly to optimize their effectiveness and minimize potential complications, confirming the importance of detailed treatment protocols (Oudheusden et al., 2023). Lymphovascular space invasion (LVSI) assessment in conditions such as endometrial cancer can have a significant impact on decision-making regarding uterine displacement and associated disorders. LVSI has been found to be an effective prognostic marker, particularly in evaluating the risk of recurrence among endometrial cancer patients. Existing studies attest to the requirement for precise measurement of LVSI in order to properly optimize recommendations for adjuvant treatment. Secondly, higher interobserver agreement for grading LVSI makes it more practical as a tool in clinical decision-making. Quantifying the volume of LVSI more reproducibly is a step towards more accurate and personalized treatment plans. This integration of enhanced prognostic evaluation into treatment algorithms can aid clinicians in deciding the most appropriate interventions for patients with complex cases of uterine displacement, thus optimizing therapeutic approaches and ensuring evidence-based treatment plans for patient outcomes.

1.6.1. Non-Surgical Management Strategies

In uterine displacement management, non-operative interventions play a vital role in symptom alleviation and enhancing the quality of life of the individuals involved. The interventions are normally focused on patient education, lifestyle modification, and pharmacotherapy. Patient education about their condition and the potential causes and effects of uterine displacement encourages them to be involved in their own care. Lifestyle changes, such as healthy weight, exercise on a regular basis, and Kegel exercises, are also crucial in alleviating symptoms. By acknowledging the merit of such non-surgical interventions, clinicians can create individualized care plans that effectively address each patient's needs without surgery. Pharmacologic treatment is also a key component of non-surgical uterine displacement. Hormone therapy, in the form of oral contraceptives or progestins, can control menstrual cycles, decrease heavy bleeding, and minimize pain-related discomfort associated with them. Analgesics can further reduce pain symptoms and improve overall patient comfort. Complementary treatments, such as acupuncture or physiotherapy, can also help improve symptoms and enhance pelvic floor function. By combining these pharmacological and adjunct approaches, medical professionals are able to offer a holistic treatment plan that minimizes the disadvantages of uterine displacement while minimizing the risks of surgery.

Also, psychological consequences of uterine displacement cannot be excluded from consideration in non-surgical interventions. Support groups or counseling, as part of mental health support, can assist patients in coping with depression or anxiety that may be caused by their condition. Emotional well-being support for patients significantly enhances the efficacy of treatment measures and fosters a supportive environment for uterine displacement patients. Furthermore, studies on non-surgical treatment are constantly evolving, and new alternatives emerge for effective management. As medical practices increasingly focus on value-based care, these non-surgical interventions enhance the likelihood of improved patient outcomes as they lower healthcare expenses, resonating with findings from sarcoma treatment where economic factors figure prominently in the determination of management plans (Schelling et al., 2024; Nicholas A Kerna et al., 2024).

1.6.2. Surgical Interventions

Surgery plays a role in the treatment of uterine displacement, particularly where non-surgical intervention is insufficient. The procedure typically depends on the cause of the displacement, such as in prolapse of the uterus or formation of fibroids, whichever may lead to significant morbidity if untreated. Surgical interventions may involve operations in repositioning the uterus, such as hysterectomy in more extreme cases, or, on the other hand, more conservative measures such as uterine suspension procedures that do not impair organ integrity. Surgical extent can further differ from minimally invasive laparoscopic methods to open abdominal surgery, impacting recovery times and levels of complications. It is important to recognize the indications for both surgical options, as this allows clinicians to personalize interventions based on the individual needs of the patient, thereby maximizing the possibility of positive outcomes and patient satisfaction.

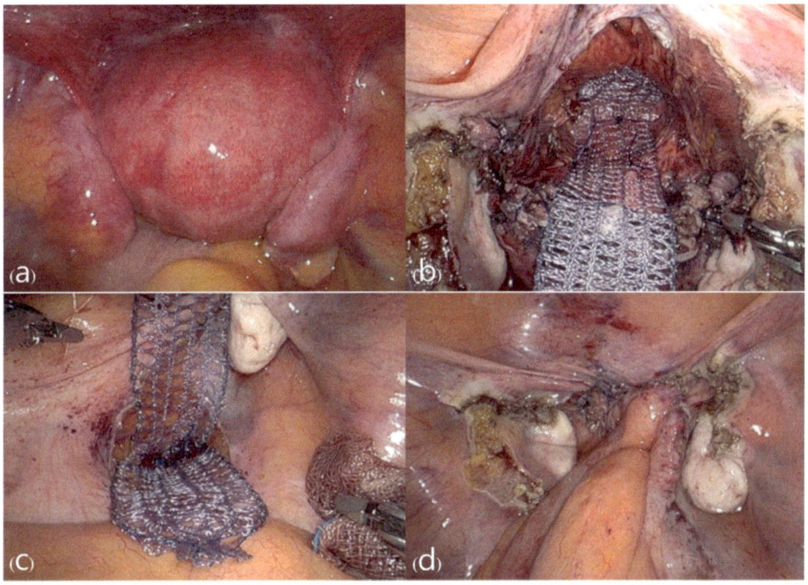

Figure 1.12. Pictures of the surgical procedure: (a) The uterine prolapse within the abdominal cavity before surgery, (b) appearance after hysterectomy with mesh fixation to the stump, (c) fixation of mesh to the sacral promontory, (d) mesh was covered by the peritoneum in the end.

Source: https://www.mdpi.com/2077-0383/13/14/4210

In the management of postpartum complications, surgical intervention also addresses problems such as intractable atonic postpartum hemorrhage (PPH) following delivery. The World Health Organization recommends Uterine Balloon Tamponade (UBT) as one of the most frequently utilized means employed in the treatment of such severe complications. Studies have proven that UBT is also able to control hemorrhaging effectively by compressing the uterine wall with success rates ranging from 84.2% to 98.3% for various UBT devices such as condom-UBT and Bakri balloon systems. These treatments are the best examples of how immediate surgical procedures can prevent life-threatening complications and save maternal lives. Also, their comparative efficacy suggests that, as the methods are different, advances in surgical intervention techniques have significantly improved the treatment of uterine displacement issues that are associated with complications during childbirth and, in the process, translate into a reduction in maternal morbidity and mortality.

Their precision and application of advanced imaging studies in preoperative planning cannot be overlooked when talking about uterine displacement. For instance, in surgeries, accurate tracking of organ motion is essential, particularly in the case of interventional MRI when high-intensity focused ultrasound is used for non-invasive treatments. The methods that utilize MR-based navigation can potentially improve the safety and efficacy of such treatments by providing real-time knowledge about organ position. Developing sophisticated imaging techniques, such as four-dimensional imaging, can improve our understanding of organ movement in living patients and, in turn, inform surgical planning and reduce displacement risks. Moreover, these developments hold promise for the future, more image-guided surgical intervention with improved surgical success as well as overall management of patients, which is critical in complicated instances of uterine displacement.

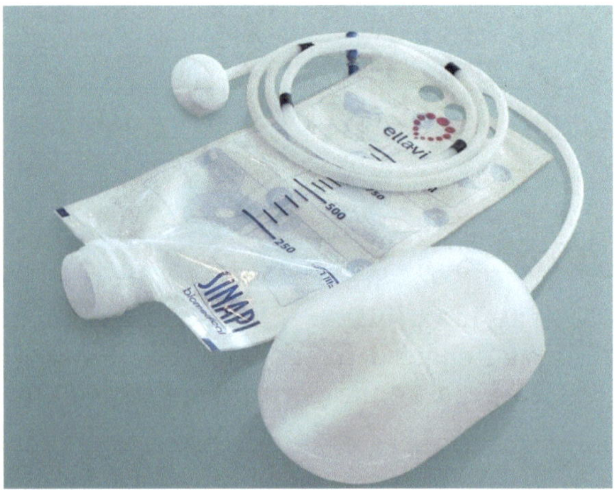

Figure 1.13. Uterine Balloon Tamponade (UBT).

Source: https://media.path.org/images/Sinapi-UBT-2-edit.max-1200x800.jpg

1.6.3. Lifestyle Modifications and Physical Therapy

These lifestyle modifications are of utmost importance in treating uterine displacement, particularly in the prevention of associated symptoms and overall enhancement in pelvic function. Consistent physical exercise not only increases muscle strength in the core and pelvic floor but also enhances blood circulation and reduces associated risks of pelvic pain and dysfunction.

Pelvic floor dysfunction-specific physical therapy may provide individualized interventions, enabling patients to take control of their bodies. With the utilization of exercises such as biofeedback and pelvic floor muscle exercises, patients can be enabled to strengthen their muscles and coordination, which can alleviate symptoms linked to uterine displacement (Abramov et al., 2016). The incorporation of these changes in lifestyle into the daily routine tends to produce more profound, long-term effects, and these are often a crucial part of women's overall care following the displacement of the uterus. In addition, dietary changes are also instrumental in maintaining pelvic health and general well-being. A diet consisting of high levels of anti-inflammatory foods, such as fruits, vegetables, whole grains, and omega-3 fatty acids, helps to manage inflammation that may exacerbate displacement-related pelvic pain and dysfunction. In addition, optimal weight status obtained via caloric balance and management of eating habits reduces pelvic area stress, leading to favorable functional outcomes. This nutritional strategy also aligns with metabolic health guidelines, as inappropriate weight can complicate additional reproductive issues and further exacerbate underlying conditions (Chavarro et al., 2024). Coupling dietary correction with regular physical therapy generates a synergistic effect that not only corrects symptoms of uterine displacement but also promotes a more holistic approach to women's health. Finally, including mental health and stress management techniques in lifestyle modifications is crucial in addressing the complex issue of uterine displacement. Stress possesses the ability to exacerbate physical symptoms and lead to a low quality of life. Mindfulness, yoga, and counseling are among the methods that have the ability to prepare women with coping mechanisms that can ultimately translate to psychological as well as physical health. These include practices that promote awareness of the body, which can enhance one's ability to recognize and attend to their symptoms before they become problematic. By creating a supportive environment that focuses on both physical and emotional health, women are likely to engage and adhere to treatment programs, thereby making lifestyle modification and physical therapy more effective in curing uterine displacement (Abramov et al., 2016; Chavarro et al., 2024). This comprehensive approach is pivotal to fostering resilience and improving the quality of life of the affected individuals.

Test Your Knowledge

1. What are common physical examination techniques used to evaluate gynecological health?
2. How does ultrasound imaging contribute to diagnosing reproductive system conditions?

SUMMARY

Uterine displacement, a condition that is multifactorial and affects many females, requires knowing the causative factors well and their ramifications. Prolapse of the pelvic organs, as mentioned in recent work done on research, is prevalent in many females, about 10% of females in regions such as Nepal. The condition can be a great change in a woman's life, with people experiencing tremendous physical as well as psychological challenges. The findings indicate that some activities performed during the particular phases of the menstrual cycle, particularly heavy lifting, may be contributing to exacerbating the tendency towards displacement. The finding recognized between increased intra-abdominal pressure and the phase of hormonal change highlights the need for increased awareness and preventive strategies among women who experience intense exertion on a daily basis during these susceptible periods (Biswokarma et al., 2016). Recognition of these factors is essential in the development of targeted interventions and education to mitigate against the risks associated with uterine displacement. The involvement of traditional practice in uterine condition management, especially in Sub-Saharan Africa, should also be addressed. The use of tonic effects with a number of plant species demonstrates a culturally rooted use of herbal medicines. While in some cases such practices may be efficacious, there is a high chance of adverse effects, given the evidence of inter-preparation variation in potency and activity of herbal preparations. Recent pharmacological evaluations have validated the uterotonic activity of numerous plants, underscoring the need for exhaustive testing for efficacy and safety (Anderson et al., 2012). Where more women in such places embrace conventional practices at delivery and labor, there is a need to make both patients and healthcare providers aware of the risks involved and the evidence-based practices that can be provided. The multifaceted issue of uterine displacement requires an interdisciplinary approach to address both the medical and social sides of it. Additional research is critically required to establish effective preventive treatment and intervention strategies, as well as to bridge the gap between modern medical technology and traditional practices. Informing women on reproductive health is able to effectively reduce the risk of disorders such as pelvic organ prolapse, thus improving their overall well-being. Besides, the healthcare systems need to incorporate culturally sensitive education regarding uterotonic agents and their suggested benefits and drawbacks. Through the creation of a complementary conversation among customary and contemporary practices in medicine, we are able to improve the care and support provided to women and, hence, deliver better health outcomes in the event of uterine displacement.

One of the phenomenal aspects of uterine displacement relates to biomechanical interactions between the developing fetus and the uterine environment. Evidence indicates that fetal movement is significant in musculoskeletal development, describing the importance of the mechanical stimuli experienced during gestation. In one particular study, cine-MRI data were utilised to track movements by the fetus, specifically kicking, and yielded mean uterine deflections of approximately 6.95±0.41 mm. These displacements were of major boundary conditions to model the uterine force dynamics, showing that each kick evoked estimated reaction forces with a mean of 0.52±0.15 N. These findings point to the advanced biomechanical environment of the fetus, concluding that the forces that occur during uterine displacement play important roles not only in fetal growth but also in understanding pathological conditions related to uterine positioning during pregnancy (Hajnal et al., 2015). In addition, the role of pulmonary surfactant proteins SP-A and SP-D provides a vital insight regarding uterine displacement, specifically towards the induction of labor. Not only are these proteins engaged in pulmonary immunity, but they also appear to have a modulatory effect on myometrial contractions at the feto-maternal interface. Through research, it was noted that recombinant proteins of SP-A and SP-D significantly enhance the contractile activity of human myometrial cells. Through increased speed of cells and overall displacement, these proteins allow for the change in the uterus from the resting state to the contractile state with the onset of labor. Scientific evidence further shows that these proteins also regulate contractile genes, once again emphasizing their pivotal position in uterine dynamics, most importantly during critical phases of gestation (Nayak et al., 2015). Finally, being aware of uterine displacement is not merely about comprehending the mechanical effects of fetal movement but also the biochemical signals that provoke labor. The interaction between mechanical stress and biochemical mediators like SP-A and SP-D is a complex interdependent system critical to fetal health and delivery processes. The ability of these proteins to control contractions and induce pro-inflammatory cytokines indicates they may be vital to prepare the uterine environment for labor. This tightrope between the mechanical and biochemical forces mirrors the sensitive balance required for healthy uterine function, illustrating how disruption in either can lead to complications in pregnancy. Accordingly, the total analysis of biomechanical and biochemical aspects is necessary for a complete understanding of uterine displacement and its effects on fetal and maternal well-being (Hajnal et al., 2015; Nayak et al., 2015).

KEY TERMS FROM THIS CHAPTER

- Anatomical relations
- Anteversion
- Bowel displacement
- Care support systems
- Clinical pregnancy rates
- Clinical vigilance
- Concomitant displacement
- Gynecological symptoms
- Intervention tactics
- Intrauterine device (IUD),
- Kegel exercises
- Lateral displacement
- Maternal-fetal medicine
- Menstrual cycles
- Menstruation mechanics
- Mortality rates
- Pelvic cavity
- Pelvic floor dysfunction

CRITICAL THINKING QUESTIONS

1. **The most common type of uterine displacement is:**
   a. Retroversion
   b. Anteversion
   c. Prolapse
   d. Lateral displacement
2. **Uterine prolapse is primarily due to weakness of which structure?**
   a. Ovaries
   b. Fallopian tubes
   c. Pelvic floor muscles and ligaments
   d. Abdominal muscles
3. **Which of the following is NOT a common symptom of uterine prolapse?**
   a. Pelvic pressure
   b. Backache
   c. Dyspnea
   d. Vaginal bulge
4. **Uterine retroversion is best diagnosed by:**
   a. Chest X-ray
   b. Pelvic ultrasound
   c. Colonoscopy
   d. Mammography
5. **Pessaries are used in the management of:**
   a. Fibroid uterus
   b. Ectopic pregnancy
   c. Uterine displacement and prolapse
   d. Ovarian cysts

Short Answer Questions

1. What are the main anatomical parts of the uterus?
2. Name two common types of uterine displacement.
3. What are some possible causes of uterine displacement?
4. List two symptoms commonly associated with uterine displacement.
5. Which diagnostic methods are used to detect uterine displacement?
6. What treatment options are available for uterine displacement?

Answer to Critical Thinking Questions

1. (a) 2. (c) 3. (c) 4. (b) 5. (c)

REFERENCES

1. Abramov, Y., Almeida, F. G., Berghmans, B., Bo, B., et al. (2016). An International Urogynecological Association (IUGA)/International Continence Society (ICS) joint report on the terminology for the conservative and nonpharmacological management of female pelvic floor dysfunction. https://core.ac.uk/download/293861075.pdf (accessed on 15th June 2025).
2. Allen, R. E., Berglas, B., Blandpied, P., Brooks, S. V., Brooks, S. V., Colombo, M., DeLancey, J. O. L., et al. (2007). Functional anatomy of the female pelvic floor. http://deepblue.lib.umich.edu/bitstream/2027.42/72597/1/annals.1389.034.pdf (accessed on 15th June 2025).
3. Anastasi, E., Ballesio, L., Bernardo, S., Fuggetta, F., et al. (2015). Endometriosis: 10 key points for MRI. https://core.ac.uk/download/54518026.pdf (accessed on 15th June 2025).
4. Anderson, F. W. J., Stanton, C., & Tripathi, V. (2012). Traditional preparations used as uterotonics in Sub-Saharan Africa and their pharmacologic effects. http://deepblue.lib.umich.edu/bitstream/2027.42/135671/2/ijgo16.pdf (accessed on 15th June 2025).
5. Barker, A., Benner, A., Cutting, G., Richter, K., Nguyen, K. H., Brezina, P., Anchan, R., et al. (2011). Genetic normalization of differentiating aneuploid human embryos. https://core.ac.uk/download/pdf/290095.pdf (accessed on 15th June 2025).
6. Bartosch, C., Bosse, T., Genestie, C., Lax, S., et al. (2019). Reproducibility of lymph vascular space invasion (LVSI) assessment in endometrial cancer. https://core.ac.uk/download/322827724.pdf (accessed on 15th June 2025).
7. Biswokarma, Y. (2016). Effect of heavy lifting with a head strap on the pelvic floor across the menstrual cycle. https://core.ac.uk/download/151739599.pdf (accessed on 15th June 2025).
8. Blake, J. R., Gadelha, H., Gaffney, E. A., Kirkman-Brown, J., et al. (2011). Mammalian sperm motility: Observation and theory. https://core.ac.uk/download/pdf/1593464.pdf (accessed on 15th June 2025).
9. Bonney, E. A., Nott, J. P., Pickering, J. D., Simpson, N., et al. (2016). The structure and function of the cervix during pregnancy. https://core.ac.uk/download/42625653.pdf (accessed on 15th June 2025).
10. Borgatta, L., & Stubblefield, P. G. (2009). *The Challenging Abortion*. https://doi.org/10.1002/9781444313031.ch13 (accessed on 15th June 2025).
11. Celicanin, Z. (2014). Respiratory organ motion in interventional MRI: Tracking, guiding and modeling. https://core.ac.uk/download/46605059.pdf (accessed on 15th June 2025).
12. Chaudhari, P., Gupta, V., Kumari, N., Nimonkar, A., et al. (2018). Displaced intrauterine contraceptive device: A prospective study at tertiary level hospital of Uttarakhand, India. https://core.ac.uk/download/539901558.pdf (accessed on 15th June 2025).
13. Chaurasia, H., Joshi, B., Moray, K. V., Sachin, S., et al. (2022). A narrative review comparing clinical effectiveness of commonly used uterine balloon tamponade devices for postpartum hemorrhage management in India. https://core.ac.uk/download/539902633.pdf (accessed on 15th June 2025).
14. Chavarro, J., Nichols, A., & Oken, E. (2024). Reproductive risk factors across the female life course and later metabolic health. https://core.ac.uk/download/643236611.pdf (accessed on 15th June 2025).

15. Chiantera, V., Cicinelli, E., Dellino, M., Etrusco, A., et al. (2023). The challenge of FIGO type 3 leiomyomas and infertility: Exploring therapeutic alternatives amidst limited scientific certainties. https://core.ac.uk/download/599093414.pdf (accessed on 15th June 2025).

16. Comin, A., Crociati, M., Floridi, C., Fruganti, G., et al. (2017). Influence of lipoproteins at dry-off on metabolism of dairy cows during transition period and on postpartum reproductive outcomes. https://core.ac.uk/download/84480889.pdf (accessed on 15th June 2025).

17. Cornillie, P., Deprez, P., Gasthuys, F., Pardon, B., et al. (2012). Left abomasal displacement between the uterus and rumen during bovine twin pregnancy. https://core.ac.uk/download/55844239.pdf (accessed on 15th June 2025).

18. Crichton, E. C. (2018). The significance of the retroverted uterus in obstetrics and gynecology. https://core.ac.uk/download/478312989.pdf (accessed on 15th June 2025).

19. Dietz, H. P. (2018). Ultrasound in the assessment of pelvic organ prolapse. *Best Practice & Research Clinical Obstetrics & Gynecology, 54*, 12–30. https://doi.org/10.1016/j.bpobgyn.2018.06.006 (accessed on 15th June 2025).

20. Drabo, S., Filippi, V., & Storeng, K. T. (2013). Too poor to live? A case study of vulnerability and maternal mortality in Burkina Faso. https://core.ac.uk/download/pdf/13598752.pdf (accessed on 15th June 2025).

21. Fischell, D. R., & Mazique, J. C. (1981). Cervix-to-rectum measuring device in a radiation applicator for use in the treatment of cervical cancer. https://core.ac.uk/download/pdf/10357708.pdf (accessed on 15th June 2025).

22. Franco, D. M., & Maya, M. V. (2017). Resuscitation of obstetric patient. https://core.ac.uk/download/322432310.pdf (accessed on 15th June 2025).

23. Göbel, J., Schmidt, M., Seifried-Dübon, T., Linden, K., Degen, L., Rind, E., Eilerts, A., et al. (2022). Higher work-privacy conflict and lower job satisfaction in GP leaders and practice assistants working full-time compared to part-time: Results of the IMPROVEjob Study. *International Journal of Environmental Research and Public Health, 19*. https://www.semanticscholar.org/paper/762d8dde82381cf67093c1b1b8b78d71ac29cff9 (accessed on 15th June 2025).

24. Godwin, R., Saxena, A., Sethi, A., & Tomar, G. S. (2015). Laparoscopic surgeries during pregnancy – related anaesthetic concerns. https://core.ac.uk/download/pdf/144770076.pdf (accessed on 15th June 2025).

25. Goldspohn, A. (1896). The proper indications for repair of pathologic lacerations of the cervix uteri, and the proper operations to meet them. *Journal of the American Medical Association, 26*, 512–512. https://doi.org/10.1001/jama.1896.02430630014002d (accessed on 15th June 2025).

26. Gorman, C. N., Grabois, E. P., Grabois, S. A., Mathur, A., et al. (2023). Dichorionic-diamniotic twin pregnancy in a bicornuate uterus with twin A affected by Ebstein's anomaly. https://core.ac.uk/download/598023232.pdf (accessed on 15th June 2025).

27. Hajnal, J. V., Hayat, T. T. A., Loo, J. H. W., Nowlan, N. C., et al. (2015). Modeling the biomechanics of fetal movements. https://core.ac.uk/download/327073069.pdf (accessed on 15th June 2025).

28. Jacquinet, A., Flasse, L., Dohet, M., Vanhaeren, R., Pendeville, H., Saunders, C., Lehman, A., et al. (2025). Variants in NR6A1 as a cause for congenital renal, vertebral and uterine anomalies.

https://www.semanticscholar.org/paper/d9fbc5a1ef927b4bb416dc666c04728a8f79ccd8 (accessed on 15th June 2025).

29. Jana, P., & Madhumithaa, V. S. (2025). Ayurvedic management of Vataja Yoni Vyapad–A case study. https://core.ac.uk/download/641551338.pdf (accessed on 15th June 2025).

30. Jousilahti, J., Grabovac, I., Licht, A., et al. (2023). Ethnic disparity in cancer mortality in adult Fijian women, 2013–17. *The European Journal of Public Health, 33*. https://www.semanticscholar.org/paper/b69dd083e12d029d3932f9c83162792a23aec2de (accessed on 15th June 2025).

31. Kerna, N. A., Carsrud, N. V., Zhao, X., Holets, H. M., Chawla, S., Flores, J. V., Ngwu, D. C., et al. (2024). The pathophysiology of scoliosis across the spectrum of human physiological systems. *European Journal of Medical and Health Research*. https://www.semanticscholar.org/paper/fd1565715d85106bf88f26c616aea4c84a675b1e (accessed on 15th June 2025).

32. Khan, B. Z., Hussain, R., Ahmad, R., & Munir, S. (2022). Amplification of environmental appraisal coordination at General Hospital Lahore and its implications to evaluate management review. *International Journal of Economic and Environmental Geology*. https://www.semanticscholar.org/paper/a95306ebab6e52a452725a24bf0c7236858a69a9 (accessed on 15th June 2025).

33. Kinsella, S., Carvalho, B., Dyer, R. A., Fernando, R., McDonnell, N., Mercier, F. J., Palanisamy, A., et al. (2017). International consensus statement on the management of hypotension with vasopressors during caesarean section under spinal anesthesia. *Anesthesia, 73*, 71–92. https://doi.org/10.1111/anae.14080 (accessed on 15th June 2025).

34. Lai, M., Chen, Y., Li, H., Li, Y., Wu, S., Li, Z., & Zhang, Q. (2022). A modified bowel displacement technique for magnetic resonance imaging–guided focused ultrasound surgery in the treatment of uterine fibroids and adenomyosis. *Journal of Computer Assisted Tomography, 46*, 379–382. https://www.semanticscholar.org/paper/adf348a7b451b72bc7bb7172b24223e0a534dcc4 (accessed on 15th June 2025).

35. Lavoie, J., Varcoe, C., Wathen, C., Ford-Gilboe, M., Browne, A., on behalf of the DeepMind Health Team. (2018). Sentinels of inequity: Examining policy requirements for equity-oriented primary healthcare. *BMC Health Services Research, 18*. https://www.semanticscholar.org/paper/d46387d946a89850a8ca40aa6db8857f21012483 (accessed on 15th June 2025).

36. Li, Q., Qi, D., Bi, T., Guo, X., & Chen, H. (2024). Case report: Uterine perforation caused by migration of intrauterine devices. *Frontiers in Medicine, 11*. https://www.semanticscholar.org/paper/4e3d5be00c1ed111db926f32dd2f4d0a83b89305 (accessed on 15th June 2025).

37. Lloyd, D., Pushparajah, K., Simpson, J., van Amerom, J., van Poppel, M. P. M., Schulz, A., Kainz, B., et al. (2019). Three-dimensional visualization of the fetal heart using prenatal MRI with motion-corrected slice-volume registration: A prospective, single-center cohort study. *The Lancet, 393*, 1619–1627. https://doi.org/10.1016/s0140-6736(18)32490-5 (accessed on 15th June 2025).

38. Macheku, G. S., Jungulu, F. C., Kiyogoma, E. K., Kagya, K., Mrutu, S. I., & Mahande, M. J. (2025). Retroperitoneal displacement of an intrauterine device (IUD): A case report. *International Journal of Innovative Science and Research Technology*. https://www.semanticscholar.org/paper/f84f32f2ae1836d38dc2ccf59397de57df5107ea (accessed on 15th June 2025).

39. Moustafa, M. (2014). Fetus safety in motor vehicle accidents. https://core.ac.uk/download/288377561.pdf (accessed on 15th June 2025).

40. Moy, J., Landon, M., Vigilante, J., Lehmann, B., DeChambeau, A., Rohlfing, F., & Marks, R. (2024). An *in-vivo* study of the safety of copper-containing intrauterine devices in 3.0 Tesla magnetic resonance imaging. *Abdominal Radiology (New York), 49*, 4592–4599. https://www.semanticscholar.org/paper/d8ef97cbe019f2812b64aaca129d8cc2e11e790f (accessed on 15th June 2025).

41. Nayak, A., Mosher, A. A., Yadav, A. K., Montalbano, A. P., Belt, A. R., Krolak-Olejnik, B., Schaub, B., et al. (2015). Surfactant proteins SP-A and SP-D modulate uterine contractile events in ULTR myometrial cell line. https://core.ac.uk/download/74409355.pdf (accessed on 15th June 2025).

42. Negruț, N., Menegas, G., Kampioti, S., Bourelou, M., Kopanyi, F., Hassan, F. D., Asowed, A., et al. (2024). The multisystem impact of long COVID: A comprehensive review. *Diagnostics, 14*, 244–244. https://doi.org/10.3390/diagnostics14030244 (accessed on 15th June 2025).

43. Padmalatha, V. V., Poornima, M., Rao, S. R., Shakuntala, A., et al. (2012). A rare case of isolated torsion of haematosalphinx presenting as acute abdomen during pregnancy. https://core.ac.uk/download/pdf/13598752.pdf (accessed on 15th June 2025).

44. Parente, M. P. L. (2008). Biomechanics of the pelvic floor during vaginal delivery. https://core.ac.uk/download/143373121.pdf (accessed on 15th June 2025).

45. Parry, J. P., & Isaacson, K. (2019). Hysteroscopy and why macroscopic uterine factors matter for fertility. *Fertility and Sterility, 112*, 203–210. https://doi.org/10.1016/j.fertnstert.2019.06.031 (accessed on 15th June 2025).

46. Pineda, D. O., Campo, M. de la C., Carballo Gutierrez, J. L., & Moreno González, I. (2025). Excessive uterine bleeding in a patient with functional thrombopathy associated with chronic kidney disease. About a case. *South Health and Policy*. https://www.semanticscholar.org/paper/c1eccc1452fee84cb0ec1ddc127bce48ccae6525 (accessed on 15th June 2025).

47. Schelling, G., Heesen, P., Tautermann, B., Wepf, M., Di Federico, B., Frei, A., van Oudenaarde, K., et al. (2024). Impact of institutional practices and surgical complexity on sarcoma surgery costs: Driving efficiency in value-based healthcare. *Cancers, 16*. https://www.semanticscholar.org/paper/1f99afb2f6dd830414db20467879a74e913f69a3 (accessed on 15th June 2025).

48. Smolarz, B., Szyłło, K., & Romanowicz, H. (2021). Endometriosis: Epidemiology, classification, pathogenesis, treatment and genetics (Review of literature). *International Journal of Molecular Sciences, 22*, 10554–10554. https://doi.org/10.3390/ijms221910554 (accessed on 15th June 2025).

49. Uccella, S., Kho, R. M., Garzon, S., Casarin, J., Zorzato, P. C., & Ghezzi, F. (2021). The Large Uterus Classification System: A prospective observational study. *BJOG: An International Journal of Obstetrics & Gynaecology, 128*, 1526–1533. https://doi.org/10.1111/1471-0528.16753 (accessed on 15th June 2025).

50. van Oudheusden, A. M. J. (2023). Surgical treatment for apical vaginal prolapse: Sacro colpopexy, Sacro hysteropexy, and sacrospinous fixation. https://core.ac.uk/download/586790240.pdf (accessed on 15th June 2025).

51. Wang, W., Sung, N., Gilman-Sachs, A., & Kwak-Kim, J. (2020). T helper (Th) cell profiles in pregnancy and recurrent pregnancy losses: Th1/Th2/Th9/Th17/Th22/Tfh cells. *Frontiers in Immunology, 11*. https://doi.org/10.3389/fimmu.2020.02025 (accessed on 15th June 2025).

52. Watad, H., Ifrach, U., Stockheim, D., Yulzari, V., Meron, O. C., Blank, M., Sredni, B., et al. (2024). The contradictive findings between ultrasound, hysteroscopy and cytokines in women with nonhormonal IUDs suffering from menorrhagia: A prospective study. *Archives of Gynecology and Obstetrics, 309*, 2057–2062. https://doi.org/10.1007/s00404-024-07457-7 (accessed on 15th June 2025).

53. Wiles, R., Hankinson, B., Benbow, E., & Sharp, A. (2022). Making decisions about radiological imaging in pregnancy. *BMJ*. https://doi.org/10.1136/bmj-2022-070486 (accessed on 15th June 2025).

54. Woodall, P. H. (1902). *Manual of Osteopathic Gynecology*. https://core.ac.uk/download/234121797.pdf (accessed on 15th June 2025).

FEMALE INFERTILITY

2

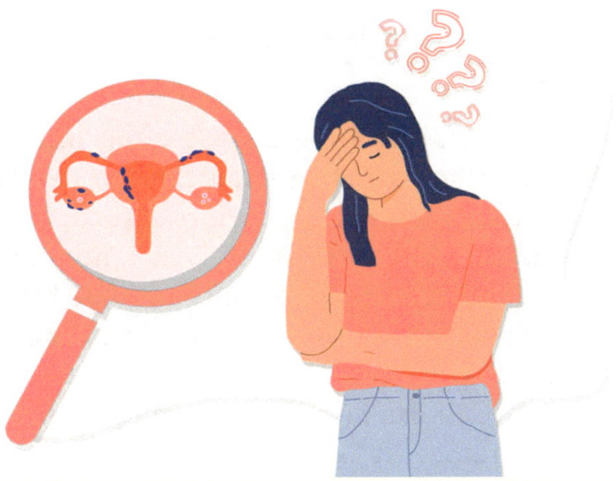

Introduction

Female infertility should be understood due to its increasing incidence and its large impact on couples and individuals. Infertility, or clinical pregnancy failure following 12 months of frequent unprotected coitus, is seen in approximately 8% to 12% of reproductive-age couples globally. The beginning of waning fertility in women typically begins in women's late twenties to early thirties and presents an enormous challenge for the majority who want conception. It is important to establish the various causes of infertility that dominate, from health complications to lifestyle variables. The importance of the knowledge is not just in the diagnosis of the condition but in the introduction of effective treatments and preventive measures, particularly those centered on lifestyle and diet interventions, as noted in recent literature (Kahan et al., 2024). A careful examination of the etiology of female infertility reveals that it is not only a biological condition but is often co-mingled with psychological and social factors. For instance, such diseases as Polycystic Ovarian Syndrome (PCOS) are known to be major

LEARNING OBJECTIVES

After studying this chapter, you will be able to:

1. Identify the various causes of female infertility
2. Explain medical conditions that are commonly associated with infertility in women
3. Analyze lifestyle factors that can affect female fertility
4. Describe diagnostic procedures used to evaluate female infertility
5. Evaluate treatment options available for managing female infertility
6. Discuss the psychological and emotional impacts of infertility

etiologies of infertility, occurring in a large number of women with issues of reproduction. The psychological toll of infertility can lead to increased stress, anxiety, and depression levels, which are often accompanied by outside pressures and internal expectations regarding motherhood. Another is the growing prevalence of obesity because it is linked to fertility, which underscores the necessity of a multidisciplinary approach to female infertility understanding and treatment. Many studies cite dietary changes, for example, improved dietary habits, as having beneficial effects on fertility levels (Ibrahim et al., 2024).

Lastly, the study of female infertility entails knowing its scope, understanding its causes, and being aware of its psychological impacts. The role of good nutrition and lifestyle becomes increasingly significant with research identifying a correlation between nutrition and reproduction. Through the presentation of these elements, scientists and healthcare professionals are better placed to support women faced with issues of infertility. This introduction provides a foundation for an elaborative discussion on diagnosing and treating female infertility successfully and emphasizes the importance of considering a wide range of causative factors from physiological status to lifestyle habits, ultimately empowering women in their reproductive experiences (Kahan et al., 2024).

Definition of Female Infertility

The condition of female infertility encompasses a complex mixture of biological, medical, and psychological factors and is the major issue for the majority of couples desiring to get pregnant. Generally, infertility can be described as the inability to conceive after a year of regular, unprotected intercourse. The condition can arise from any of a variety of causes, such as disorders of ovulation, congenital abnormalities in the reproductive tract, or hormonal imbalance. Of greatest concern is the role of age, as women's fertility significantly reduces after 35. The definition of infertility must also move beyond basic medical formulations to include societal and cultural conceptions that may influence how women view and respond to infertile conditions. Studies emphasize the extent to which there is a need for more information regarding infertility as well as the surrounding issues. Youth, both medical and non-medical students, were revealed to possess varying levels of knowledge about the definition and causes of infertility, with non-medical students having significantly lower knowledge (Adlani et al., 2024).

This variation suggests the likelihood of ignorance and bad education on reproductive health, leading to behaviors that could pose the risk of infertility. Moreover, ignorance about various causes of infertility can hide individuals' awareness of reproductive options for them, leading to excessive reliance on less effective conventional methods or fertility control myths. Therefore, it is necessary to fill the gaps in knowledge to empower individuals to control their reproductive life effectively. Furthermore, recent progress in assisted reproductive technology has augmented the awareness of infertility by facilitating more successful embryological and clinical assessment. Statistical modeling has identified certain infertility endophenotypes, extremely fine differences in fertility capacity that are not necessarily evident in the natural conception environment (Ottolini et al., 2024). These advances have highlighted the complex genetics and biology of infertility, where the disease is revealed to always include complex developmental deficits tailored to an individual case. As the field prospers, infertility shall not only be characterized in its holistic form of clinical presentation but also by a depth of insight into its diverse biological heterogeneity in the context of female reproductive health. This sophisticated understanding underscores the need for personalized treatment approaches, demonstrating that female infertility is not a singular condition but a continuum of reproductive pathology controlled by gene and environmental determinants.

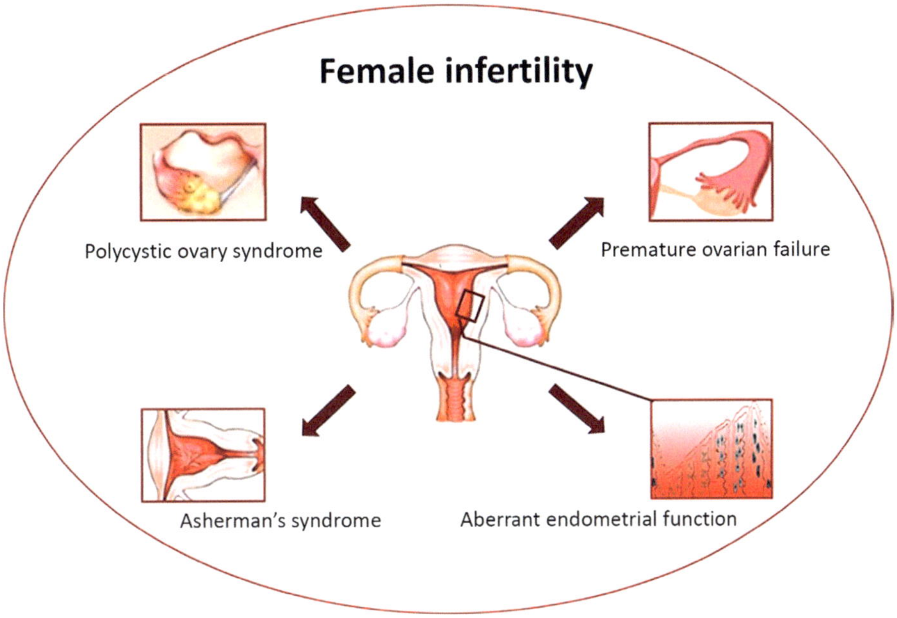

Figure 2.1. The common types of female infertility issues.

Source: https://www.researchgate.net/figure/The-common-types-of-female-infertility-issues_fig2_359587273

Importance of Addressing Infertility Issues

The need to resolve fertility issues extends beyond personal despair, entwining with broader social implications. Infertility affects approximately 15% of couples globally, and this can engender psychological pain, marital issues, and public shame. Women are most frequently the victims of this condition, not only experiencing physical barriers to conception but also cultural forces that equate womanhood with motherhood. As the Global Burden of Diseases, Injuries, and Risk Factors Study emphasized, infertility is a significant aspect of women's health that is usually overlooked in public health issues. By touching on reproductive health and infertility specifically, healthcare systems can improve general well-being and ease associated mental illness among women. To this end, the function of curing and diagnosing infertility enhances empowerment by enabling women to make informed reproductive choices. This ultimately resonates as a matter of individual and public health. The cure for infertility also has major effects on population dynamics and economic stability. For most societies, a fall in birth rates has important effects on the composition of the workforce and national economic production. As seen in the outcomes of extensive global studies, for instance, GBD 2017, countries experiencing fertility decline are likely to face issues of aging and shrinking workforces. This can lead to greater inequality in social support systems from an economic perspective and even shortages of labor. In this way, through the encouragement of infertility treatment and research, policymakers are helping stabilize current and future populations in harmony with demographic transformation. These measures not only increase the chances of family building but also go a long way in promoting sustainable economic development, reflecting the broader social benefit of tackling infertility. Additionally, there is a critical need to raise awareness and education about infertility to demystify myths and clear common misconceptions as well as lower stigma. Despite the uprise in medical technology advancements and changes in societal values, myths surrounding infertility continue, causing many women to delay coming forward. Through promoting comprehensive, inclusive reproductive health education, healthcare workers can empower the citizenry with data on fertility decisions and the importance of early treatment. GBD evidence emphasizes that longevity and quality of life are not separable from reproductive health, showing that infertility treatment promotes family formation but also improves general health outcomes for women. Heightened awareness can foster a sensitive community where it is acceptable to talk about infertility, thus helping towards increased availability of treatment processes and psychological counseling among sufferers.

2.1. Causes of Female Infertility

Learning Outcome

1. Explain the impact of hormonal imbalances on female infertility
2. Identify structural abnormalities that contribute to female infertility
3. Analyze how age-related factors affect female fertility

The multifactorial pathogenesis of female infertility consists of multiple biological, environmental, and lifestyle factors that can undermine reproductive function. Hormonal fluctuations typically have a causative role, disrupting the delicate interaction between the hypothalamus, pituitary gland, and ovaries, resulting in infertility conditions such as polycystic ovary syndrome (PCOS) and irregular menstrual cycles. Furthermore, anatomical abnormalities, such as uterine fibroids or congenital abnormalities, contribute significantly to causing infertility by affecting implantation or development of a fertilized egg. 31.5% of infertilities have been attributed specifically to result from female factors alone, showing a huge proportion of the population suffering from such conditions (Amininezhad et al., 2020). The quality and quantity of oocytes in women also decline with advancing age, making conception even more challenging. Taken together, these points underscore the need for comprehensive evaluations in order to identify specific causes of infertility among these individuals. In addition to biological points, lifestyle and environmental factors uniquely affect women's fertility. Exposure to environmental toxins, such as pesticides, heavy metals, and endocrine-disrupting chemicals, has also been associated with decreased reproductive success. Further, lifestyle elements, including smoking and alcohol consumption, adversely affect fertility by altering hormonal balance and egg quality. The assessment of these elements is important because it has been proven in studies that alterations in lifestyle can improve fertility outcomes. Surprisingly, male partners' occupation and socioeconomic status also emerge as contributing factors, since it has been proven that there is a high degree of correlation between a husband's profession and spontaneous pregnancy (Amininezhad et al., 2020). These findings suggest that the holistic treatment of infertility must consider both partners' profiles, e.g., occupational exposures and lifestyle, and thus provide an actual diagnostic scenario for treatment.

Psychological effects of infertility cannot be overemphasized because it has a profound impact on women's psychological state. Women who are undergoing fertility treatment have been reported to have high levels of anxiety and depression, which further results in a cycle of stress that can further weaken reproductive functioning. Tossed on top of this is social pressure to get pregnant, which captivates the people involved with sensations of isolation and desperation. Research indicates that the fear of potential health effects of assisted reproductive technologies, such as increased susceptibility to cancer, is most specifically influencing these women. The complexity involved in the connection between treatments for infertility and future health outcomes complicates decision-making for both patients and health professionals. As awareness of the numerous causes of female infertility grows, thought must be given to the psychological implications in offering comprehensive care and support to those affected.

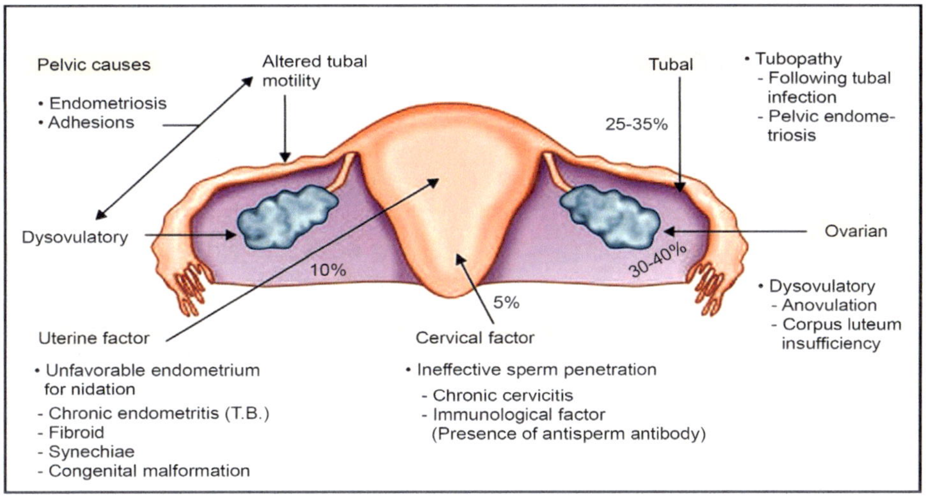

Figure 2.2. Common causes of female infertility.

Source: https://oshimu.com/wp-content/uploads/2021/07/Gynaecology-DC-Dutta.pdf

2.1.1. Hormonal Imbalances

The role of hormonal imbalances in female infertility is vast, as such imbalances can disrupt the delicate endocrine system that regulates reproduction. These hormones include estrogen, progesterone, luteinizing hormone (LH), and follicle-stimulating hormone (FSH), and are crucial in ovarian function and menstrual cycles. A hormonal disruption can lead to a myriad of conditions, such as polycystic ovary syndrome (PCOS) and hypothalamic amenorrhea, both of which are causes of infertility. Elevated androgen levels in PCOS, for instance, result in irregular ovulation or anovulation and hence compromised fertility potential. Also, the inability of proper hormonal communication may impair embryo implantation, illustrating the way in which hormonal health is inextricably linked with reproductive success. Thus, correction of the hormonal imbalance must ensue if fertility is to be gained and the likelihood of conception maximized. Further, the complexity of endocrine interplay demands a multidimensional approach to female infertility diagnosis and therapy. Endocrine function measurement tests and their function testing are a critical component of determining underlying issues. For example, elevated prolactin levels can indicate pituitary gland abnormalities, which may impair menstrual cyclicity predictability and ovulation. Similarly, low progesterone concentrations can inhibit endometrial maturation for implantation. All these treatment modalities, ranging from lifestyle modifications to pharmacologic treatment, are capable of restoring hormonal balance. However, the hormonal treatments may involve the administration of drugs such as clomiphene citrate to stimulate ovulation or hormonal replacement therapies that regulate levels of some hormones. Although the treatments show promise, there needs to be an arrangement of treatments based on each patient's hormonal pattern and overall well-being, as evidenced by current research.

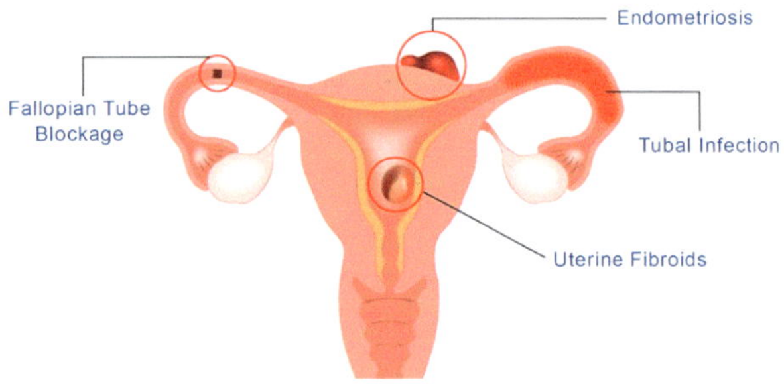

Figure 2.3. Female infertility can arise from a wide variety of factors.

Source: https://risaaivf.com/female-fertility-causes-and-treatment/

In studying female infertility, new studies also suggest potential genetic links and new diagnostic tests, both of which further establish hormonal imbalance as understood today. As an example, dermatoglyphics studies have proposed intriguing correlations between unique skin ridge patterns and fertility-pertaining genetic diseases such as Turner syndrome and polycystic ovary syndrome (PCOS) (Anjankar et al., 2024). These trends, encouraging as they are, require more stringent study to ascertain any ultimate causal connections with infertility. In addition, increased emphasis on holistic practices—like lifestyle adjustments, stress management, and comprehensive medical assessment—can make favorable contributions toward balancing hormones. Integrative care is rewarded in clinician-patient collaboration, providing targeted methods for enhanced reproductive health. With advancing research, understanding the intricacies of hormonal imbalances in female infertility will be key in developing effective treatment plans and supporting optimistic parents every step of the way to conception.

2.1.2. Structural Abnormalities

The impact of structural defects on female infertility is complex, often necessitating a comprehensive assessment and treatment. The defects can be in one of a variety of forms, such as congenital uterine malformations like a septate uterus or a unicornuate uterus, that compromise implantation and sustain early pregnancy. Structural defects can also extend to the fallopian tubes, which can lead to blockages to prevent the egg and sperm from uniting, severely compromising fertility. It is necessary to identify these conditions since they are not always easy to note during routine examination. Correction of structural issues through surgical intervention, such as hysteroscopic or laparoscopic surgery, can correct normal anatomical function and increase chances for fertility.

As per the literature, optimal medical care and surgical intervention aimed at correcting such abnormalities can significantly promote reproductive success in these women (Dalis, 2024). The complexity of structural anomalies extends to the realm of genetic predispositions that can disrupt reproductive anatomy. Mutations and genetic inclinations have a profound effect on organogenesis and the function of the reproductive organs. Recent studies have recognized the significance of specific genes responsible for oocyte maturation, of which the zona pellucida (ZP) is particularly vital. Abnormalities of the zona pellucida can be representative of oocyte maturation defects, resulting in direct fertility. Interestingly, researchers isolated a new mutation of the ZP1 gene for the disease, emphasizing the genetic basis of some structural issues. This gives insight into how delicate the relationship between genetics and anatomy is, whereby treating genetic defects may be as crucial as addressing physical flaws. Thus, incorporating genetic screening into fertility testing could enhance diagnosis and tailor treatment options better for women with structural causes of infertility (Cao et al., 2024).

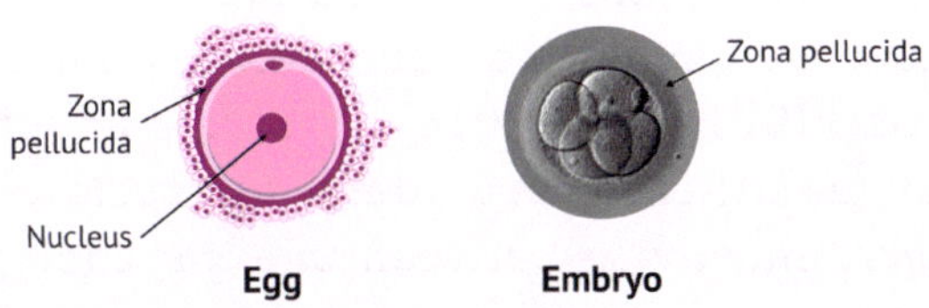

Figure 2.4. Zona pellucida.

Source: https://www.invitra.com/en/zona-pellucida/

Further, the combination of structural defects with other causative factors renders female infertility a multifactorial entity. Endocrine disorders, hormonal imbalance, and lifestyle can combine with structural defect-related issues to further aggravate problems, rendering it a multifactorial condition. A woman with a structural defect, for instance, might have co-existing issues due to disorders such as polycystic ovary syndrome (PCOS) that can influence ovarian function and hormonal control.

Thus, an integrative treatment of infertility is necessary, wherein the resolution of individuals' specific mix of structural and physiological issues is of utmost significance. Advances in reproductive technologies, like in vitro fertilization (IVF) and genetic counseling, offer efficient methods for minimizing these issues. As reproductive medicine continues to evolve, extending our understanding of how structural anomalies disrupt numerous elements will be crucial to achieving improved fertility rates among women (Dalis, 2024).

2.1.3. Age-Related Factors

The influence of age on the fertility of women is profound and intricate, exerting a significant influence on the probability of conception. When women's age progresses, their number of oocytes decreases along with their quality, making it challenging to conceive. When they are 35, they begin to lose their fertility in a more striking way, and at 40, natural conception becomes an offshore idea. This decline in fertility is caused by natural mechanisms of aging, which include an increase in aneuploidy rates of embryos, ultimately resulting in implantation and pregnancy.

Younger women are more likely to report more sexual distress and emotional distress related to infertility because they may feel a larger desire to become pregnant, and therefore may feel an even greater psychological burden of their illness (Group IOPP et al., 2016). Against these background considerations, physicians must take into account the effect of age on fertility when they counsel patients who are trying to conceive.

Another dimension that needs mention is the relationship between age and endometrial receptivity, particularly in women of older reproductive age. Research has shown that advances in reproductive technology, such as in vitro fertilization (IVF), are unable to overcome the inherent obstacles that come with age changes in the endometrium. Aging influences the balance of embryo and endometrial receptivity for development to establish conditions adverse to implantation. Infertility in women due to endometrial factors is more difficult with age, underlining the need to probe endometrial status in reproductive checks (Kravtsova et al., 2020).

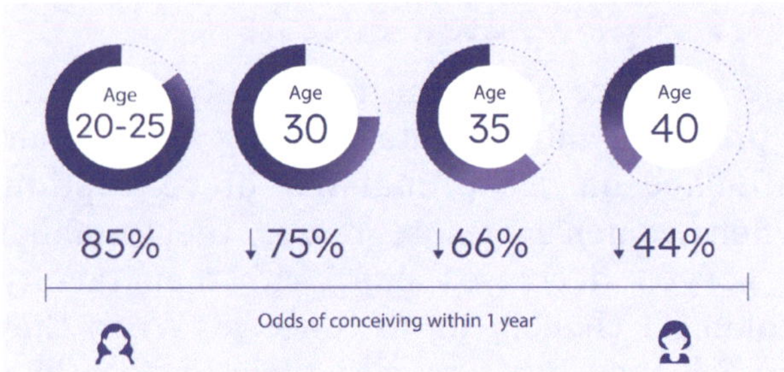

Figure 2.5. Age Affects Fertility.

Source: https://cdn.shopify.com/s/files/1/0038/5417/2275/files/2_9.png?v=1682526398

Early diagnoses and targeted treatments of endometrial ailments can improve fertility prospects, which points to the importance of comprehensive approaches considering age as well as concomitant reproductive well-being. Furthermore, age affects not only physical fertility but also has psychological implications that contribute to stress arising from infertility. The psychological pressure of wanting to have a child can lead to greater anxiety and depression, particularly in younger women who may have difficulties with family planning and social expectations. The psychological pressure is added where there is perceived female-factor infertility because women's self-esteem and sexual well-being may be adversely impacted (Group IOPP et al., 2016). It is thus important that healthcare providers appreciate the interconnectivity between age, psychological health, and fertility outcomes. Offering assistance that covers mental health alongside medical therapies can result in a more holistic, integrated framework, enabling greater support structures for women experiencing infertility complications as they progress in age.

Test Your Knowledge

1. How do hormonal imbalances contribute to female infertility?
2. What structural abnormalities can affect female fertility?

2.2. Medical Conditions Associated with Infertility

Learning Outcome

1. Define polycystic ovary syndrome (PCOS)
2. Explain the endometriosis
3. Discuss uterine fibroids

The spectrum of medical conditions causing female infertility is wide and heterogeneous, involving a complex interaction of structural, hormonal, and genetic conditions. Conditions such as polycystic ovary syndrome (PCOS) are extremely prevalent among infertile women, with endocrine disturbance and insulin resistance causing derangement of metabolic and reproductive function. Similarly, endometriosis involves the growth of endometrial tissue outside the uterus with resultant chronic scarring and pain, and it can prevent conception. Structural abnormalities, like uterine or fallopian tube obstruction, are also very problematic. It is significant to learn about these health disorders because they are the cause of nearly half the cases of infecundity among couples, emphasizing the need for targeted medical management strategies for the improvement of reproductive outcomes (Vakili et al., 2024). In addition to the disorders mentioned, premature ovarian failure (POF) has also been in the limelight as it has drastic consequences for women's fertility. It takes place when the ovaries are not able to function properly prior to 40 years of age, resulting in fewer eggs being generated and also irregular menstruation. POF may be triggered by hormonal imbalances, genetic factors, and autoimmune diseases, among other reasons, resulting in not just infertility but also other complications. Advances in assisted reproductive technologies (ART), e.g., in vitro fertilization (IVF), hold promise for patients afflicted by such conditions; however, efficacy and potential risks remain ongoing concerns. Foraying into new treatment modalities, e.g., using mesenchymal stem cells (MSCs), is a promising avenue to address POF-induced infertility, thereby broadening the arsenal of therapeutic interventions (Dalis, 2024). The most recent breakthroughs in understanding female infertility have emphasized the necessity of combining clinical interventions with the most recent developments in molecular and developmental biology. Through the deciphering of the biological mechanisms of diseases such as endometriosis and PCOS, researchers are poised to develop more effective interventions that treat the root causes and not mere symptoms. Improved understanding of genetic susceptibility is also a dominant factor in making treatment protocols more individualized, thereby increasing the success rates of ART methods. In addition, proposed applications of MSC therapy to regenerate reproductive tissues and restore balance to the immune response indicate a vision-directed strategy for the treatment of infertility. With emerging studies bringing more clarity to the complexities of female infertility, health professionals must remain up to date about these advances so that they may optimally care for their patients through personalized management strategies (Vakili et al., 2024).

2.2.1. Polycystic Ovary Syndrome (PCOS)

Polycystic Ovary Syndrome (PCOS) is a multifaceted endocrine disease that contributes significantly to female sterility, and it occurs in about 5-10% of women of reproductive age. One of the major features of PCOS is coexistence with anovulation, which inhibits normal ovulatory function and inhibits conception from occurring. This imbalance of hormones is usually followed by hyperandrogenism, leading to evidence such as hirsutism, acne, and obesity. Furthermore, women with PCOS are at risk of metabolic disturbances, including insulin resistance and low-grade inflammation, which contribute to reproductive health complexities. Management of the symptoms by modifiable lifestyle factors and medications is crucial to improve fertility in women with PCOS, since a well-rounded treatment approach can enable the restoration of ovulation as well as reproductive function.

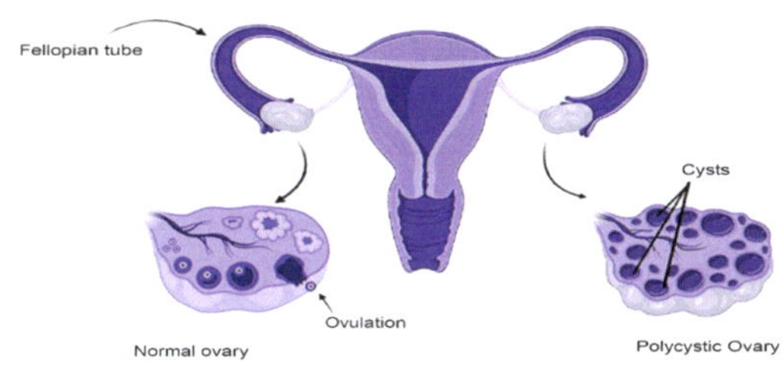

Figure 2.6. PCOS can cause infertility in some women.

Source: https://kiranivfgenetic.com/blog/wp-content/uploads/2023/07/Can-Polycystic-Ovary-Syndrome-PCOS-Cause-Infertility-621x309.jpeg

The dietary nutrients, particularly the intake of some of the fatty acids, have emerged as key determinants in managing PCOS. Diets that are very rich in n−6 polyunsaturated fatty acids, i.e., linoleic acid (LA), have proved to be harmful to the hormonal and metabolic homeostasis in women with PCOS. Increased consumption of LA has been correlated with increased systemic inflammation, which in turn exacerbates symptoms of PCOS and can potentially lead to complications during fertility procedures. Interestingly, the need for strict control of diet is evident in consideration of the fact that inappropriately adjusted dietary fatty acids not only exacerbate symptoms but also diminish the efficacy of ART protocols. Therefore, it is necessary to consider the role of nutrition in relation to PCOS while fighting female infertility by using holistic health approaches (Zhang et al., 2025).

Recent research has explored potential therapeutic agents to counteract the effects of PCOS on fertility, including novel molecules such as Mogroside V (MV). MV, in animal models, was shown to be anti-inflammatory and insulin-sensitizing in action, thereby addressing some of the fundamental pathophysiological mechanisms of PCOS. By suppressing the markers of hyperandrogenism and insulin resistance, MV administration demonstrated significant improvement in hormone secretion and ovarian function. Restoration of estrous cycles and reduced inflammation highlighted the therapeutic potential of the compounds as a viable treatment strategy for the induction of fertility in females suffering from PCOS. The observations highlight the importance of continued research into pharmacological therapy in association with dietary adjustment since the two are of utmost importance in mitigating the reproductive challenge posed by PCOS (Yang et al., 2025).

2.2.2. Endometriosis

The relationship between endometriosis and infertility in women is a complicated and multifaceted problem that affects many women worldwide. Endometriosis is a disease where endometrial-like tissue grows in locations outside the uterus, and it may lead to various complications such as pain and infertility. Endometrial tissue in abnormal locations could disrupt normal reproductive function by the formation of anatomical distortions that affect the ovaries, fallopian tubes, and uterus. Women with endometriosis are able to form adhesions or scarring, which can impede the ovulation process and interfere with embryo implantation, thereby playing a huge part in their inability to conceive. New genetic studies have witnessed the discovery of positive associations between endometriosis and female infertility of all causes, whereby it is emphasized that for fertility outcomes to be improved in such patients, the understanding of causative biological mechanisms is important (Venkatesh et al., 2024).

Also, the impact of endometriosis on fertility is compounded by its often asymptomatic nature at early stages, leading to late treatment and diagnosis. Because most women are symptomatic, such as pelvic pain, heavy menstrual bleeding, and fatigue, the vagueness of endometriosis might mask more severe reproductive conditions until infertility becomes apparent. Studies indicate that the etiology and pathogenesis of endometriosis include genetic influences, making female infertility even more complex. For instance, genome-wide association studies identified genetic loci for both endometriosis and infertility, which suggests a shared genetic susceptibility (Venkatesh et al., 2024).

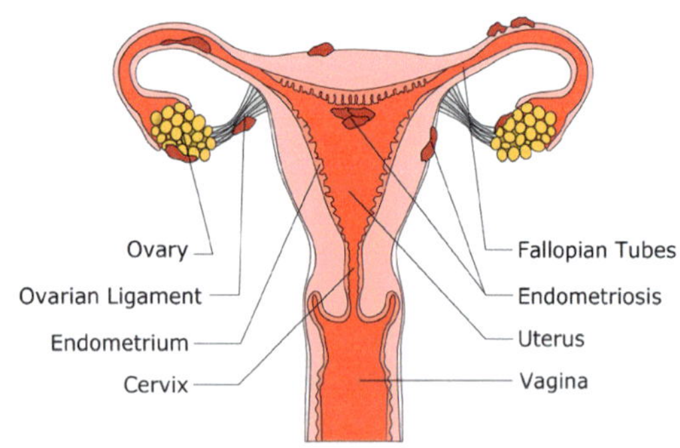

Figure 2.7. Endometriosis.

Source: https://hayatmedtour.com/wp-content/uploads/2020/06/endometriosis-treatment-in-Iran.jpg

This discovery mandates a multidisciplinary treatment, including both medical and surgical treatments, and considering the psychological implications of the illness and how it contributes to the relationship patterns between the parties concerned. Additionally, the interaction between allergic conditions and fertility has also been recently brought into question, specifically regarding endometriosis. It is possible, according to some research, that women suffering from endometriosis may also suffer from high levels of allergies and sensitivities, making it even more difficult for them to conceive. An interesting case report described a patient experiencing unexplained infertility that was diagnosed with human seminal plasma allergy, raising the question of how such allergic responses interface with endometriosis. This new link raises the call for additional research to break down these complex relationships and provide holistic interventions. Since knowledge on endometriosis is continuously evolving, clinicians are required to unravel the disease's challenges, its capacity to complicate or co-occur with other health conditions hindering fertility, thus enabling more effective, personalized care interventions.

2.2.3. Uterine Fibroids

Uterine fibroids or leiomyomas are a significant pathology of the female reproductive system, namely fertility. They are benign smooth muscle tumors that arise from the uterine smooth muscle and may be highly variable in number and dimension. Their presence may disrupt the normal function of the uterus in a variety of ways, including occluding the fallopian tubes, distorting uterine form, and preventing implantation. As is suggested by recent studies, uterine fibroid prevalence has a significant association with female infertility and complicates the reproductive health scenario. Moreover, a total incidence estimate of uterine abnormality, such as fibroids, necessitates the thorough consideration of their role in fertility assessments since treatment protocols are reliant on the detection and characterization of these underlying abnormalities in reproductive health (Starodubova et al., 2025). Diligent etiologic examinations of female infertility usually find intrauterine disease to be the foremost cause, among which uterine fibroids are most common. The findings of a study conducted on 383 infertile women showed that conditions like uterine abnormalities are the primary causes of infertility, thereby making the condition of fibroids all the more crucial in this category (Thatipelli et al., 2024).

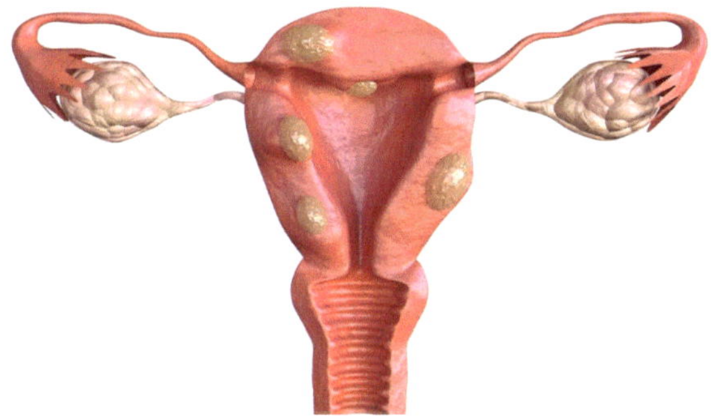

Figure 2.8. Uterine Fibroids.

Source: https://www.inovifertility.com/wp-content/smush-webp/2024/11/Fibroids-1400X700.jpg.webp

The implication of untreated fibroids can culminate in a variety of complications, including chronic pelvic pain and irregular bleeding, which can impede a woman's overall reproductive potential. The psychological impact of infertility can also tend to be amplified by fibroids, creating emotional distress and added complications for treatment. Treatment of such fibroids by medical or surgical methods may enhance the life of women who are trying to conceive, thus the importance of a holistic reproductive healthcare package. Treatment of uterine fibroids greatly impacts the fertility and quality of life of a woman. Numerous therapeutic modalities, from minimal intervention such as myomectomy to very aggressive treatments such as hysterectomy, depend on the size and location of the fibroids. The aim of such interventions is to eliminate or minimize the fibroids without damaging the uterus, thus allowing for the potential of conception. Studies have shown that women undergoing successful treatment for fibroids tend to exhibit better menstrual function and fertility rates after surgery. The need to monitor and strengthen reproductive health cannot be overemphasized, especially considering the increasing rates of infertility brought up in state health reports and policies (Starodubova et al., 2025). As the awareness of fibroids in the uterus and how they affect fertility increases, proactive steps towards diagnosis and care can lead to better reproductive outcomes for most women who are struggling with infertility.

Test Your Knowledge

1. What are the common symptoms of polycystic ovary syndrome (PCOS)?
2. How does endometriosis affect the female reproductive system?

2.3. Lifestyle Factors Impacting Fertility

Learning Outcome

1. Evaluate the influence of nutrition and diet on fertility.
2. Assess the role of exercise and physical health in reproductive function.
3. Analyze the effects of substance use and environmental factors on fertility.

Lifestyle components play a significant role in affecting the fertility of women, with habits directly affecting the health of the reproductive system. Factors such as obesity, smoking, and alcohol consumption have been demonstrated to provide lower levels of fertility in women. Obesity, for instance, leads to hormonal disorders that disrupt ovulation, while smoking is associated with decreased ovarian reserve and unfavorable reproductive outcomes. In addition, studies show that excessive alcohol consumption might influence fertility by manipulating estrogen and progesterone levels essential for maintaining a healthy menstrual cycle. Studies indicate that these lifestyle choices not only impact fertility in the short term but can also have long-term effects on reproductive health and overall health, and therefore it is essential that women modify their lifestyle anticipating conception (Murani, 2024). Furthermore, awareness of lifestyle risks of infertility continues to be extremely low among the majority of young women. In 2022, a survey was taken, which pointed out that students possessed moderate knowledge about infertility causes; however, lifestyle issues such as possessing multiple sex partners and use of psychoactive substances were common, particularly among young women (Wellington, 2024). This ignorance can lead to behaviors that not only compromise their fertility but also increase the risk of sexually transmitted diseases (STIs), which are proven to have adverse effects on reproductive health. Therefore, enhancing education on how lifestyle considerations impact fertility is instrumental in empowering women to make effective choices and promoting healthier behavior that can lead to better reproductive health. Finally, preconception counseling and lifestyle education should be promoted as the key to improving fertility levels in women. A multi-disciplinary intervention that involves diet suggestions, physical activity, and the effects of poisonous behaviors can profoundly increase women's awareness about their reproductive health. Every healthcare practitioner must prioritize holistic options in their fertility intervention modalities because research identifies the need for multiplex interventions specific to situations.

Such training programs can assist women in comprehending the inter-relationship between aspects of lifestyle and fertility, thereby maintaining more proactive health management. As indicated in recent literature, the effect of chronic disease and lifestyle on fertility is immense, further suggesting the necessity of focused interventions and education programs to prevent infertility risks (Murani, 2024).

2.3.1. Nutrition and Diet

The intricate interrelation between nutrition and women's infertility is better and better understood in contemporary reproductive health medicine. Proper balanced nutrition with sufficient essential nutrients is very important for optimal reproductive function. Some vitamins and minerals, like folate, iron, and vitamin D, have been proven to affect levels of reproductive hormones and ovarian function. For instance, deficiencies in folate can impair ovulation, while anemia due to iron deficiency has a link with anovulation and compromised egg quality. Furthermore, consumption of antioxidants found in fruits and vegetables is crucial, as they combat oxidative stress, which has adverse effects on oocytes. It was discovered that nutritional deficiencies impact not only hormone homeostasis but also fertility capacity. Understanding these food dynamics is valuable for health professionals who design comprehensive fertility treatment programs that consider dietary needs alongside medical treatment. In addition to the attention afforded to specific nutrients, total eating patterns also play a significant role in female fertility.

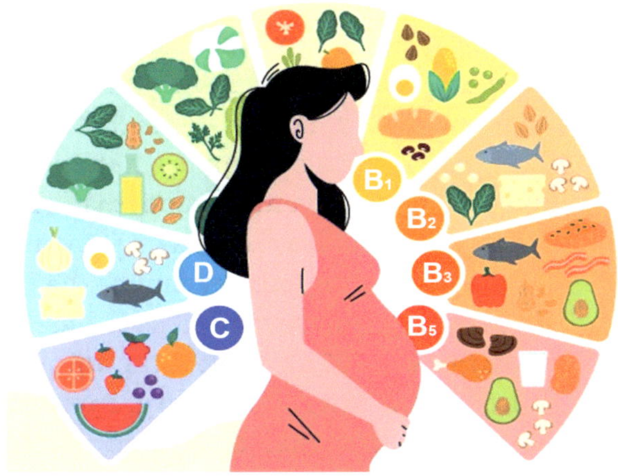

Source: https://oasisindia.in/wp-content/uploads/2023/09/Oasis-blog-banner-sep-7-2.jpg

Dietary habits of high glycemic index food and processed sugars have also been associated with insulin resistance, which can interfere with ovarian function and hormonal regulation. In contrast, a Mediterranean-type dietary pattern including whole grains, healthy fats, legumes, and lean proteins has been associated with improved fertility outcomes. This eating plan not only guarantees proper nutrients are taken into the body but also helps in maintaining a healthy weight, a significant factor in influencing fertility, particularly in women with polycystic ovary syndrome (PCOS). This emphasis on healthy nutrition triggers sustainable and long-term lifestyle changes that promote total health. Participation in dietary counseling and education can enable women to be in control through making rational decisions that optimize their reproductive health. Secondly, the impact of diet on female infertility is not just individual food intake but also society and culture that dictate eating habits. In certain regions, traditional diets lack essential nutrients needed in reproduction, and therefore, pose a challenge in the regulation of infertility that is closely interwoven with diet. Community education on balanced diets and nutrient intake can play a vital role in promoting reproductive well-being. Lessons from health interventions, such as those developed within multi-partner programs in India, affirm the need to adopt strategy modifications that value cultural practices but also support nutritional consciousness and intervention tactics (Kurz et al., 2006). These efforts are essential in providing an environment that supports women's health and fertility through improved access to healthy food (Aboua et al., 2013). In general, the way forward lies in an interdisciplinary approach that combines nutritional education, health policy, and cultural competence to tackle female nutritional infertility issues.

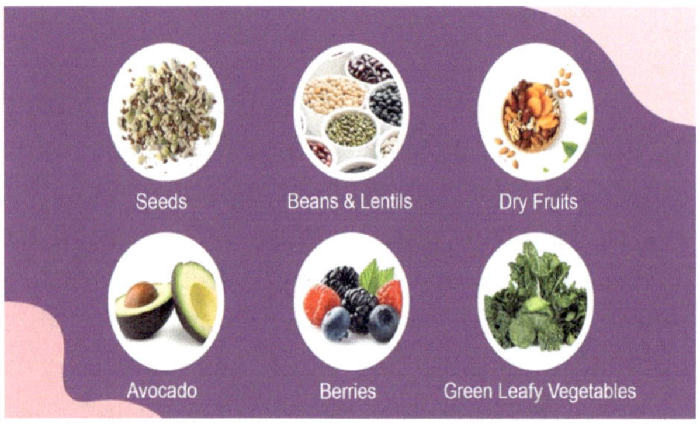

Figure 2.9. Food impact egg quality.

Source: https://oasisindia.in/blog/10-foods-that-will-boost-female-egg-quality/

2.3.2. Exercise and Physical Health

Involvement in regular exercise has significant implications for bodily health, influencing a multitude of physiological processes that play critical roles in reproductive function. Physical activity has been determined to maintain a healthy body weight, which is significant when it comes to hormonal balance and reproductive health. Women who engage in moderate to intense exercise have been found to experience normal menstrual cycles, as sustained activity can help govern hormonal fluctuation. In contrast, excessive exercise, as is typical in various sports or exercise regimes, may lead to amenorrhea, a condition in which menstruation ceases due to low energy availability. This disruption can have long-term implications for fertility, and therefore it is imperative that women are in a position to create an ideal exercise routine that optimizes overall health and also reproductive health, demarcating the delicate balance between body weight, physical exercise, and endocrine regulation of female fertility. Additionally, the intensity and type of exercise have a drastic impact on reproductive outcomes. Aerobic exercise, for example, has been discovered to improve cardiovascular function and enhance blood circulation, both of which are essential components of reproductive function. However, excessive training or excessive endurance exercise could result in a detrimental effect on the pituitary-ovarian axis, which can lead to endocrine imbalances that disrupt ovulation. This phenomenon is particularly prevalent in women with eating disorders such as, for instance, anorexia nervosa (AN), where insufficient caloric intake along with inappropriate exercise may result in severe disturbances of menstrual health and fertility. Understanding these dynamics is critical for women who wish to become pregnant, as customized exercise regimens that focus on modest gains in physical health at the cost of limited energy availability can lead to a more welcoming environment for reproductive wellness, with exercise habits directly correlated to fertility outcomes (Maheshwari et al., 2010).

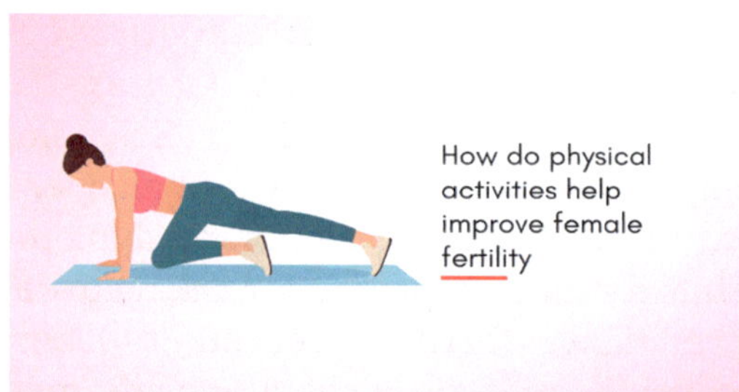

Source: https://www.ferty9.com/wp-content/uploads/2025/04/How-Do-Physical-Activities-Help-Improve-Female-Fertility1.png

Lastly, the psychological benefits of physical exercise cannot be overlooked, especially regarding female infertility. Chronic physical exercise has been associated with reduced anxiety, improved mood, and better body image, all of which can indirectly promote reproductive well-being. State of mind and stress both have critical roles in the hormone balance necessary for creating ovulation and fertility. For infertile women, the addition of exercise can also be an outlet for healing that counteracts the emotional load of their conditions. Furthermore, as outlined in contemporary literature, endocrine dysfunctions caused by conditions such as anorexia nervosa highlight that physical and mental health must be treated (Ciobanu et al., 2020). Collectively, a comprehensive plan that includes an exercise routine that is maintainable can promote not only greater physical health but also a healthier mental perspective, in turn helping to improve reproductive outcomes for women who opt to stick it out through the struggle of infertility.

2.3.3. Substance Use and Environmental Factors

Substance use, particularly among women, carries significant impacts on reproductive health and is closely linked with the problem of infertility. Environmental factors play a significant role in shaping substance use behaviors and also the risk and timing of initiation. For instance, exposure to risky social environments can amplify the risk of substance use, alcohol and marijuana. Studies indicate that teenagers who are clustered with problematic peers are likely to become victims of these drugs, which may result in reproductive issues in adulthood. This finding indicates the importance of addressing conditions in the environment that allow for substance use so that an environment that supports reproductive health is developed, particularly for those whose risk for infertility comes about through social environment and behaviors (Wood et al., 2024). In addition, the relationship between drug use and women's infertility is further confounded by the impact of lifestyle elements and environmental toxins. Stress and chronic chemical exposure have been linked with reproductive impairment, further complicating women's challenge with infertility. For example, smoking is linked to impaired ovarian reserve and hormonal dysregulation, both of which are harmful to conception. Similarly, obesity, generally due to lifestyle reasons, has beenproven to be detrimental to endometrial receptiveness and the efficiency of implantation. All these points highlight the necessity for treating as well as preventing both substance abuse and environmental etiological factors as interrelating causal determinants of female infertility through a comprehensive prevention and treatment method (Gonnella et al., 2024).

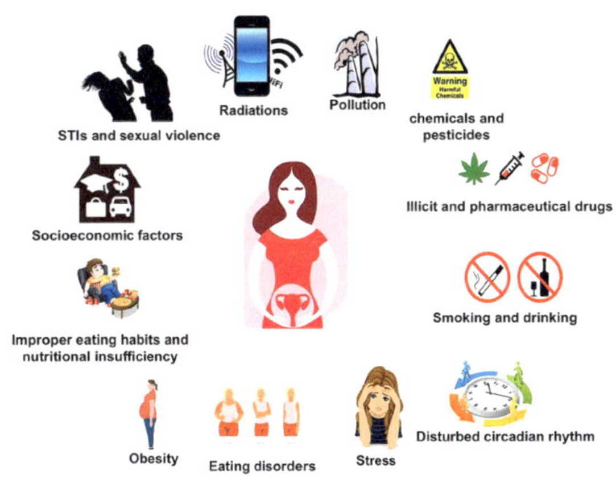

Figure 2.10. Environmental factors affecting female infertility.

Source: https://zivafertility.com/important-factors-affecting-fertility/

Awareness of the interlink between substance use, environmental conditions, and female infertility can inform practical interventions in reducing infertility. Public health programs informing people about the risks of substance use and a healthy lifestyle are essential. Such programs will help counteract the impacts of negative environmental factors and encourage healthier attitudes among reproductive-age women. Moreover, an awareness of the intricate interdependence of social support networks, substance abuse, and reproductive well-being can lead to more targeted interventions that not only address individuals' behavior but also enhance the efficacy of community support systems. Through the resolution of these interdependent issues, we can facilitate improved outcomes for women suffering from infertility challenges (Wood et al., 2024; Gonnella et al., 2024).

Test Your Knowledge

1. How does nutrition and diet influence female fertility?
2. What role does regular exercise play in maintaining reproductive health?

2.4. Diagnostic Procedures for Infertility

Learning Outcome

1. Discuss the hormonal testing
2. Explain the imaging techniques (ultrasound, hysterosalpingography)
3. Define laparoscopy

Female infertility is a multifactorial condition, and the process is typically initiated by taking a full medical history and physical examination. The initial step is crucial in determining potential contributory factors as well as guiding further tests. Subsequently, various laboratory investigations can be performed in order to measure levels of hormones such as follicle-stimulating hormone (FSH), luteinizing hormone (LH), estradiol, and progesterone. Alterations in these hormone levels can indicate the occurrence of conditions like ovarian dysfunction or hyperprolactinemia. A semen analysis of the male partner is also typically added because male factors contribute to infertility in approximately 30% of instances. These initial tests lay a foundation on which more invasive diagnostic procedures can be warranted, such as hysterosalpingography (HSG) or laparoscopy, enabling individualized therapy. Advanced diagnostic techniques play a significant role in diagnosing the etiology of female infertility with minute accuracy. Hysterosalpingography is an X-ray examination where a dye is injected through the uterine cavity. This helps evaluate the patency of the fallopian tubes and the uterine shape. The test could uncover abnormalities such as obstruction, fibroids, or polyps blocking conception. Furthermore, laparoscopy, being a minimally invasive surgical procedure, offers direct visualization of the reproductive organs to make a diagnosis of symptoms such as endometriosis or pelvic adhesions, which are not necessarily visible by other means. Through a retrospective study, laparoscopy and hysteroscopy combined effectively diagnosed and treated cases of infertility in a high number of women, which summarizes the potential of the technologies to maximize fertility outcomes (Donthu et al., 2024).

Moreover, developments in reproductive medicine keep improving the diagnostic spectrum of female infertility. The development of technologies such as One4Two®, stringently tested, is proof of how translational research can significantly influence clinical practice. This prototype is tailored to specific needs in reproductive diagnostics with an efficient mechanism for testing factors of infertility. The use of such devices not only enables enhanced diagnostic accuracy but also imposes timely and effective treatment, critical for infertile couples. With ongoing convergence of laboratory proof and clinical practices, there is a need to adopt comprehensive diagnostic practices that leverage these advances to optimize fertility treatment (Cariati et al., 2020).

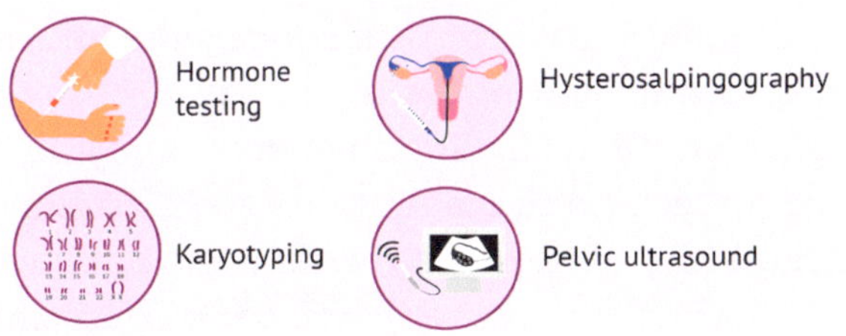

Figure 2.11. Female Fertility Tests.

Source: https://www.invitra.com/en/wp-content/uploads/2015/02/female-infertility-test.png

2.4.1. Hormonal Testing

Hormonal evaluation is also crucial in the diagnosis of female infertility since it offers a way of establishing several vital reproductive-function-controlling hormones. An important component of this establishment is hormones such as estrogen, progesterone, and luteinizing hormone (LH), which play a crucial role in ovulation, implantation, and normal pregnancy. Hormonal imbalance can disrupt the menstrual cycle and lead to anovulation or luteal phase dysfunction, hindering conception. Blood tests at some points within the menstrual cycle are typically employed in hormonal testing to accurately quantify levels. By identifying hormonal abnormalities earlier, clinicians can tailor therapeutic regimens for the correction of these specific conditions, thereby improving the chance of successful conception in infertile women. In addition to informing us about hormone levels, analysis of hormones also tells us about interactions between hormonal imbalance and immune response throughout the process of implantation. Current evidence has found that hormonal levels might be related to immune cell invasion of the endometrium and human leukocyte antigen (HLA) expression, which creates a complicated association that defines success with infertility. A case in point is HLA-F protein levels, which are controlled by progesterone, and have been found to have varying associations with immune cell populations in recurrent implantation failure (RIF). Hormone level evaluation together with immune markers provides valuable information on receptivity and the potential for successful embryo implantation, which is essential for achieving pregnancy. A combination of hormonal testing with immunological assessments is a significant development in identifying the parameters of female infertility processes, emphasizing the need for thorough evaluation procedures (Papuchova et al., 2022).

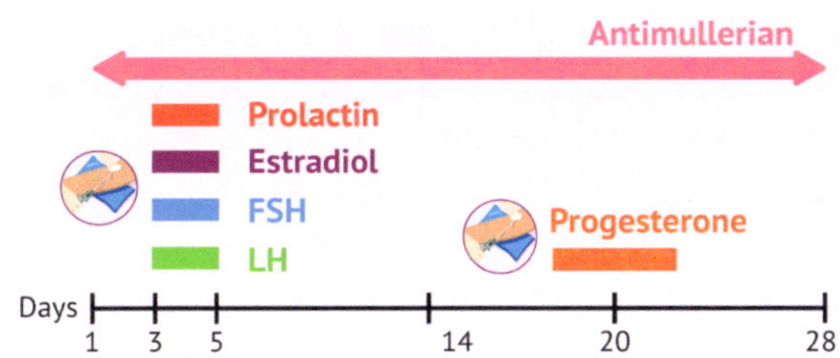

Figure 2.12. Hormone blood tests for female fertility.

Source: https://www.invitra.com/en/female-infertility-tests/

Besides, the history of infertility work-up procedures has placed focus on hormonal testing in an extensive diagnostic process. Thorough conventional approaches have been found to provide higher pregnancy success rates than short assessments, suggesting that extensive hormonal evaluation can enhance diagnostic accuracy and guide treatment decisions. For example, thorough work-ups always include extensive hormonal profiling by which doctors can identify unique underlying causes of infertility.

On the other hand, shortened tests may be missing crucial hormonal imbalances that are crucial for success with treatment. As shown in recent studies, restoring expanded hormonal testing may lead to increased rates of ongoing pregnancy. Therefore, refining hormonal test protocols throughout work-ups for infertility can have the potential to maximize treatment pathways and thus positively impact more women towards achieving their goals in fertility therapy (Hamilton et al., 2021).

2.4.2. Imaging Techniques (Ultrasound, Hysterosalpingography)

The diagnosis of female infertility is primarily done using different imaging methods to identify any anatomical and functional defects in the reproductive tract. Two common methods that are utilized are HSG and ultrasound, where each one provides information that is crucial in diagnosis as well as therapy. HSG is specifically valuable in creating views of the fallopian tubes and uterine cavity so that any seeming obstruction or structural abnormality can be easily determined. While two-dimensional ultrasound (2D US) has been a traditional method used for the assessment of abnormalities, its accuracy has been questioned. Some recent research has shown that more modern imaging modalities, such as sonohysterography (SHG) and three-dimensional ultrasound (3D US), are capable of providing increased diagnostic accuracy, particularly in the diagnosis of congenital uterine anomalies, which have been reported to be more prevalent in women who are facing infertility or recurrent pregnancy loss (Cocksedge et al., 2008).

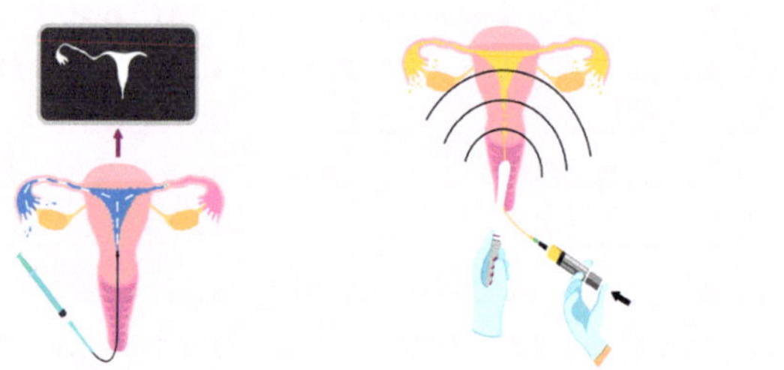

Figure 2.13. Types of hysterosalpingography.

Source: https://www.invitra.com/en/female-infertility-tests/hysterosalpingography-hysterosalpingosonography/

Sonohysterography utilizing saline infusion under ultrasound offers a less invasive option compared to HSG. Sonohysterography is an imaging technique that obtains good results for intrauterine abnormality, with high sensitivity and specificity rates compared to HSG (Lakshmi et al., 2017). In a comparison study between the two methods, sonohysterography proved to be an excellent diagnostic tool with a sensitivity rate of 97% and a specificity rate of 94%. These statistics indicate its potential as a first-line tool for diagnosing tubal patency, given the prevalence of ultrasound machines in the majority of health institutions. Not only does it improve patient comfort with less invasive technologies, but earlier and more accurate diagnoses become attainable, allowing clinicians to adequately customize infertility treatments. Furthermore, the significance of using advanced imaging techniques extends beyond diagnostic implications. Detection of uterine abnormalities, for instance, a septate uterus, which is reportedly more prevalent in women seeking help with infertility, can actually alter the treatment plan radically. Once such abnormalities are detected by such imaging equipment, physicians can recommend certain interventions or surgery to correct these abnormalities and enhance reproductive success. Proper assessment of tubal patency and uterine shape is crucial, as both are essential for successful conception as well as pregnancy maintenance. The increased precision and decreased invasiveness of methods like SHG and 3D US render them valuable tools in the comprehensive analysis of female infertility, which ultimately leads to more astute clinical decisions and improved patient results (Cocksedge et al., 2008).

2.4.3. Laparoscopy

Laparoscopy has emerged as a breakthrough diagnostic and therapeutic mode to treat female infertility because it is minimally invasive and offers broad-based insights into reproductive health. Laparoscopy enables gynecologists to probe the pelvic cavity, identify anatomical defects, and assess the health status of reproductive organs accurately.

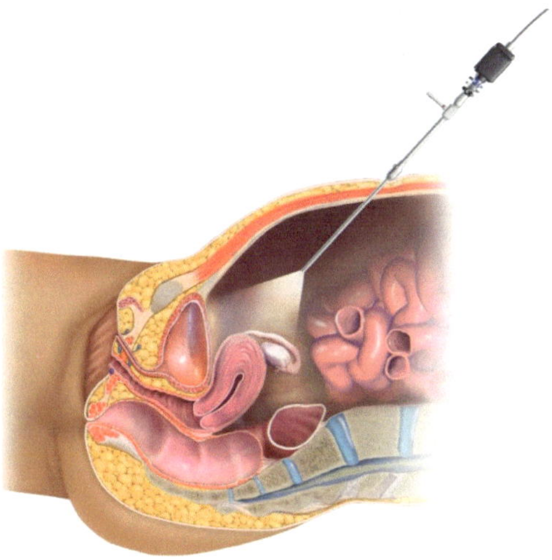

Figure 2.14. Laparoscopy for infertility.

Source: https://www.gaudiumivfcentre.com/blog/wp-content/uploads/2016/02/Laparoscopy-1.jpg

These are significant observations, particularly in women with unexplained infertility, as laparoscopy allows direct visualization of suspected underlying issues such as endometriosis, adhesions, or ovarian cysts. Laparoscopic results direct targeted interventions that enhance fertility outcomes, justifying its role as not just a diagnostic tool but also as an important component in the treatment of infertility. Therefore, it is crucial to know where laparoscopy stands in the big scheme of female infertility in order to further improve patient treatment and maximize reproductive outcomes.

Its importance is also highlighted by the use of laparoscopy in the treatment of conditions leading to female infertility. A case was reported about a 36-year-old woman with a unicornuate uterus, a congenital defect diagnosed by diagnostic laparoscopy and magnetic resonance imaging (MRI). Despite the challenges of her condition and four consecutive intrauterine insemination (IUI) cycle failures, follow-up laparoscopic surgery created the possibility for a customized in vitro fertilization (IVF) protocol. With controlled ovarian stimulation, mature oocyte retrieval, and success through intracytoplasmic sperm injection (ICSI), a healthy blastocyst formation and eventual confirmed pregnancy ensued. This figure shows how laparoscopy allows treatment protocols to be personalized to the individual patient, with clinicians being able to treat specific patient conditions while maximizing the chances of conception with anatomical anomalies (Mahajan et al., 2025). Laparoscopy is also very relevant in addressing male factors leading to female infertility, as evidenced by advancements in the methods of preserving sperm. In one case with extreme oligozoospermia, laparoscopy was used to assess the female partners' reproductive capacity while novel sperm vitrification protocols were employed to circumvent male factor infertility. Following rigorous hormonal screening and ovarian stimulation, the recovery of healthy oocytes and resultant successful fertilization with ICSI resulted in the creation of two blastocysts, one of which was transferred.

The above case identifies the necessary synergy between assisted reproductive technologies and laparoscopic diagnosis, illustrating how a comprehensive approach can lead to satisfactory results even in complex infertile cases. Their overlap is a signal that multidimensional aspects of infertility are better acknowledged today, adding emphasis to the position of laparoscopy in modern reproductive medicine (Wadhe et al., 2025).

Test Your Knowledge

1. What are the common diagnostic tests used to evaluate female infertility?
2. What role does imaging, such as ultrasound or hysterosalpingography, play in diagnosing infertility?

2.5. Treatment Options for Female Infertility

Learning Outcome

1. Define medications and hormonal therapies
2. Explain the assisted reproductive technologies (ART)
3. Discuss the surgical interventions

The treatment setting for female infertility is also complicated, as the variations in causes that can result in it make the situation complex to handle. The initial examinations are normally detailed assessment of both partners with particular attention given to the female's reproductive system. The investigations employed may vary from hormonal testing, imaging studies such as ultrasounds or hysterosalpingograms, to laparoscopic examinations in order to assess anatomical factors. Understanding the specific cause of infertility is essential since it determines the subsequent treatment protocol. Women with ovulatory disorders, for instance, can be treated using pharmacological therapy including clomiphene citrate and gonadotropins to stimulate ovulation. Additionally, controlling lifestyle factors such as diet and exercise has emerged as a central component of treating infertility, with increasing support to embrace a holistic treatment paradigm (Kahan et al., 2024). Once underlying etiologies are diagnosed, treatment regimens can range from minimally invasive treatments to very complex assisted reproductive technologies. Intrauterine insemination (IUI) is usually used as first-line therapy for unexplained or mild male factor infertility. By directly placing sperm into the uterus during the time of ovulation, IUI increases the chance of fertilization. For women with more severe infertility, in vitro fertilization (IVF) may be warranted. IVF involves egg extraction, sperm fertilization in the lab, and the implantation of embryos into the uterus at a later date. The procedure is best suited to women with blocked fallopian tubes, advanced maternal age, or those who have failed with milder therapy. Success with IVF relies greatly on age, health, and some diagnosed causes of infertility (Group IOPP et al., 2016).

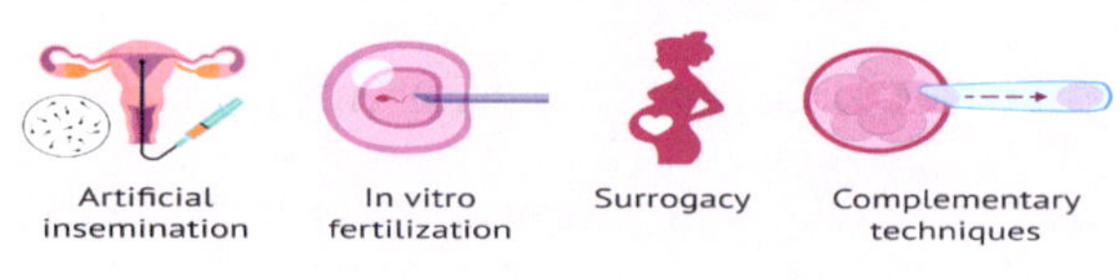

Figure 2.15. Infertility Treatment Options.

Source: https://drbhupendrabathla.com/images/services/infer.png

In recent decades, advancements in reproductive technology have progressively expanded women's options for those experiencing infertility. Genetic testing of embryos, or preimplantation genetic testing (PGT), enables doctors to identify chromosomal defects prior to implantation, increasing the likelihood of a successful pregnancy. In addition, novel treatments such as ovarian tissue cryopreservation and egg donation have opened new doors for infertile women seeking treatment for premature ovarian insufficiency or certain medical conditions. Psychological stress and emotional states are generally affected during fertility treatments, and therefore, healthcare providers need to provide supportive counseling and psychological assistance in addition to medical treatments. This integrative approach not only addresses the physical aspects of fertility treatment but also the emotional and psychological challenges faced by women who are working towards settling down their families (Kahan et al., 2024).

2.5.1. Medications and Hormonal Therapies

Female infertility treatment involves an understanding of many drugs and hormone treatments that are directed towards enhancing reproductive success. Hormonal imbalance, which is often linked to conditions such as PCOS or hypothalamic insufficiency, can cause ovulation to be significantly impaired and, by proxy, fertility. To treat this, hormonal therapy using drugs such as Clomiphene citrate, a selective estrogen receptor modulator, has been widely used to stimulate ovarian activity through gonadotropin release stimulation. In addition, the use of aromatase inhibitors provides a second line, typically recommended in the event of anovulatory infertility in women. Aromatase inhibitors allow for follicular development and can lead to higher ovulation rates, thereby indirectly having the potential to increase conception chances. The efficacy of the treatments has proved the critical role of pharmacological treatment in the proper management of female infertility. Drugs for infertility in obesity have also attracted increasing attention, with excessive weight capable of aggravating reproductive disorders. For instance, their use with agents like metformin and other anti-obesity drugs has been promising in the improvement of fertility in obese women, particularly those with insulin resistance conditions like PCOS. Gradual weight reduction has been found to improve the female reproductive hormonal profile, ovulating more frequently, and correcting for menstrual irregularity. In particular, Glucagon-Like Peptide-1 receptor agonists (GLP-1 RAs) represent a potential breakthrough, which has evidenced promising outcomes not only in weight management but also in the enhancement of fertility via several mechanisms of action. The efficacy of these new treatments in the improvement of reproductive function will require more studies in order to obtain full protocols in females with weight-related infertility (Pavli et al., 2024).

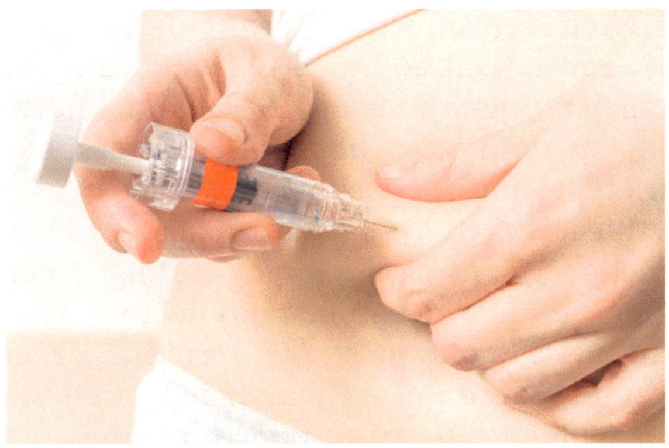

Figure 2.16. Hormone Treatments.

Source: https://www.repromedfertility.com/editor-uploads/website-786/hormone-treatments-1573642187.jpg

The multiaxial nature of female infertility demands a holistic approach that combines hormonal therapies with traditional modalities of treatment. Hormonal therapies, especially in disorders such as endometrial cancer, have also illustrated the delicate interrelationship between cancer and reproductive health. Estrogen and progesterone wind up controlling the endometrium lining, and extreme hormonal imbalances can predispose females to resultant malignancies, thus complicating infertility treatment options. Hormonal therapies with progestin can modulate such an imbalance and hence potentially reduce the risks of cancers as well as infertility. Moreover, individualized hormonal therapies are now the norm, in consideration of the variability of hormonal profiles in individuals and their effect on fertility. By facilitating personalized medicine, healthcare professionals can optimize reproductive outcomes while safeguarding women's overall well-being and, thus, emphasize the invaluable character of targeted hormonal interventions in female infertility (Mehboob, 2024).

2.5.2. Assisted Reproductive Technologies (ART)

Assisted reproductive technologies (ART) have revolutionized how female infertility has been managed, infusing millions of infertile couples with new hope. ART refers to a variety of interventions comprising in vitro fertilization (IVF), intracytoplasmic sperm injection (ICSI), and embryo freezing, among others. As knowledge of reproductive health continues to advance, ART procedures are currently more precisely intended to address established causes of infertility, including disorders of ovulation, structural abnormalities, or decline in fertility with increasing age. The application of transvaginal sonography (TVS) was key in this regard, providing a non-invasive diagnostic technique that improved the capacity for detection of abnormalities such as polycystic ovary syndrome (PCOS) and uterine anomalies. In general, ART represented a paradigm shift in the field of reproductive medicine, transitioning away from generalized care and towards more individualized strategies based on personal assessment and need (Babita et al., 2025). The psychological and emotional impact of infertility typically reflects the physical, thus complicating the ART procedure. Females who have been subjected to ART are likely to demonstrate elevated stress and anxiety rates, which further impact treatment outcomes. It has been identified that socio-economic status and overall psychological well-being are pivotal success determinants for fertility therapy. Stress related to persistent domestic conflict or dissatisfaction with sexual relationships is one of the contributing factors that could exacerbate the challenges experienced during ART. In particular, the co-occurrence of infertility with symptoms accompanying conditions like long-COVID-19 has been of interest, affecting the mental state of females and potentially compromising the efficacy of ART. It is essential to address these psychological complications for enhancing treatment success, suggesting the necessity for a multidisciplinary treatment involving mental health support in treating females receiving ART treatment (Boichuk et al., 2024).

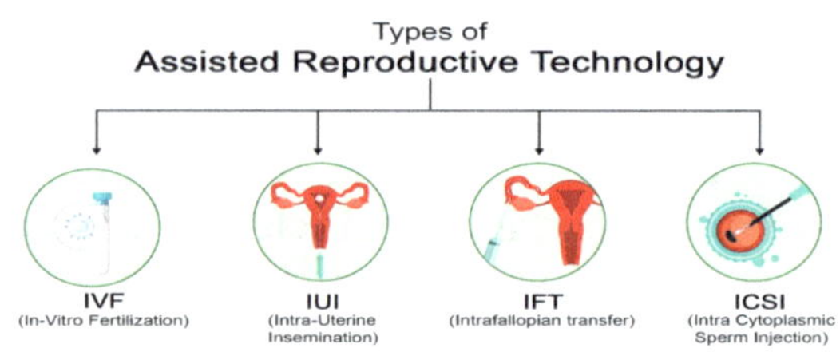

Figure 2.17. Types of Assisted Reproductive Technology (ART).

Source: https://aurawomen.in/wp-content/uploads/2024/08/What-are-the-different-types-of-assisted-reproductive-technology-ART.jpg

With future outlooks of ART on female infertility, research and development will play a pivotal role. The advancement in genetic screening techniques, such as preimplantation genetic testing, will allow the selection of genetically healthy embryos free of some genetic disorders, thus maximizing the possibility of successful conception. Furthermore, incorporating personalized medicine into ART grows increasingly viable; therapy can be customized based on individual reproductive health status, age, and comorbidities. New studies continue to explore the implications of physical and psychological health in women undergoing ART on ART outcomes, emphasizing the importance of careful evaluation before initiating treatment. With both medical and psychosocial therapy of infertility, ART can move forward to grow, ushering in new avenues for enhancing reproductive success in such women, bringing their journey toward motherhood to a newer level.

2.5.3. Surgical Interventions

Surgical interventions play an important role in the management of some of the root causes of female infertility. One such condition, endometriosis, is one of the most frequent and recalcitrant conditions and affects an estimated 10% of women of childbearing age. Surgical interventions for endometriosis can vary from excisional surgery to eliminate endometriotic lesions to ablative procedures that destroy the tissue. These operations can minimize pain and improve fertility outcomes, particularly when performed laparoscopically. The literature indicates that an individualized strategy based on the location and the severity of endometriosis needs to be employed to achieve maximum benefit from the operation. Minimally invasive techniques, such as electrosurgery and laser ablation, are now producing favorable results in the preservation of ovarian function and the elimination of lesions, thereby enhancing the likelihood of conception for the majority of women with this condition (Tsuei et al., 2025).

Aside from endometriosis, there are also other surgical interventions that are intended to correct anatomical flaws responsible for inhibiting a woman's conception. Uterine fibroids, polyps, or structural abnormalities of the uterus may necessitate as little as hysteroscopic intervention to as much as more extensive surgery like myomectomy. Treatment with hysteroscopy is an option for fibroid and polyp removal without invasion, typically resulting in a brief convalescence period and minimal complications. Myomectomy offers the option for the management of these larger or more complicated fibroids and the preservation of the uterus intact, a consideration for women desiring future conception. Not only do these surgeries address the acute problem of infertility, but they also contribute to improved reproductive outcomes by optimizing the uterine environment. According to research, the appropriate surgery can significantly improve pregnancy rates in women undergoing assisted reproductive technologies and thus is in favor of the holistic approach needed in treating female infertility (Buzzaccarini et al., 2025).

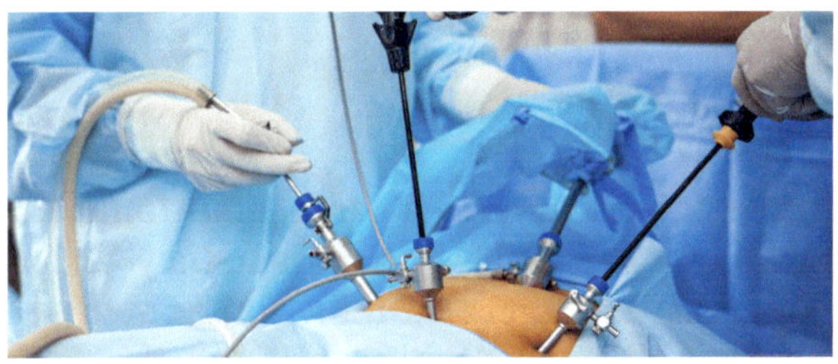

Figure 2.18. Laparoscopy for infertility.

Source: https://www.nufertility.com/blog/wp-content/uploads/2024/01/Shutterstock_525787207-compressed.png

Furthermore, surgical correction of tubal ligation as a cause of infertility remains an integral component of therapy in presentations to women who are infertile. Surgical interventions, such as tubal reanastomosis, aim to open closed fallopian tubes, which have inherent significance for conception. It is undertaken in tubal ligation cases or when adhesions make the tubes non-functional. Laparoscopy becomes simpler with greater accuracy in treating these issues without adding to the overall recovery period. In cases where extensive damage or disease of the fallopian tubes has ensued, assisted reproductive technologies like in vitro fertilization (IVF) may be recommended as a substitute, but can be rendered more effective by treating any surgically related problems, which can be resolved first. Outcomes of these procedures again highlight the necessity for an all-around, individualized approach to surgical interventions in female infertility, eventually providing means of increasing the chances of successful conception (Tsuei et al., 2025).

Test Your Knowledge

1. What are the common medical treatments used to address female infertility?
2. How do assisted reproductive technologies (ART) like IVF help in treating infertility?

2.6. Psychological and Emotional Impact

Learning Outcome

1. Define stress and anxiety related to infertility
2. Understand the coping mechanisms and support systems
3. Identify the impact on relationships and family dynamics

Female infertility has a large emotional and psychological impact, with a tendency to lead to distress that alters an individual's own self-concept and relationship with other people. Being unable to have children often leads to feelings of inadequacy and failure, as society defines womanhood in terms of motherhood. Women suffering from infertility are likely to have higher levels of anxiety due to both internal demands and pressure exerted by society. This has a tendency to lead to a cycle of negative thoughts, with women internalizing their challenges and feeling depression and isolation. Overuse of social media, particularly in young adults, has been associated with increased anxiety and depression, showing the danger that external factors can contribute to the emotional burden of infertility (Karim et al., 2025). This virtual world can perpetuate a negative self-concept as individuals compare themselves with others who appear to have more traditional or socially desirable lifestyles. In addition to psychological impacts on the individuals, infertility can strain interpersonal relationships between couples and families. Emotional impact may generate conflict and misunderstanding in relationships as couples mourn in different ways. Women may have difficulty communicating their hopelessness or frustration, resulting in withdrawal of emotions or increased tension in family interactions. This tension can extend into social groups, where child-rearing-centered meetings can create exclusionary sentiment among those who have difficulty reproducing. In addition, research indicates that women who have undergone female genital cutting present with higher incidences of anxiety and depression, which implies that intrinsic psychological trauma can be exacerbated further by infertility (Ifeanyi, 2024). These results illustrate the complex interplay between psychological well-being and social support mechanisms essential to resilience in such a life-altering experience. The psychological effects of infertility can even affect a woman's overall quality of life and lead to severe emotional distress. Recurrent stress built up during the course of infertility also affects physical health, and a recursive process sets in when mental and physical states of well-being are intertwined. Women have reported symptoms like insomnia and fatigue, which are typically associated with anxiety and depressive disorders. This highlights the urgent necessity of mental health education and counseling interventions targeting specifically women facing issues of infertility. The impact of emotional health on treatment outcome cannot be overruled; hence, interventions need to focus on providing holistic care incorporating the psychological in addition to the physiological aspect of infertility. This integrated approach can even empower women to cope better with their experiences, yielding strength and improving their overall psychological well-being at this challenging time.

2.6.1. Stress and Anxiety Related To Infertility

The psychological stress of infertility runs deep and is complicated, and manifests itself generally as heightened anxiety and stress among infertile women. Conceiving can turn into an overbearing task, with the majority of women being reminded of their failure all the time. In a variety of studies, it has been proposed that nearly 78.7% of women undergoing conception are subject to extreme anxiety and distress. These feelings are reinforced by societal pressures regarding motherhood and the perceived stigma of being infertile. High levels of mood and anxiety are prevalent, particularly among individuals with distress due to infertility, underscoring the need for psychological intervention and effective coping mechanisms. The psychological stress impinges not only on mental health but also on the overall well-being of women attempting to overcome infertility issues (Hecht et al., 2024). In addition, the psychological effect of infertility is likely to be compounded by additional extrinsic stressors. Current uncertainties, such as socioeconomic uncertainty and global conflicts, can enhance the sense of powerlessness in women with infertility. For instance, studies have proven increased anxiety toward fear of war and increased international tensions, thereby contributing to the emotional climate of patients with infertility. The overlap of these broader social concerns with personal trouble conceiving introduces in a tangled web of stressors, a compounding of the mental illness problems women are already facing. Particularly in times of crisis, women may find their distress and worry increased as they are forced to contend not only with their infertility but with the unstable nature of the world in general. This multi-dimensional stress underlines the need to treat not just the patient's experience of infertility but also the more general contextual factors that could influence mental health outcomes (Regnoli et al., 2024).

Stress and anxiety due to infertility must be addressed by specialized interventions and overall support systems. Mental health professionals play an important role in providing therapy and specialized resources for women with infertility. Such interventions not only help to alleviate symptoms of depression and anxiety but also seek to build resilience and coping skills. Additionally, networks and groups in the community can also introduce helpful interventions in terms of emotional validation and shared experiences with others, which can offset the sense of isolation. As determined from other studies, severe mental health issues amongst women can be addressed by taking positive actions such as counseling and peer support. Thus, a holistic framework that encapsulates social support and psychological care becomes essential in optimizing the emotional well-being of women navigating through the rugged terrain of infertility (Hecht et al., 2024).

2.6.2. Coping Mechanisms and Support Systems

Coping with the emotional distress of female infertility provokes an urgent need for healthy coping strategies and effective support systems. Infertility is likely to induce isolation, loss, and fear, which require interventions that enable women to process these concerns in a helpful way. Coping strategies are likely to be very heterogeneous but can include psychological interventions like cognitive restructuring, wherein one rephrases negative thoughts about their experience with infertility into a more constructive format. Evidently, the provision of coping mechanisms, as well as learning key life skills, is critical in relieving stress-related, challenges as argued in Karagiannis et al. (2014).

Through the enhancement of resilience by such interventions, women can best cope with the psychological chaos that accompanies infertility, leading to improved mental well-being and heightened perceived mastery over their lives. Support systems play an important role in the women's coping process with infertility. Support systems can be many forms, such as support groups, family, and friends who provide emotional support. Stigma around infertility in certain societies is a contributing factor to feelings of loneliness that make it hard for individuals with infertility to seek assistance. This cultural stigma, as recognized in Singh et al. (2021), intrudes significantly on coping strategies as women run the risk of being judged or misunderstood by those around them. This can thus make the development of open discussions on infertility a significant move towards alleviating stigma, which allows women to access the help they seek. Because each woman's circumstance is distinct, the efficacy of support systems typically hinges on their ability to address customized needs, so the women feel heard in their experience. The intersection of coping strategies and support systems underscores the need for integrative approaches to addressing female infertility.

Health professionals must not only guarantee medical treatments but also establish supportive environments that guarantee unencumbered discussions around infertility. This includes the inclusion of the talk of reproductive health education and access barriers, as per (Singh et al., 2021). Increased education and awareness of infertility can empower women, decrease emotional burdens, and facilitate understanding among the community. In creating an accommodating and inspiring environment, infertile women can develop a sense of solidarity, hence improving their coping strategies. Therefore, an integrated strategy that pairs effective coping strategies with robust support networks is needed to facilitate the empowerment of women on their infertility journeys, enabling them to navigate the turbulences of their experience with dignity and hope.

2.6.3. Impact on Relationships and Family Dynamics

The intra-family relationship dynamics are highly influenced by the experience of female infertility and tend to leave couples in a maze of emotional challenges. Since the burden of infertility is shared by both partners, couples usually feel more stressed, which can put a tremendous amount of pressure on their relationship. Research has indicated that the perception of stress about infertility is strongly intertwined with relationship satisfaction in a way that decreasing levels of satisfaction can be used to predict higher levels of stress among women facing the prospect of infertility. This implies that the psychological well-being of couples is closely tied to their ability to cope as a unit. When couples are experiencing infertility, the delicacy of their relationship can either contribute to their personal resilience or increase feelings of frustration and loneliness, which themselves lead to complex changes in family dynamics worthy of extensive research (Fernandes et al., 2023). Beyond emotional distress, infertility can also disrupt communication patterns in relationships and families. The difficulty of conceiving is likely to provoke feelings of inadequacy, shame, or guilt, which inhibit open communication between the couple. While the couple navigates their disappointment and sorrow, they unconsciously construct emotional defenses that hinder mutual support. Complexity of emotions may manifest in different ways, e.g., defensiveness or denial, hence making fertility treatment or future family planning hard to discuss. Moreover, families may feel obligated to provide support, and this can thereby unintentionally create tension if there are different perceptions regarding coping with infertility (Fernandes et al., 2023). Therefore, the experience of going through infertility not only tests the union of partners but also affects the general family dynamics surrounding them (Fernandes et al., 2023). Finally, the experience of going through female infertility can reshape not only intimate relationships but also family forms and support networks. The need for children can trigger a rededication to traditional family roles and expectations, as well as relationship tensions if situations do not fit individual or societal expectations. Psychological therapy that focuses on emotional support and relationship quality could assist couples to overcome such challenges, a potential element in minimizing the harmful effects of infertility on both partners. The interconnectedness of relationship satisfaction and social support is realized in research showing that a protective relational context can act as a buffer against the stress of infertility. Such findings reinforce the importance of promoting healthy communication and mutual understanding to maximize resilience against the overwhelming emotional terrain that infertility affords.

Test Your Knowledge

1. How can infertility contribute to increased stress and anxiety in affected individuals?
2. What coping mechanisms are effective for managing the emotional impact of infertility?

SUMMARY

In Conclusion, a foray into female infertility, it is imperative to integrate the complex issues that confront those experiencing the condition. Not merely impacting reproductive function, but with substantial emotional and psychological consequences, infertility ravages the individual as a whole. Women struggling with infertility tend to suffer at the hands of societal judgments and internal anguish, which can further amplify feelings of loneliness and incompetence. The acknowledgment of these emotional implications is an acknowledgment of the demand for comprehensive support structures engaging both the medical and psychological aspects of infertility. Support structures have the potential to empower women to walk through their complex journeys and make informed decisions regarding treatment and lifestyle adjustments. The comprehensive method underscores the importance of infertility as a condition requiring multidimensional treatment rather than as an individual medical condition. Also, with advances in reproductive technology continuing, the implications of these advances must be adequately assessed. The use of assisted reproduction technologies (ART) raises significant concerns over health risks, such as the potential for increased cancer risk from hormone treatment. It is crucial to comprehend the cancer-risk relationship of infertility because delay in conception or prolonged exposure to infertility has been identified as risk factors in other cancers among women. Current literature depicts a multifaceted picture of these risks and calls for the necessity of well-informed consultations between health care givers and patients regarding the pros and cons of ART interventions (Codacci-Pisanelli et al., 2018). This risk-treatment interaction therefore demands ongoing research and clinical debate to ensure that women are properly informed about their choices. Finally, the role of diagnostic modalities in approaching female infertility cannot be overlooked, particularly regarding the use of diagnostic laparoscopy. The surgical procedure has posed controversy due to various evidence for or against its use in addressing infertility. Despite evidence from some trials that diagnostic laparoscopy reveals treatable pelvic conditions, its routine use is questionable. The evidence available is that laparoscopic surgery can optimize fertility outcomes in some cases, such as correcting hydrosalpinges before in vitro fertilization (IVF) treatment. As the practice is going on, it is clear that randomized controlled trials are required in order to develop standardized recommendations for using laparoscopy in infertility diagnosis and treatment (Bosteels et al., 2007). Therefore, a balanced view of such factors can end up leading to improved management strategies based on individual women's individual needs.

Women's infertility demands a thorough understanding of the aetiology and its relevance to women's health and social well-being. Decline in reproductive ability due to age is one of the most significant causes of infertility, and most profoundly affects women over 35 years old. As ovarian function declines, the chances of conception reduce steadily, and this accompanies the rise in demand for fertility conservation strategies. This has led to an increase in awareness about such choices as in vitro fertilization (IVF), oocyte cryopreservation, and ovarian tissue cryopreservation (OTC) that have been devised to assist women suffering from infertility problems. The recommendations of guidelines highlight the importance of giving clear information about these alternatives, which can empower women in making proper choices about their reproductive lives. As suggested by existing research, greater awareness and availability of fertility treatment can significantly constrain the physical and emotional cost of infertility (Anderson et al., 2020). The psychological and emotional dimensions of infertility are also significant in defining a woman's experience during this challenging process. Experiences have revealed that women suffering from infertility typically encounter distress, worry, and isolation, which exacerbate their situations. The efficacy of treatments, medical as well as psychological, is crucial in addressing these underlying emotional issues. In response, health professionals are encouraged to develop supportive frameworks that include counseling and peer support. Recommendations are to incorporate psychological assessments as components of fertility treatment for stress relief and enhancing overall well-being. These steps are not just encouraging emotional resilience but can also have beneficial impacts on the physical outcomes of fertility treatment, allowing women to better deal with their infertility experience (Anderson et al., 2020).

It is important to realize that female infertility is addressed beyond isolated treatments, as it is an extended health care narrative. Inclusion of evidence-based approaches, as illustrated in the guidelines of ESHRE, is fundamental in the determination of options for management of infertile women. Secondly, ongoing exploration of innovative methods of fertility preservation serves to underscore that reproductive health is dynamic and there must be constant progress. Practitioners are called upon to balance old-established practices and recent evidence to cater to the unique needs of patients. As highlighted by experts, considering the intricacy of preserving fertility not only contributes to enhancing patients' results but also aids in addressing social dimensions of infertility, improving women's control over reproductive choices and eventually promoting healthier family planning in society (Anderson et al., 2020).

KEY TERMS FROM THIS CHAPTER

- Anorexia nervosa (AN)
- ART interventions
- Diagnostic modalities
- Endometriosis
- Female infertility
- Follicle-stimulating hormone (FSH)
- Hormonal imbalance
- Human leukocyte antigen (HLA) expression
- Hypothalamic amenorrhea
- Integrative care
- Leiomyomas
- Assisted reproductive technologies (ART)
- Congenital abnormalities
- Endocrine regulation
- Fallopian tubes
- Fertility treatment programs
- Gonadotropin release stimulation
- Hormonal testing
- Hyperandrogenism
- In vitro fertilization (IVF)
- Laparoscopy
- Linoleic acid (LA)

CRITICAL THINKING QUESTIONS

1. **The most common cause of female infertility is:**
   a. Tubal blockage
   b. Ovulatory dysfunction
   c. Uterine fibroids
   d. Endometriosis
2. **Which of the following hormonal tests is commonly used to evaluate ovarian reserve in women?**
   a. Prolactin
   b. Anti-Müllerian hormone (AMH)
   c. Thyroid-stimulating hormone (TSH)
   d. Luteinizing hormone (LH)
3. **A woman with primary infertility has normal ovulation and patent fallopian tubes. The next best investigation to evaluate is:**
   a. Hysterosalpingography (HSG)
   b. Semen analysis of partner
   c. Laparoscopy
   d. Endometrial biopsy
4. **Endometriosis can cause infertility by:**
   a. Increasing estrogen levels
   b. Causing pelvic adhesions and distorted pelvic anatomy
   c. Stimulating excessive ovulation
   d. Preventing implantation in the uterus
5. **Which of the following conditions is NOT typically associated with female infertility?**
   a. Polycystic ovarian syndrome (PCOS)
   b. Hypothyroidism
   c. Premature ovarian failure
   d. Gestational diabetes

Short Answer Questions

1. What are common causes of female infertility?
2. Name two medical conditions that can contribute to infertility in women.
3. Which lifestyle factors can negatively impact female fertility?
4. What diagnostic procedures are typically used to evaluate female infertility?
5. What are some common treatment options for female infertility?
6. How can infertility affect the psychological and emotional well-being of women?

Answer to Critical Thinking Questions

1. (b) 2. (b) 3. (b) 4. (b) 5. (d)

REFERENCES

1. Aboua, G., Oguntibeju, O. O., & Stefan, S. (2013). Can lifestyle factors of diabetes mellitus patients affect their fertility? https://core.ac.uk/download/322420013.pdf (accessed on 15th June 2025).
2. AlAsmi, R. (2025). Hormonal dysfunction and male infertility: A comprehensive review of current treatment options. https://core.ac.uk/download/640070691.pdf (accessed on 15th June 2025).
3. Amininezhad, F. S., Nikbakht, R., Saadati, N., Sattari, M., et al. (2020). Spontaneous pregnancies and determinant factors in infertility: A cross-sectional study. https://core.ac.uk/download/417410070.pdf (accessed on 15th June 2025).
4. Anderson, R. A., Amant, F., Braat, D. D. M., D'Angelo, A., Chuva de Sousa Lopes, S. M., Demeestere, I., Dwek, S., et al. (2020). ESHRE guideline: Female fertility preservation. *Human Reproduction Open, 2020*. https://doi.org/10.1093/hropen/hoaa052 (accessed on 15th June 2025).
5. Anjankar, V. P., Chimurkar, V., More, A., Rauniyar, R., et al. (2024). Exploring dermatoglyphics as a potential indicator of female infertility: A review of current evidence and future directions. https://core.ac.uk/download/622174057.pdf (accessed on 15th June 2025).
6. Boichuk, O., Golovchak, I. S., & Kolomiichenko, T. (2024). The influence of neurovegetative and psychological characteristics of infertile patients with long-term COVID-19 on the effectiveness of assisted reproductive technologies. *Ukrainian Journal Health of Woman*. https://www.semanticscholar.org/paper/4f13f06be25996dd3990917e0b55249a5ca5b320 (accessed on 15th June 2025).
7. Bosteels, J., D'Hooghe, T., Van Herendael, B., Weyers, S., et al. (2007). The position of diagnostic laparoscopy in current fertility practice. https://core.ac.uk/download/55795844.pdf (accessed on 15th June 2025).
8. Buzzaccarini, G., Degliuomini, R., De Rosa, L., Villa, S., Messina, S., Siesto, G., Candiani, M., et al. (2025). A road map through the multi-faceted world of female genital cosmetic surgical techniques. *International Journal of Gynaecology and Obstetrics: The Official Organ of the International Federation of Gynaecology and Obstetrics*. https://www.semanticscholar.org/paper/77bde9a256440c1e37a8e06daf4b895753a6f037 (accessed on 15th June 2025).
9. Cao, G., Yu, L., Fang, J., Shi, R., Li, H., Lu, F., Shen, X., et al. (2024). ZP1-Y262C mutation causes abnormal zona pellucida formation and female infertility in humans. *Frontiers in Genetics, 15*. https://www.semanticscholar.org/paper/a84d0b7a1f6850b951f0a0451f53788f35f0c3ff (accessed on 15th June 2025).
10. Cariati, F., D'Argenio, V., Izquierdo, R., Tomaiuolo, R., et al. (2020). From laboratory bench to benchmark: Technology transfer in laboratory medicine. https://core.ac.uk/download/pdf/323187997.pdf (accessed on 15th June 2025).
11. Ciobanu, C., Fica, S., Poterasu, M., Rowland, N., et al. (2020). Anorexia nervosa and reproduction: Connecting brain to gonads. https://core.ac.uk/download/304672903.pdf (accessed on 15th June 2025).
12. Cocksedge, K. A., Li, T. C., & Saravelos, S. H. (2008). Prevalence and diagnosis of congenital uterine anomalies in women with reproductive failure: A critical appraisal. https://core.ac.uk/download/50624.pdf (accessed on 15th June 2025).

13. Codacci-Pisanelli, G., Del Pup, L., Levi-Setti, P. E., Patrizio, P., et al. (2018). Risk of cancer after assisted reproduction: A review of the available evidences and guidance to fertility counselors: https://core.ac.uk/download/188830441.pdf (accessed on 15th June 2025).

14. Dalis, N. S. (2024). Female infertility: Exploring biological causes and advanced therapeutic approaches. *Academia Open*. https://www.semanticscholar.org/paper/dc35be2e0347bade98ddcafa18fdcdf3e97dbb8c (accessed on 15th June 2025).

15. Dev, B. K. (2025). The role of transvaginal ultrasound in assessing ovarian function and guiding treatment in infertility management. *International Journal of Research in Medical Sciences*. https://www.semanticscholar.org/paper/92f9f234b16e3f515c92a91e364c4582ce7d381f (accessed on 15th June 2025).

16. Didziokaitė, G., Kuznecovaite, A., Biliute, G., & Kvedarienė, V. (2024). Case report: Human seminal plasma allergy diagnosis for a woman with unexplained infertility. *Frontiers in Medicine, 11*. https://www.semanticscholar.org/paper/51b90db0e5a6b3feb03fc3d8d6b54f6a8baba82a (accessed on 15th June 2025).

17. Donthu, K., Dubey, A., Himabindu, Y., Rakholia, M., et al. (2024). Efficacy of combined hysteroscopy and laparoscopy in the evaluation and management of female infertility at a tertiary care center. https://core.ac.uk/download/620836163.pdf (accessed on 15th June 2025).

18. El Adlani, S., Benksim, A., & Cherkaoui, M. (2024). The impact of knowledge to optimize attitude and behaviour about infertility: Perspectives from students in Morocco. *African Journal of Reproductive Health, 28*(8), 22–29. https://www.semanticscholar.org/paper/263a936337c5e33141513aad7f089fe9cdfc0ccb (accessed on 15th June 2025).

19. Fernandes, M., Martins, M., & Pedro, J. (2023). P-578 Interactive effects of relationship satisfaction and social support on stress: A dyadic study. *Human Reproduction*. https://www.semanticscholar.org/paper/d4379c3edcaaac781a2e746d761a610353473878 (accessed on 15th June 2025).

20. Gonnella, F., Konstantinidou, F., Donato, M., Gatta, D. M., Peserico, A., Barboni, B., Stuppia, L., et al. (2024). The molecular link between obesity and the endometrial environment: A starting point for female infertility. *International Journal of Molecular Sciences, 25*. https://www.semanticscholar.org/paper/7ca88d62b58efa0419a52f9494afe99cf5843443 (accessed on 15th June 2025).

21. Hamilton, J. A. M., van der Steeg, J. W., Hamilton, C., & de Bruin, J. D. (2021). A concise infertility work-up results in fewer pregnancies. *Human Reproduction Open, 2021*. https://www.semanticscholar.org/paper/674a877149676f87e9b2c14b8f4748c953f0dedf (accessed on 15th June 2025).

22. Hecht, L. M., Joseph-Mofford, G., Iacobelli, R., Ahmed, M., Haley, E. N., Loree, A. M., & Miller-Matero, L. (2024). Anxiety, depression, and infertility-specific distress among women with female factor infertility. *Journal of Health Psychology, 30*, 32–39. https://www.semanticscholar.org/paper/4d9409894a669aeccf6711f1e5a9e3c7b0e18f1a (accessed on 15th June 2025).

23. Ibrahim, R. O., Khorsheed, T. H., & Bahram, K. A. (2024). Investigating infertility causes, obesity rates, and mental status of infertile females attending the infertility center at Azadi Teaching Hospital in Kirkuk City, Iraq. *Journal of Advances in Medical and Pharmaceutical Sciences*. https://www.semanticscholar.org/paper/a076cb735f35a6944c53111d3c904e6881e29534 (accessed on 15th June 2025).

24. Ifeanyi, N. H. (2024). Female genital mutilation's effects on women's physical, mental, and social health. *Journal of Clinical Case Reports & Studies*. https://www.semanticscholar.org/paper/8fd403c3cc4ba573f3bf97b395e3c70dc47c02c7 (accessed on 15th June 2025).

25. Infertility Outcomes Program Project Group, Katz, P. P., Rowen, T. S., Smith, J. F., et al. (2016). The sexual impact of infertility among women seeking fertility care. https://core.ac.uk/download/323063639.pdf (accessed on 15th June 2025).

26. James, S. L., Abate, D., Abate, K. H., Abay, S. M., Abbafati, C., Abbasi, N., Abbastabar, H., et al. (2018). Global, regional, and national incidence, prevalence, and years lived with disability for 354 diseases and injuries for 195 countries and territories, 1990–2017: A systematic analysis for the Global Burden of Disease Study 2017. *The Lancet, 392*, 1789–1858. https://doi.org/10.1016/s0140-6736(18)32279-7 (accessed on 15th June 2025).

27. Kahan, W., Kosińska, A., Kras, M., Lelek, M., et al. (2024). Impact of pre-conception diet on female infertility. https://core.ac.uk/download/620863233.pdf (accessed on 15th June 2025).

28. Kahan, W., Poborowska, D., Szafrańska, W., Polańska, K., Wojaczek, M., Niedbał, P., Kosińska, A., et al. (2024). Impact of pre-conception diet on female infertility. *Quality in Sport*. https://www.semanticscholar.org/paper/5f1d57ed1794251dd3cd3b08f058eae78c2cb0b7 (accessed on 15th June 2025).

29. Karagiannis, C., Mills, D., & Zulch, H. (2014). Stress–its effects on health and behavior: A guide for practitioners. https://core.ac.uk/download/20320967.pdf (accessed on 15th June 2025).

30. Karim, S., Bibi, A., Nazik, A., & Karim, R. (2025). Impact of social media on mental health of young adults in Pakistan. *Insights–Journal of Life and Social Sciences*. https://www.semanticscholar.org/paper/2b074c59019582667d42bb1b399944f20e85ba7a (accessed on 15th June 2025).

31. Kravtsova, E. I., Kravtsov, I. I., Kutsenko, I. I., Kudlai, J. V., & Uryupina, K. V. (2020). Endometrial infertility in patients of late reproductive age (a review). https://core.ac.uk/download/441242527.pdf (accessed on 15th June 2025).

32. Kurz, K., MacQuarrie, K., Pande, R., Jain, S., & Walia, S. (2006). Improving the reproductive health of married and unmarried youth in India. https://core.ac.uk/download/71352223.pdf (accessed on 15th June 2025).

33. Lakshmi, C. S., Sampath, K., & Vardani, P. (2017). Evaluation of tubal patency by sonosalpingography is as good as hysterosalpingography in infertile women. https://core.ac.uk/download/539899875.pdf (accessed on 15th June 2025).

34. Mahajan, S. S., More, A., Shrivastava, D., Anjankar, N., Mamankar, D., & Nawale, N. (2025). Navigating infertility in unicornuate uterus: Clinical management and success with assisted reproductive techniques. *Journal of Pharmacy and Bioallied Sciences*. https://www.semanticscholar.org/paper/5c2247c207cb59eacccb030f404eca58fd0c90d5 (accessed on 15th June 2025).

35. Maheshwari, A., Ayyad, B., Balen, A., Bellver, J., et al. (2010). The impact of female obesity on the outcome of fertility treatment. https://core.ac.uk/download/4193248.pdf (accessed on 15th June 2025).

36. Mehboob, R. (2024). Hormonal therapy and endometrial cancer: Latest advancements. *Pakistan Biomedical Journal*. https://www.semanticscholar.org/paper/de84e51c28ae90702a6290d813f6d205ab44d5d3 (accessed on 15th June 2025).

37. Murani, S. (2024). Navigating the maze of female infertility: A review of factors affecting young women across cultures and conditions. *Indian Journal of Applied Research*. https://www.semanticscholar.org/paper/42c6589f6d5d13d49fd0a1477f5a4e8cf761648e (accessed on 15th June 2025).

38. Murray, C. J. L., Ikuta, K. S., Sharara, F., Swetschinski, L. R., Robles Aguilar, G., Gray, A. P., Han, C., et al. (2022). Global burden of bacterial antimicrobial resistance in 2019: A systematic analysis. *The Lancet, 399*, 629–655. https://doi.org/10.1016/s0140-6736(21)02724-0 (accessed on 15th June 2025).

39. Ottolini, C., Mulas, F., Picchetta, L., Caroselli, S., Cruz Palomino, M., Ferrando Llobell, R., Vergara Bravo, V., et al. (2024). O-071 Stringent statistical analysis of 108,684 oocyte donation cycles identifies 2.6% of donors with specific oocyte/embryo developmental arrest phenotypes for genome association studies. *Human Reproduction*. https://www.semanticscholar.org/paper/e145b6ab7667b877c39a9651ed279f0fc32b892c (accessed on 15th June 2025).

40. Papuchova, H., Saxtorph, M. H., Hallager, T., Jepsen, I., Eriksen, J., Persson, G., Funck, T., et al. (2022). Endometrial HLA-F expression is influenced by genotypes and correlates differently with immune cell infiltration in IVF and recurrent implantation failure patients. *Human Reproduction*. https://www.semanticscholar.org/paper/eb3410c18d360c0019b19b4b494fe28545d23277 (accessed on 15th June 2025).

41. Pavli, P., Triantafyllidou, O., Kapantais, E., Vlahos, N., & Valsamakis, G. (2024). Infertility improvement after medical weight loss in women and men: A review of the literature. *International Journal of Molecular Sciences, 25*. https://www.semanticscholar.org/paper/1692ef096d55c5990027f678a49543a1bbf641b6 (accessed on 15th June 2025).

42. Regnoli, G. M., Tiano, G., & De Rosa, B. (2024). How is the fear of war impacting Italian young adults' mental health? The mediating role of future anxiety and intolerance of uncertainty. *European Journal of Investigation in Health, Psychology and Education, 14*, 838–855. https://www.semanticscholar.org/paper/009a583e6698b68506b6eb100299309dc5aa5b61 (accessed on 15th June 2025).

43. Roth, G. A., Abate, D., Abate, K. H., Abay, S. M., Abbafati, C., Abbasi, N., Abbastabar, H., et al. (2018). Global, regional, and national age-sex-specific mortality for 282 causes of death in 195 countries and territories, 1980–2017: A systematic analysis for the Global Burden of Disease Study 2017. *The Lancet, 392*, 1736–1788. https://doi.org/10.1016/s0140-6736(18)32203-7 (accessed on 15th June 2025).

44. Singh, D. (2021). Female infertility in the United States and India: An analysis of treatment barriers and coping strategies. https://core.ac.uk/download/479046417.pdf (accessed on 15th June 2025).

45. Starodubova, D. A., & Mamaeva, M. E. (2025). Female reproductive health after treatment of intrauterine pathologies: Uterine synechiae and fibroids. *Glavvrač (Chief Medical Officer)*. https://www.semanticscholar.org/paper/c4c4e3d40bf26bce1e4352d26c4c5fc46497a49f (accessed on 15th June 2025).

46. Thatipelli, R. C., Parunandi, Y., Nousheen, S., Shenkeshi, H. F., & Anitha, A. (2024). An observational study on causes of female infertility. *International Journal of Reproduction, Contraception, Obstetrics and Gynecology*. https://www.semanticscholar.org/paper/62d939b58e8253207a3c29382b10666f91ea2f63 (accessed on 15th June 2025).

47. Tsuei, A., Nezhat, F., Amirlatifi, N., Najmi, Z., Nezhat, A., & Nezhat, C. (2025). Comprehensive management of bowel endometriosis: Surgical techniques, outcomes, and best practices. *Journal of Clinical Medicine, 14*. https://www.semanticscholar.org/paper/cb413885467979b75f2e8069717b00caaac2ac1c (accessed on 15th June 2025).

48. Vakili, S., & Jafarinia, M. (2024). Advances in mesenchymal stem cell research applications for female infertility: Mechanisms, efficacy parameters, challenges and future roadmap. *Galen Medical Journal, 13*. https://www.semanticscholar.org/paper/464dafc1eb5b1ead7ce23ff78627d61ee2c6cf7d (accessed on 15th June 2025).

49. Venkatesh, S. S., Wittemans, L., Palmer, D., Baya, N., Ferreira, T., Hill, B., Lassen, F., et al. (2024). Genome-wide analyses identify 21 infertility loci and over 400 reproductive hormone loci across the allele frequency spectrum. *medRxiv*. https://www.semanticscholar.org/paper/deb8337639cd8259948d143de3293c60c95d8b67 (accessed on 15th June 2025).

50. Wadhe, T., More, A., Choudhary, N., Naik, N., Chaudhary, A., & Dhamija, P. (2025). Optimizing assisted reproductive outcomes using a sperm vitrification device in severe oligozoospermia: A breakthrough in male infertility treatment. *Journal of Pharmacy and Bioallied Sciences*. https://www.semanticscholar.org/paper/b6859d237ea604aae8a71f89c6355903664ca46b (accessed on 15th June 2025).

51. Wellington, O. A. (2024). Investigating fertility health knowledge and lifestyle risk factors among Nigerian university students: A cross-sectional survey. *International Journal of Adolescent Medicine and Health, 36*, 251–258. https://www.semanticscholar.org/paper/0c64f3ef74c158358055a0b4195cbb71f785770a (accessed on 15th June 2025).

52. Wood, E. E., Liang, Y., Moon, T., Hill-Kapturczak, N., Wasserman, A., Roache, J., Mathias, C. W., et al. (2024). Social and environmental predictors of youth alcohol and cannabis initiation risk: The moderating role of family history of substance uses disorders. *Substance Use & Misuse, 60*, 403–413. https://www.semanticscholar.org/paper/ccae54a4aa39a4ba31cd20be279eee414c6ed963 (accessed on 15th June 2025).

53. Woodhouse, C. (2023). Liebe in Zeiten von Corona. *Uro-News, 27*, 35–39. https://www.semanticscholar.org/paper/efbc408165471fc1bcde1f5671b5e3c7377496c3 (accessed on 15th June 2025).

54. Yang, W., Ma, Y., Wu, Y., Lei, X., Zhang, J., & Li, M. X. (2025). Study on the effects of Mogroside V in inhibiting NLRP3-mediated granulosa cell proptosis and insulin resistance to improve PCOS. *Journal of Ovarian Research, 18*. https://www.semanticscholar.org/paper/11e1a664d92766832a7014460e3a2af553ce4dc9 (accessed on 15th June 2025).

55. Zhang, W., & Wu, F. (2025). Elevated linoleic acid intake becomes a risk factor for polycystic ovary syndrome by affecting ovarian granulosa cells. *The FASEB Journal, 39*. https://www.semanticscholar.org/paper/604e4ee9fe01d86a8213d07308b7f170bbfcee7a (accessed on 15th June 2025).

CONTRACEPTIVE METHODS

3

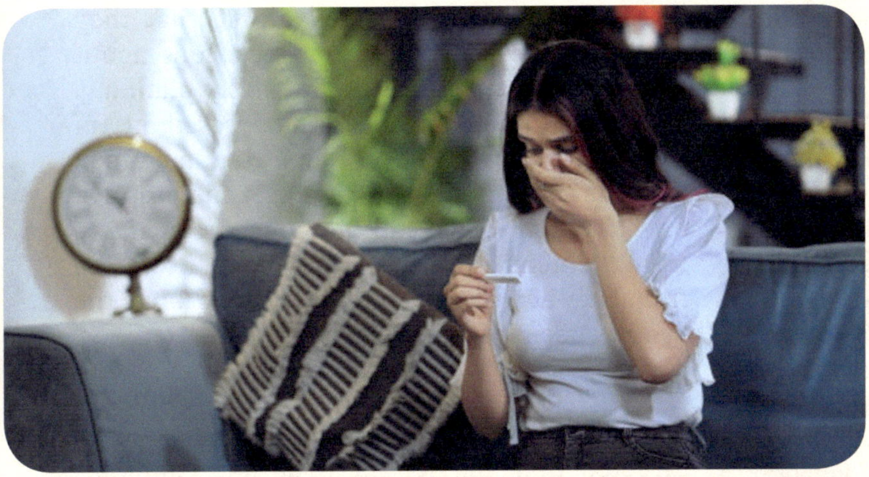

LEARNING OBJECTIVES

After studying this chapter, you will be able to:

1. Describe the various hormonal contraceptive methods
2. Explain the use and effectiveness of barrier contraceptive methods
3. Discuss the types and functions of intrauterine devices (IUDs)
4. Identify permanent contraceptive methods
5. Evaluate natural family planning techniques

Introduction

The detection of contraceptive methods in women is an essential part of reproductive health since it provides women with control over their reproductive lives and the prevention of unwanted pregnancies. Contraceptive history ranges from ancient methods to modern pharmacy findings that have transformed family planning. All of this occurs at a time when the world population is still on the increase, and the number is projected to increase to 10.1 billion by the end of the current century. The need for reliable methods of contraception demonstrates the significance of continuous research and development in this area to provide women with easy and reliable access to fertility control. It is therefore important to learn about existing methods of contraception as well as those being developed, as the latter directly affects women's health, roles within society, and family relationships. The current contraceptive options for women are diverse, varying in hormonal contraceptives like birth control pills, patches, and long-acting reversible contraception such as IUDs. These offer women autonomy over their fertility with varying degrees of user intervention and efficacy. Additionally, non-hormonal methods like barrier devices and fertility awareness-based methods offer other alternatives that do not interfere with the hormonal balance of the body. The importance of education and availability of these practices cannot be overstated; disparities in availability and knowledge can lead to the misuse of contraceptives, which results in higher rates of unintended pregnancy. Further, constant innovation in contraceptive technologies is equally crucial to addressing unmet needs, underlining further the necessity for a comprehensive understanding and usage of these practices in society. Recent advances in contraceptive research point to both hormone and non-hormone alternatives being researched, in line with the changing options in family planning. Of particular note among these is the development of contraceptive vaccines, which is a novel field for this research, integrating immunological approaches with reproductive health (Delves et al., 2002). While few trials have been undertaken, the promise for safe and effective substitutes remains a focus for future study. Additionally, as studies persist to prioritize barriers to the application of contraceptives in addition to their efficacy, it is important that the contribution of both women and men towards shared responsibility within family planning be factored into consideration. Information regarding such practices will not only be utilized for educational purposes but also empower people, which will ultimately result in healthier reproductive outcomes and well-informed decision-making of family planning measures (Alsaadi et al., 2013).

Definition of Contraceptive Methods

The description of contraceptive methods is used to denote a wide range of techniques and devices adopted to avoid pregnancy, making them fundamental components in reproductive health care. Contraceptive methods have been classified on a wide scope into two categories: reversible and irreversible methods. Reversible methods, such as hormonal contraceptives such as pills, patches, and intrauterine devices (IUDs), grant women control over their fertility without being subjected to permanent procedures. These methods act by regulating hormonal cycles or physically preventing sperm from reaching an egg. Irreversible methods, such as tubal ligation, offer a one-time solution for those individuals who are sure they never wish to be pregnant. Women should be made aware of the various options available so that they can make their own educated decisions about their reproductive health and family planning. Moreover, the effectiveness and accessibility of means of contraception are important factors in their definition and application. Contraceptive effectiveness is typically defined through the measurement of failure rate, which shows the frequency at which pregnancy occurs despite the use of specific types of contraceptive methods.

For instance, hormonal birth control methods are less likely to fail when used as directed than barrier methods like condoms. Availability of such methods of contraception may vary significantly based on socioeconomic, legal, and cultural factors. Disparities in availability limit women's autonomy to make choices about family planning, underscoring the significance of education and policy that enhances accessibility. Knowing these differences is essential since they define women's control over reproductive health decisions. Another dimension to incorporate into the definition of contraceptive methods is the sociocultural context in which they are used. Societies may hold different beliefs or approaches to doing things regarding contraception that affect women's access and use of available options. For example, how contraception is understood tends to cut across cultural femininity and motherhood beliefs and values, and these may have an impact on women's use of specific methods. Besides, issues such as contraceptive sabotage, where one of the partners may encroach on the use of contraceptive methods without informing their partner, illustrate the complexity of reproductive autonomy and safety (Plunkett et al., 2014). These social determinants must be addressed to understand the broader function of contraceptive methods on women's welfare and rights, necessitating inclusive and culturally responsive policies in reproductive health (Behnke et al., 2013).

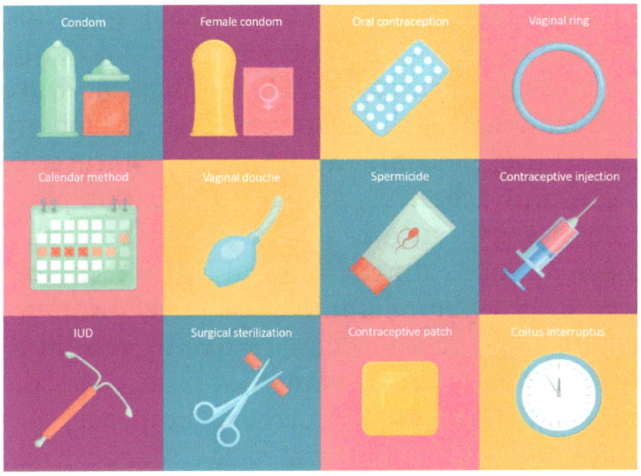

Source: https://blog.drhc.ae/hubfs/Family%20 Planning%20Methods%20-%20Dubai%20 Gynecology%20Clinic.png

Importance of Contraception in Women's Health

The value of contraception to women's health extends beyond merely birth control; it can be a significant aspect of allowing women to control their reproductive lives by being able to effectively control whether and when they get pregnant, women are better positioned to seek out education, careers, and personal goals. This empowerment is not just individually beneficial but also socially beneficial because it is conducive to increased economic security and general public health. Furthermore, access to contraceptive techniques has the potential to avoid unwanted pregnancies and, therefore, reduce the health risks to both mothers and infants. Studies show that increasing access to contraception can even be linked with lower prematurity rates, pointing to its overall impact on maternal and child health outcomes, as evidenced by various lines of proof on women's empowerment and reproductive health (Bermúdez-Millán et al., 2017). Moreover, contraception is also linked directly to improved maternal health through its role in spacing pregnancies. Appropriate interpregnancy intervals are vital in reducing pregnancy and childbearing-related risks. Inadequate spacing aggravates health conditions and leads to negative consequences, including maternal mortality. The application of contraceptive methods allows women to space pregnancies, which improves nutritional status, lowers domestic violence rates, and improves psychological well-being. By making sure that women are able to control the timing of their pregnancy, health systems are able to reduce the risk of prematurity and pregnancy-related complications significantly (Bermúdez-Millán et al., 2017). The capability to make informed decisions is a landmark change in women's health that benefits both individual and community health. Additionally, the political and historical framework of reproductive rights highlights the general implications of contraception for women's health results. The ratification of the 19th Amendment in the U.S. was a milestone win for women's rights, providing a backdrop for future healthcare activism and the call for access to contraceptives. Women's political involvement has been central to the formulation of policies that regulate reproductive health, reflecting growing awareness of the hazardous conditions surrounding pregnancy and childbirth. This evolution reflects the imperative need for contraceptive habits, which demonstrate how they are involved in health and wellbeing in the long run. As women demand ownership of their bodies, the interconnection of contraception, women's empowerment, and health continues to be unequivocally necessary.

3.1. Hormonal Contraceptive Methods

Learning Outcome

1. Discuss the birth control pills
2. Define hormonal IUDs
3. Explain the contraceptive implants

Hormonal methods of contraceptives such as oral contraceptives, implants, and injectables primarily function by regulating the levels of hormones within a woman's system to inhibit ovulation and, consequently, pregnancy. They employ synthetic hormones—largely estrogen and progestin—that act against the menstrual process. Oral contraceptives, the most common form, are usually taken in a cycle for uniform hormone levels. In addition to preventing pregnancy, they can also relieve premenstrual syndrome (PMS) symptoms, regularize menstrual cycles, and suppress acne, so they are extremely popular among women who desire both contraceptive and therapeutic effects. The attractiveness of these methods, however, must be weighed against some understanding of their potential side effects, including weight gain, mood swings, and heightened risk of blood clots, and thus the requirement of informed choice on the user's part regarding their reproductive health (Ferenczy et al., 2020). Though hormonal contraceptive methods have numerous advantages, access and information are significant barriers, particularly in young women in developing countries, as qualitative findings highlighted. Conventional family planning methods are mostly dominant in most of these regions due to limited exposure to modern types like hormonal. Young women may be discouraged by factors such as a lack of information on side effects and fear of harmful long-term effects on health, even to the extent of infertility. Also, negative beliefs that accompany existing contraceptives might lead to the use of less effective traditional practices or unsafe abortive methods. These are some of the problems to be tackled; community-based strategies that ensure awareness, education, and youth-friendly services can establish a better knowledgeable and enabling environment for adolescent girls, making their reproductive choices (Harden et al., 2009). The moral implications of hormonal contraceptive modes also deserve close attention, with the mechanism of action playing a role in informing consent. Some operate by suppressing ovulation and others by altering the endometrial lining, disrupting implantation if fertilization were to occur. Given the controversies in society about the possible abortifacient nature of these contraceptives, adequate education plays a crucial role in informing women about how these methods function to guide their choices according to personal values and beliefs. Notably, while the status of women's health continues to evolve, providing women accurate, specific information regarding hormonal contraception allows them to have informed choices regarding their reproductive life, improving autonomy and knowledge of the implications of the chosen contraceptive method (Ferenczy et al., 2020).

3.1.1. Birth Control Pills

Birth control pills are perhaps the most popular method of birth control among women, primarily because they work so well and are so easy to use. Hormone pills, including the pill, usually work by preventing ovulation, thereby reducing the risk of becoming pregnant to virtually nothing. They can also regulate menstrual periods and suppress premenstrual syndrome (PMS) symptoms and conditions such as endometriosis. Studies indicate that the majority of women who adopt this practice have positive attitudes towards the contraceptive impact of this practice, which is a predictor of increased acceptance of hormonal methods among the younger generation, particularly college women (Heisler et al., 2012). This highlights the necessity of well-designed sexual education programs that consider the benefits and potential side effects of birth control pills. Though they have advantages, birth control pills are not free from risks and are accompanied by some side effects. Side effects of these drugs, like nausea, headache, or mood changes, can result in the discontinuation of the method in women. Also, there is an urgent necessity for education regarding the health consequences of hormonal contraceptives, particularly for diseases like blood clots, which could be exacerbated in certain groups. College health center-specific education can increase student knowledge so that they can make decisions regarding their contraceptive use (Heisler et al., 2012).

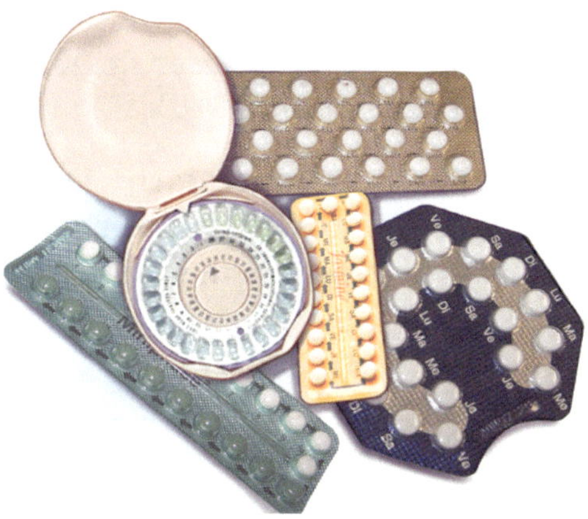

Figure 3.1. Birth Control Pill.

Source: https://my.clevelandclinic.org/-/scassets/images/org/health/articles/3977-birth-control-the-pill

Besides, this pedagogical focus is necessary, as, apart from passing on the physiological consequences of pills, it fosters a culture of healthy practice in sustaining sexual health. Beyond the medical concerns, physical aspects of such forms of birth control affect the moral dimensions of such forms of birth control, like birth control pills as well. A rather alarming phenomenon known as birth control sabotage defines situations in which a partner interferes with another's use of contraceptive methods, to the detriment of the victim. This points toward respecting individuals' choices regarding contraception and reaffirms the value of personal authority in sexual activity. Making such acts criminalized is one step society can advance toward safeguarding women's rights in choosing their method of contraception without coercive influences from others. Addressing these issues within the overall context of contraceptive education not only gives women power but also encourages healthier relational patterns overall and thus results in improved sexual health outcomes.

3.1.2. Hormonal IUDs

Hormonal intrauterine devices, or IUDs, have been a highly effective option among the many forms of birth control for women.

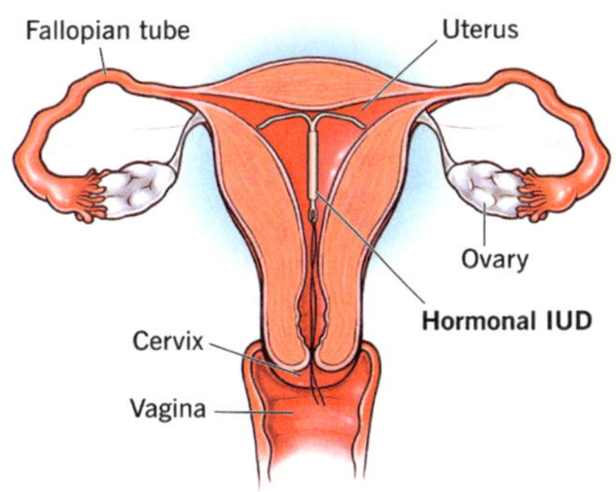

Figure 3.2. Hormonal IUDs are T-shaped devices containing progestin that you wear inside your uterus to prevent pregnancy.

Source: https://my.clevelandclinic.org/-/scassets/images/org/health/articles/hormonal-iud-mirena

The IUDs release the hormone levonorgestrel and work mostly by thickening cervical mucus, preventing sperm from traveling and fertilizing an egg. Hormonal IUDs also inhibit ovulation and thin the lining of the endometrium, making it more difficult for an embryo to implant if fertilization occurs. Thus, their multiple mechanisms of action result in a failure rate of below 1%, and they are among the safest choices for long-term contraception. More and more, health care providers are advising the use of hormonal IUDs because they offer long-term protection for 3 to 7 years, depending upon type, as well as the less frequent need for daily maintenance involved with other contraceptive devices (Greydanus et al., 2010; Greydanus et al., 2012).

Besides their effectiveness, hormonal IUDs have various non-contraceptive health benefits that enhance women's well-being. Many consumers have fewer menstrual symptoms, e.g., lighter menstrual periods and reduced dysmenorrhea. These benefits can greatly improve women's quality of life if they have heavy or painful menses. Moreover, the hormonal IUDs will also be useful in managing endometriosis symptoms and may be used in the treatment of such diseases as pelvic inflammatory disease (PID).

The ability of hormonal IUDs to provide these additional health benefits makes them a preferred choice among other birth control forms, complementing the objectives of health care providers to promote proper use of contraceptives as well as address the overall health requirements of female patients (Greydanus et al., 2010; Greydanus et al., 2012). Even though they possess many advantages, it is also crucial that users comprehend the risks and side effects of hormonal IUDs. Women can experience certain side effects such as abnormal bleeding, changes in hormones, or a chance of expulsion. Moreover, like every other medical device, there are slight chances of complications while inserting it or a risk of pelvic infection. To make effective decisions, women should see their physicians so they are well aware of the merits and demerits of the insertion of hormonal IUDs. Ultimately, contraceptive selection must be individualized, about medical history, lifestyle, and preference, so that women select what is appropriate for them and their circumstances (Greydanus et al., 2010; Greydanus et al., 2012).

3.1.3. Contraceptive Implants

Contraceptive implants are a fresh option among long-acting reversible contraceptives (LARCs) in the area of women's contraception. They are small, flexible rods implanted subdermally in the upper arm and deliver hormones that suppress ovulation very efficiently over a long period, typically for three years. The American College of Obstetricians and Gynecologists (ACOG) acknowledges implants as a first-line contraceptive for sexually active women because they are both highly effective and allow tremendous levels of user flexibility and convenience (Anna et al., 2018).

This aspect is particularly useful for women who may experience issues with daily contraceptive adherence, therefore reducing the risk of unintended pregnancies, which still account for around 45% in America (Anna et al., 2018). Despite all the benefits, the acceptability of contraceptive implants by certain groups, particularly young women, has been considerably lower than anticipated. Research indicates that while LARCs, including implants, are safe and effective among individuals below the age of 25, fewer youths still use these methods. A Seattle-based initiative at the Orion Clinic identifies this disparity, which reveals that among youths, there is limited awareness and knowledge of LARC availability, directly proportional to lower demand for such practices. Education among this population can have a significant impact on correcting misinformation and boosting overall acceptance and utilization of contraceptive implants.

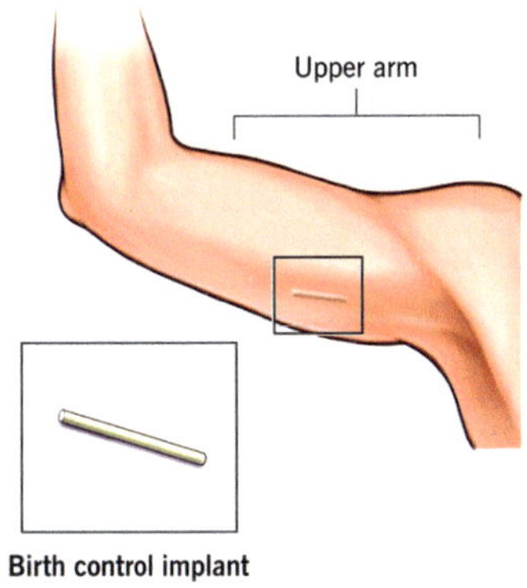

Figure 3.3. A birth control implant is a small, thin rod-like device you wear under the skin in your upper arm to prevent pregnancy.

Source: https://my.clevelandclinic.org/-/scassets/images/org/health/articles/24564-contraceptive-implant

Understanding drivers of contraceptive decision-making is an important step in increasing access and education on implants. The use of intensive counseling strategies, e.g., those outlined by the World Health Organization Decision-Making Tool, can assist providers in referring clients to effective services like contraceptive implants (Anna et al., 2018). These teaching interventions can assist women in making informed choices based on their unique health needs and life choices. Through the emphasis on access and awareness, hospitals, particularly in marginalized communities, can contribute towards minimizing the endemic levels of unplanned pregnancies as well as improving reproductive health outcomes by promoting effective methods of contraception such as implants (Anna et al., 2018).

Test Your Knowledge

1. What hormones are commonly found in birth control pills, and how do they prevent pregnancy?
2. How do hormonal IUDs work to provide long-term contraception?

3.2. Barrier Methods

Learning Outcome

1. Define male and female condoms
2. Explain the diaphragms and cervical caps
3. Discuss the spermicides

Barrier methods are a significant portion of the infrastructure for female contraception, which avoids pregnancy by creating a real barrier between the sperm and egg. The most widely used of these are male condoms and female condoms, diaphragms, and cervical caps. All these methods function on the same fundamental principle of denying sperm access to the uterus, thus maintaining reproductive autonomy while providing other health benefits, such as protection against sexually transmitted diseases (STIs). Among all of these means, male condoms are most prevalent since they are easily accessible and provide a double protection factor, thus being an inexpensive option for the majority of couples. By providing a physical barrier, these methods present a non-hormonal choice over hormonal contraceptive methods, which are attractive to those who prefer to avoid systemic hormonal effects for other health-related reasons. The effectiveness and acceptance of barrier methods may be influenced by various factors, including correct application and user acceptability. For instance, while female condoms offer more control to the woman and may be inserted ahead of sex, their application is limited by inconvenience and additional cost in comparison to male condoms. Further, the cervical cap and diaphragm need to be carefully fitted by medical practitioners, adding a factor of commitment on the part of the user. While barrier methods have a failure rate of 12% to 24% under typical use, they can be even more effective with proper and regular use. Of particular note is the observation that increased access to education and contraceptives remains vital in order to make these methods even more effective, hence addressing the unmet need for safe and effective contraceptive arrangements on the part of men and women (Alsaadi et al., 2013). Amidst the changing landscape of contraceptive technologies, the position of barrier methods continues to hold prominence, especially in view of new contraceptive technologies and research endeavors. As research into male contraceptives continues, an appreciation of the interplay between different methods can enhance discussion around contraceptive options. Studies have indicated that the use of both barrier methods and hormonal types in an integrated method can counteract world population increase as well as meet reproductive health needs effectively (Appleton et al., 2006). Moreover, dual functionality for STI prevention also indicates the suitability of barrier methods in public health interventions aimed at augmenting sexual health. Lastly, continuing promotion and evaluation of barrier methods will be crucial as society works towards ensuring access to diverse contraceptive methods that strike a balance between personal choice and public health.

3.2.1. Male and Female Condoms

In the consideration of contraceptive options, male and female condoms are an unusual case of balance between accessibility and user control. Male condoms are well known to be effective in the prevention of pregnancy and STIs. Even though they are readily available, most women still prefer a wide range of contraceptive choices. Research shows that in some countries, like Angola, the male condom is the most commonly used contraceptive, with around 32.1% of women using them. There are, however, enormous barriers to this, one of which is the low level of awareness of other forms, including long-acting reversible contraceptives (LARCs), where women's knowledge is still low, with fewer than 40% of women having heard of these (Bell et al., 2017). This inequality underscores the necessity for extensive education and available resources to enable individuals, especially women, to take control of their reproductive well-being and make informed decisions regarding their sexual health. The female condom, on the other hand, presents a new approach by putting the control of contraception in the hands of women. This practice not only enables women to take control of their sexual well-being but also prevents STIs. Evidence has proven that female condoms may play a key role in family planning, particularly in societies where cultural gender norms reinforce men's dominance in making contraceptive decisions. In spite of high levels of awareness of family planning methods, there are couples who have inconsistent practices because of pressures and attitudes within society about intentions for fertility (Capurchande et al., 2017).

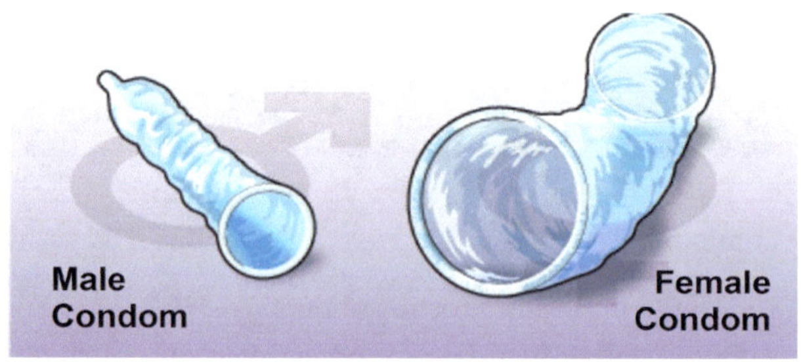

Figure 3.4. Male and female condoms.

Source: https://healthfacts.ng/wp-content/uploads/2016/12/male-and-female-condoms.jpg

Encouraging the use of female condoms can soften these pressures and further enhance women's choice in reproductive health issues. If so done, these issues can foster a culture where both parties freely discuss the use of contraceptives and share family planning responsibilities. Condom integration programs for males and females together can significantly enhance women's likelihood of selecting their preferred methods. In Angola and Mozambique, specifically, concerted efforts are needed to close the knowledge-practice gap. Availability remains an important concern, with limited facilities that offer a range of methods, including female condoms. The importance of gender-sensitive counseling and service delivery cannot be overstressed. Women are subjected to societal norms regarding childbearing that constrain their choices and knowledge about available contraceptives (Capurchande et al., 2017). By surmounting these structural and educational barriers, health policies can better provide women's needs, ultimately leading to a more educated and empowered citizenry who can make decisions that suit their reproductive health agendas.

3.2.2. Diaphragms and Cervical Caps

Diaphragms and cervical caps are barrier contraceptive techniques that do not contain hormones but provide women with a choice in avoiding unwanted pregnancy. Both devices are put into place to physically obstruct sperm from the cervix, so sperm are unable to enter the uterus. The diaphragm is a silicone or latex dome-shaped cup that must be inserted into the vagina before intercourse and can be used in conjunction with spermicide for better effectiveness. On the other hand, since the cervical cap is smaller and closer to the natural fit, it could be trickier to insert correctly, requiring caution in insertion. Both are women's control measures over their reproductive lives that make them attractive options for those who want to have less hormonal interference over family planning. Diaphragm and cervical cap effectiveness differ from one another, with typical use documenting a higher failure rate than with hormonal contraceptives. Studies have demonstrated that diaphragms can have a failure rate ranging from 12% to 24% based on proper use, while cervical caps also have similar figures, particularly among birth-given women. It is therefore critical for users of such methods to understand the proper use and limitations. Furthermore, despite protection against STIs, such protection is far less than that of condom use. Women must take all of these factors, including efficacy and convenience, into account when selecting the most suitable method for their life and family planning purposes, as discussed in the recent literature on contraceptive utilization (Greydanus et al., 2010).

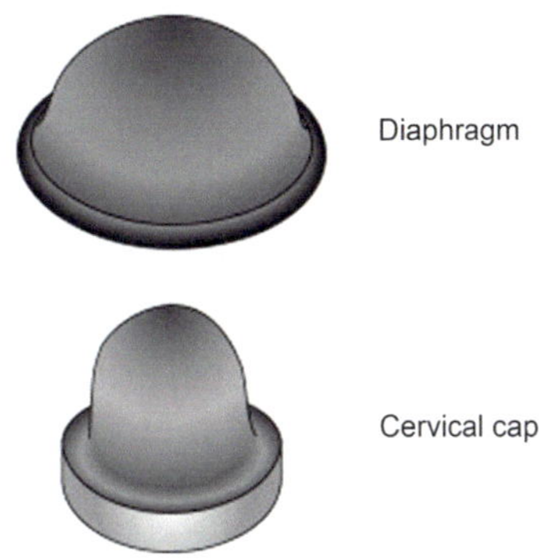

Figure 3.5. Diaphragm and cervical cap.

Source: https://ars.els-cdn.com/content/image/3-s2.0-B9780128036785001557-f00155-04-9780128036785.jpg

In the broader context of contraceptive options available to women, among diaphragms, cervical caps, and so on, one's convenience, accessibility, and learning center must be considered. Health care providers play a significant role in informing patients about these methods, calling for sexual education as well as the individual's choice when it comes to reproduction. According to the literature, awareness promotion and effective management of non-hormonal methods can lead to better adolescent and young adult outcomes (N/A). The choice to use cervical caps or diaphragms extends beyond prevention of simple pregnancy; it involves a significant aspect of women's health that needs to be discussed and considered with much thought and debate between practitioners and patients.

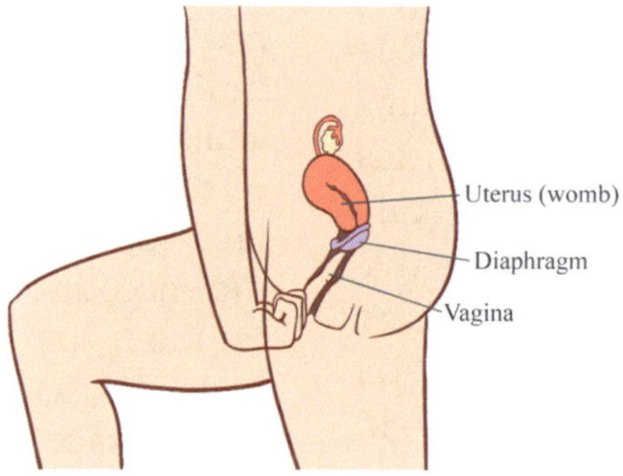

Figure 3.6. Illustration of the diaphragm being inserted into vagina.

Source: https://www.saintlukeskc.org/health-library/birth-control-diaphragm-and-cervical-cap

3.2.3. Spermicides

Among all the contraceptive options available to women, spermicides are a valuable but often neglected choice. Spermicides are chemical substances that kill or inactivate sperm and are generally contained in preparations such as gels, foams, and films. Their action is primarily through interference in sperm cell membranes, such that the sperm remain inactive upon exposure. While spermicides can be used alone as birth control, they are usually used in conjunction with barrier methods such as condoms or diaphragms. Combining them enhances overall effectiveness through the physical barrier while chemically halting sperm movement. However, despite their potential, the use and knowledge of spermicides are low, as indicated in research that demonstrates that only 5% of women know of this type of contraceptive (Abimbola et al., 2013).

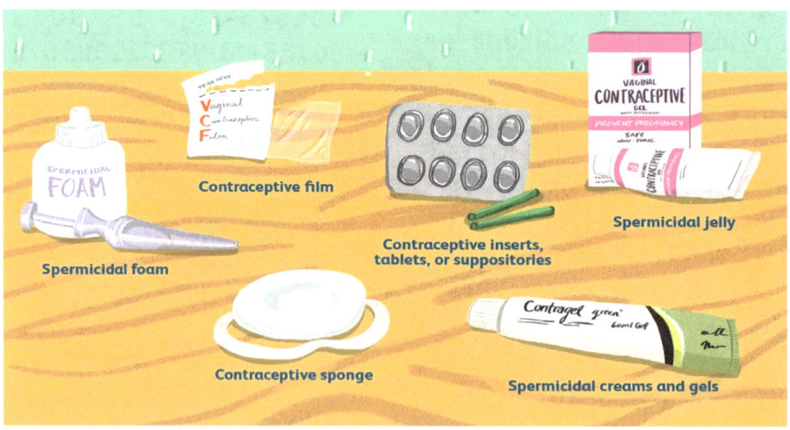

Figure 3.7. Types of spermicides.

Source: https://www.verywellhealth.com/thmb/BhCp-Cv9tVxM9QSKA2S1CFA6TFs=/1500x0/filters:no_upscale():max_bytes(150000):strip_icc()/types-of-spermicide-906824-v3-9f5cbfdf7c6c4bc7b4b9730a4d179ddd.png

The effectiveness of spermicides, though valuable, is different among products and application methods. To be most effective, spermicides need to be applied correctly and within a certain time frame before sex. Research shows that when spermicides are properly used, the failure rate can range from 15% to 30%. The fact that it is between 15% and 30% emphasizes the need for user education and for healthcare providers to counsel women on correct application. Parameters such as timing, frequency of application, and anatomical individual variation can all influence the effectiveness of spermicides. Additionally, side effects in the form of irritation or allergic reactions to users can deter the continued application of the product. Therefore, utilization of spermicides should be enjoyed in its technicalities if rates of undesired pregnancies are to be reduced, particularly within the context of an overall framework of contraceptive education. Under family planning, adding spermicides to overall contraceptive measures has advantages as well as disadvantages. Public health interventions for encouraging safe use of contraceptives through sensitization and education on the types of contraception should involve comprehensive consideration of spermicides. This is especially so in populations where there are low rates of contraceptive use due to cultural barriers and myths about modern contraceptives, for example, in sub-Saharan Africa. Education efforts towards awareness of women's access to contraceptives serve as a critical factor for increasing contraceptive prevalence, with them made aware of the benefits and limitations of products like spermicides (Abimbola et al., 2013). By providing women with information, health interventions can empower them to make informed decisions about their reproductive lives, hence contributing to improved maternal and child health status.

Test Your Knowledge

1. How do male and female condoms function to prevent pregnancy and reduce the risk of sexually transmitted infections?
2. What is the role of diaphragms and cervical caps in contraception, and how are they used?

3.3. Intrauterine Devices (IUDs)

Learning Outcome

1. Discuss various types of IUDs
2. Define the mechanism of action for female contraceptive methods
3. Explain the benefits and risks of contraceptive methods

Intrauterine devices (IUDs) are an extremely effective form of long-acting reversible birth control, becoming increasingly popular for their high effectiveness and low maintenance needs. Unlike other forms of birth control, however, IUDs can be effective in preventing pregnancy for several years, depending on the type of device utilized—copper or hormonal. Such long-lasting protection for IUDs makes them very attractive to women who require a steady source of birth control without the day-to-day involvement of pills. Interestingly, the introduction of newer LARC (long-acting reversible contraception) products has been at the root of a sharp decline in teen pregnancy rates, abortion, and unwanted pregnancy, being a significant reproductive health step forward (Glantz et al., 2018). Also, the variety of IUDs offered in different types implies women can choose the best type to fit their health needs and lifestyle preferences. Despite being effective, IUDs have been met with resistance through misperceptions and access constraints. Evidence has indicated that the majority of women are ill-informed about IUDs, and this does not motivate them to use this form of contraception. Inhibitors to the use of IUDs universally include lack of knowledge among healthcare professionals, ignorance among prospective users, and systemic impediments to healthcare, e.g., affordability and narrow insurance coverage. A side effect review of long-acting reversible contraceptives indicates that the majority of women discontinue IUDs early, most commonly due to pain or ignorance, thus emphasizing the necessity of complete education and awareness of these devices (Glantz et al., 2018). Such concerns are essential for increased utilization rates of IUDs so that women may make optimal choices concerning their reproductive health. To encourage greater successful use of IUDs, policy change and focused intervention are required. Expansion of insurance coverage of IUD insertion and removal, particularly through public programs like Medicaid, is a key step toward alleviating economic barriers. Furthermore, health clinics must go out of their way to establish an environment conducive to non-coercive and confidential delivery of IUDs, particularly among vulnerable groups where they may also face other types of barriers to receiving contraceptive services. Empirical studies have shown that with the right resources and support, the barriers to IUD use can be effectively circumvented, resulting in improved reproductive outcomes (Allina et al., 2016). Ultimately, the development of an informed conversation about IUDs will empower women to take control of their reproductive lives, allowing them to make good and certain choices on their birth control strategy.

3.3.1. Types of IUDs

Intrauterine devices (IUDs) are among the most prevalent long-acting reversible contraceptive methods, which are highly effective and easy to use. These are inserted inside the uterus by a healthcare provider and remain there for years, providing continuous pregnancy prevention without daily effort. There are various types of IUDs, which are primarily categorized as hormonal and non-hormonal types. Hormonal IUDs that release a form of progestin work by making mucus thicker on the cervix, thinning the uterine lining, and also preventing ovulation. The method not only prevents pregnancy but may also cause less menstrual bleeding, which makes it attractive to many users. Non-hormonal IUDs, however, which are made of copper, can create a toxic place for sperm so that fertilization is prevented. The appropriateness of the use of an IUD is determined based on an individual's health, lifestyle, and personal principles. In teenagers, the insertion of IUDs would decrease unintended pregnancy and sexually transmitted diseases substantially, as seen through the increase in contraceptive usage among this age group. Research indicates that a significant proportion of sexually active teens face challenges with effective contraception, and thus, the clinicians' responsibilities become essential in resolving comprehensive information about numerous methods, including IUDs (Greydanus et al., 2012). Hormonal IUDs are especially helpful among youth as they offer a dual benefit of contraceptive effectiveness and menstrual regulation. In contrast to this, copper IUDs have also provided a hormone-free alternative for those who may be predisposed towards not using the hormonal method, thus reaching more individuals. Use of IUDs has been found to be far less prevalent within specific ethnic and socioeconomic groups, highlighting a call for increased outreach and education initiatives targeted towards these particular groups (Meese et al., 2016). Increased familiarity and access to IUDs can enable youths and women to make knowledgeable choices in reproductive health. Further, the launch of no-cost contraception schemes has been promising to enhance access as the sharp increase in IUD use among some groups indicates (Meese et al., 2016). By expanding understanding of the distinct advantages of both copper and hormonal IUDs, clinicians are better positioned to address varied populations' needs for contraception, ultimately lowering unintended pregnancy and total reproductive health.

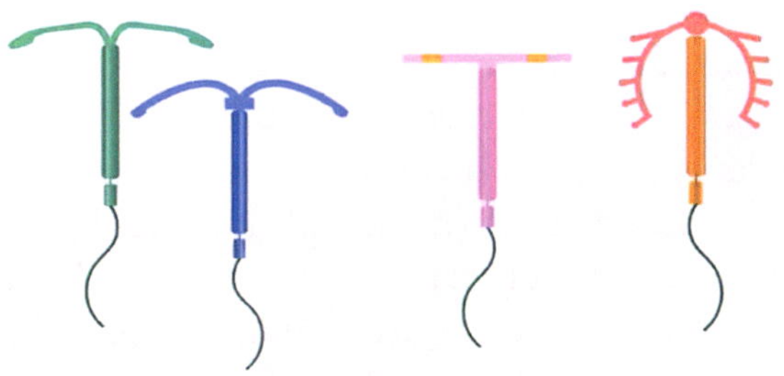

Figure 3.8. IUD types.

Source: https://www.thehealthsite.com/pregnancy/are-intra-uterine-devices-painful-heres-what-you-need-to-know-about-the-safest-method-of-contraception-1076615/

3.3.2. Mechanism of Action

In examining the mechanism of action of female contraceptive options, it is essential to understand how the methods work to avoid pregnancy. Hormonal contraceptives, for instance, do so largely through the manipulation of the hormonal environment in order to inhibit ovulation. By the provision of synthetic forms of estrogen and progestin, such methods introduce an artificial hormonal environment, one that talks to the body in an effort to suppress the secretion of hypothalamic gonadotropin-releasing hormone (GnRH).

Consequently, there is a reduction in the secretion of luteinizing hormone (LH) and follicle-stimulating hormone (FSH), eventually inhibiting the maturation and release of an egg from the ovaries. This process not only reduces the chances of fertilization but also modifies the cervical mucus, which becomes less sperm-permissive. These hormonal manipulations illustrate the extreme biological manipulation with contemporary contraception technology. In addition to hormonal approaches, non-hormonal alternatives also have specific mechanisms of action. Barrier methods, including condoms and diaphragms, act physically to block sperm from accessing the egg, thus decreasing the likelihood of fertilization. These are the first line of defense, keeping sperm from entering the reproductive tract. Another example is intrauterine devices (IUDs), specifically the copper-based IUDs, which take advantage of the presence of copper to generate a localized inflammatory response within the uterus. This is an anti-egg and anti-sperm reaction, significantly inhibiting fertilization and implantation. Through explanations of these varied mechanisms, one may also observe the many methods employed in contraceptive technology, adjusting to changing preferences and physiological behaviors among women.

Research also examines emerging contraceptive technologies that are continually enhancing in effectiveness and utilization. Advances in non-hormonal contraceptives, such as immunocontraceptive agents interfering with specific sperm proteins, are a new frontier in reproductive well-being. Such mechanisms aim to invoke an immune response against sperm and thereby prevent fertilization without the reliance on hormones (Alsaadi et al., 2013). Further evidence shows the potential of agents that disrupt sperm-associated mechanisms, which would expand the menu of contraceptive options. As evidenced by participatory practice in reproductive health discourse, these advances recognize that there is a necessity for sound strategies that adapt to women's evolving needs (Malhotra et al., 2004). Lastly, understanding the complex mechanisms involved in various types of contraceptives ensures sound decision-making in female reproductive health.

3.3.3. Benefits and Risks

The evaluation of contraceptive measures is a cautious study of both their risks and benefits, which usually has a bearing based on the perception of society and individual experience. The perceptions of risk and benefit, in the majority of situations, particularly in developing countries like Nigeria, are highly critical in the adoption and use of contraceptive measures. Research has also indicated that side effects, which are normally experienced in terms of fear and misperception, tend to be the major causes of non-use of contraceptives among women. The Ibadan and Kaduna qualitative research revealed that the participants had a wide range of concerns, ranging from health-related risks, such as cancer and fertility myths, to perceived advantages of family planning, which is not only comprised health advantages but also socio-economic benefits, for instance, empowerment and improved family well-being. These perceptions need. to be tackled for the enhancement of contraceptive use and informed decision-making women's part. Among all the available forms of contraception, the combined oral contraceptive pill, or COCP, is a significant one due to its efficacy and additional health advantages. The pill, introduced during the early part of the 1960s, has been modified to include decreased doses of hormones, specifically ethinylestradiol in combination with various progestogens, fine-tuning the preparations in such a manner as to minimize side effects while maximizing contraceptive effectiveness. The benefits of the COCP extend beyond mere pregnancy prevention; ovarian and endometrial cancer risk has been demonstrated to be reduced in trials, which can greatly enhance a woman's overall long-term health. These effects have no risk; however, venous thromboembolism and stroke have been noted as being serious complications, but only in specific populations with contraindications. Hence, healthcare professionals must balance these benefits with the risks while prescribing this method to ensure safe and successful use (Brincat et al., 2006).

Policies to promote family planning must take into account various perceptions of the pros and cons of various contraceptive methods. By working on the identified specific issues via qualitative assessments, healthcare initiatives can correct misconceptions and provide special information to prospective users. For instance, in Nigeria, myth correction regarding the use of contraceptives significantly influences women's willingness to use them. In addition, highlighting the advantages, for example, better reproductive health and social empowerment, is also very important in eliminating misconceptions and bringing a better attitude towards the use of contraceptives. These specific strategies can promote knowledge and ease dialogue regarding the advantages and risks of all the available methods. Finally, by integrating family planning contraceptive health programs with community values, the barriers to adoption can be reduced, and enhanced education and access can be encouraged in family planning (Hebert et al., 2015).

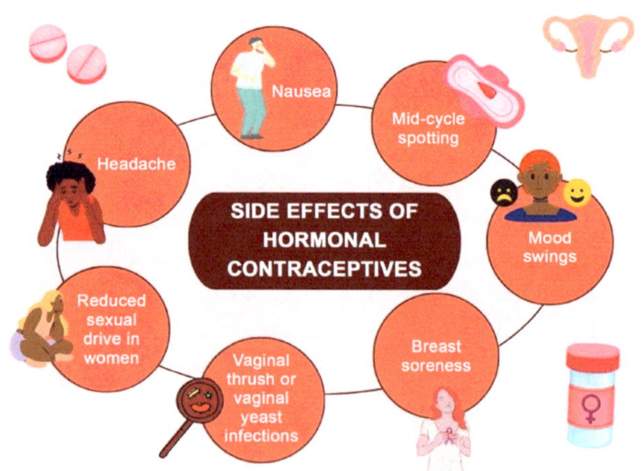
SIDE EFFECTS OF HORMONAL CONTRACEPTIVES
Nausea
Mid-cycle spotting
Mood swings
Breast soreness
Vaginal thrush or vaginal yeast infections
Reduced sexual drive in women
Headache

Figure 3.9. Side Effects of hormonal contraception.

Source: https://www.icliniq.com/articles/womens-health/hormonal-contraception

Test Your Knowledge

1. What are the main types of intrauterine devices (IUDs) used for contraception?
2. How do female contraceptive methods generally work to prevent pregnancy?

3.4. Permanent Contraceptive Methods

Learning Outcome

1. Discuss the tubal ligation
2. Understand the essure procedure
3. Define considerations for permanent methods

Long-term contraceptive methods, also referred to as sterilization, provide a woman with a permanent method of avoiding pregnancy. Tubal ligation and hysteroscopic sterilization are the only two procedures that come under this category and are done through surgery to close off or destroy the fallopian tube, thereby preventing the sperm from accessing the egg. According to recent data, close to 41.6% of users of contemporary contraceptives in some locations, such as Dadra and Nagar Haveli, opt for female sterilization, bringing out its popularity as a long-lasting method among individuals who have already given birth or do not want to give birth to any child. Such methods are attractive because of their efficacy, which is over 99%, and the lack of necessity for continuous user compliance as with reversible methods. In assessing the adoption of such methods, it is important to look at the impact on women's reproductive health and agency. The decision to go for permanent contraceptive methods most often relies on different social and individual factors, including health concerns, family size, and economic standing. Women's view of reproductive health and access to family planning knowledge often leads to the decision to be sterilized. As per research, education and awareness have a significant impact on decisions regarding contraceptive use. One study on adopters' quality of life showed a statistically significant difference between adopters and non-adopters in terms of life satisfaction, suggesting that permanent method adoption can contribute to the quality of a woman's overall life and enable them to pursue other life objectives, e.g., work or education. Therefore, access to counseling and educational materials is central to promoting informed family planning choices. Despite the benefits associated with long-term contraceptive methods, there remain problems regarding access to healthcare and social attitudes. Even though these methods present a final solution to preventing pregnancy, stereotypes associated with sterilization, particularly in certain cultural contexts, can deter women from trying them. In addition, health facilities may be inadequately prepared to provide extensive counseling on these options, as evidenced by statistics that indicated 85% of college-age women surveyed were not well-educated regarding contraception in general. Education efforts that serve to raise awareness, such as offering the effects and benefits of long-term methods, are essential to empower women to make healthy decisions regarding their reproductive lives. This is to complement the contraceptive situation and increase coverage for women to reach autonomy in family planning (Dhodi et al., 2024; Pandey et al., 2023).

3.4.1. Tubal Ligation

Tubal ligation is a permanent form of contraception for women who want to avoid pregnancy in the future. It is a medical procedure by which the fallopian tubes are either blocked or severed, thereby ending the passageway through which eggs travel from the ovary to the uterus. Tubal ligation is extremely effective, with a calculated less than 1% failure rate. The majority of women opt for the tubal ligation as a last measure if they are certain that they will never have more children or in instances where other reversible methods of birth control are not ideal for them. One should, however, consider well the implications of undertaking such a permanent procedure, including the risk of post-surgery regret. Discussions of tubal ligation also exist very much in tandem with broader socio-cultural implications, such as women's autonomy over reproductive healthcare choices and family size pressures. In addition, demographic facts often come into play when deciding on tubal ligation.

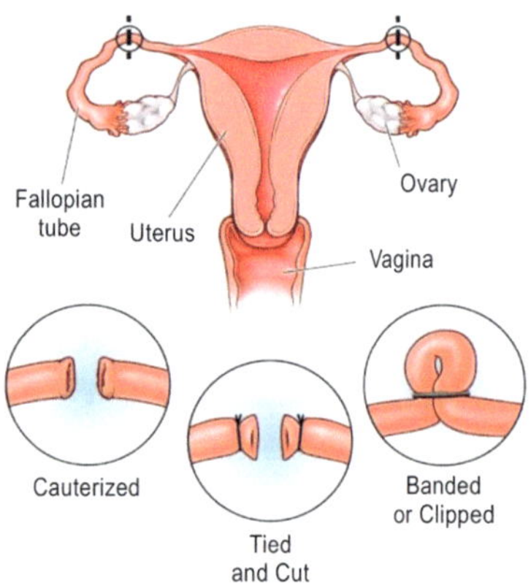

Figure 3.10. The fallopian tubes can be blocked several ways during tubal ligation surgery (getting your tubes tied).

Source: https://images.ctfassets.net/yixw23k2v6vo/7xpamPR9OKitqD9slyHFtx/cddcf0591770c69464fa6a8897a06fa5/large-GettyImages-1133181391-tubal-ligation.jpg?fit=thumb&w=492&h=328

Research has shown that couple dynamics, particularly education levels and domestic responsibilities, are a significant factor in determining contraceptive choice. Studies indicate that in couples in which women have more control over decision-making or both men and women equally share domestic duties, there are increased chances of selecting female sterilization, such as tubal ligation, over traditional reversible methods. This kind of association indicates how the gender role dynamics in relationships translate to contraceptive method selection. As suggested by recent studies, educational attainment of both partners is the most significant predictor of the choice in contraceptive selection, which shows that even now, reproductive health choices are influenced by social structures (Bracke et al., 2017).

Opening educational opportunities and fostering equitable domestic relationships can allow women to make informed decisions in their reproductive futures. While tubal ligation is extremely advantageous, the disadvantages and constraints of this procedure need to be considered. In contrast with reversible procedures that can easily be halted, tubal ligation involves surgery and is generally considered irreversible for women who may in the future desire to be fertile, alternatives such as *in vitro* fertilization exist, but are expensive and logistically complex. International context of choice of contraceptive is still challenging, with public health efforts to limit unplanned pregnancy set against the double danger of sexually transmitted disease (Agudelo et al., 2017). It is important that healthcare providers give proper counseling on the spectrum of available contraceptive methods and the long-term consequences of tubal ligation. This will enable them to inform women completely and make the best choice for their individual reproductive health.

3.4.2. Essure Procedure

The Essure procedure is significant in the advancement of female sterilization procedures by taking advantage of a minimally invasive approach that is far from the traditional surgical way of sterilization. Initially approved by the FDA in 2002, Essure is a technique whereby small metal coils are placed inside each of the fallopian tubes through a hysteroscopic procedure, which can be performed in a physician's office rather than an operating room. This technology contributes to women's access to permanent contraception since it reduces hospitalization and general anesthetic usage. Up to 2015, approximately 750,000 women had opted for the Essure procedure, which highlights its popularity and convenience compared to conventional sterilization methods (Mahoney et al., 2021). This trend reflects the greater popularity of non-invasive reproductive health procedures and a focus on education of the various contraceptive methods for women. While the advantages of the Essure procedure are apparent, it is appropriate to comment on its safety profile and complications. While many women have successful outcomes, others do have side effects ranging from discomfort to severe reactions that necessitate device removal. The metal content in Essure is a source of concern for compatibility with medical imaging equipment such as MRI. Studies indicate, however, that devices such as Essure are marked as MR Conditional by the FDA, which means they can safely receive MRI procedures subject to certain conditions (Correia et al., 2012).

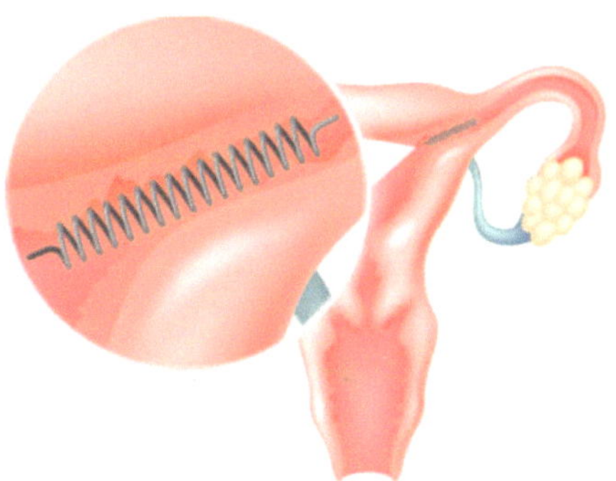

Figure 3.11. Essure procedure.

Source: https://www.drugwatch.com/wp-content/uploads/essure-uterus-tort.jpg

This classification is relevant for females who may be in need of imaging for health reasons after sterilization. By enlightening patients to the potential risks, practitioners can render the choice for contraception more informed.

The Essure procedure also initiates the discourse regarding the more significant role of long-term contraception choices in women's health. The hysteroscopic sterilization alternative is of particular importance in a global environment where women's empowerment to make the right reproductive choices is paramount. Even so, women who consider undergoing such a procedure have to weigh the benefits against the potential for unforeseen complications. It is crucial that doctors provide extensive counseling with options and potential side effects considered. The Essure debate, as one of the gamut of contraceptive methods, upholds individualized healthcare that places women's autonomy at the forefront in making health decisions. In the end, the procedure is more than a method for contraception, but also the ongoing evolution of women's reproductive health and rights (Mahoney et al., 2021).

3.4.3. Considerations For Permanent Methods

The choice of using permanent family planning methods, particularly among women, is dependent on a range of factors, from personal circumstances to societal culture. Permanent methods such as female sterilization offer women a long-term solution for individuals who have completed childbearing or do not wish to have any more children at all. However, the use of such methods can be hampered by various factors like poor awareness and knowledge about such options, as was largely evident in Ethiopia. On this note, although a high overall knowledge of family planning behavior was felt, only 0.1% of women utilized long-acting and permanent forms of contraception like female sterilization. This disparity highlights the need for both closing knowledge gaps as well as shaping attitudes towards such practices, particularly in regions where such decisions remain untapped (Alemayehu et al., 2012).

Furthermore, cultural attitudes strongly contribute to women's decisions towards permanent contraceptive practices. LAPMs' attitudes are often reflective of broader societal norms and stigmas regarding female sexuality and conception. It has been found through research that women may hold a negative perception towards permanent methods, and this could be attributed to the absence of proper information or fear of potential health complications arising from the procedures. For instance, 53.6% of married Ethiopian women had a negative attitude towards the use of LAPMs, which consequently led to their underutilization despite being good options for curbing family planning demands. This negative attitude can present barriers to both personal preference and to public health interventions encouraging comprehensive contraceptive education (Alemayehu et al., 2012).

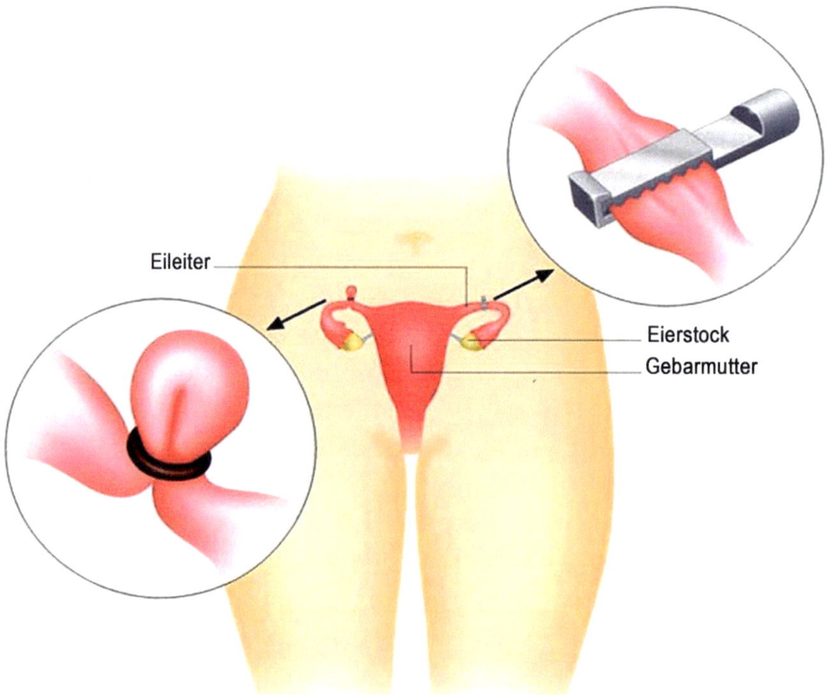

Figure 3.12. Permanent Female Contraception.

Source: https://www.indiaparenting.com/sterilisation-permanent-female-contraception.html

In addition to addressing knowledge and attitude problems, the reinforcement of contraceptive education targeted at specific groups can also result in significant gains in the use of permanent methods. Raising awareness through targeted education could best help women in their younger years and college students, where risky sexual behavior remains a source of concern. A study of undergraduate students demonstrated that the sample had a positive attitude towards contraception and that educational interventions could draw upon this to promote levels of contraceptive use and reduce the number of unwanted pregnancies and sexually transmitted diseases (STDs). By enabling individuals with rightful information and instilling a positive attitude towards LAPMs, public health workers can promote an informed decision-making process for family planning options among women.

Test Your Knowledge

1. What is tubal ligation and how does it serve as a permanent contraceptive method?
2. How does the Essure procedure work to provide permanent birth control?

3.5. Natural Family Planning

Learning Outcome

1. Explain the calendar method as a natural contraceptive technique.
2. Describe the basal body temperature method and its role in fertility awareness.
3. Analyze the cervical mucus method for tracking fertility and natural contraception.

Natural Family Planning (NFP) is a collection of practices undertaken by couples in order to regulate conception according to observation of fertile and infertile periods of a woman's menstrual cycle. NFP is based on the understanding of the biological indicators of ovulation that can be observed with the aid of various methods, including calendar methods, basal body temperature checking, and observing cervical mucus. NFP is distinct from other contraceptive methods in its emphasis on self-awareness and the body's natural biological processes to allow couples to make informed decisions regarding having a family. Unlike the use of hormonal contraceptives, which can carry side effects, NFP poses no health danger, making it a safer choice for certain women. Apart from this, it also encourages free communication and collaboration between partners in order to know each other's reproductive health better, which is essential in making sound decisions (Alsaadi et al., 2013). Natural Family Planning relies on the willingness, education, and commitment of the couples to monitor the fertility signs accurately. Evidence shows that with regular use, NFP can yield pregnancy rates comparable to hormonal contraceptives and is therefore an effective family planning option. It becomes less effective with irregular usage and in the absence of proper education, and that's why it is all the more critical to receive full training and instruction from medical experts. NFP also aligns with certain religious and ethical doctrines that esteem natural methods of planning a family and are not predisposed towards artificial means. As the world is becoming more conscious of the importance of reproductive freedom, NFP becomes a popular option among women seeking to hold on to their values while being allowed to manage their reproductive health (Shah et al., 2016). While having several benefits, Natural Family Planning is not without challenges. The majority of women will discover that the tracking process is tedious or difficult to read, particularly if they have irregular menstruation. Such intricateness might deter potential consumers who are afraid of the need to adhere stringently to time and watchfulness. Societal and cultural taboos surrounding fertility awareness might also be a deterrent to wider social acceptance and use of NFP as a valid contraceptive practice. Training courses and data are of the highest significance in neutralizing these types of barriers, ensuring correct information and support to potential users. Secondly, increased collaboration with healthcare providers can demystify the methods, making NFP an easier option for those prepared to use good family planning (Alsaadi et al., 2013).

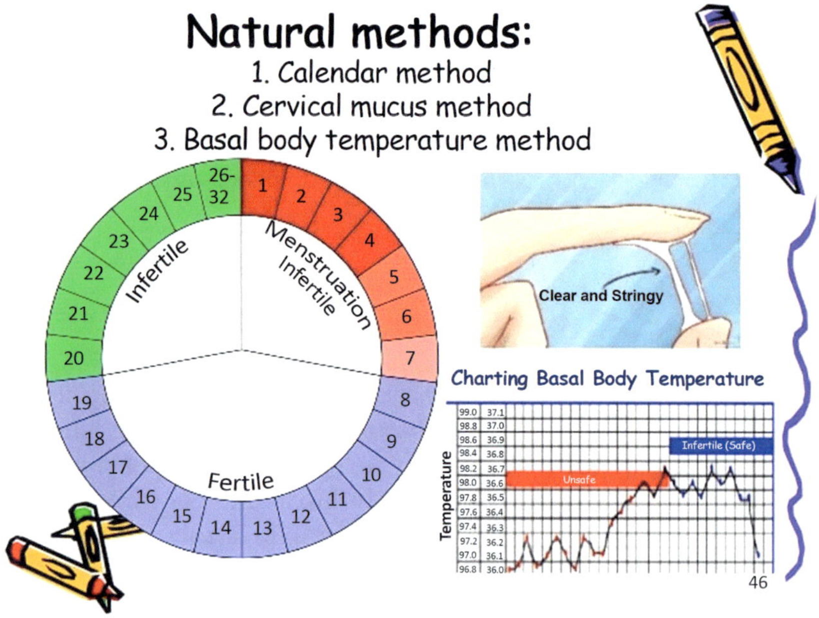

Figure 3.13. Different natural methods.

Source: https://americanpregnancy.org/wp-content/uploads/2020/08/family-planning-46-638.jpg

3.5.1. Calendar Method

The Calendar method, or rhythm method, is a natural birth control that relies on the monitoring of a woman's menstrual cycle to predict fertile days. Through the tracking of the length of the cycle through different months, one may identify patterns that distinguish fertile and infertile periods. The system is premised on the consideration that ovulation is usually 14 days prior to the onset of menstruation. Interestingly, it relies on correct monitoring and consistency, and as such, it is important that users maintain extremely careful records of their cycles. Although this self-regulation can bring some empowerment to individuals, the method's effectiveness is often defeated by irregular cycles, which will conceal correct prediction and lead to more chance pregnancies. Although easy, the Calendar method is both beneficial and disadvantageous, and should be taken into account. One of its primary benefits is the lack of interference from hormones or mechanical devices, allowing women to exercise family planning without drugs and associated side effects or invasive penetrating methods. Furthermore, for individuals who desire to be more in touch with their reproductive health, this practice evokes awareness and encourages a closer connection to their bodies. However, the failure rate of the methods is high, at a quoted 25% among typical users, according to calculations and natural variation of menstrual cycles. This everyday context emphasizes the necessity of honest sexual education that would counsel women on the potential benefits but also the constraints of the Calendar method as a means of contraception, allowing informed choice. In addition, the sociocultural environment where the Calendar method is used can have a powerful impact on its uptake and success rates.

Where modern contraceptive methods are not available or in short supply in a region or community, like sub-Saharan Africa, women tend to resort to traditional methods of family planning. A study observed that the adoption of new contraception is still very low in such areas, and only 29.6% women utilized advanced contraception to avoid pregnancy (Ahinkorah et al., 2021). In contrast, immediate educational campaigns about reproductive health and accessible contraception would make the Calendar method more effective among women in such areas. Also, among youth in these communities, the ability to make reproductive health choices goes along with increased contraceptive use (Ahinkorah et al., 2020). These findings underscore the need for culturally sensitive education programs to empower women in family planning choices regardless of the contraceptive type they use.

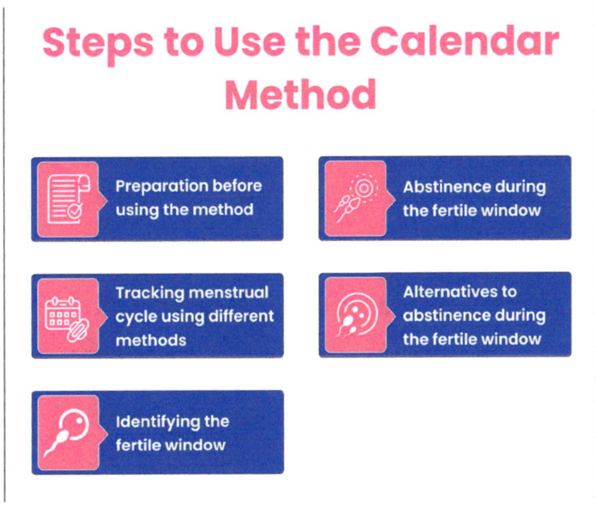
Steps to Use the Calendar Method
Preparation before using the method
Abstinence during the fertile window
Tracking menstrual cycle using different methods
Alternatives to abstinence during the fertile window
Identifying the fertile window

Figure 3.14. Steps to use the calendar method.

Source: https://www.primeivfcentre.com/assets/media/how-to-use-calendar-method-to-prevent-pregnancy-info.webp

3.5.2. Basal Body Temperature Method

The basal body temperature (BBT) method is one of the most significant natural family planning techniques used by women to monitor their fertility. This entails observing the change in a woman's body temperature throughout her menstrual cycle, i.e., identifying ovulation. Generally, a woman's basal body temperature is lowest just before ovulation and then increases—normally by about 0.5 to 1 degree Fahrenheit—shortly after the expulsion of an egg from the ovary. This change in temperature is due to increased progesterone levels after ovulation, which means that the window of fertilizability is now closed. By plotting BBT from time to time over long durations, women can learn to recognize their own temperature patterns; thus, it is easy to predict ovulation and, by extension, the fertile windows during their cycle. Such predictability allows one to make informed decisions regarding sexual intercourse, thereby playing an important role in family planning efforts. Although the BBT method is an effective contraceptive strategy, consideration should be given to its weaknesses. Irregularities in menstrual cycles could lead to inaccuracies in the prediction of ovulation, particularly in a woman with fluctuation in basal temperature caused by illness, stress, or sleep disturbances. Besides, the BBT method requires diligent daily observation, commonly before any bodily movement in the morning, and the consumption of alcohol or certain medications can further distort accurate readings. Above all, vaginal infections also impact the reliability of basal body temperature readings, and again, this emphasizes the necessity of observing regularly over a series of cycles in order to make any meaningful conclusions regarding one's rhythm. That said, many users report a similar degree of effectiveness in avoiding pregnancy when applying this method in conjunction with other natural methods of family planning, especially within a systemized regime of observation and awareness of one's own body (Aznar et al., 2020).

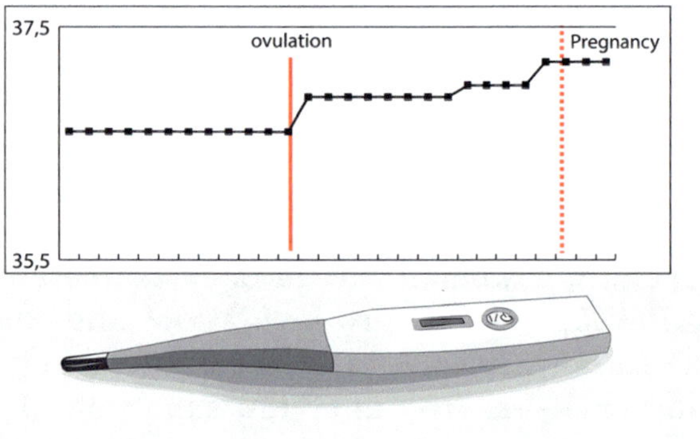

Figure 3.15. Birth Control Affect Basal Body Temperature.

Source: https://fleurhealth.com/blog/does-birth-control-affect-basal-body-temperature/

Partners using the BBT technique tend to report that its implementation in their partnership adds to communication and cooperation when it comes to reproductive health. Through careful basal temperature charting, partners are more attentive to signs of fertility, encouraging discussions about a planned family that puts a high value on mutual understanding and consent. As has been observed in the wider field of natural family planning, which may be offered as an alternative to hysterectomy under medically justified circumstances, the BBT method affirms the ethical and moral implications that some couples observe in the event of conception (Hosogaya et al., 2021). In essence, the BBT technique is not just a method of contraception; it is a total reproductive health strategy that educates women and men to actively become involved in their family planning, as well as contributing to the broader discourse of contraceptive techniques of female reproductive health.

3.5.3. Cervical Mucus Method

The cervical mucus method is a natural form of birth control that capitalizes on cervical mucus variation throughout the menstrual cycle to mark fertile and non-fertile periods. Women who have knowledge of their own physiology can track the variation to ensure conception or conception avoidance.

Cervical mucus tends to be stiff and pale during the follicular phase of the cycle due to low estrogen levels. As ovulation approaches, increased estrogen secretion causes an alteration in the mucus by making it more abundant, transparent, and elastic. It is this "fertile mucus" that indicates that the body is prepared for ovulation, and this is when conception is most likely if intercourse is engaged in. Being knowledgeable about these cyclical changes, therefore, gives the general principle behind the effectiveness of the cervical mucus method in achieving reproductive goals. Research has cited the correlation of sexual intercourse and menstrual cycle characteristics and the fact that sexual intercourse may affect the quality of cervical mucus as well as overall fertility. Results from research suggested that cycles involving sexual intercourse were found to have a longer luteal phase and better quality of cervical fluid. Sexless cycles had shorter cycle lengths and increased probability of luteal phase defect, particularly. These findings underscore the importance of interpreting cervical mucus patterns more as active factors influenced by sexual behavior and health rather than as fertility signs. In discussing contraception in the context of the cervical mucus method, it is important to consider how behaviors correlate with reproductive physiology because such a correlation might improve the accuracy of fertility awareness and boost rates of contraceptive efficacy (Najmabadi et al., 2022).

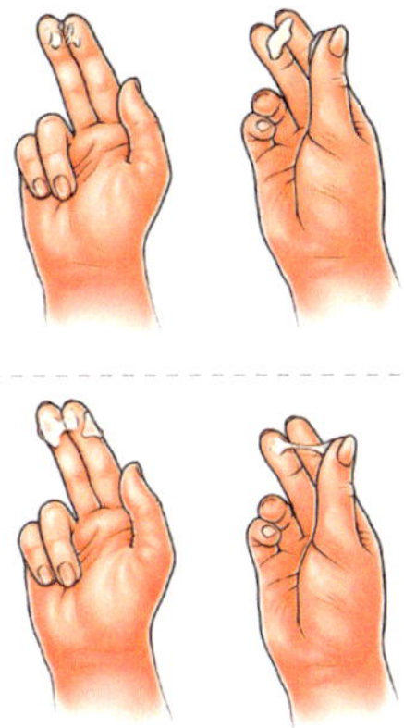

Figure 3.16. Cervical Mucus.

Source: https://my.clevelandclinic.org/-/scassets/images/org/health/articles/21957-cervical-mucus

With the growing need for various forms of contraceptive methods, techniques such as the FemCap arrive with new means of associating with the cervical mucus technique. The FemCap is a non-hormonal sperm-blocking condom for contraception, but also one that allows a woman's natural mucus cycle. By observing cervical mucus without leakage of other body fluids, the FemCap solves fertility awareness and contraceptive needs. This dual function is useful for those women who may be hesitant with respect to hormonal contraception or prefer something more natural in the way of family planning. Supplementing one's fertility awareness method with the FemCap may make the cervical mucus method more reliable, leading to better outcomes as far as contraception and awareness in the area of reproductive health is concerned (Alfred et al., 2021).

Test Your Knowledge

1. What is the basic principle behind the calendar method of natural family planning?
2. What changes in cervical mucus indicate the most fertile days during the menstrual cycle?

SUMMARY

The study of the various methods of contraception plays a significant role in empowering women to make the right choice for their reproductive lives. While the discussion regarding the kind of contraceptives shifts, it is certain that efficacy, along with side effects, goes a long way in the decisions of women. Surprisingly, progestin-only contraceptives have been found to be equally effective in stopping pregnancy when compared to combination birth control. Even though they have a reduced risk of acute venous thromboembolism, they present a safer alternative for the majority of women. This finding underlines the significance of medical practitioners engaging in extensive consultations with patients regarding contraceptive options so that they are fully aware of the benefits and drawbacks of each option presented to them. The significance of good communication cannot be overstated, as it enables women to make decisions most appropriate for their health requirements and choice of life (Smith et al., 2024). Additionally, the significance of understanding the social dynamics of contraceptive use cannot be emphasized enough. Research done has emphasized the fact that sexual acceptability is a key factor to make the methods of contraception effective in practice. The development of questionnaires such as the Sexual Acceptability of Contraceptive Methods Questionnaire gives evidence of women's preferences and experiences and their regulation by factors such as placement, side effects, and intimate relationships with partners. With these factors incorporated, healthcare providers are in a position to tailor their recommendations to satisfy not only the biological demands but also the affective dimensions of contraceptive use. Last but not least, recognizing the nuanced nature of contraceptive acceptability can lead to higher consumer satisfaction and compliance in the use of contraceptives, thereby resulting in an overall improvement in the efficacy of contraceptive interventions (Díaz Vega et al., 2024). The discussion on contraceptive choices for women is filled with reverberations for individual and public health. As women traverse their reproductive terrain, questions of effectiveness, safety, and personal autonomy have to be reckoned with. The progestin-only contraceptive data highlights a promising potential for enhancing women's health outcomes, particularly for individuals at higher risk of developing thromboembolic events. In addition to improved efficacy, implementing the findings from the Sexual Acceptability of Contraceptive Methods Questionnaire into practice has the potential to render healthcare interventions more tailored. It is therefore important for medical professionals to not only offer the options but also establish an educational platform of communication that is sensitive to women's diverse needs and values in the selection of contraception. This well-integrated system can eventually translate into better health outcomes and contentment with the methods of contraception employed (Smith et al., 2024; Díaz Vega et al., 2024).

The landscape of contraceptive options among women is varied and complex, spanning a wide diversity in reproductive health needs. Traditional choices are hormone-based methods, such as the birth control pill, patches, and injectables, which primarily function by suppressing ovulation and thereby reducing pregnancy risk. Other common methods include intrauterine devices (IUDs), hormonal or non-hormonal, which are effective for extended periods. Barriers, including male and female condoms, also help by providing physical barriers against sperm penetration. Other forms of contraceptive methods, such as natural fertility awareness, are popular among some women but require adequate monitoring and training to be effective. It is therefore important to understand the unique mechanisms and user types of each contraceptive method in order to offer well-informed choices. In the past several years, new technologies in contraceptives have been created and launched to expand the range of options for women and address unmet reproductive health demands. Research activities have been focused on participatory approaches to identify and learn women's specific issues regarding contraception, as discussed in the study undertaken by ICRW, EngenderHealth, and their Nepali collaborators (Malhotra et al., 2004). These developments are important in the evolution of contraceptive options to match altered needs and tastes, as well as the health needs of various groups. Furthermore, ongoing development and innovation in contraceptive technology strive to provide better and safer options, so family planning can be accessed by more individuals. This changing world not only guarantees the importance of safety and efficacy but also that of individual choice in determining the most suitable method of contraception for personal needs. In addition, population growth considerations and reproduction decisions are an urgent challenge to expand the availability of contraceptives. According to current estimates, the human population count can be up to 10.1 billion by the turn of the century, taking into account that there is an urgent need for effective contraceptive methods (Alsaadi et al., 2013). The requirement lies in having a two-pronged emphasis on female and male contraceptives, with newer studies probing hormonal and non-hormonal methods specifically for men. Hence, the conversation regarding the application of means of contraception should involve not only the acknowledged female-oriented methods but also the strides in male contraception aimed at encouraging shared responsibility in family planning. Such progressive awareness necessitates comprehensive education on the available means to help everybody be properly aware so that they can make active decisions over their reproductive lives.

KEY TERMS FROM THIS CHAPTER

- Cervical mucus method
- Contraceptive implants
- Contraceptive services
- Endometrial lining
- Ethinylestradiol
- Female condoms
- Gonadotropin-releasing hormone (GnRH)
- Hysteroscopic sterilization
- Infertile periods
- Condom integration programs
- Contraceptive methods
- Contraceptive technologies
- Essure procedure
- Family planning
- Follicular phase
- Hormonal methods
- Hysteroscopic sterilization alternative
- Luteinizing hormone (LH)

CRITICAL THINKING QUESTIONS

1. **Which of the following contraceptive methods provides protection against both pregnancy and sexually transmitted infections (STIs)?**
   a. Oral contraceptive pills
   b. Male condom
   c. Intrauterine device (IUD)
   d. Injectable contraceptives
2. **The most effective long-acting reversible contraceptive (LARC) method is:**
   a. Oral contraceptive pill
   b. Copper intrauterine device (IUD)
   c. Male condom
   d. Diaphragm
3. **Which hormone is primarily responsible for preventing ovulation in combined oral contraceptive pills?**
   a. Estrogen
   b. Progesterone
   c. Follicle-stimulating hormone (FSH)
   d. Luteinizing hormone (LH)
4. **Which contraceptive method is contraindicated in a woman with a history of deep vein thrombosis (DVT)?**
   a. Copper IUD
   b. Combined oral contraceptive pills
   c. Barrier methods
   d. Progestin-only pills
5. **Emergency contraception is most effective when taken within:**
   a. 24 hours after unprotected intercourse
   b. 3 days after unprotected intercourse
   c. 5 days after unprotected intercourse
   d. 7 days after unprotected intercourse

Short Answer Questions

1. What are the common types of hormonal contraceptive methods?
2. How do barrier contraceptive methods prevent pregnancy?
3. What are the main types of intrauterine devices (IUDs)?
4. Name two permanent contraceptive methods.
5. What is natural family planning, and how does it work?

Answer to Critical Thinking Questions

1. (b) 2. (b) 3. (b) 4. (b) 5. (c)

REFERENCES

1. Abimbola, O. H., Adekeye, O. A., Adeusi, S. O., Idowu, A., et al. (2013). Proximate determinants of women's use of birth control methods in Ota, Ogun State. https://core.ac.uk/download/18294874.pdf (accessed on 15th June 2025).

2. Agudelo, J., Burns, J., Gonzalez, J. A., Nuñez, M., et al. (2017). An introduction and high yield summary of female contraceptive methods. https://core.ac.uk/download/141737218.pdf (accessed on 15th June 2025).

3. Ahinkorah, B. O., Budu, E., Aboagye, R. G., Agbaglo, E., Arthur-Holmes, F., Adu, C., Archer, A. G., et al. (2021). Factors associated with modern contraceptive use among women with no fertility intention in sub-Saharan Africa: Evidence from cross-sectional surveys of 29 countries. *Contraception and Reproductive Medicine, 6*. https://doi.org/10.1186/s40834-021-00165-6 (accessed on 15th June 2025).

4. Ahinkorah, B. O., Hagan, J. E., Seidu, A. A., Sambah, F., Adoboi, F., Schack, T., & Budu, E. (2020). Female adolescents' reproductive health decision-making capacity and contraceptive use in sub-Saharan Africa: What does the future hold? *PLoS ONE, 15*, e0235601–e0235601. https://doi.org/10.1371/journal.pone.0235601 (accessed on 15th June 2025).

5. Alemayehu, M., Degfie, T. T., & Lema, T. B. (2012). Factors associated with utilization of long acting and permanent contraceptive methods among married women of reproductive age in Mekelle town, Tigray region, North Ethiopia. https://core.ac.uk/download/55845106.pdf (accessed on 15th June 2025).

6. Allina, A., Borkowski, L., Couillard, M., Strasser, R., et al. (2016). *Bridging the Divide White Paper: Long-Acting Reversible Contraception (LARC) in the United States.* https://core.ac.uk/download/230831315.pdf (accessed on 15th June 2025).

7. Alsaadi, M., Ferro, V., Garside, D. A., Gebril, A., et al. (2013). An update on the potential for male contraception: Emerging options. https://core.ac.uk/download/9843862.pdf (accessed on 15th June 2025).

8. Appleton, J., Brooks, F., Bunn, F., Magnusson, C., et al. (2006). Contraception advice and provision for the prevention of under 18 conceptions and STIs: A rapid review. https://core.ac.uk/download/29841254.pdf (accessed on 15th June 2025).

9. Aznar, J., & Tudela, J. (2020). The use of NFP when pregnancy is contraindicated? *The Linacre Quarterly, 87*, 171–181. https://www.semanticscholar.org/paper/8a8c998fe4a90359d61b1be5c10fe2b0b1b84413 (accessed on 15th June 2025).

10. Behnke, B., Craig, P., Ghate, D., Gillies, M., Hall, J., et al. (2013). *Supporting Fathers in Multi-Ethnic Societies: Insights from British Asian Fathers.* [No DOI or weblink provided].

11. Bell, S., Fedorova, A., Fidel, E., Nieto-Andrade, B., et al. (2017). Women's limited choice and availability of modern contraception at retail outlets and public-sector facilities in Luanda, Angola, 2012–2015. https://core.ac.uk/download/323081973.pdf (accessed on 15th June 2025).

12. Bermúdez-Millán, A., Prost, A., Singh, A., Al-Riyami, A. A., Picklesimer, A. H., Donovan, B., et al. (2017). Conceptualizing pathways linking women's empowerment and prematurity in developing countries. https://core.ac.uk/download/323079918.pdf (accessed on 15th June 2025).

13. Bertrand, J. T., & Brown, J. E. (2025). Family planning success in two cities in Zaire. https://core.ac.uk/download/pdf/6719632.pdf (accessed on 15th June 2025).
14. Bracke, P., Buffel, V., & Dereuddre, R. (2017). Power and the gendered division of contraceptive use in Western European couples. https://core.ac.uk/download/55803463.pdf (accessed on 15th June 2025).
15. Brincat, M. P., & Calleja-Agius, J. (2006). "Conceiving" the pill: The 45th birthday of the oral contraceptive pill in Europe. https://core.ac.uk/download/46602091.pdf (accessed on 15th June 2025).
16. Capurchande, R., Coene, G., Meulemans, H., Roelens, K., et al. (2017). 'If I have only two children and they die, who will take care of me?': A qualitative study exploring knowledge, attitudes and practices about family planning among Mozambican female and male adults. https://core.ac.uk/download/91389519.pdf (accessed on 15th June 2025).
17. Correia, L., Machado, A. I., Marques, C., Ramos, J., et al. (2012). Magnetic resonance imaging and gynecological devices. https://core.ac.uk/download/71736242.pdf (accessed on 15th June 2025).
18. Delves, P. J. (2002). The development of contraceptive vaccines. https://core.ac.uk/download/1669590.pdf (accessed on 15th June 2025).
19. Dhodi, U. J., & Prajapati, A. (2024). A study to determine the quality of life among the permanent contraceptive adopters and non-adopters at selected rural areas of Dadra and Nagar Haveli. *International Journal for Multidisciplinary Research*. https://www.semanticscholar.org/paper/65ce902e402b42410ec2c95b6ba5487eba664950 (accessed on 15th June 2025).
20. Díaz Vega, M., Jurado López, A. R., Juárez Vela, R., Lahoz Pascual, A., et al. (2024). A reliable and valid tool to assess the sexual acceptability of contraceptive methods. https://core.ac.uk/download/611941717.pdf (accessed on 15th June 2025).
21. Ferenczy, T. (2020). Contraceptive methods in the United States: The question of abortive mechanisms. https://core.ac.uk/download/362657422.pdf (accessed on 15th June 2025).
22. Glantz, J. C., Jacobson, J., & Nasso, J. (2018). Use of an evidence-based guideline for management of side effects from long-acting reversible contraceptives: A quality improvement report. https://core.ac.uk/download/213034060.pdf (accessed on 15th June 2025).
23. Greydanus, D. E., Lentzsch-Parcells, C. M., & Omar, H. A. (2012). Contraception in adolescents. https://core.ac.uk/download/232583672.pdf (accessed on 15th June 2025).
24. Greydanus, D. E., Matytsina, L. A., Omar, H. A., Tsitsika, A., et al. (2010). Contraception. https://core.ac.uk/download/232583897.pdf (accessed on 15th June 2025).
25. Harden, A., Gage, A. J., Blanc, A. K., Fort, A. L., Parkes, A., Wang, B., Paterson, B. L., et al. (2009). Limits to modern contraceptive use among young women in developing countries: A systematic review of qualitative research. https://core.ac.uk/download/pdf/8266300.pdf (accessed on 15th June 2025).
26. Hebert, L. E., Saad, A., Schwandt, H., Skinner, J., et al. (2015). Perceived risks associated with contraceptive method use among men and women in Ibadan and Kaduna, Nigeria. https://core.ac.uk/download/232697581.pdf (accessed on 15th June 2025).
27. Heisler, K., & Van Eron, D. M. (2012). A descriptive study of undergraduate contraceptive attitudes among students at the University of New Hampshire. https://core.ac.uk/download/72047922.pdf (accessed on 15th June 2025).

28. Hosogaya, N., Miyazaki, T., Fukushige, Y., Takemori, S., Morimoto, S., Yamamoto, H., Hori, M., et al. (2021). Efficacy and safety of nelfinavir in asymptomatic and mild COVID-19 patients: A structured summary of a study protocol for a multicenter, randomized controlled trial. *Trials, 22*. https://www.semanticscholar.org/paper/dc43bdef25adf4e9ec0ab87b4c9639cbd0dfc90f (accessed on 15th June 2025).

29. Kim, A. (2018). *World Health Organization Decision Making Tool for Family Planning–Can We Increase IUD Use?* https://core.ac.uk/download/236388302.pdf (accessed on 15th June 2025).

30. Mahoney, J. (2021). Essure: The IUD story we should have seen coming. https://core.ac.uk/download/475696315.pdf (accessed on 15th June 2025).

31. Malhotra, A., Mehta, M., & Mathur, S. (2004). *Youth Reproductive Health in Nepal: Is Participation the Answer?* https://core.ac.uk/download/71356010.pdf (accessed on 15th June 2025).

32. Meese, H. K. (2016). Characteristics of long-acting reversible contraception users presenting to a pediatric emergency department. https://core.ac.uk/download/142066210.pdf (accessed on 15th June 2025).

33. Najmabadi, S., Schliep, K., Simonsen, S., Porucznik, C., Egger, M., & Stanford, J. (2022). Characteristics of menstrual cycles with or without intercourse in women with no known subfertility. *Human Reproduction Open, 2022*. https://www.semanticscholar.org/paper/fb4ec4b4beef314e0006587cd8add11f07cea452 (accessed on 15th June 2025).

34. Pandey, L., Gupta, P., Sen, P., Anjum, S., Satyarthi, S., Yadav, S., Shrestha, S., et al. (2023). A study to assess the effectiveness of video assisted teaching programmed on knowledge regarding temporary contraceptive methods among college going females in selected college at Lucknow, Uttar Pradesh. *International Journal of Science and Research (IJSR)*. https://www.semanticscholar.org/paper/297e526897b7215fb14b20969d88ce01595637f4 (accessed on 15th June 2025).

35. Plunkett, L. A. (2014). Contraceptive sabotage. https://core.ac.uk/download/72051969.pdf (accessed on 15th June 2025).

36. Shah, H. (2016). Aftermath of the Hobby Lobby decision: Implications for women in the workforce. https://core.ac.uk/download/130354088.pdf (accessed on 15th June 2025).

37. Shihata, A., Brody, S., & Linderoth, B. (2021). Non-hormonal contraceptive device with multiple uses: Increases the effectiveness of fertility awareness methods and controls stress incontinence. *Japan Journal of Clinical & Medical Research*. https://www.semanticscholar.org/paper/2e9280d5f4dac10b016c62a3522f601428fd96bf (accessed on 15th June 2025).

38. Simon, L. (2021). Long-acting reversible contraception education for street-involved youth: Impact on knowledge, attitudes, and behaviors. https://core.ac.uk/download/478564876.pdf (accessed on 15th June 2025).

39. Smith, H. (2024). Safety and efficacy of progestin only and combination oral contraceptives. https://core.ac.uk/download/619691381.pdf (accessed on 15th June 2025).

40. Weber, M. M. (2021). The ways in which women's suffrage affected healthcare. https://core.ac.uk/download/430559893.pdf (accessed on 15th June 2025).

ENDOMETRIOSIS AND ADENOMYOSIS

4

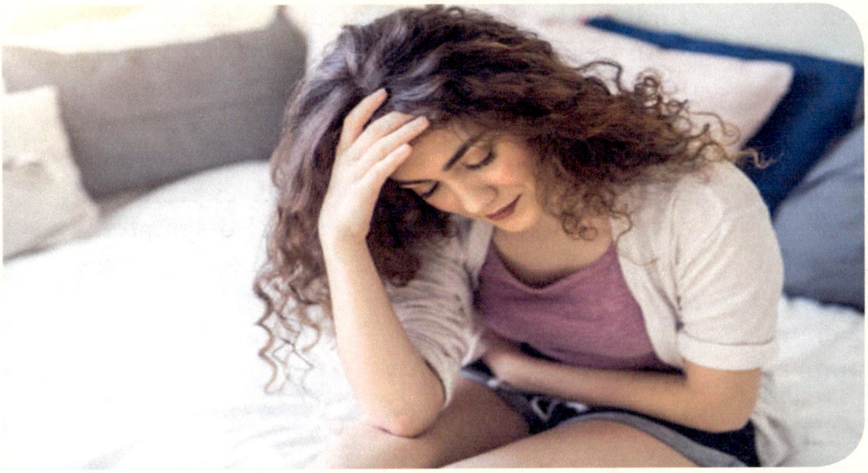

LEARNING OBJECTIVES

After studying this chapter, you will be able to:

1. Explain the epidemiology of endometriosis and adenomyosis
2. Describe the pathophysiology of endometriosis and adenomyosis
3. Identify the symptoms and diagnostic methods for endometriosis and adenomyosis
4. Evaluate the treatment options available for endometriosis and adenomyosis
5. Assess the impact of endometriosis and adenomyosis on quality of life

Introduction

The issue of endometriosis and adenomyosis is an important and sometimes neglected aspect of women's health. Endometriosis, or the growth of endometrial-like tissue outside the uterus, and adenomyosis, or the growth of endometrial tissue in the uterine muscle, are both multifactorial in etiology and affect millions of women worldwide. Both diseases have superimposable symptoms of chronic pelvic pain, heavy periods, and infertility. Their prevalence highlights an acute need for enhanced awareness and comprehension among the medical fraternity and society at large, as misdiagnosis and late treatment can result in worsening health outcomes. The consequences of these disorders extend beyond the physical to include mental health and quality of life and thus warrant a comprehensive study of their biological, psychological, and socio-economic aspects. Understanding the complexity of endometriosis and adenomyosis entails a multidisciplinary approach that involves gynecological, psychological, and sociocultural perspectives. Research has established that the pathogenesis of these diseases is due to impaired immune responses, hormonal dysregulation, and genetic factors, hence rendering diagnosis and management a complicated process. Women are prone to find themselves in a medical environment that is full of stigma and misinformation. This framework both affects their medical interactions and is able to misplace their symptoms within cultural narratives of women's health and femininity. Additionally, given the history of resistance to treating women's health comprehensively, the controversy surrounding endometriosis and adenomyosis can benefit from a critical analysis in order to sort through these elements. The interface between medical science and society's attitudes affects the lived reality of the affected, and hence, advocacy and education become essential. As the discourse around endometriosis and adenomyosis evolves, it is necessary to address these diseases with an eye on improved healthcare outcomes. Awareness-raising efforts, support for research, and medical education are needed to de-stigmatize these diseases. This transition not only ensures an educated patient population but also encourages practitioners to take seriously women's symptoms and pain. As interest arises in advocacy and support groups, the potential exists for across-the-board improvement in management and treatment. Emphasizing the collaborative effort among patients, practitioners, and researchers will lead to a better understanding of these conditions, ultimately enhancing the quality of life of affected individuals. Facing the multifaceted challenges of endometriosis and adenomyosis and their accompanying health problems is a pivotal horizon in women's health research and practice.

Definition of Endometriosis

Endometriosis is a complex reproductive medical condition in which endometrial tissue proliferates outside the uterus, causing extreme inflammation and a multitude of debilitating symptoms. It is an inflammatory, hormone-dependent benign disorder that is most common among women of childbearing age and is characterized by symptoms such as agonizing menstrual cramps, chronic pelvic pain, and infertility. The ectopic growth of endometrial-like tissue typically occurs on organs within the pelvis, including the ovaries, fallopian tubes, and peritoneum, thereby creating a condition that not only complicates diagnosis but also aggravates the symptoms of those affected by it. The multifactorial etiology of endometriosis renders finding its etiology particularly challenging, with delays in diagnosis ranging from 7 to 12 years from the onset of symptoms to definite diagnosis (Gabriel et al., 2021). The economic burden of endometriosis on healthcare systems is considerable, as it not only involves prolonged investigation for diagnosis but also symptoms causing loss of quality and productivity in the affected individuals.

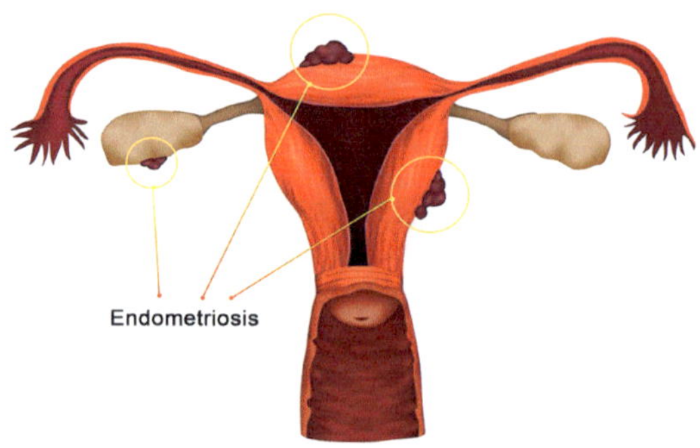

Figure 4.1. Endometriosis.

Source: https://media.healthdirect.org.au/images/inline/original/endometriosis-illustration-fcc644.jpg

The treatment available is poor, consisting largely of hormonal therapy and surgical interventions aimed at symptom management rather than curative treatment. While hormonal treatments do have the ability to minimize symptoms, they do have side effects, of which weight gain and disturbance in mood are prominent, so treatment for most women is a complex procedure. Thus, treatment of endometriosis is usually multifold with both medical and surgical treatments that must be tailored to the particular need and context of the patient (Gabriel et al., 2021).

In addition, it is essential to understand the psychosocial impacts of endometriosis so that proper support systems can be established for the victims. Indecisiveness regarding diagnosis and treatment can cause tremendous stress and anxiety that can affect one's mental health. Research has indicated that the emotional burden of endometriosis-related infertility and chronic pain has the tendency to instill feelings of distress and isolation among women, which underlines the need for comprehensive healthcare interventions addressing both the physical and psychological dimensions of the disease. By identifying the key nursing diagnoses relevant to this disorder, healthcare professionals are able to design particular interventions that consider the unique challenges confronting women with endometriosis, thus establishing a more helpful environment for addressing this complex disorder.

Definition of Adenomyosis

Adenomyosis is a complex gynecologic condition in which endometrial tissue invades the myometrium, or muscle of the uterus. It thickens the uterine walls and can cause a variety of symptoms like heavy menstrual flow, severe pelvic discomfort, and painful intercourse. The pathophysiology of adenomyosis is not yet completely understood and has been theorized to be due to hormonal imbalance, trauma at delivery, or hormonal influence. Unlike endometriosis, which is outside the uterus, adenomyosis occurs within the uterus, making it challenging to treat and diagnose. The accurate diagnosis includes certain imaging techniques such as transvaginal ultrasound or magnetic resonance imaging, both of which may further define the extent of the disease and its influence on surrounding organs or tissues (Exacoustos et al., 2014).

The distinction between adenomyosis and endometriosis is particularly critical from the clinical presentation and treatment perspectives. Although both conditions involve endometrial tissue, adenomyosis is surrounded by the walls of the uterus, which presents different symptoms and potential complications. The condition tends to affect women of childbearing age, and its prevalence has been documented among as many as 30% of women undergoing hysterectomy for non-neoplastic reasons. Adenomyosis tends to be hard to diagnose since it presents symptoms similar to other conditions, such as fibroids or endocrine disorders. Thus, health care professionals are forced to adopt an all-inclusive approach of a total clinical history, imaging studies, and, in some cases, histological examination to make the diagnosis (Damodaran et al., 1956).

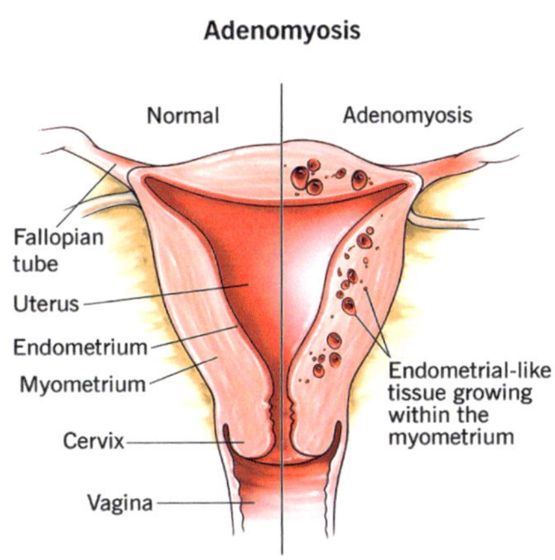

Figure 4.2. Adenomyosis is when tissue that lines your uterus grows into the muscular walls of your uterus.

Source: https://my.clevelandclinic.org/-/scassets/images/org/health/articles/14167-adenomyosis

It is not only crucial to achieve appropriate patient management but also to advance the broader dialogue regarding reproductive health to realize adenomyosis. As research remains evolving, the exploration of potential treatment modalities—spanning from hormonal therapy to surgery—is and continues to remain a high priority in clinical practice. Current research emphasizes the importance of higher awareness and knowledge of adenomyosis among healthcare providers and patients, as misdiagnosis can lead to inappropriate treatment regimens and persistent symptoms. Mentioning adenomyosis within the context of other diseases of the female reproductive tract, endometriosis, offers a comprehensive platform for the understanding of the complexities of women's health and underscores the role of accurate diagnosis and customized treatment planning (Exacoustos et al., 2014).

Importance of Understanding Both Conditions

The multifaceted character of endometriosis and adenomyosis serves to emphasize the importance of both conditions in the broad context of women's health. Endometriosis is characterized as an ongoing illness by the presence of endometrial-like tissue outside the uterus, whereas adenomyosis is characterized as being due to the invasion of endometrial tissue into the uterine muscle. Both of these conditions have the ability to dramatically affect a woman's quality of life by the production of debilitating pain, excessive menstrual bleeding, and infertility. Such a comprehensive understanding of the diseases allows medical professionals to apply more individualized methods of treatment that are sensitive to patients' specific needs and histories. Additionally, it will assist in the eradication of misdiagnosis, which is very critical in the correct treatment and management of diseases. Proper classification and comprehension will also enhance research that will assist in explaining the pathophysiologic mechanisms of both disorders. Further, the recent advancements in medical imaging, particularly MRI, underline the significance of distinguishing between endometriosis and adenomyosis.

The application of grading systems such as the mr#Enzian enhances the radiologists' ability to identify the specific features of these conditions with a high degree of accuracy (Benli et al., 2024). This assumes greater significance because of the shift to medical therapy for endometriosis and adenomyosis, which requires clear-cut identification of their presentations. For instance, the accuracy of MRI in delineating such conditions can be applied to inform surgical planning and improve more efficient treatment options. Further, understanding the nuances of each condition assists in more informed discussions regarding prognosis and treatment outcomes. The integration of imaging techniques into practice highlights the importance of not only diagnosing both conditions but also understanding their complexities to provide better care to patients. In line with these developments, the incorporation of information from radiomics—a relatively new field that analyzes quantitative features derived from medical images—further enhances the understanding of these conditions as well as their differentiation (Burla et al., 2024). Radiomics promises potential in the development of non-invasive methods of distinguishing adenomyosis-present from adenomyosis-absent uteri. With a combination of feature analysis using state-of-the-art imaging modalities, researchers have begun to develop machine learning models capable of reliably diagnosing adenomyosis from MRI data. These advancements underscore the need to understand both endometriosis and adenomyosis as they increase the diagnostic accuracy level and enable treatment methods that are individually tailored. As there is further progress in the field of research, the findings achieved through radiomics are soon to be an impactful determining factor in the growth of clinical practices, improved patient outcomes, and indirectly, to more overall healthcare solutions for women's reproductive health.

4.1. Epidemiology

Learning Outcome

1. Define the prevalence of endometriosis and adenomyosis
2. Explain the demographic factors influencing incidence

Endometriosis and adenomyosis epidemiology present a multifaceted challenge to disease understanding and management with universal implications. Endometriosis most frequently occurs in reproductive-aged women, with an estimated 10% to 15% prevalence in this group, leading to significant physical and emotional morbidity. The chronic pain of the disease typically manifests as dysmenorrhea, chronic pelvic pain, and infertility, each of which significantly diminishes quality of life and work-related productivity. Interestingly, they are found to co-occur with other comorbidities such as irritable bowel syndrome and chronic fatigue syndrome, hence complicating diagnosis and treatment. Information regarding their prevalence is vital to enable proper healthcare provision of resources and plan accordingly with specific intervention for the affected individuals. This epidemiological background supports health professionals to address the multifaceted implications of endometriosis and adenomyosis in an efficient manner, encouraging greater awareness of their widespread influence on women's health (Anastasi et al., 2015). Recent advancements in diagnostic instruments have come a long way in demystifying the epidemiology of endometriosis and adenomyosis. Among these, magnetic resonance imaging (MRI) has emerged as a key modality, offering high levels of accuracy in detecting and evaluating the extent of these conditions. The ability of MRI to unveil the intricate manifestations of endometriosis assists gynecologists in implementing appropriate treatment strategies. Furthermore, the recent adoption of Fusion Imaging—a technique that integrates ultrasonography and MRI—represents a pivotal advancement in diagnostic accuracy. In spite of all these technological advancements, there remains an ongoing need for more studies that focus on refining diagnostic processes and improving patient outcomes within the domain of gynecological wellbeing. With this changing diagnostics landscape comes the demand for an effective epidemiologic foundation in controlling and treating endometriosis and adenomyosis optimally (Bellati et al., 2018).

The impact of endometriosis and adenomyosis extends to individual health and spreads into significant societal issues. Economically, they incur considerable healthcare costs in the form of repeated consultations with physicians, diagnostic procedures, and treatment for symptom control. The value of loss of productivity in terms of lost workdays and suboptimal work output is an additional burden imposed on the patients as well as the economy. Education and awareness about the epidemiology of such disorders need to be promoted so that early diagnosis and comprehensive treatment plans can be made. For instance, the recognition of the extensive prevalence of endometriosis among infertile women might lead to augmented screening and early intervention strategies. By addressing the economic and psycho-social issues that are intertwined with the epidemiology of endometriosis and adenomyosis, medical care systems can establish more effective support mechanisms for women, and hence a better quality of life and improved health outcomes (Anastasi et al., 2015).

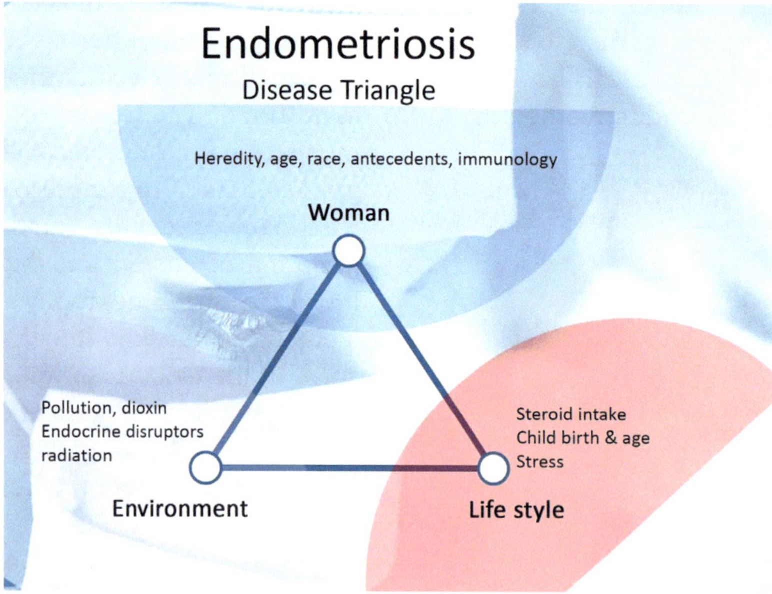

Figure 4.3. Endometriosis disease triangle: etiology and epidemiology

Source: https://i0.wp.com/www.gynsurgery.org/wp-content/uploads//endom-disease-triangle.png

4.1.1. Prevalence of Endometriosis

Endometriosis occurrence is a critical matter for women's health that has been approximated to occur in 10% of women of reproductive age across the globe. Diagnosis tends to be delayed when symptoms are mistakenly linked to other causes, leading to prolonged pain and misery. Studies have shown that endometriosis leads to chronic pain, affecting day-to-day activities and mental well-being. Also, the chronic condition can have long-term health consequences like infertility, so awareness and early diagnosis are paramount. Being aware of the prevalence of endometriosis is not only imperative for health professionals but also for women who may be symptomatic but unaware of its cause. The complexity of the condition and also the attitudes of society towards menstrual pain, by and large, lead to the secrecy around the scope of its prevalence, which is why more educational efforts have to be undertaken in order to allow women to visit doctors when they have symptoms. The cross-talk between endometriosis and adenomyosis also complicates analyzing prevalence statistics further. Both conditions are characterized by endometrial-like tissue outside the uterine lining, but differently. Women with adenomyosis have a higher risk of recurrence of endometriosis following surgery, and recent studies that have examined the shared lymphatic drainage pathways for the two conditions have shown this. The findings suggest lymphatic vessels play a part in the dissemination of endometrial tissue and, by extension, adenomyosis as a causative agent of exacerbating endometriosis. This association is what underscores the necessity of comprehensive evaluation and management plans that address adenomyosis and endometriosis concomitantly to improve patient outcomes and quality of life, pointing to the need for more research on concordant prevalence and pathophysiological pathways for both diseases (Bonaccorsi et al., 2019). The application of cutting-edge imaging modalities, such as MRI and ultrasound, has revolutionized the diagnostic landscape for endometriosis with the promise of earlier detection and treatment. MRI, in particular, has proven to be an extremely valuable tool due to its excellent contrast and resolution characteristics, thus facilitating better visualization of endometriotic lesions and associated abnormalities. These imaging technologies enhance the ability to estimate the extent of the disease and differentiate between adenomyosis and endometriosis, a necessity given their shared prevalence. Effective diagnoses not only advance treatment efficacy but also have effects on healthcare resource management and quality of life among these women to a large degree. Through increased awareness of their incidence and by employing advanced diagnostic methods, therapists can better ensure increased understanding of endometriosis and adenomyosis, ultimately to create improved care and support for women with these chronic conditions (Anastasi et al., 2015).

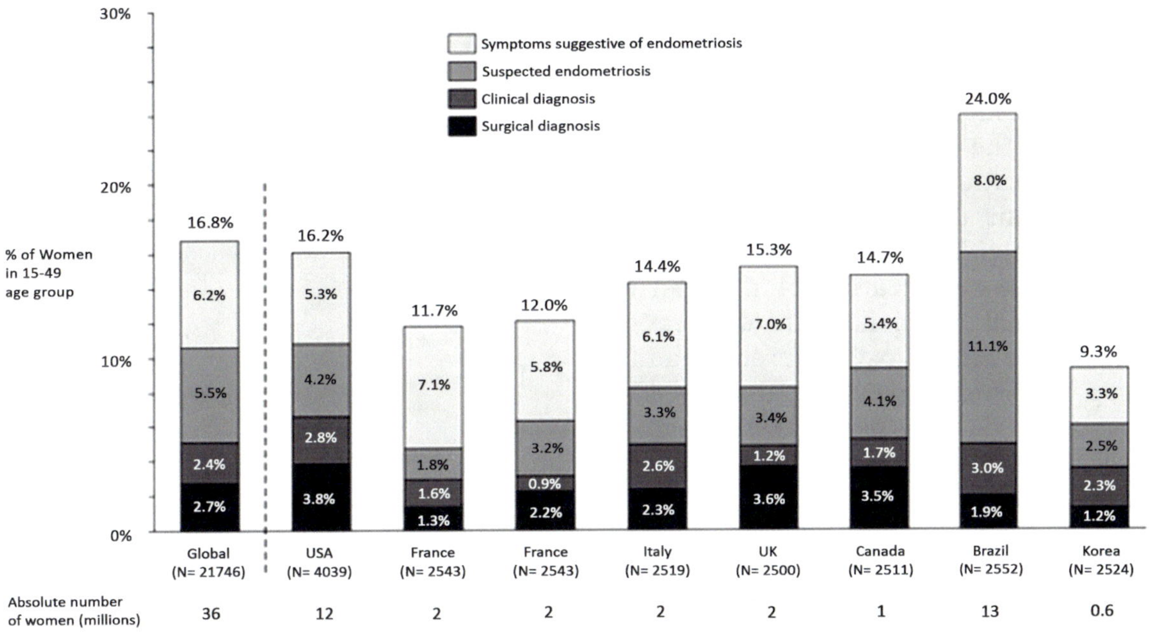

Figure 4.4. Prevalence of endometriosis categories across countries vs. global population.

Source: https://www.researchgate.net/profile/Thomas-Faustmann/publication/225107632/figure/fig4/AS:393842982441000@1470910892981/Prevalence-of-endometriosis-categories-across-countries-vs-global-population.png

4.1.2. Prevalence of Adenomyosis

The prevalence of adenomyosis, that is, the presence of endometrial tissue in the muscular uterine wall, has in recent decades been of greater interest, primarily because of its association with serious reproductive and gynecological morbidity. Epidemiological studies indicate adenomyosis may be present in up to 20-30% of women undergoing gynecological surgery, a figure that raises an eyebrow to its prevalence amongst women's health. This co-occurrence is notably significant in endometriosis cases, in which the concurrent occurrence of these two conditions will complicate their diagnosis and treatment. Additionally, as the evolution of knowledge in gynecology progresses, clinicians are increasingly identifying adenomyosis among young women, expanding the range of affected groups' ages and demonstrating the need for improved diagnostic equipment capable of specifically identifying adenomyosis in combination with endometriosis. These results highlight the necessity of further research into the clinical relevance of this disorder. In a bid to better determine the prevalence of adenomyosis, an understanding of the methods used for diagnosis in its identification must be taken into consideration. As noted, magnetic resonance imaging (MRI) is playing a vital role in the identification of adenomyosis as well as endometriosis due to its capacity for the generation of high-definition images. Not only does MRI offer visualization of the uterine architecture, but it also helps in delineating the extent of adenomyosis, thereby leading to therapy in women with the disease. The effectiveness of imaging methods in depicting the occurrence of adenomyosis has prompted a more cautious approach among healthcare providers and consequently raised awareness about the disease. Furthermore, improvements in imaging protocols suggest the incidence of adenomyosis may have been underestimated due to previous diagnostic imprecision, further justifying the need for novel research techniques to accurately represent the real incidence of the disease. The co-existence of adenomyosis with endometriosis suggests that both these conditions may potentially share common pathways in pathophysiology, and therefore may be contributing to the higher rates of recurrence after surgery in patients with adenomyosis. Interestingly, studies have found that women with adenomyosis are at a greater risk of recurrence of endometriosis after surgery, which suggests some inter-relationship between these two conditions that needs to be investigated. Research by Bonaccorsi et al. (2019) documents the function of ectatic lymphatics in endometrial tissue dispersal, which may be behind the interfering prevalence rates of adenomyosis and endometriosis. Both, in reality, have strong implications on women's quality of life as well as their reproductive performance, therefore increasing the necessity to amplify awareness, develop better diagnostic criteria, and create specific therapeutic modalities to combat the challenges introduced by adenomyosis in healthcare facilities. Therefore, an awareness of the prevalence and impacts of adenomyosis within the wider framework of reproductive health remains paramount.

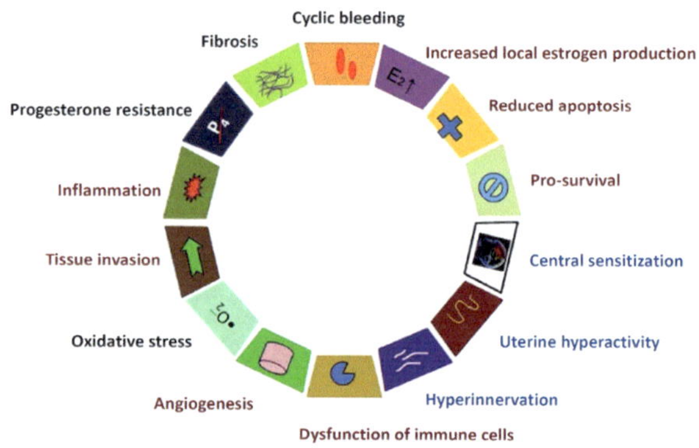

Figure 4.5. Endometriosis: mechanism for the effect of pollution, food intake, chemical disruptors and stress.

Source: https://i0.wp.com/www.gynsurgery.org/wp-content/uploads//guo.png

4.1.3. Demographic Factors Influencing Incidence

The incidence of such diseases as endometriosis and adenomyosis is largely defined by various demographic factors, such as educational attainment, ethnicity, and socioeconomic status. Research has shown that women from low socioeconomic backgrounds may be at risk of a higher prevalence of such disorders due to variables such as limited access to adequate healthcare and inadequate health education.

For example, women from poor economic status may not receive early medical treatment or counseling, leading to delayed diagnosis and complications. Intersecting with the education level of economic status may further exacerbate the risk because less educated individuals may be ignorant of the symptoms and effects of these diseases. Therefore, awareness of these demographic factors is crucial in the identification of risk groups and in the alleviation of healthcare disparities that persist among populations. Ethnically, another significant demographic factor that affects the prevalence of endometriosis and adenomyosis is ethnicity. It has been revealed in epidemiological research that the prevalence and severity of the conditions vary exceedingly with various ethnic populations. For example, some studies highlight that African women may be diagnosed with endometriosis at higher frequencies, while Caucasian women may present dissimilar symptomatology and disease course. These differences may be a result of a combination of genetic, environmental, and sociocultural determinants that influence disease expression and reporting tendency. Moreover, cultural stigma and beliefs related to menstruation and women's reproductive health may also play a role in how women access care and perceive their symptoms. Therefore, culturally appropriate health education and healthcare can facilitate better understanding and control of these diseases and ultimately lead to better health outcomes. In addition to ethnic and socioeconomic determinants, age and reproductive history are also important demographic variables associated with endometriosis and adenomyosis prevalence. Clinical studies have reported both diseases to be prevalent in women within the reproductive age bracket, i.e., 25 to 40 years old. Hormonal fluctuations during this age range may predispose them to these conditions. Moreover, reproductive history, for instance, age at menarche, parity, and history of uterine operations, could have a significant impact on risk. Lower parity and greater infertility are commonly seen with a higher incidence of endometriosis, indicating the complex relationship between reproductive factors and these conditions. Therefore, a complete analysis of age and reproductive history is required in the demography of endometriosis and adenomyosis with preconditions for future prevention and treatment strategies.

Test Your Knowledge

1. What is the estimated prevalence of endometriosis among reproductive-aged females?
2. How common is adenomyosis, and which age group is most affected?

4.2. Pathophysiology

Learning Outcome

1. Define mechanisms of endometriosis development and adenomyosis development
2. Explain the differences in tissue behavior between the two conditions

The pathophysiology of endometriosis and adenomyosis entails a complex interaction between cellular and molecular mechanisms underlying their symptomatology. Endometrial tissue in the ectopic location in endometriosis leads to an ongoing inflammatory process, producing cytokines, adhesion molecules, and prostaglandins, which have systemic effects on surrounding tissues. This inflammatory process forms the background for the symptoms of dysmenorrhea, chronic pelvic pain, and infertility. Conversely, adenomyosis arises after the endometrial cells are seeded within the myometrium, and the resultant effect is an increase in the number of smooth muscle cells and hypertrophy. The tissue maljunction is the cause of heavy menstrual flow and debilitating pain. It is critical to understand these intricate pathogenic mechanisms in unmasking the disorders and developing effective treatment protocols that do not merely address symptoms but assail the underlying pathophysiology. More detailed examination of adenomyosis reveals some mechanisms possibly underlying its pathophysiological nature. According to one hypothesis, microtrauma at the border of the endometrium and myometrium leads to invasion of endometrial cells into the myometrium, creating an adenomyotic lesion. This dysregulation results in local inflammation, neurogenesis, and vascularization, which exacerbates symptoms like dysmenorrhea and menorrhagia. Additionally, recent evidence has made estrogen responsible for the growth and survival of adenomyotic as well as endometrial tissues, making hormonal regulation even more important in these diseases. Understanding such interactions not only adds to adenomyosis pathophysiology knowledge but also directs targeted interventions that can improve patient care and regulate symptoms (Giudice et al., 2020). Furthermore, the involvement of environmental factors, particularly the impact of endocrine disruptor exposure, necessitates studying their role in the pathophysiology of endometriosis and adenomyosis. Implications from animal studies provide evidence that developmental chemical exposure to substances such as 2,3,7,8-tetrachlorodibenzo-p-dioxin (TCDD) has lasting repercussions on reproductive well-being, influencing disease development and progression. Epigenetic remodeling caused by such exposures can be responsible for transgenerational susceptibility to reproductive disorders, including endometriosis. The role of environmental influences emphasizes the need for a multidisciplinary research approach, combining toxicology with studies of reproductive health. Through an understanding of the interaction between genetic predispositions and environmental influences, researchers are able to continue to deconstruct further the pathophysiological intricacies involved in endometriosis and adenomyosis (Adachi et al., 2017).

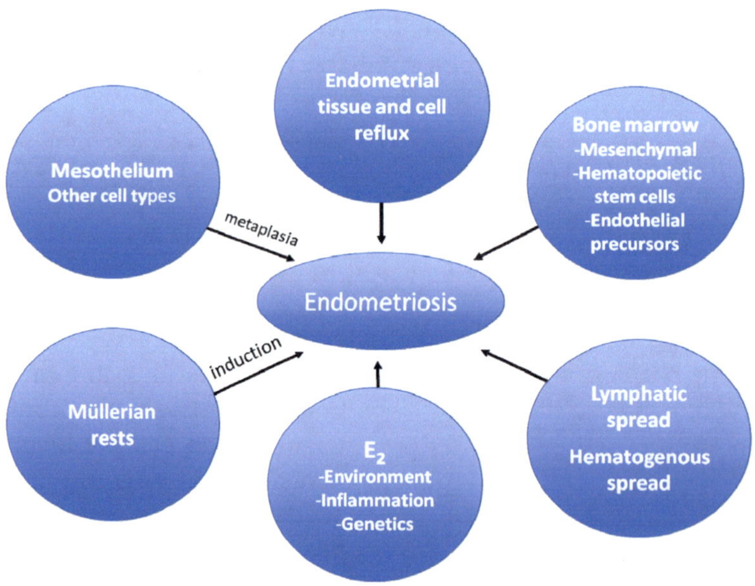

Figure 4.6. Theories regarding endometriosis pathogenesis.

Source: https://www.fertstert.org/cms/10.1016/j.fertnstert.2012.06.029/asset/78dcf8fb-0ebd-4687-9209-494872ffa0a7/main.assets/gr1_lrg.jpg

4.2.1. Mechanisms of Endometriosis Development

Unveiling the causation mechanisms of endometriosis reveals a complex interplay of genetic, hormonal, and immunological factors. Central to this is genetic susceptibility, whereby women with a family history of endometriosis are at a significantly higher risk of developing the condition themselves. It is currently thought that several genes contribute to the susceptibility to endometriosis, affecting hormone regulation and immune response. Additionally, hormonal actions, particularly estrogens, have important roles to play in endometriosis' etiopathogenesis, promoting the growth and survival of endometrial-like cells beyond the uterus. Knowledge of these hormonal and genetic pathways provides the basis for the targeted treatment regimens that are able to at least cure the symptoms and enhance individuals' quality of life (Horne et al., 2022).

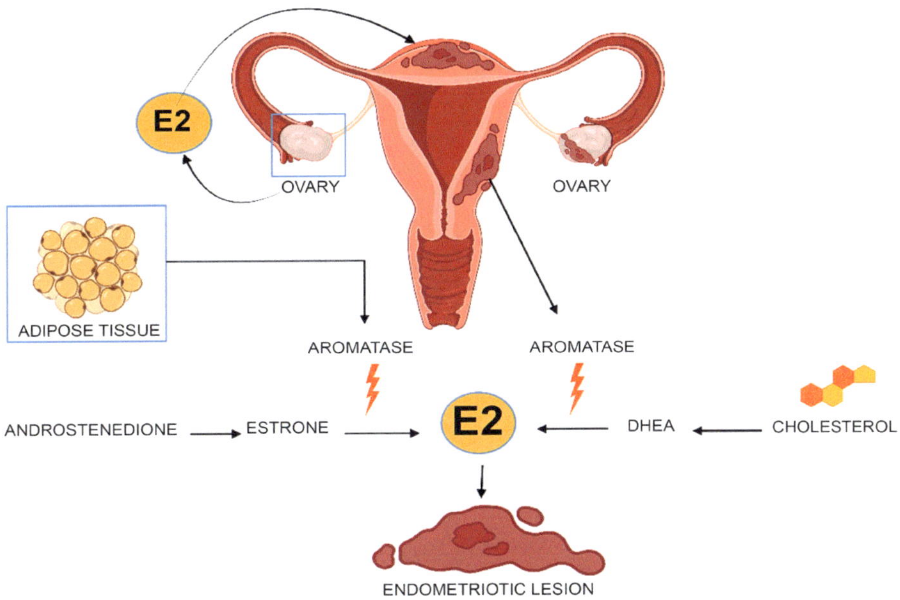

Figure 4.7. The three major sources of estradiol (E2) within endometriosis.

Source: https://www.mdpi.com/ijms/ijms-25-05815/article_deploy/html/images/ijms-25-05815-g002.png

Furthermore, immunological factors play a significant role in the formation and perpetuation of endometrial tissue outside the uterine environment. In the healthy case, the immune system functionally identifies and eliminates abnormal cells. However, in individuals who will develop endometriosis, there seems to be an interference with successful immune surveillance, possibly allowing for the survival and growth of ectopic endometrial cells. Immune cell population shifts, such as elevated macrophages and altered cytokine profiles, account for the inflammatory environment of endometriosis. The endometriosis develops not only through localized inflammation but also worsens pain, making symptoms debilitating to the afflicted. Uncovering the subtle interactions between immunologic and hormonal factors will provide crucial information regarding the multifactorial nature of endometriosis etiology and can guide future research into directions of novel therapeutic uses to combat this challenging illness (Horne et al., 2022). Moreover, new findings have ascertained the role of environmental determinants, predominantly endocrine-disrupting chemicals (EDCs), in the causation of endometriosis. EDCs could interfere with hormonal function, leading to alterations in reproductive health and fertility. Exposure to a myriad of EDCs through industrial and agricultural practices has become an extensive public health concern with the potential to be associated with a variety of reproductive illnesses. As most of these chemicals pervade daily life, from contaminated water sources to domestic products, their role in endometriosis is crucial to understand. This environmental perspective is supplementary to the growing evidence indicating that EDC exposures might either promote or initiate endometriosis, a point that underscores the value of collaborative action in reducing environmental risk as a preventive measure to prevent endometriosis formation.

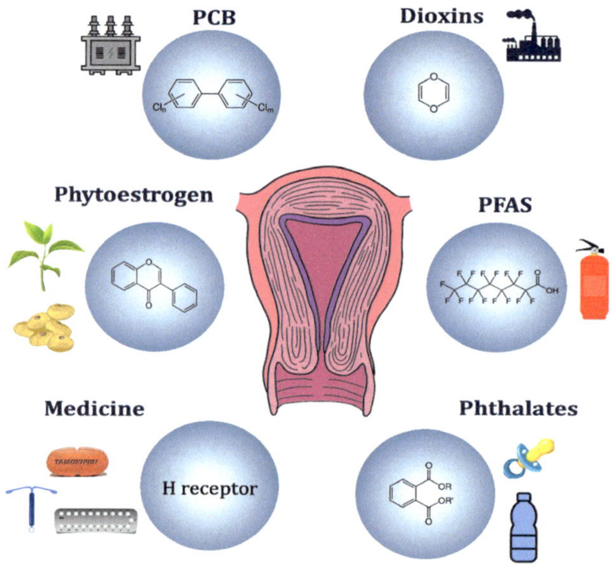

Figure 4.8. Potential endocrine pathogenic causes of adenomyosis.

Source: https://www.preprints.org/manuscript/202401.1528/v1

4.2.2. Mechanisms of Adenomyosis Development

Pathogenesis of adenomyosis is inextricably linked with an array of physiological and pathological processes that remain at the center of ongoing study. Although the exact cause of adenomyosis remains to be established, a pertinent hypothesis is that inflammatory processes are key to the pathogenesis of adenomyosis. Women with endometriosis, who are also prone to systemic inflammation, have been found to develop adenomyosis as a secondary disease frequently. This inflammatory milieu dysregulates the endometrial microenvironment to result in abnormal cellular growth and stimulates endometrial tissue invasion of the uterine myometrium. Associated complications, such as chronic pain and menstrual bleeding, exacerbate the condition, underscoring the imperative for greater insight into the mechanisms of adenomyosis development within the broader context of endometriosis.

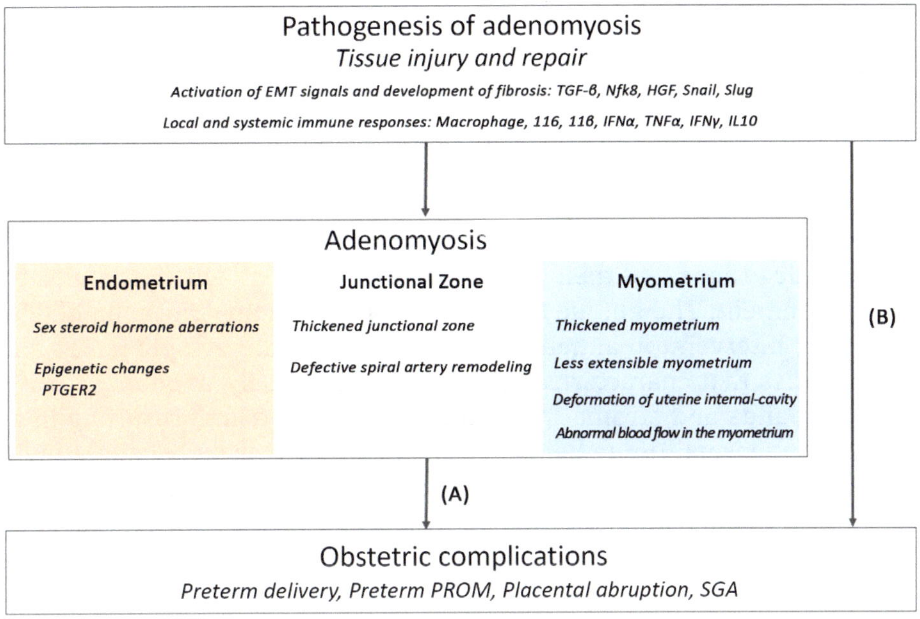

Figure 4.9. Proposed mechanisms of obstetric complication in patient with adenomyosis (A) alterations in the uterus affected with adenomyosis lead to obstetric complications; (B) obstetric complications arise in the pathogenesis of adenomyosis.

Source: https://www.researchgate.net/figure/Proposed-mechanisms-of-obstetric-complication-in-patient-with-adenomyosis-A-alterations_fig1_361852659

Another one of the etiologies for the occurrence of adenomyosis is hormonal imbalance, particularly estrogen dysregulation. Estrogens are pivotal controllers of growth of endometrial tissue; therefore, their alterations or fluctuations in levels may cause adenomyosis. Estrogen-regulated processes such as those of adhesion and invasion of cells become functionally abnormal and cause implantation of endometrial cells within the uterine muscular layers. Besides, endometrial stem cell function has emerged as a key point, in which differentiation and migratory activities might be affected by altered estrogen signaling to facilitate the development from eutopic to ectopic endometrial tissue. This hormonal deregulation can be augmented by environmental factors, complicating even more the etiology and pathmechanisms of adenomyosis (Anastasi et al., 2015). In addition to inflammatory and hormonal factors, environmental stimuli, particularly endocrine-disrupting chemicals (EDCs), have also been suggested to be involved in the mechanistic pathogenesis of adenomyosis. These toxicants can mimic or interfere with the body's hormonal functions and subsequently lead to further dysregulation of the endocrine system. Evidence supports that exposure to EDCs is linked to the pathogenesis of both endometriosis and adenomyosis because these chemicals can lead to a state of pro-inflammatory status and cellular growth. Given the prevalence of concomitant endometriosis and adenomyosis among the affected women, the link between the two conditions and environmental toxicants deserves serious consideration. Mechanistic elucidation of how EDCs facilitate the conditions is important to the design of targeted interventions that can mitigate risks and improve patient outcomes (Anastasi et al., 2015).

4.2.3. Differences in Tissue Behavior Between the Two Conditions

The pathologic tissue behavior of adenomyosis and endometriosis highlights distinctive features that are essential for identifying these diseases. In endometriosis, the proliferation of ectopic endometrial tissue induces an ongoing inflammatory process that results in tissue remodeling and increased angiogenesis. This abnormal tissue behavior may result in the formation of fibrous scarring tissue and adhesions that penetrate nearby organs, generating a significant amount of pelvic pain and dysmenorrhea. Consequently, the disease is an active interaction between the pathological cellular activities of endometriotic lesions and their host microenvironment, which sustains and exacerbates the inflammatory environment. The unique tissue reaction of endometriosis highlights the necessity of particular therapeutic intervention aimed at decreasing both the ectopic tissue and the resultant tissue remodeling activities that characterize the disease. Conversely, adenomyosis is defined by the finding of endometrial glands and stroma invaded in the myometrium, resulting in another kind of similar manifestation of abnormal tissue behavior. The disorder is usually coupled with hypertrophy of the myometrial tissue due to the proliferative action of the ectopic endometrium combined with hormonal effects. Clinical manifestations of adenomyosis can include menorrhagia and pelvic pain, which are caused by the deranged endometrial architecture and resultant myometrial changes. Surprisingly, investigations have proved a potential link between hyperprolactinemia and adenomyosis, in which altered uterine levels of prolactin may be the causative factor for aberrant growth patterns and tissue response within the uterus. This correlation underscores the significance of hormonal regulation in the etiology of adenomyosis and necessitates rigorous research on treatment avenues such as dopamine agonists for the management of symptoms (Andersson et al., 2021).

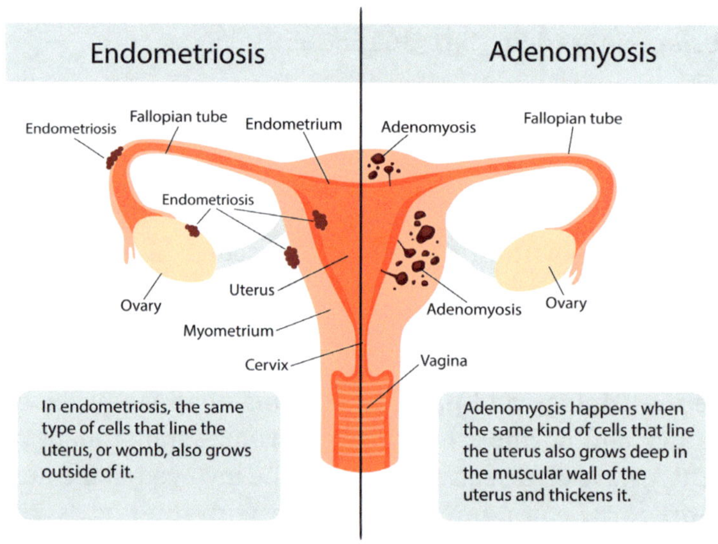

Figure 4.10. Endometriosis and adenomyosis are two distinct medical conditions that affect the uterus and can cause similar symptoms, but they are not the same.

Source: https://www.pantai.com.my/images/pantaihospitalmalaysialibraries/specialties/o-g-fertility/pantai-endometriosis-vs-adenomyosis.webp?sfvrsn=e2d92db_1

Furthermore, epigenetic alterations in tissue function that are associated with both endometriosis and adenomyosis necessitate a complex strategy in diagnosis and therapy. Recent studies have indicated that exposure to endocrine disruptors such as 2,3,7,8-tetrachlorodibenzo-p-dioxin can explain the epigenetic signature associated with reproductive diseases such as endometriosis and can even lead to transgenerational consequences (Adachi et al., 2017). These findings suggest that gene expression changes caused by the environment can contribute to the pathophysiology of these diseases. In adenomyosis, the tissue reaction of the endometrium to hormone fluctuations can produce novel patterns of gene expression that are distinct from what is seen in endometriosis, contributing further to difficulties of diagnosis and treatment strategies. Hence, the investigation of these distinctions in tissue behavior provides critical information that enhances our awareness and therapy of the two disorders.

Test Your Knowledge

1. What are the proposed mechanisms behind the development of endometriosis?
2. How does adenomyosis develop within the uterine wall?

4.3. Symptoms and Diagnosis

Learning Outcome

1. Identify the common symptoms of endometriosis and adenomyosis
2. Discuss the diagnostic methods for both conditions

The symptoms of endometriosis and adenomyosis often overlap, making diagnosis challenging. The patients will most commonly complain of chronic pelvic pain, dysmenorrhea, and dyspareunia, with a significant negative impact on their quality of life. The period pain becomes disabling in endometriosis, while the pain is similar in severity but concurrent with menses in adenomyosis. Heavy bleeding is also a common complaint in most women, contributing to the challenge in characterizing the cause of the suffering. Identification of the subjective nature of these symptoms is crucial, as they will lead clinicians down different lines of diagnosis. These symptoms are frequently misdiagnosed or delayed because they can easily be misdiagnosed as other common gynecologic disorders, hence the need for complete assessment involving patient history and symptomatology in the diagnosis of potential cases of endometriosis and adenomyosis. Endometriosis diagnosis usually relies on imaging techniques, which are most frequently ultrasound and magnetic resonance imaging (MRI). Imaging techniques assist in visualizing the lesions and adhesions of endometriosis, enabling more accurate staging and treatment. Ultrasound, especially performed by endovaginal technique, is able to detect endometriotic cysts and uterine pathology, while MRI possesses high contrast resolution and can yield good images of the pelvis. This capability is crucial, as MRI can distinguish between endometriosis and adenomyosis so that targeted treatment interventions can be planned. Furthermore, being aware of the various imaging findings allows clinicians to plan a more individualized approach to symptom management. Thus, the role of imaging in diagnosis cannot be exaggerated, as it acts as the bridge between clinical signs and symptoms and potential surgical interventions that might be necessary for further diagnosis and management of such ailments (Anastasi et al., 2015). Histological examination remains the gold standard for the diagnosis of endometriosis and adenomyosis, but is not always necessary in initial diagnosis due to concurrent clinical symptoms and imaging data. Recent research has outlined a significant correlation between adenomyosis and endometriosis in that patients with adenomyosis are at increased risk for recurrence of endometriosis following surgery (Bonaccorsi et al., 2019). The pathophysiologic relationship between these two conditions suggests a shared etiology in uterine tissue, further making the process of diagnosis challenging. Clinicians are thus keenly cautioned to monitor patients for both of these conditions, particularly after surgical intervention, in order to individualize treatment and improve patient outcomes. By means of clinical evaluation, imaging studies, and histologic correlation, a proper understanding of a patient's condition is made possible, allowing for an improved management plan.

4.3.1. Common Symptoms of Endometriosis

Endometriosis symptoms are widespread and can significantly affect a woman's way of life. For the most part, the most common symptom of this condition is pelvic pain, which tends to be heavy and might even be crippling. This kind of pain typically occurs at the same time as the menstrual cycle, but also sometimes happens at other times, creating constant pain that makes daily activities difficult. Dysmenorrhea, or pain connected to menstruation, is especially linked with endometriosis and is further exacerbated by the presence of endometrial-like tissue outside the uterus, causing inflammation and scarring. Notably, the severity of pain does not always correlate with the size of the disease, an observation that captures the complex nature of endometriosis symptoms and their variability from patient to patient (Piriyev et al., 2025).

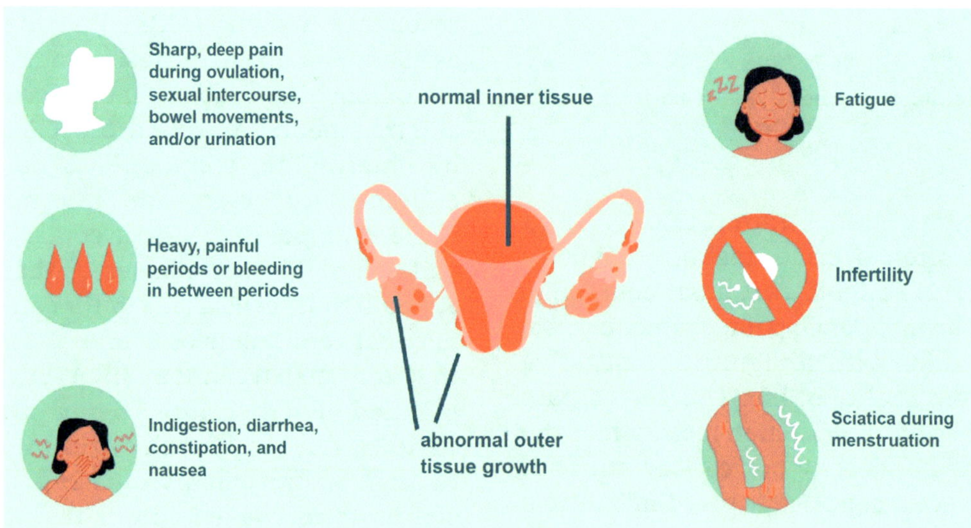

Figure 4.11. Signs and symptoms of endometriosis.

Source https://ik.imagekit.io/d7t01fhx21/Ovum_Hospitals/Blogs/Endometriosis%20symptoms%20and%20treatment-01.jpg?updatedAt=1698650199303

Other than pelvic pain, the majority of women with endometriosis are also infertile. Infertility is a sign that generates the need for further medical studies and leads to an endometriosis diagnosis. Endometrial-like tissue outside the uterus may interfere with the usual physiology of the female reproductive organs by making ovulation impossible or inducing adhesions, which can obstruct the fallopian tubes. As such, the link between endometriosis and infertility constitutes a concern for women who wish to conceive, underscoring the value of early diagnosis and effective therapy protocols to alleviate both pain as well as reproductive complications. Moreover, psychological consequences of infertility may compound the pain caused by the physical effects of endometriosis, symbolizing the interdependence between physiological and emotional health in affected women (Li et al., 2025).

Gastrointestinal symptoms also often accompany endometriosis since most patients report diarrhea, constipation, bloating, and nausea, especially during menstruation. These are commonly mistaken for irritable bowel syndrome (IBS), and thus, it becomes tricky to diagnose. Shared symptoms because of the close anatomical relationship between the reproductive and gastrointestinal systems further make it challenging for medical practitioners. Additionally, inflammatory response from endometrial lesions can influence gut motility and function and lead to additional discomfort. The presence of gastrointestinal symptoms stresses the necessity for close examination of patients who have suspected endometriosis because detection and treatment of all manifestations can contribute significantly to patient management and treatment success (Piriyev et al., 2025).

4.3.2. Common Symptoms of Adenomyosis

Adenomyosis can only be properly understood by its intense analysis of its common occurrence, which is the same as endometriosis, and thus rendering it hard to diagnose. Dysmenorrhea is one of its most frequent symptoms, which involves very painful and aching cramping menstrual pains that can incapacitate the individual during menstruation. This pain is brought about by the proliferation of endometrial tissue in the uterus muscle, resulting in a superimposed pressure and inflammation. Moreover, the majority of patients suffer from menorrhagia or heavy menstrual bleeding, which could lead to significant loss of blood and potentially anemia in the long term. Detection of such symptoms is crucial as they indicate the aetiological disease and may decide to treat individuals with adenomyosis and related disorders like endometriosis (Piriyev et al., 2025). Another prominent symptom of adenomyosis is pelvic pain that is chronic, extending even beyond the duration of the menstrual cycle itself, reflective of the chronic nature of the disease. The pain is generally dull, but sometimes it is severe enough to affect quality of life, disrupt normal activities, and produce mental ill-being. Females with adenomyosis may also have a host of gastrointestinal disturbances, including bloating, constipation, or diarrhea, that may further exacerbate the clinical presentation. The combination of pelvic pain and gastrointestinal symptoms accounts for the complexity of adenomyosis and its overlap with the physiological functions of the body. A proper knowledge of these symptoms helps in the differentiation of adenomyosis from other gynecologic pathologies and emphasizes the targeted therapy (Li et al., 2025). In addition to this, adenomyosis may result in evident modifications in a female's reproductive well-being, such as infertility. Numerous women can experience difficulty in getting pregnant, as the ectopic endometrial tissue can interfere with regular implantation and pregnancy patterns. Also, some women describe a pelvic pressure or feeling of fullness, and in some instances, especially with intercourse, this can be significant and cause sexual dysfunction. The emphasis on these symptoms is vital in the development of a complete clinical picture of adenomyosis since these symptoms not only impact physical well-being but also have an emotional impact. A correct diagnosis and awareness of all the symptoms can lead to improved management plans and improved outcomes for women who are grappling with these interconnected conditions, adenomyosis and endometriosis (Piriyev et al., 2025).

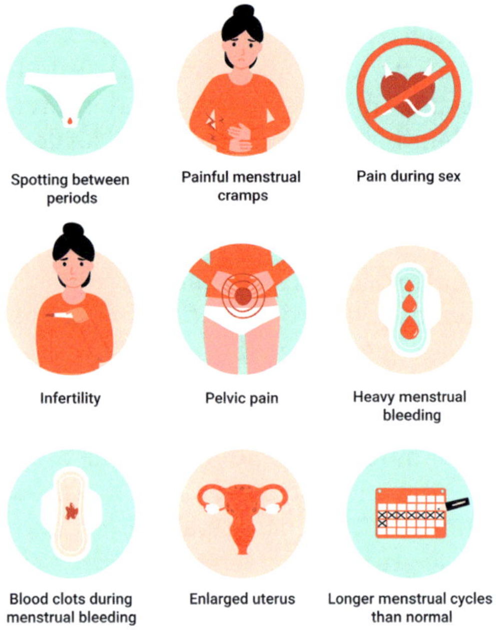

Figure 4.12. Symptoms of Adenomyosis.

Source: https://ufefibroidspecialist.com/wp-content/uploads/2024/02/endometriosis-adenomyosis-3943636.webp

4.3.3. Diagnostic Methods For Both Conditions

The diagnostic methods for endometriosis and adenomyosis are becoming more advanced, a reflection of the pathology of these conditions. Pelvic examination remains a commonly employed initial diagnostic method in endometriosis; however, its sensitivity is low. Transvaginal ultrasound (TVUS) is being used more often to describe endometriotic cysts and pelvic masses, offering a non-invasive option. Magnetic resonance imaging (MRI) is a powerful tool, giving precise anatomical information about the extent of endometriotic lesions. In addition, innovations such as Fusion Imaging, which fuses ultrasonography with MRI, hold out the potential for improved diagnostic precision by unifying functional and structural information, potentially unmasking features that cannot be distinguished by conventional imaging alone (Bellati et al., 2018). These developments emphasize the requirement of multidisciplinary approaches in the detection of gynecological diseases, paving the way for effective and timely intervention.

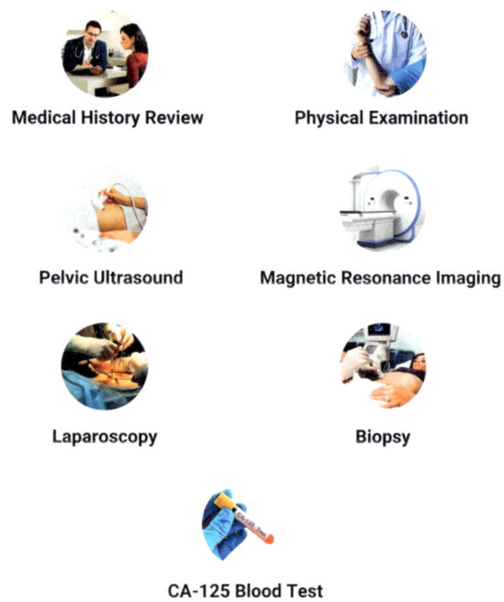

Figure 4.13. Endometriosis and adenomyosis diagnosis tests.

Source: https://images.drlogy.com/assets/uploads/img/admin/health_blog/editor-img/endometriosis_diagnosis_-_drlogy_diagnosis-1.webp

Transvaginal sonography is the gold standard in diagnosing adenomyosis, with consensus agreement from a number of studies regarding its high sensitivity and specificity. Emerging evidence indicates that sonographic findings of asymmetry of uterine walls and hyperechoic striae are highly correlated with histology, making them all the more diagnostic

(Zannoni et al., 2017). New markers, such as the physical examination sign of a question mark and uterine tenderness on transvaginal exam, have become available through more recent research, introducing new dimensions of diagnostic utility. Inclusion of these new markers is a significant step forward in the assessment of adenomyosis. This improves the capacity for early diagnosis, ultimately having implications on treatment in women with often disabling symptoms, and enhancing the quality of care provided. Both endometriosis and adenomyosis can share similar symptoms, and hence, differential diagnosis is complex. Because of this complexity, a general strategy for evaluation is necessary. Clinicians typically employ a combination of history, physical examination, and advanced imaging modalities in arriving at a proper differential diagnosis between the two conditions. Although the gold standard test for diagnosing endometriosis is laparoscopy because it offers direct visualization of lesions, histological evidence could be necessary in cases of doubt. In adenomyosis, concordance of clinical presentation with imaging findings also favors the diagnosis. As research continues to unveil the nuances of such disorders, a multimodal approach to diagnosis will remain essential to equipping patients with correct diagnoses and appropriate treatment regimens tailored to their unique requirements.

Test Your Knowledge

1. What are common symptoms experienced by individuals with endometriosis?
2. List typical symptoms associated with adenomyosis.

4.4. Treatment Options

Learning Outcome

1. Discuss the medical treatments for endometriosis and adenomyosis
2. Explain the surgical interventions for both conditions

The treatment landscape of endometriosis and adenomyosis is characterized by an array of choices that depend on the specific patient requirements, symptoms, and disease severity. Initial care usually involves pharmacologic management, with a first-line focus on symptom control and pain relief. Non-steroidal anti-inflammatory drugs (NSAIDs) are frequently employed to relieve pain. In contrast, hormonal therapies such as oral contraceptives and progestins are employed to regulate menstrual cycles and reduce endometrial tissue growth. These therapies have a high potential to impact quality of life, but they are not always able to fix underlying conditions completely. In response, their success frequently needs careful observation and reassessment, particularly in patients with severe or refractory symptoms, suggesting the potential necessity of more aggressive treatment. Surgical options are a valuable possibility for patients whose symptoms remain out of control despite conservative therapies alone. Laparoscopy, as the most minimally invasive surgical procedure, is referred to as the gold standard for the diagnosis and management of endometriosis. Under laparoscopy, lesions of the endometrium can be removed or ablated by surgeons, providing both diagnostic reliability and symptomatic relief. Evidence is beginning to identify the correlation of surgical outcomes with adenomyosis, such that patients suffering from this disease are likely to experience increased rates of postoperative recurrence of endometriosis (Bonaccorsi et al., 2019). Surgical treatment is most appropriate for patients suffering from infertility due to endometriosis, as results show that the successful resection of endometriotic lesions may enhance reproductive capacity and thus modify the therapeutic approach from symptom relief to fertility restoration (Alexander et al., 2020).

The topic of adjunct treatments, including lifestyle modification and complementary therapies, becomes increasingly frequent in endometriosis and adenomyosis therapy. Dietary changes, physical therapy, and acupuncture can benefit patients and complement mainstream medical treatments. Additionally, psychotherapy is essential because chronic pain related to these conditions can cause enormous emotional distress. Mental health care must become part of treatment plans not only to assist with overall wellness but also to enhance the effectiveness of medical interventions. As ongoing research uncovers more about the complex underlying processes in such disorders, a multidisciplinary treatment approach incorporating both mainstream and complementary therapies takes center stage in optimizing outcomes and facilitating patients' active role in their management.

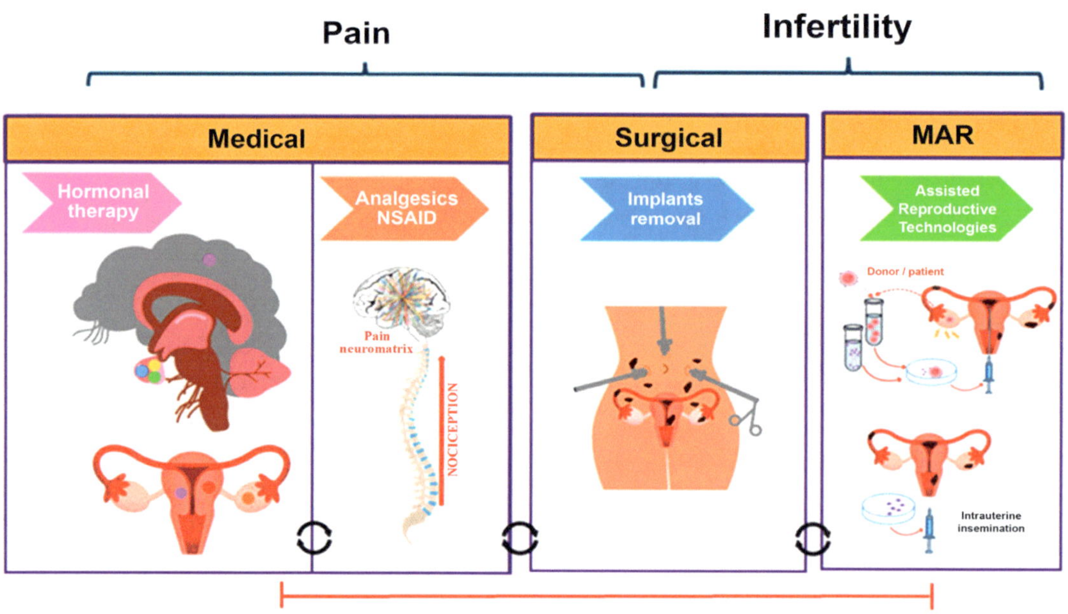

Figure 4.14. Current options for management of endometriosis symptoms. Pain is the main symptom associated with EM and is currently treated with medical (hormonal therapy, analgesics and NSAID) or surgical strategies.

Source: https://www.mdpi.com/ijms/ijms-25-07068/article_deploy/html/images/ijms-25-07068-g001.png

4.4.1. Medical Treatments For Endometriosis

Endometriosis treatment is multidimensional, with both medical and surgical options to manage the symptoms and quality of life. Hormonal treatments remain an important area of treatment, with the aim of blocking the production of estrogen, thus reducing endometrial tissue growth. Combined oral contraceptives (COCs) and progestins are two of the most popular methods that may cure pain in the pelvic area and dysmenorrhea. While COCs are universally prescribed, they may not be equally effective for every woman, which is why individualized treatment regimens are called for. GnRH agonists have increasingly been employed; these medications induce a short-term menopausal state, significantly reducing estrogen levels. Continuous use, though, leads to profound side effects, such as bone loss in density. Thus, the most important aspect of treatment of endometriosis is the balancing act between symptom relief and the reduction of side effects, a challenge that persists in the management of endometriosis.

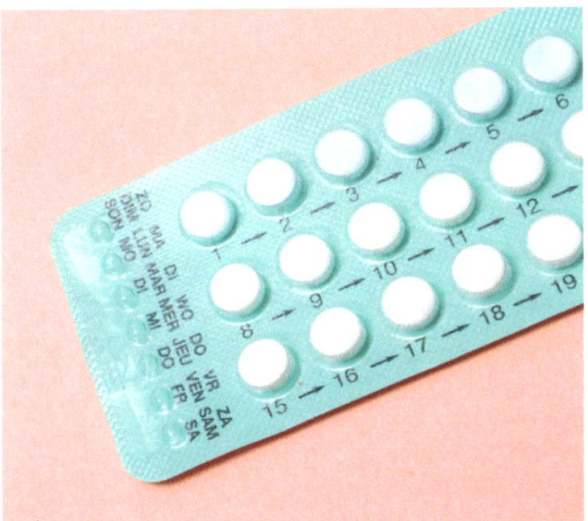

Source: https://cdn.sanity.io/images/0vv8moc6/contobgyn/130b25f02f306356db2507b578bffd02940e9821-3938x2544.jpg?fit=crop&auto=format

Apart from the hormonal treatments, other pharmaceutical treatments such as NSAIDs play an additive role as an option for the management of pain associated with endometriosis. Though NSAIDs, such as ibuprofen, are increasingly recommended due to their analgesic property, their efficacy varies with different patients. Most women continue to experience debilitating pain in the presence of NSAID use, and this means that this strategy is not sufficient as an isolated treatment. Moreover, interdisciplinary interventions, including acupuncture and physical therapy, have been evaluated in an attempt to further enhance symptom alleviation. The use of different modalities reflects the need for multifaceted care strategies, particularly because the annual prevalence of conditions like dysmenorrhea shows that many women require more than one line of treatment.

Other studies have shown that adding NSAIDs to hormonal therapy can yield a better outcome, and further studies on optimal regimens for endometriosis are needed. Newer therapeutics include the exploration of new drugs such as aromatase inhibitors, which have proven to be useful for targeting the hormonal pathways of endometriosis pathophysiology. These medications work by estrogen blockade and cause pain relief and reduction in lesion size; yet, long-term safety profiles are dubious. This trend towards new therapies is a shining future for treating endometriosis. As emphasized in the current literature, it is critical to have clearly established clinical guidelines because the disease is often linked with adenomyosis, again complicating treatment algorithms. Subsequent research will need to set evidence-based recommendations that consider unique patient presentations, including symptom severity and fertility goals. The complexity of endometriosis calls for ongoing investigation into the effectiveness of treatments, ultimately maximizing patient outcomes and quality of life in this often-overlooked population setting (Barra et al., 2023; Holland et al., 2024).

4.4.2. Medical Treatments For Adenomyosis

The management of adenomyosis is also a complex and evolving issue, primarily due to the many symptoms with which the disease presents, such as abnormal uterine bleeding (AUB) and crippling dysmenorrhea. The therapy of medical professionals most often aims to alleviate these symptoms and improve overall quality of life. Amongst the available choices, nonsteroidal anti-inflammatory medications (NSAIDs) are routinely employed to treat pain, though their efficacy is often less than ideal for women experiencing more severe symptoms. The management within the realm of medicine is the cornerstone upon which hormonal therapies are based, and the levonorgestrel-releasing intrauterine system (LNG-IUS) has been shown to be highly effective in reducing uterine volume and improving symptoms, even as the lack of standardized treatment options complicates decision-making. These initial treatments, although helpful to relieve symptoms, emphasize the importance of continued research to optimize treatment modalities for adenomyosis (Barra et al., 2023). In addition to LNG-IUS, hormonal contraceptives and progestins are important in the treatment of adenomyosis. COCs can regulate menstrual bleeding and dysmenorrhea; however, efficacy can be outweighed by others like progestin-only treatments. For those patients who require successful management, Dienogest (DNG) is an available therapy, but with the limited data supporting its use, it needs clinical caution in prescribing. Danazol is another that is typically limited by its androgenic side effects, which may discourage some from using it long-term. The need for personalized treatment strategies is the first priority, with every woman's response to medication dramatically differing based on unique health profiles and symptom severity (Holland et al., 2024).

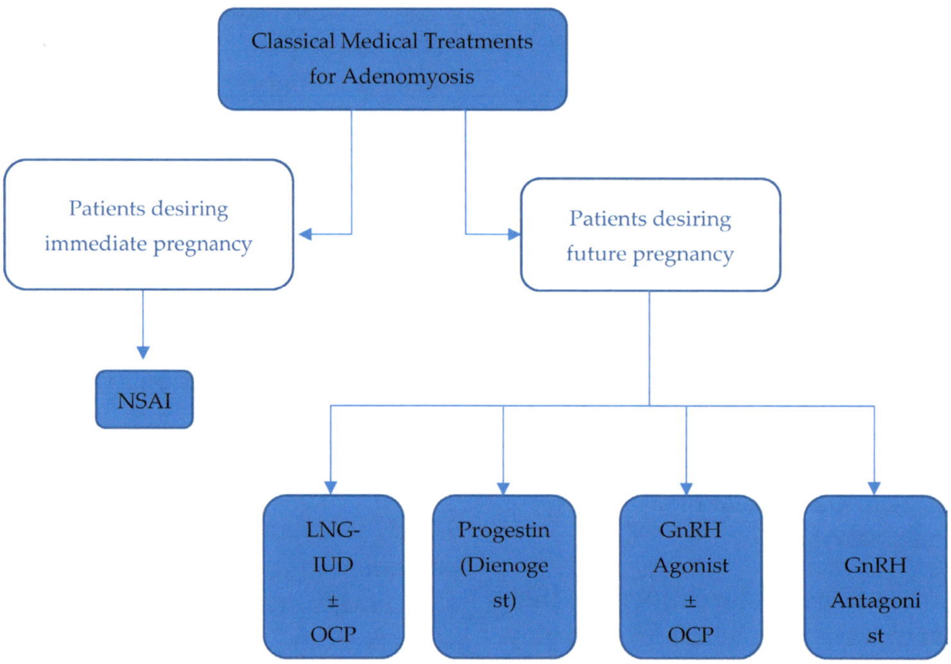

Figure 4.15. https://www.mdpi.com/2077-0383/12/19/6130

Source: https://www.mdpi.com/jcm/jcm-12-06130/article_deploy/html/images/jcm-12-06130-g002.png

Research on newer therapeutic medicine has expanded the options for treating adenomyosis. Gonadotropin-releasing hormone (GnRH) agonists are to be remembered for having a great symptom reduction but often induce menopausal symptoms after long-term use, a significant trade-off. Recent developments have also put GnRH antagonists on center stage, yet their safety and efficacy profile are still under investigation to define guideline criteria. Aromatase inhibitors (AIs) are promising in their ability to reduce AUB and pelvic pain but are still in trial phases for use in cases of refractoriness. Lastly, awareness of how to interpret the subtle interplay of adenomyosis with other gynecologic conditions like endometriosis is crucial to establishing an integrated treatment strategy. As it keeps on conducting research, establishing clear evidence-based guidelines shall be crucial to improving patient outcomes and rendering effective targeted care to increase adenomyosis-impacted persons (Barra et al., 2023).

4.4.3. Surgical Interventions For Both Conditions

Surgical intervention in adenomyosis and endometriosis is an essential method of treating these often incapacitating conditions. If conservative treatments fail or symptoms persist, surgery is then required. Laparoscopic resection is a widely practiced technique used to treat endometriosis, aiming to excise endometrial lesions and adhesions without compromising ovarian function. This minimally invasive technique not only eradicates discomfort but also enhances fertility potential among women wishing to conceive children. In addition, surgical processes include ablation of endometriotic lesions or, in the worst cases, hysterectomy. These processes are credited with significant symptom relief and improvement in quality of life, thus suggesting the importance of customized surgical planning to patient needs as established by clinical practice guidelines (Ball et al., 2020). Adenomyosis is especially challenging when it involves surgical management since it typically adds to the difficulty of the treatment process for women with endometriosis and adenomyosis. Deep endometriosis (DE), in 15-30% of endometriosis patients, is often associated with adenomyosis in 25-49% of patients, which complicates surgical intervention (Carmona et al., 2022). Surgery for adenomyosis is most commonly hysterectomy as the definitive procedure, particularly in women who have completed childbearing. But a conservative operation can be endometrial ablation or uterine artery embolization, depending on the severity of symptoms and the patient's reproductive intentions. Thus, successful intervention is largely contingent on accurate preoperative diagnosis and individualized planning for treatment, both of which are crucial for effective treatment. It has been demonstrated that the presence of adenomyosis has a significant influence on operative results in women who are undergoing intervention for DE, with adenomyosis patients having a higher reported complication rate than non-adenomyosis patients (Carmona et al., 2022).

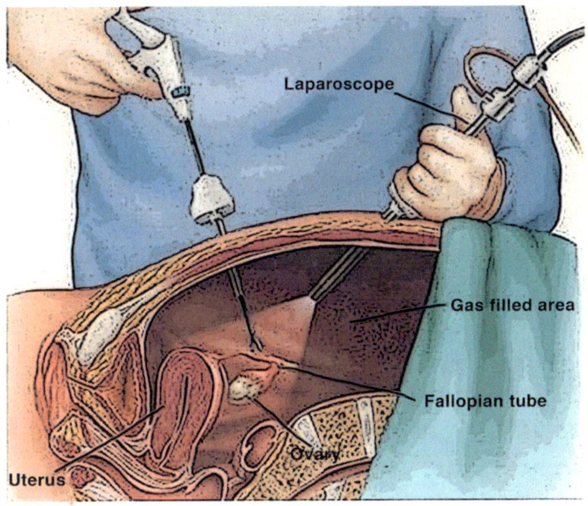

Figure 4.16. Laparoscopic Surgery for Endometriosis.

Source: https://images.squarespace-cdn.com/content/v1/5ac5219289c1722c939a13c3/1557866276022-2RNMJY0ZLRDC2BG57REY/lapx.jpg

In a retrospective cohort study, the incidence of surgical complications was found to be highly elevated in patients with adenomyosis, yielding a 4.56-fold higher risk of the adverse outcome related to the procedure (Carmona et al., 2022). The correlation is a reminder that multidisciplinary teams of caregivers have to assess risks and manage patient expectations carefully. Last but not least, understanding the interplay between endometriosis and adenomyosis is essential to optimize surgical interventions, treating not just the palpable characteristics of these pathologies but also their profound impact on patients' lives.

Test Your Knowledge

1. Which medications are typically used in the treatment of adenomyosis?
2. What surgical interventions are available for endometriosis and adenomyosis?

4.5. Impact on Quality of Life

Learning Outcome

1. Describe the physical effects on daily activities
2. Define emotional and psychological effects
3. Explain the social implications and support systems

The impact of endometriosis and adenomyosis on quality of life is extensive and far-reaching, encompassing physical, emotional, and social well-being. Women with these conditions often report disabling symptoms such as severe pelvic pain, heavy menstrual bleeding, and gastrointestinal disturbances that lower activities and productivity dramatically. The chronic conditions not only make life more difficult day-to-day, but also impose huge burdens at the workplace, leading to absenteeism and degraded work performance. The symptoms have been shown to not only be physically exhausting but also lead to chronic stress and anxiety, further perpetuating the cycle of suffering from the diseases (Anastasi et al., 2015). Hence, a very clear understanding of the effects of endometriosis and adenomyosis on quality of life is called for in the process of developing optimal therapeutic strategies. The chronic pain that accompanies these conditions is a major factor determining overall quality of life. Classified as pain of durations three to six months or more, chronic pelvic pain (CPP) is identified as an important problem that requires a variety of management modalities (Ball et al., 2020). Although endometriosis is one of the most frequent structural causes of CPP, its occurrence reinforces the necessity to use comprehensive care strategies that go beyond the consideration of just the physical symptoms. Interventions such as lifestyle change, counseling, and complementary therapy—namely meditation and physiotherapy—are fundamental treatment components that form part of the enhanced quality of life outcomes. It not only seeks to diminish pain but to maximize levels of emotional resilience and social support networks, thus reinforcing the interdependence of physical status and well-being. Moreover, the social impacts of adenomyosis and endometriosis cannot be ignored since the prevalence of symptoms affects not just the patient but also the family and community. The physical limitations and unpredictability of symptoms strain relationships and lead to social isolation as well as decreased quality of life. The need for increased knowledge and education on such disorders is high in terms of creating empathy and compassion within society. Moreover, ongoing research on diagnostics and treatments, including high-level diagnostic procedures such as MRI that enhance diagnostic precision, is crucial (Anastasi et al.,

2015). By being aware of the complete effect of endometriosis and adenomyosis, medical staff can further assist their patients, gaining access to necessary resources and improving overall quality of life.

4.5.1. Physical Effects on Daily Activities

The bodily manifestations of adenomyosis and endometriosis dramatically disrupt everyday functioning, presenting in varied forms that undermine women's best functioning. Chronic pelvic pain is among the most debilitating symptomatology of these conditions, affecting approximately 4%–25% of women of reproductive age as cited by recent literature.

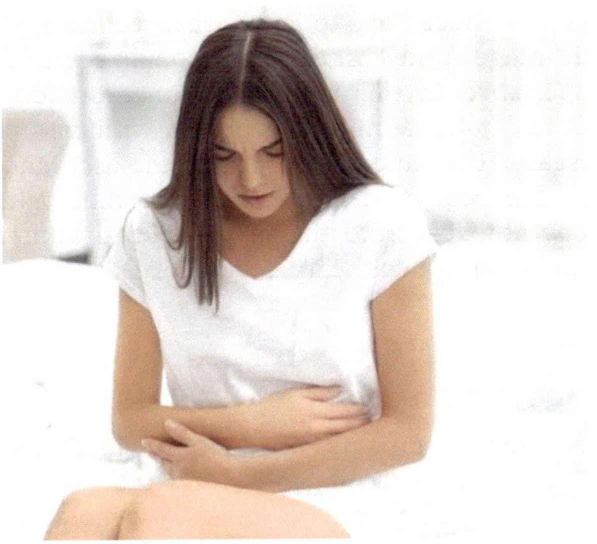

Source: https://sa1s3optim.patientpop.com/assets/images/provider/photos/1935684.jpg

This ongoing discomfort can lead to decreased activity at work, social function, and exercise, leading to a cycle of frustration and stress. The disabling nature of pelvic pain often leads women to modify or abandon normal activities, which results in an overall worse quality of life. Thus, the experience of these physical limitations and routine aspects needs a deeper insight into the way endometriosis and adenomyosis limit women's lives, in addition to the health implications of the diseases. Additionally, the psychological effect of managing these long-term illnesses cannot be overstated because it coincides with the physical load that disrupts daily life. Endometriosis and adenomyosis primarily affect female patients, and they typically have anxiety and depression because of their chronic pain and the uncertainties surrounding their health.

The symptom variability from dysmenorrhea to chronic pelvic pain leads to interference with work and personal life, which is normally reflected in lost working days or decreased productivity. Under such a situation, the application of such treatment modalities as hormonal therapies or even surgery can provide relief, but has secondary complications attached as well. Taking into consideration the physical presentations of both these conditions and their impact on psychology, a complete picture of how they affect everyday living is presented, with the focus laid on better systems of support. The choice of treatment available can also have an effect on the physical effects of endometriosis and adenomyosis on everyday living.

Options available for treatment range from non-invasive medical interventions such as the combined oral contraceptive pill to more invasive surgical interventions such as hysterectomy. While the latter provides a more tangible management for severe cases, it has significant reproductive health and hormonal balance ramifications, as put forward in the literature. An appreciation of the nuances of management approaches, including less invasive alternatives like LNG-IUS, is essential for women attempting to find a balance between maintaining their quality of life and managing symptoms effectively. As documented, the impacts of pelvic pain transcend physical pain; they can have pervasive lifestyle changes, pointing to the intricate relationship between physical well-being and functional daily activities among women with these syndromes.

4.5.2. Emotional and Psychological Effects

The emotional and psychological effect of endometriosis and adenomyosis seriously distorts the quality of life among victims. Victims of these conditions are usually exposed to ongoing pain, which further generates debilitating stress and anxiety. The chronic nature of their conditions usually equates to feelings of hopelessness, loneliness, and frustration as the ability to undertake normal activities is greatly compromised. Evidence indicates that such physical pain often results in mental issues, including depression and anxiety disorders, and tends to interfere not just with emotional wellbeing but also with interpersonal relationships. People suffering from endometriosis are likely to have feelings of being judged or not understood, which adds to their emotional suffering. This emotional distress then leads to their social lives deteriorating, generating a cycle of isolation and heightened symptomatology, hence indicating the symbiotic relationship between physical health and emotional stability. Apart from that, the psychological impacts of endometriosis and adenomyosis extend beyond individual suffering to affect overall life outcomes, for example, professional and academic achievements. Women are likely to complain of losing focus, leading to issues within working or learning environments. The stress and tiredness of long-term conditions can weaken cognitive function, resulting in reduced productivity and reduced self-worth. These issues were echoed in a study that revealed psychological factors like mobility impairments and depression affect academic functioning in students, illustrating the significant influence mental health can have in many situations (Azubuike et al., 2024). Consequently, the impact extends throughout a woman's course of life to her long-term results, redefining career and personal objectives, illuminating the long-reaching effects these issues have over and above physical symptomatology. Lastly, the marrying of these emotional concerns and advanced medical technologies, namely artificial intelligence (AI), reveals a complex realm of potential benefits and risks. The application of AI in medicine, especially in conditions such as endometriosis and adenomyosis, holds the promise to enhance patient care by making diagnoses and treatment plans easier (Cetera et al., 2024). But applying technology in healing emotional and psychological suffering could also spark fear of obsolescence among healthcare practitioners and concerns about the security of information. As much as AI technology is desired to enhance efficiency and interaction with patients, it becomes necessary to counteract technology's advantage at the cost of a depersonalized health experience. In this respect, an understanding of the emotional nuances entailed with chronic diseases continues to be core to the assurance that the incorporation of advanced technologies does not desecrate the much-needed human touch within healthcare settings.

4.5.3. Social Implications and Support Systems

The social impacts of endometriosis and adenomyosis extend far beyond the physical symptoms, impacting women's psychological well-being, relationships, and general quality of life. Socially stigmatised and often poorly understood, both conditions contribute to heightened levels of isolation amongst victims. Hard to articulate for many women tormented by the widespread pain and exhaustion that characterise these conditions. This challenge can be linked with a lack of support from family and friends, who are not aware of the debilitating nature of the disease. As stated, the incapacities for women suffering from endometriosis and adenomyosis can lead to real social disability, exacerbating exclusion and isolation. Awareness campaigns for the diseases are crucial in order to minimize stigma and maximize comprehension, thereby providing a supportive environment for individuals with these conditions. Support networks are critical for dealing with the social consequences of endometriosis and adenomyosis. Women are likely to benefit from support group networks, both in-person and on the internet, in which they can exchange messages regarding experiences, concerns, and coping strategies. These support groups are able to provide emotional support and advice, both of which are crucial to overcoming the intricacies of having a chronic disease. Secondly, medical practitioners have a crucial role in providing a welcoming environment where women are heard and recognized. The incorporation of psychological care in treatment protocols is also of utmost importance; focusing on the psychological effects of such illnesses as much as the physical can result in comprehensive well-being. Educational interventions to enhance the awareness of clinicians regarding endometriosis and adenomyosis become increasingly important in order to deliver more empathetic and informed care. The comorbidity overlap, such as migraine with endometriosis and adenomyosis, adds to social complexity for these women. Research finds adenomyosis exacerbates pain and disability, and therefore, its effective treatment is crucial (Albanese et al., 2024). Also, women who have endometriosis and migraine endorse more severe pain, as well as more days of migraines per month. Not only do these symptoms' interaction enhance physical challenge, but can further put pressure on relationships and work responsibilities. What the intricate nature of these illnesses signifies is the necessity for holistic care approaches that address physical as well as social elements. By providing them with robust support systems and advocacy, we are able to empower women to improve their health conditions, hence their overall quality of life and integration into communities.

Test Your Knowledge

1. How can endometriosis and adenomyosis physically impact a person's daily activities?
2. What are the common emotional and psychological effects associated with these conditions?

SUMMARY

The intricate interaction of adenomyosis and endometriosis warrants proper elucidation of the two pathologies to ensure proper management. As medical research now indicates the co-existence of the two pathologies, clinicians need to ensure diagnosis of both pathologies during the assessment of a patient, particularly because similar symptoms overlap. The findings of the research are that a high percentage of patients who present with fibroids also have concomitant uterine pathologies, including adenomyosis and endometriosis, which highlights the need for thorough diagnostic procedures (Konda et al., 2020). By identifying such concomitant conditions at an early level, healthcare professionals can implement treatment methods case-wise that address the variability of patients' symptoms and thus lead to improved quality of life. Moreover, the therapeutic results for women with endometriosis of the ovaries underscore the importance of preoperative and postoperative management protocols. Findings indicate that initiating treatment procedures such as the preoperative use of dienogest can significantly alleviate symptoms of pelvic pain and lead to less complicated surgery (Choijiljaw et al., 2021). This evidence addresses the importance of preventive and symptom-directed strategies in addressing endometriosis and adenomyosis. Therefore, the combination of pharmacologic interventions with surgical therapies may yield enhanced patient outcomes, highlighting the necessity for ongoing interdisciplinary collaboration among healthcare professionals to achieve maximal therapeutic regimens for individualized patient demands. Finally, the constantly evolving nature of endometriosis and adenomyosis research highlights the pressing need for ongoing investigation into these debilitating disorders. With the increasing availability of data concerning their pathophysiology and reaction to various treatment regimens, practitioners will have the ability to provide more integrated care based on the complex interplay of factors influencing each disease. A focus on multidisciplinary treatment utilizing application of surgical expertise, medical therapy, and psychological guidance is critical to facilitate individuals suffering from these illnesses (Konda et al., 2020). Future studies will try to understand endometriosis and adenomyosis mechanisms more clearly and bring revolutionary treatments that will alleviate the suffering of millions of women all around the world.

A critical examination of adenomyosis and endometriosis identifies divergent but related pathologies with profound impact on women's health. Each is characterized by the proliferation of uterine tissue outside its normal site; endometriosis by the formation of endometrial-like tissue at sites outside the uterus, and adenomyosis by the invasion of endometrial glands and stroma into the myometrium. The interfacing of these illnesses with a wide range of symptoms, including painful menstruation, abnormal uterine bleeding, and infertility, underscores their clinical significance. These pathologies are also important to know in order to establish useful treatment protocols, as they tend to co-occur and influence one another, making diagnosis and treatment complicated. The need for more awareness among patients and the healthcare community is evident, given the extent to which such conditions can drain quality of life and disrupt well-being altogether. The relationship between abnormal uterine peristalsis and adenomyosis points to an intricate interaction within the female reproductive tract. Abnormalities of the uterus, such as adenomyosis, appear to influence uterine motility, reinforcing the symptoms of dysmenorrhea and abnormal bleeding, studies indicate. An overview of available literature shows that the menstrual phase significantly affects the mentioned effects of these pathologies on uterine contractions and leaves open the possibility of a menstrual phase-dependent relationship, which should be explored further. While research suggests that adenomyosis may impact uterine function, conclusive findings for its overall impact on fertility and on other clinical parameters remain significant but elusive. Therefore, a comprehensive grasp of uterine peristalsis in the setting of adenomyosis can prove useful for creating targeted interventions that take into consideration symptomatology as well as potential reproductive implications. Endometriosis and adenomyosis remain all too frequently under-diagnosed despite advances in diagnostic technologies and growing understanding of their pathophysiology. Histopathologic definitions, most notably those of adenomyosis, still create controversy with greater diagnostic specificity based on the identification of specific molecular markers. Recent literature is symptom-oriented, instead of etiologically-driven, and calls for a multidimensional treatment model. Except this, greater diagnostic criteria and solid clinical research are needed to break down the mysteries behind these disorders. Ultimately, the treatment of the subtle pathophysiologic factors of endometriosis and adenomyosis not only enhances patient outcomes but also aids in the ongoing discourse regarding women's reproductive health conditions that deserve greater focus and investment in medical research.

KEY TERMS FROM THIS CHAPTER

- Endometriosis
- Acupuncture
- Adenomyosis therapy
- Chronic pelvic pain (CPP)
- Dienogest (DNG)
- Endocrine-disrupting chemicals (EDCs)
- Gynecological diseases
- Hormonal dysregulation
- Immune system
- Lymphatic drainage pathways
- Multifactorial etiology
- Endometriosis formation
- Adenomyosis
- Aromatase inhibitors (AIs)
- Diagnostic precision
- Dysmenorrhea
- Endometrial-like tissue
- Healthcare resource management
- Hormone fluctuations
- Irritable bowel syndrome (IBS)
- Magnetic resonance imaging (MRI)
- Patient management

CRITICAL THINKING QUESTIONS

1. **Which of the following best describes endometriosis?**
   a. Growth of endometrial tissue inside the uterus only
   b. Growth of endometrial tissue outside the uterus
   c. Inflammation of the endometrium due to infection
   d. Thickening of the uterine wall during pregnancy
2. **Adenomyosis is characterized by:**
   a. Endometrial glands growing on the ovaries
   b. Endometrial tissue invading the uterine muscle wall (myometrium)
   c. Inflammation of the cervix
   d. Endometrial hyperplasia confined to the endometrial lining
3. **Common symptoms shared by both endometriosis and adenomyosis include:**
   a. Weight loss and increased appetite
   b. Irregular heartbeat and chest pain
   c. Pelvic pain and heavy menstrual bleeding
   d. Cough and shortness of breath
4. **Which diagnostic tool is most commonly used to detect adenomyosis?**
   a. Chest X-ray
   b. Pap smear
   c. Transvaginal ultrasound or MRI
   d. Liver function test
5. **Which of the following statements is TRUE about endometriosis?**
   a. It always resolves after menopause without treatment.
   b. It can cause infertility in some women.
   c. It only affects women over 50 years old.
   d. It is caused by a bacterial infection.

Short Answer Questions

1. What is the epidemiology of endometriosis and adenomyosis?
2. Describe the pathophysiology of endometriosis and adenomyosis.
3. What are common symptoms of endometriosis and adenomyosis?
4. Which diagnostic methods are used to identify endometriosis and adenomyosis?
5. What treatment options are available for managing endometriosis and adenomyosis?
6. How do endometriosis and adenomyosis impact a patient's quality of life?

Answer to Critical Thinking Questions

1. (b) 2. (b) 3. (c) 4. (c) 5. (b)

REFERENCES

1. Abbott, J., & Won, H. R. (2010). Optimal management of chronic cyclical pelvic pain: An evidence-based and pragmatic approach. https://core.ac.uk/download/pdf/8490679.pdf (accessed on 15th June 2025).
2. Adachi, S., Andersson, J., Andrieux, M., Anh, N., Anway, M. D., Archibong, A., et al. (2017). Exposure to the environmental endocrine disruptor TCDD and human reproductive dysfunction: Translating lessons from murine models. https://core.ac.uk/download/46564969.pdf (accessed on 15th June 2025).
3. Albanese, M., Della-Morte, D., Exacoustos, C., Martire, F., et al. (2024). Correlation between endometriosis and migraine features: Results from a prospective case-control study. https://core.ac.uk/download/621339760.pdf (accessed on 15th June 2025).
4. Alexander, P., Popov, A., Koval, A., Fedorov, I., et al. (2020). Benefits of surgical intervention in women with endometriosis-related infertility. https://core.ac.uk/download/322580722.pdf (accessed on 15th June 2025).
5. Anastasi, E., Ballesio, L., Bernardo, S., Fuggetta, F., et al. (2015). Endometriosis: 10 keys points for MRI. https://core.ac.uk/download/54518026.pdf (accessed on 15th June 2025).
6. Andersson, J. (2021). *Adenomyosis: Imaging Features for Diagnosing the Disease and Treatment Effects of Bromocriptine*. https://core.ac.uk/download/427718038.pdf (accessed on 15th June 2025).
7. Azubuike, R. N., & Nwakire, A. O. (2024). Psychological effects of physical and emotional challenges on academic achievement of impaired business education students in the South East Nigeria. *International Journal of Research and Innovation in Social Science*. https://www.semanticscholar.org/paper/b77058184eaa221e155c7cfe3a21d7c582a8c462 (accessed on 15th June 2025).
8. Ball, E., & Khan, K. S. (2020). Recent advances in understanding and managing chronic pelvic pain in women with special consideration to endometriosis. https://core.ac.uk/download/305120038.pdf (accessed on 15th June 2025).
9. Barra, F., Bogliolo, S., Ceccaroni, M., Chiantera, V., et al. (2023). Current medical therapy for adenomyosis: From bench to bedside. https://core.ac.uk/download/590920564.pdf (accessed on 15th June 2025).
10. Bellati, F., Caserta, D., Costanzi, F., De Marco, L., et al. (2018). Real-time virtual sonography in gynecology & obstetrics: Literature's analysis and case series. https://core.ac.uk/download/195777140.pdf (accessed on 15th June 2025).
11. Benli, M., Filleböck, V., Hötker, A. M., Pausch, J., et al. (2024). MRI of pelvic endometriosis: Evaluation of the MR#Enzian classification and the importance of adenomyosis subtypes. https://core.ac.uk/download/611957491.pdf (accessed on 15th June 2025).
12. Bonaccorsi, G., Greco, P., Noventa, M., Pesci, F., et al. (2019). Dye diffusion during laparoscopic tubal patency tests may suggest a lymphatic contribution to dissemination in endometriosis: A prospective, observational study. https://core.ac.uk/download/286075797.pdf (accessed on 15th June 2025).
13. Burla, L., De Wilde, R. L., Imesch, P., Krentel, H., et al. (2024). MRI-based radiomics as a promising noninvasive diagnostic technique for adenomyosis. https://core.ac.uk/download/646220909.pdf (accessed on 15th June 2025).

14. Carmona, F., de Guirior, C., Gracia, M., Martínez-Zamora, M. A., Matas, I., Quintas, L., Rius, M., et al. (2022). Adenomyosis is an independent risk factor for complications in deep endometriosis laparoscopic surgery. https://diposit.ub.edu/dspace/bitstream/2445/206277/1/Adenomyosis%20is%20an%20independent%20risk%20factor%20for%20complications%20in%20deep%20endometriosis%20laparoscopic%20surgery_ScientificReports.pdf (accessed on 15th June 2025).

15. Cetera, G., Tozzi, A. E., Chiappa, V., Castiglioni, I., Merli, C., & Vercellini, P. (2024). Artificial intelligence in the management of women with endometriosis and adenomyosis: Can machines ever be worse than humans? *Journal of Clinical Medicine, 13*. https://www.semanticscholar.org/paper/91107e7387860f8cab63f42ec0eb347f36a2c3dd (accessed on 15th June 2025).

16. Choijiljaw, M., Darmaa, Y., & Sonomjamts, M. (2021). Results of surgical treatment of ovarian endometrioma. https://core.ac.uk/download/617921809.pdf (accessed on 15th June 2025).

17. Damodaran, V. N. (1956). Endometriosis: Clinical and pathological review of 279 personal cases. https://open.bu.edu/bitstream/2144/4431/1/Damodaran_1956_web.pdf (accessed on 15th June 2025).

18. de Boer, A., Huirne, J., Mischi, M., Rees, M., et al. (2023). The influence of uterine abnormalities on uterine peristalsis in the non-pregnant uterus: A systematic review. https://core.ac.uk/download/598997831.pdf (accessed on 15th June 2025).

19. Dedes, I., Eberhard, M., El-Hadad, S., Haeberlin, A., et al. (2023). Physical activity in women with endometriosis: Less or more compared with a healthy control? https://core.ac.uk/download/586766074.pdf (accessed on 15th June 2025).

20. Esmark, A. (2020). *Rediscovering Technocracy. The New Technocracy*. https://www.semanticscholar.org/paper/a3770a246168be923ff74d01e7449965edd6276c (accessed on 15th June 2025).

21. Exacoustos, C., Manganaro, L., & Zupi, E. (2014). Imaging for the evaluation of endometriosis and adenomyosis. https://core.ac.uk/download/pdf/53867255.pdf (accessed on 15th June 2025).

22. Gabriel, M. (2021). ENDOMET database–A means to identify novel diagnostic and prognostic tools for endometriosis. https://core.ac.uk/download/481513731.pdf (accessed on 15th June 2025).

23. Gao, M. (2021). Life course determinants of women's health: From reproductive age to menopause. https://core.ac.uk/download/421727044.pdf (accessed on 15th June 2025).

24. Giudice, L. C., Petraglia, F., Vannuccini, S., Zhai, J., et al. (2020). Adenomyosis: Mechanisms and pathogenesis. https://core.ac.uk/download/573398972.pdf (accessed on 15th June 2025).

25. Guo, Y., Liu, Z., Pan, X., Yang, X., et al. (2023). Histopathological characteristics of adenomyosis: Structure and microstructure. https://core.ac.uk/download/588775825.pdf (accessed on 15th June 2025).

26. Haindl, B. (2011). Belastende Erfahrungen und Ungewissheit bei Endometriose-Patientinnen. https://core.ac.uk/download/11596069.pdf (accessed on 15th June 2025).

27. Hansen, A. (2016). Book review: Elizabeth Lunbeck, *The Americanization of Narcissism. Theory in Action, 9*, 117–124. https://www.semanticscholar.org/paper/9d8ad0f852ba00a114a88daa325c9f7e1db70036 (accessed on 15th June 2025).

28. Holland, M. (2024). Comparing effectiveness of intrauterine devices versus oral contraceptives for management of dysmenorrhea. https://core.ac.uk/download/617013133.pdf (accessed on 15th June 2025).

29. Horne, A. W., & Missmer, S. A. (2022). Pathophysiology, diagnosis, and management of endometriosis. *BMJ*. https://doi.org/10.1136/bmj-2022-070750 (accessed on 15th June 2025).

30. Konda, A., & Kumbhalwar, M. J. (2020). Prevalence of uterine lesions associated with leiomyomas and role of endometrial biopsy in management. https://core.ac.uk/download/539898142.pdf (accessed on 15th June 2025).

31. Kumar, M., Sarma, D. K., Shubham, S., Kumawat, M., Verma, V., Prakash, A., & Tiwari, R. (2020). Environmental endocrine-disrupting chemical exposure: Role in non-communicable diseases. *Frontiers in Public Health, 8*. https://doi.org/10.3389/fpubh.2020.553850 (accessed on 15th June 2025).

32. Li, C., Xu, X., Zhao, X., & Du, B. (2025). The inconsistent pathogenesis of endometriosis and adenomyosis: Insights from endometrial metabolome and microbiome. *mSystems*. https://www.semanticscholar.org/paper/ff184d4c0bc2d913a66da6df48b7f3853dc0db08 (accessed on 15th June 2025).

33. Modak, B. S., Roy, D., Ghosh, T., & Nag, A. C. (2024). Comparison between LNG IUS vs hysterectomy in management of endometriosis. https://core.ac.uk/download/616974710.pdf (accessed on 15th June 2025).

34. Piriyev, E., Schiermeier, S., & Römer, T. (2025). Hormonal treatment of endometriosis: A narrative review. *Pharmaceuticals, 18*. https://www.semanticscholar.org/paper/31f90d96c0484ac5478693a2a256bd4e26336008 (accessed on 15th June 2025).

35. Rumph, J. T., Bruner-Tran, K. L., Osteen, K. G., Ameli, S., et al. (2022). The potential relationship between environmental endocrine disruptor exposure and the development of endometriosis and adenomyosis. https://core.ac.uk/download/492056137.pdf (accessed on 15th June 2025).

36. Zannoni, L. (1982). *Accuratezza Di Nuovi Marker Ecografici Nella Diagnosi di Adenomiosi*. https://core.ac.uk/download/86546557.pdf (accessed on 15th June 2025).

FEMALE GENITAL FISTULAE

5

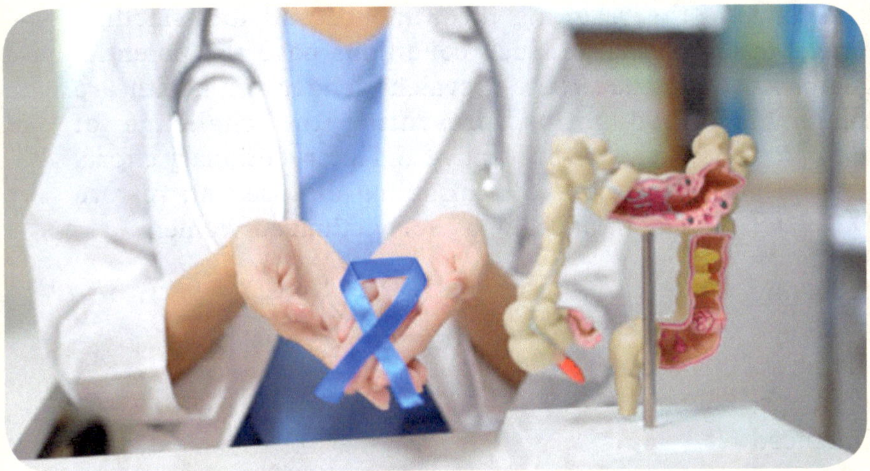

LEARNING OBJECTIVES

After studying this chapter, you will be able to:

1. Analyze the causes of female genital fistulae
2. Identify the symptoms and diagnostic approaches for female genital fistulae
3. Examine the societal and cultural implications of female genital fistulae
4. Evaluate treatment options for female genital fistulae
5. Discuss prevention strategies for female genital fistulae

Introduction

The condition of female genital fistulae is a significant public health issue, and it affects women in low-resource settings primarily. Often resulting from prolonged obstructed labor, fistulas have ruinous health consequences for those with this condition. As much as the medical field is working towards understanding more about the condition, sociocultural factors at play need to be looked into as well. Women suffering from fistulae typically experience stigma and isolation, heightened by inadequate education and a shortage of proper healthcare facilities. Awareness and education are a necessary requirement; failure to follow these will allow the sufferings and neglect to continue uninterrupted. Holistic care of women's healthcare is essential because it guarantees the health and dignity of women who are otherwise relegated to the margins in society. The health implications of female genital fistulae are not only immediate physical agony but also emotional damage. The constant leakage of urine or feces with fistulas tends to lead to social ostracism and decreased quality of life. There are surgical solutions available, but they are frequently not accessible to the individuals who would most benefit from them, especially in rural communities lacking proper medical facilities. As more research continues to shed light on the intricacies of fistula formation and repair, it grows in importance to translate these findings into health care policy. In addition, knowledge about the impact of underlying conditions—such as nutrition and gut microbiome health, as outlined in research that examines skin disorders—can provide rich insights. This data could be used to guide innovative solutions to both the immediate and circumventing impacts of this incapacitating condition (Pessemier et al., 2021).

Creating effective community-based programs and increasing accessibility to healthcare are essential measures in resolving female genital fistulae. Through empowering a collaborative model involving local healthcare workers and worldwide organizations, sustainable solutions can be created. Enhanced training of healthcare professionals and midwives is at the core of prevention against the occurrence of fistula during labor, as early treatment can prevent delivery complications. Second, increased public awareness can demystify the condition and eliminate the stigmatization that has encroached on it. Lastly, any attempt to combat and prevent female genital fistulae must engage all segments of society, with particular emphasis on education and global access to proper health care services. These interventions not only promote the well-being of affected women but also facilitate a better understanding of women's health issues in general (Ingram et al., 2018).

Definition of Female Genital Fistulae

Female genital fistulae, specifically obstetric fistulae, occur as a tragic consequence of prolonged obstructed labor and lead to a tract between the vagina and the bladder or the rectum. The condition occurs predominantly in environments with limited resources, where delayed and appropriate obstetric care is not accessible. It is a pathological connection between the two organs. Female genital fistulae induce severe physical morbidity as well as severe social and psychological disability. Obstetric fistula patients are more likely to endure stigmatization, exclusion, and rejection by their families and communities due to the resulting incontinence and foul-smelling discharge. Such conditions have the potential to exacerbate prevalent gender and healthcare inequalities, presenting the challenge of extensive preventive and interventionary efforts to correct this disabling disease and restore health and dignity for victimized women.

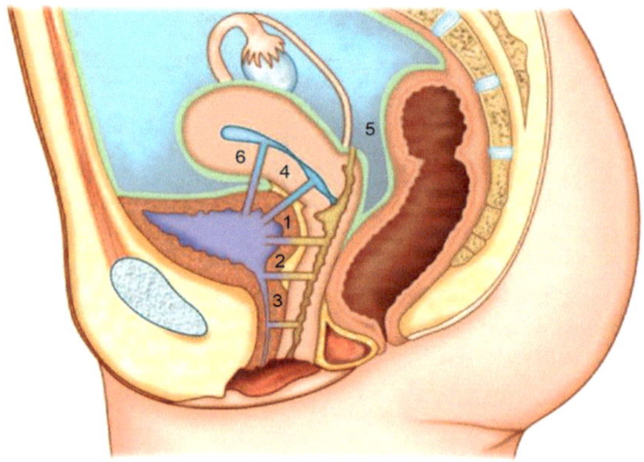

Figure 5.1. Types of genitourinary fistula—(1) Vesicovaginal (2) Vesicourethrovaginal(3) Urethrovaginal (4) Vesicocervical (5) Ureterovaginal (6) Vesicouterine.

Source: https://oshimu.com/wp-content/uploads/2021/07/Gynaecology-DC-Dutta.pdf

The impact of female genital fistulae reaches beyond the individual to families and communities in general. The original complications of this condition significantly disable women's participation in social and economic life. For instance, fistula women lose their employment due to a lack of ability to maintain hygiene, which disempowers their economic autonomy and independence. Additionally, the presence of a fistula may deter potential husbands, resulting in diminished marriage opportunities, perpetuating poverty, and gender inequalities. Treatment of female genital fistulae is not only the diagnosis and treatment of the affected women but also a greater social dedication to enhancing women's health care, maternity services, and community education to avert this avoidable disorder.

These integrated strategies highlight the necessity for social support systems to be merged with health interventions in order to offset the ill effects of obstetric fistula. Prevention of female genital fistulae depends on having trained healthcare professionals and easy access to obstetric care at the time of delivery. As highlighted in more recent studies, effective interventions can significantly reduce the incidence of this condition, especially where the issue is most prominent. For instance, well-informed birth attendants can identify women at risk during childbirth and facilitate the timely use of medical care to prevent obstructed labor, the primary cause of fistulae. Community-based programs focusing on maternal health education and access to timely medical care are also central to prevention. Additionally, alleviation of poverty and improvement in access to healthcare overall can enable a scenario under which outcomes of maternal health are optimized. Lastly, prevention and management of female genital fistulae call for a response that is multidimensional and involves education, socio-economic support, and accessible healthcare to protect and empower vulnerable groups (Al-Riyami et al., 2013; Ngoma et al., 2011).

Historical Context and Prevalence

The history of women's genital fistula is a complex intersection of socio-economic factors, healthcare access, and cultural practices. Female genital fistula is most frequently associated with complications at delivery, a condition that is highly endemic in low- and middle-income environments. In these environments, the unavailability of professional birth attendants and inadequate health infrastructure guarantees prolonged labor and the development of fistula. Historical records validate that obstetric fistulas have been an enduring issue through generations, predominantly among rural women, where culturally fostered birth traditions take priority over medically facilitated deliveries. As more world attention is devoted to improving maternal health, particularly through initiatives like the Sustainable Development Goals, further disparities between high and low-income nations emerge that must be addressed through context-specific interventions based on history and current realities in healthcare. The prevalence of female genital fistulae is a direct indicator of healthcare disparities within different regions. In poor settings, studies have shown that 1-2% of women who have survived prolonged obstructed labor are likely to develop a fistula, which dramatically affects their quality of life. However, a different etiologic pattern in better-income settings has been observed where fistulae predominantly arise as a consequence of surgical interventions rather than obstetric complications. This latter prevalence suggests the advances in medical care and surgery that are not present in resource-limited settings. Success rates in systematic reviews are indicated to be around 80% to 90% in low-income settings but as high as 95% in affluent settings, indicating differential access to quality care and efficient surgical techniques, thus highlighting the need for improved training and healthcare facilities in underdeveloped regions (Hilton et al., 2019). Recent efforts to address female genital fistulae have gained momentum through policy reforms and medical programs to ensure reproductive health services. One such example is Kenya's National Adolescent Sexual and Reproductive Health Policy, which is a joint initiative to integrate the needs of adolescent women into the national health agenda in recognition of the importance of reproductive health training and access. They aim not only to reduce the incidence of fistulae but also to promote the empowerment of women by way of education and wealth generation as laid out in Vision 2030. By emphasizing the link between socio-economic determinants, education, and health outcomes, the stakeholders are challenged to integrate a broader strategy to address fistulae and reproductive health-related complications, thereby working towards a world where all women have access to necessary healthcare services and the opportunity for a successful pregnancy (Ministry of Kenya, 2015).

Importance of Addressing the Issue

Treating the female genital fistulae condition is significant not only for the physical well-being of the individuals affected but also for the social well-being of communities. The disabling disorder, most often resulting from obstructed labor prolonged over a period of time, has devastating physical and social consequences on a woman's life. Women with fistulae are typically shunned and stigmatized, and this leads to psychological trauma and economic loss. Understanding the social determinants of this health condition is essential because it draws attention to the necessity of integrated healthcare solutions in the form of eradicating poverty and providing education for women. Through expanding health agendas that place maternal health at the top, such as ending female genital fistulae and advancing girls' secondary education, societies must benefit from improved overall well-being and greater resilience within communities (Temin et al., 2009). Furthermore, prevention interventions for preventing female genital fistulae are of utmost significance in ending this public health condition. The research conducted on Vesicovagina Fistula (VVF) in nations like Zambia highlights the importance of professional caregivers during childbirth. By identifying vulnerable women and introducing education at the community level, doctors can significantly reduce the prevalence of fistulae. According to these studies, prevention should shift towards making maternity services and emergency obstetric care stronger. As societies invest in health care and education that increase the accessibility of health care, they are also combating the root causes of fistulae. All this highlights that an interdisciplinary method, involving health care and social education, is necessary to address the complexity within this issue (Ngoma et al., 2011). Lastly, the discussion around female genital fistulae cannot rule out addressing the contribution of community engagement and increased awareness. Efforts aimed at addressing this issue have to involve not just health systems but also surrounding communities, as evidenced by the importance of community members and leaders in promoting women's health rights. This involves striving to create such enabling environments where women can seek medical care without stigma. It is important to mobilize communities around sexual and reproductive health issues in order to promote a culture of prevention and care. Through learning and sensitization, the cycle of silence on fistulae can be broken, leading to improved health and social rehabilitation of the affected women. The eradication of female genital fistulae is therefore not a matter of medicine but a social issue that needs to be addressed urgently with concerted effort.

5.1. Causes of Female Genital Fistulae

Learning Outcome

1. Discuss the obstetric complications of female genital fistulae
2. Define sexual violence and trauma
3. Understand the surgical errors and medical negligence

The causes of female genital fistulae are numerous and can significantly impact women's health in low-resource settings. Of the significant causes, obstructed labor of several hours is common, frequently in the form of a woman not receiving early treatment when delivering. This can cause extensive tissue damage to create an open tract between the vaginal canal and bladder or rectum. In addition, intraoperative and postoperative monitoring are augmented in the case of hemorrhage. Complications of surgery after procedures such as cesarean sections also result in fistula formation, thus requiring competent health care workers. Sociocultural dynamics that typically precede high maternal morbidity rates also complicate issues, with minimal access to obstetric care enhancing the likelihood of hazardous birthing routines.

Thus, knowledge about the complexity of causative factors is very important in devising potent interventions. Other than obstructed labor, other forms of trauma are also involved in genital fistula causation. Trauma related to rape and injury from accidents accounts for extremely high rates of fistula occurrence among the affected individuals. Traumatic injury caused by traditional healers, with which some societies are well-endowed, has been noted to be a leading risk factor for fistula formation (Barr-Walker et al., 2025). These practices may be informed by extremely entrenched beliefs regarding childbearing and health, which stress the importance of culturally effective education in healthcare.

Further, unsafe abortion and the infection complications, including those comprising HIV-related infections, can generate severe reproductive health complications, including fistulae development. The extensive understanding of such traumatic causes is consequently fundamental to targeted preventative measures. Female genital fistulae are also linked to a number of socio-economic factors, including poverty and illiteracy. Women living in poor areas are prone to their access to quality care restricted, thus increasing the rate of fistula from preventable causes.

The psychological impacts that arise from stigma in fistula tend to worsen the issues faced by such women, such as social isolation and diminished economic support prospects (Barr-Walker et al., 2025). Furthermore, the convergence of gender, disability, and economic insecurity demonstrates the range of addressing this public health condition. Education-focused and health-care-access-supporting interventions are important in deterring fistulae incidence. Overall, the answer to female genital fistulae causes is multi-dimensional and involves healthcare, education, and community participation for improving the women's quality of life with this condition.

5.1.1. Obstetric Complications

The incidence of obstetric complications, in this case, obstetric fistulae, is a major maternal health and quality of care indicator across various regions in the world. Obstetric fistula is a condition that turns a woman's life for the worse after prolonged labor, typically exacerbated by poor access to quality obstetric care. The challenge of diagnosing and treating obstetric fistula is also worsened by scarce data, which previously limited our understanding of its incidence and impact. A systematic review gives a pooled prevalence of 0.29 per 1,000 women of childbearing age in all regions in aggregate, and data, especially in sub-Saharan Africa, give a high incidence of 1.57 per 1,000 women. Such incidences give testimony to the need for improved access to healthcare and preventatives to diminish the chances of such life-threatening complications (Al-Riyami et al., 2013).

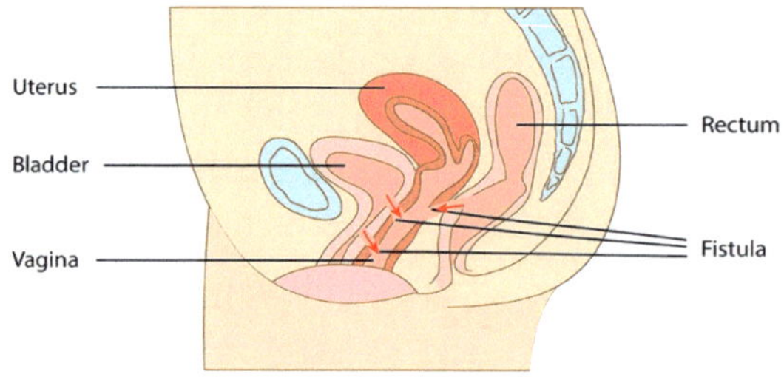

Figure 5.2. Obstetric Fistula.

Source: https://strapi.merillife.com/uploads/diz_E_Fkp5_OGH_0v_RLI_Ku_PJ_b2931bf48d.jpg

In other cases, the diagnosis and management of obstetric complications, including fistulae, are often a precursor to issues that are indicative of systemic vulnerabilities within the healthcare system. Despite improved facility-based births, a Mozambican study reported an incidence of 1.1 cases per 1,000 recently pregnant women. It supports evidence that even when there is improved birth rates at facilities, diagnostic delays and referral for surgical repair remain issues. The findings point to the need to address third delays in care urgently, where efficient health delivery systems can significantly contribute to maternal outcomes.

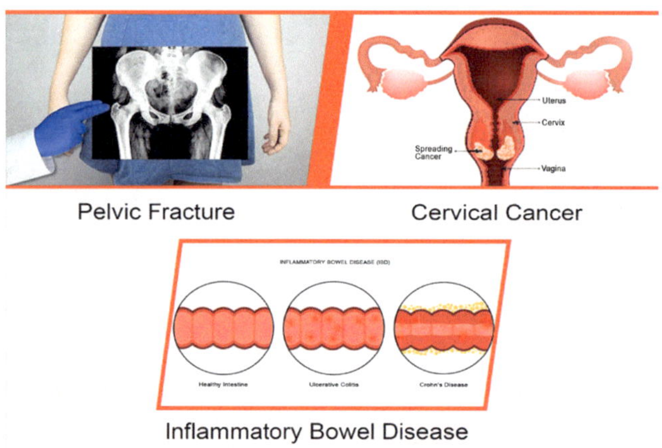

Figure 5.3. Causes of obstetric fistula.

Source: https://images.medindia.net/patientinfo/950_400/obstetric-fistula-causes.jpg

As in the above cases, the incidence of obstetric fistulae calls for an integrated response involving effective training of health workers, early referral systems, and more awareness of obstetric complications (Bergström et al., 2017). Finally, resolving obstetric complications is imperative in order to improve maternal health outcomes and in relation to the occurrence of conditions like obstetric fistulae. Notwithstanding increased access to healthcare services in certain areas, systemic barriers put women at risk during delivery. Complications, normally resulting from the failure of timely and appropriate medical treatment, speak volumes about the necessity of integrated maternal healthcare strategies. Making skilled birth attendants and high-level obstetric services available can sharply limit the incidence of disabling effects like fistulae. Thorough education and training of the health workers, along with the creation of support systems within the community, are essential strategies. It becomes achievable with these measures to reduce the obstetric complication workload and ultimately ensure healthier futures for women at risk (Al-Riyami et al., 2013; Bergström et al., 2017).

5.1.2. Sexual Violence and Trauma

The interaction of trauma and sexual violence in the context of female genital fistulae is an urgent public health issue that needs close scrutiny. Fistula most commonly results from obstructed labor of prolonged duration, a frequent occurrence in settings with a lack of adequate emergency obstetric care, particularly in sub-Saharan Africa. Women who experience such traumatic births tend to endure not only physical injury but also the psychological weight of rape, either during labor or as a consequence of stigma in society once a fistula develops. The evidence highlighted indicates the enormous mental health consequences, including higher levels of anxiety and depression, that affect about 65% and 52% of fistula patients, respectively (Barr-Walker et al., 2025). These traumatic events underscore the importance of health system interventions that are one and treat both the physical and psychological dimensions of any intervention that seeks to remove the burden of fistula from affected women. Stigma related to female genital fistulae further accumulates trauma among survivors. This stigma manifests in numerous ways, such as enacted, internalized, and anticipated stigma, each of which is part of a horrific cycle of social rejection and psychological distress. The stigma effect is high, with reported 35% divorce rates, illustrating the way in which social attitudes lead to deterioration in family and support systems (Barr-Walker et al., 2025). Women thus turn to such coping mechanisms as withdrawal into themselves, increasing hopelessness, as well as inviting more contact with the health service. In a bid to limit such effects, community-based services that target education and support are necessary. Such strategies can help dismantle existing stigmas and promote social acceptability, hence promoting recovery and reintegration of fistula-affected women. Secondly, prevention of female genital fistulae must be addressed as part of the comprehensive prevention of sexual violence and trauma. Prevention of obstetric fistula demands integrated solutions that include, for example, enhanced education of mothers, enhanced access to health services, and raised awareness of the necessity for early obstetric intervention. As demonstrated in some research from Zambia, medical workers play a crucial role in identifying risk-carrying women during delivery, and this can frequently reduce the incidence of fistula. Interventions must extend far beyond the clinic walls to encompass community-based education programs that combat poverty and champion women's health rights. When properly carried out, these will not only relieve physical suffering but have the capacity to restore hope and dignity to sexually victimized women, thus healing physical and psychological trauma caused by sexual violence and its impacts.

5.1.3. Surgical Errors and Medical Negligence

The issue of surgical errors and medical negligence is particularly relevant in the context of female genital fistulae, an illness that normally arises due to substandard obstetric care. Women experiencing prolonged obstructed labor often require surgery for fistula closure, but issues may arise as a result of errors in such interventions. These errors not only endanger the immediate well-being of the patients but also can exacerbate the long-term psychological and social sequelae of the disease. In poorer settings, as in Niger, where the prevalence of obstetric fistula is very high due to poverty compounded by reduced availability of skilled birth attendants, the risk of surgical errors is significantly increased. Hence, addressing the systemic issues of healthcare, like the training of healthcare workers and the implementation of safety protocols, is crucial to lowering the incidence of surgical negligence and enhancing the outcomes of patients (Heller et al., 2015).

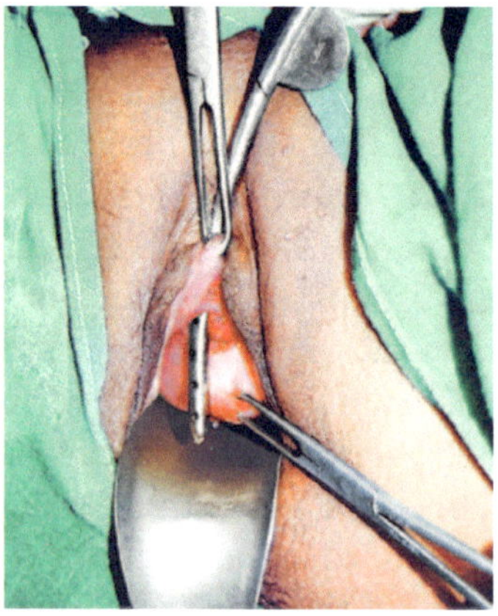

Figure 5.4. Midvaginal obstetric fistula (VVF). It was of moderate size to allow a metal catheter which is clearly visible.

Source: https://oshimu.com/wp-content/uploads/2021/07/Gynaecology-DC-Dutta.pdf

Further, the complexity of surgical errors, in this instance, of female genital fistulae, extends beyond individual events to encompass general systemic loopholes in the health system. A case in point is women's facilities and infrastructural shortfalls leading to rushed or improperly performed surgeries. These shortfalls, in turn, are typically supplemented by a lack of interdisciplinary comprehension, which is essential in addressing the multidimensionality of obstetrics. As in recent medical discourse, multidisciplinary teams can significantly enhance patient care through the provision of integrated solutions tailored to the subtle issues the patient with multiple comorbidities poses (N/A, 2022). In obstetric fistula, however, inadequate communication among medical professionals results in lost chances at early intervention and successful repair through surgery, thereby keeping the cycle of medical error and inadequacy going. The social effect of iatrogenic surgical failure should not be exaggerated, particularly among women who have fistulae. Ignorance on the part of surgeons may lead to long-term health problems, like repeated incontinence, which not only has physical repercussions but also a significant number of social implications. Women may be ostracized or secluded due to their condition, a situation that brings mental suffering as well as physical suffering. This conflation of medical negligence and social impact underscores the necessity of an integrated healthcare model that identifies the psychological, social, and medical components of patient care. Educating communities about fistulae and empowering women who have been affected by surgical negligence are key components of a broader system to develop resilience and restore dignity in the lives of such women (Heller et al., 2015).

Test Your Knowledge

1. What are common obstetric complications that can lead to female genital fistulae?
2. How is sexual violence and trauma related to the development of genital fistulae?

5.2. Symptoms and Diagnosis

Learning Outcome

1. Explain the physical symptoms of female genital fistulae
2. Define the psychological impact
3. Discuss the diagnostic procedures

The clinical presentation of female genital fistulae is often characterized by a range of troublesome signs and symptoms that are bound to undermine the quality of life of a woman. Some of the most common symptoms are persistent urine or fecal leakage, likely to lead to penetration of moisture through clothing and skin irritation, thus further causing social stigma and psychological morbidity. Other women may also experience recurrent urinary tract infections or pelvic chronic pain that can complicate diagnosis. Because the signs of these fistulae can be confused with other gynecologic disorders, healthcare workers face difficulties in accurately diagnosing female genital fistulae without rigorous investigations and accurate evaluation. The spectrum of symptom presentation varies with the type of fistula and its location, and hence, thorough evaluation must be done to rule out other pathologies such as pelvic inflammatory disease or sexually transmitted diseases. Diagnosis is typically a combination of clinical assessment and high-technology imaging techniques. A thorough gynecologic exam is necessary, where the clinician assesses the pelvic area for abnormal discharge, inflammation, or previous surgical scars that might suggest fistula formation. Imaging modalities such as ultrasonography and magnetic resonance imaging (MRI) have crucial roles to play in making a firm diagnosis, particularly in determining the extent of the injury and its impact on adjacent organs. Diagnostic interventions may also involve urinalysis and cystoscopy to determine urinary function and the presence of fistulous tracts. These subtle diagnostic methods should be employed to provide a correct picture of the patient's status, directing subsequent management plans towards healing the fistula and restoring function.

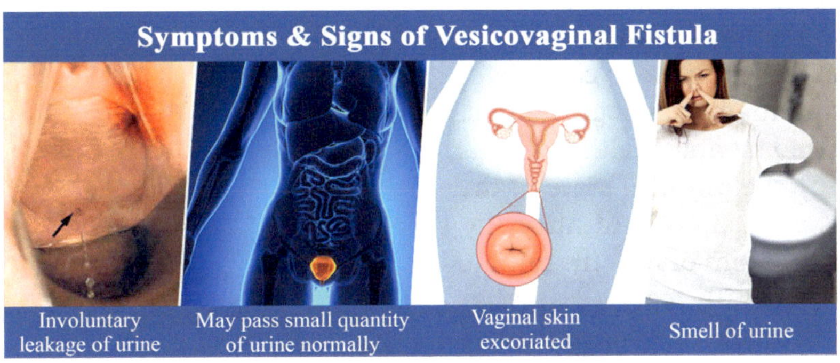

Figure 5.5. Symptoms and signs of vesicovaginal fistula.

Source: https://www.medindia.net/images/common/patientinfo/950_400/symptoms-and-signs-of-vesicovaginal-fistula.jpg

Comorbid condition filling data complicates the diagnostic picture for female genital fistulae still further. The overlapping of female genital schistosomiasis and fistula formation, for instance, indicates the challenge of diagnosing these disorders in the context of global health. The underdiagnosis of female genital schistosomiasis and its comorbidities with sexual health disorders such as HIV and HPV puts a premium on creating dynamic diagnostic systems that cure multiple disorders simultaneously. Misunderstanding the burden of female genital fistulae and comorbidities can lead to delayed diagnoses and treatment failures, thus accelerating patient morbidity and obstructed recovery channels. Thus, creation of awareness and enhancing diagnostic capabilities are essential in addressing infected women's health needs and improving overall reproductive health outcomes.

5.2.1. Physical Symptoms

The physical symptoms resulting from female genital fistulae are expressed as severe and painful conditions with a great effect on the quality of a woman's life. Persistent leakage of urine or fecal content is one of the primary symptoms due to the pathological fistulous communication between the genital tract and the urinary or gastrointestinal tracts. This leakage most commonly leads to shame and social isolation due to the smell and the personal hygiene problems that the condition creates. In addition to its physical effects, these symptoms may create extreme psychological distress, typically with the social stigma of the condition. Based on reports, health and gender cross over with stigma, enhancing the psychological effect and negatively impacting mental health, which is usually exacerbated by the physical state of the fistula itself (Richens et al., 2004). Additionally, the physical symptoms involved in female genital fistulae are generally carried further than leakage alone. Women may be suffering from chronic urinary tract infections due to the continuous introduction of pathogens into the vaginal environment. In addition, there may be a disruption in the menstrual cycle, affecting a woman's reproductive health and causing inadequacy and hopelessness. Painful sexual intercourse can also occur, further hampering intimacy and relationships. Severe long-term consequences in the form of bladder and kidney damage can occur if prompt intervention is not taken. The complex interaction of such bodily symptoms has a significant impact on women's social relationships and their ability to engage meaningfully in their societies, requiring the imperative medical care as well as social support interventions for treating not only the medical but also the psychological dimension of the disease (Richens et al., 2004).

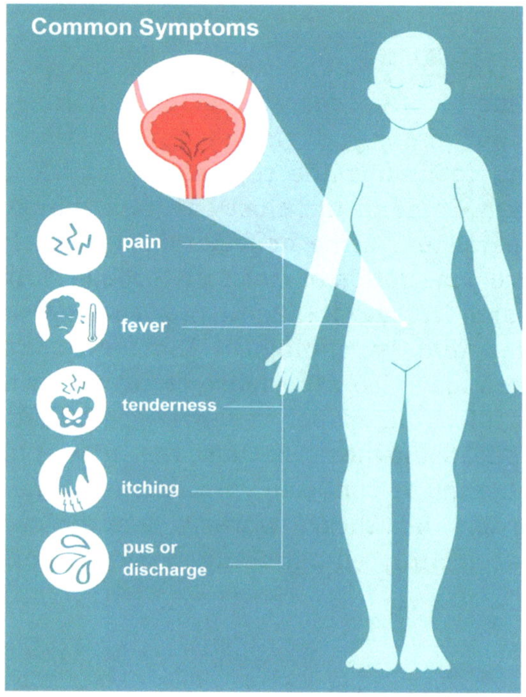

Figure 5.6. Common Symptoms of fistulae.

Source: https://www.verywellhealth.com/what-is-a-fistula-1941776

The treatment of the combination of physical symptoms needs an integrated treatment approach that incorporates medical treatment, psychological therapy, and community-level education. Clinical interventions that address the obstetric injuries causing fistulae can ease the severe physical symptoms. It is also crucial, however, to include mental health interventions to counteract the stigma and discrimination found in patients as a result of the disease. Epidemiological studies suggest that social support plays a protective role against physical symptoms of fistula and its stigma (Barr-Walker et al., 2025). Therefore, intervention of the impact of physical symptoms on female genital fistulae should include collaboration between healthcare providers, mental health professionals, and the community at the local level to enhance resilience and empower traumatized women to heal and emotionally rehabilitate.

5.2.2. Psychological Impact

The psychological impact of female genital fistulae is profound and intricate, pervasively affecting a woman's overall mental health and quality of life. Women with this affliction frequently experience not only the physical repercussions of their wounds but also heightened levels of stigma and discrimination by their communities. The prevalence of such mental illnesses as depression and anxiety among the victims is appalling, with depression at 65% and anxiety at 52% (Barr-Walker et al., 2025). The psychosocial distress is primarily due to loneliness owing to social misconceptions about fistulae, which further leads to emotional suffering that might disrupt social interaction and economic empowerment. With women presenting to have fistula repair, the trajectory of their psychosocial health is a relevant area to study. Findings indicate that while most experience significant improvement in both physical and psychosocial health following surgery, there are some residual psychological challenges. For instance, overall quality of life and self-esteem notably improve in the first six months following surgery, yet some women continue to experience negative self-image and the residue of stigma (Barageine et al., 2019). What these findings suggest is that while physical correction in the form of surgery is essential, an integrated approach that looks to the psychological impact is also needed for complete healing. Interventions that deconstruct the psychological burden of female genital fistulae are necessary to enhance the quality of life of affected women. According to research, social support has an important effect in minimizing feelings of stigmatization and enhancing mental well-being during recovery (Barr-Walker et al., 2025). This notwithstanding, existing literature shows that targeted interventions that have been designed to minimize clinical and community-level stigma of fistulae do not exist. Through developing programs based on psychological support and reintegration into communities, healthcare professionals can offer essential services outside of physical healing, creating a conducive environment for resilience and recovery in affected groups (Barageine et al., 2019). All this is needed to make sure that women with fistulae are physically healed but also equipped with the necessary psychological care to thrive.

5.2.3. Diagnostic Procedures

Diagnosis of female genital fistula is typically a problematic procedure, primarily due to the multifaceted nature of the condition and the diversity of presenting symptoms. The first investigations may involve a thorough clinical history and general physical examination, with a focus on eliciting relevant obstetric history, especially labor complications. Urinary incontinence or fecal seepage, along with chronic vaginal discharge, are often encountered. However, such symptoms can be common with other gynecologic diseases, and hence, the diagnosis is cumbersome. Advanced imaging modalities such as ultrasound and MRI are of critical significance in determining the extent and the point at which the fistula extends, thus assisting in a proper diagnosis. While tests in the laboratory are not as definitive in fistula diagnosis, they do serve to rule out concomitant infections or complications that are common in obstetric practice, so that a treatment plan that considers the patient's overall condition and health may be developed. In certain cases, female genital tuberculosis may cause similar symptoms to a fistula, resulting in a diagnostic challenge. For instance, upon evaluating a patient with nonspecific symptoms such as abdominal pain and weight loss, clinicians can initially examine malignancy, as was highlighted in a case study where the woman came in with abnormal cancer antigen levels and ascites (Alves et al., 2016). However, subsequent diagnostic procedures like CT scan and MRI concluded that a biopsy was necessary to determine the underlying causative organism – *Mycobacterium tuberculosis*, in this case. This is critical in ensuring that appropriate diagnostic procedures are employed to differentiate fistulae from other concomitant confounding lesions. A proper estimation of the root cause is not only important for effective treatment but also for preventing subsequent complications, underscoring the significance of competent practitioners in regions hardest affected by fistula prevalence. The consequences of incompetent diagnosis on women suffering from fistulae extend beyond their health and have implications for broader public health outcomes.

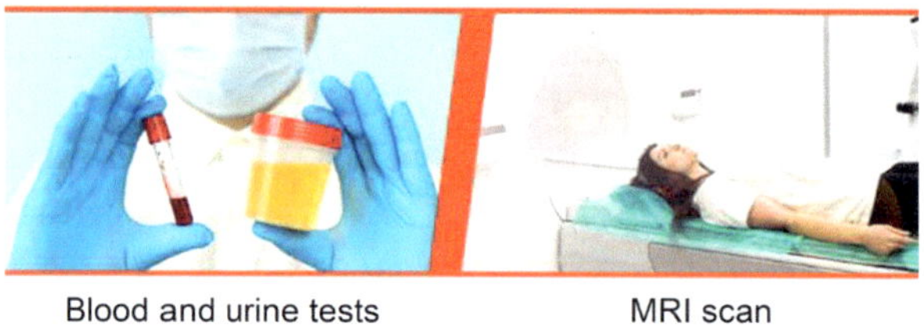

Figure 5.7. Diagnosis of Obstetric Fistula.

Source: https://www.medindia.net/health/conditions/obstetric-fistula.htm

A Guinean longitudinal study has revealed that recurrent fistulas are perilous even after repair, and recurrence and complications such as residual urinary incontinence rates are alarmingly high (Barry et al., 2017). This confirms the extreme importance of ongoing assessment and post-op follow-up within the diagnostic process. Additionally, the association of the occurrence of fistula with other adverse pregnancy outcomes like stillbirth and maternal mortality creates further burdens to healthcare systems in resource-poor settings. Thus, having integrated diagnostic approaches, alongside preventive measures, will most probably be the core to successful addressing of female genital fistulae, in that women affected by the condition have their well-being safeguarded and subsequent generations are endowed with better maternal health experiences.

Test Your Knowledge

1. How does female genital fistula affect the psychological well-being of patients?
2. What diagnostic procedures are used to identify female genital fistulae?

5.3. Societal and Cultural Implications

Learning Outcome

1. Discuss the stigmatization of affected women
2. Identify the impact on family and community dynamics
3. Define cultural beliefs and misconceptions

The cultural and social implications of female genital fistulae are vast, highly gendered, and entrenched in health disparities. In the majority of regions, particularly in sub-Saharan Africa and parts of Asia, community perceptions of women's bodies have a powerful influence on their health. Fistulae, typically resulting from obstructed labor or female genital mutilation, are stigmatized conditions that affect not only the physical health but also the long-term social status of women. The afflicted women are typically confronted with social isolation, marital problems, and limited access to healthcare, representing a dire crossroads of gender and health. Interventions to address these issues must consider the cultural discourses on women's health, and the stigmas that surround diagnoses such as fistulae, which can add to the mental and emotional distress that ensues for those who suffer from them (Broussard et al., 2008). Culturally, female genital cutting (FGC), but more widely known as female genital mutilation (FGM), can be simply accounted for by traditions and beliefs long established that prioritize male authority over female bodies. FGM comes with many health complications, including obstetric fistula, further solidifying its ruinous nature. Although prevalence is gradually declining in some areas, particularly in nations like Nigeria, where social norms still reinforce the same, it is a denial of women's rights and healthcare. The controversy surrounding FGM and its aftermath depicts the necessity for cultural competence in empowering interventions that also challenge adverse traditions. Understanding the cultural roots of fistulae can facilitate the creation of targeted public health interventions that not only treat but also prevent the onset of these disabling conditions (Emelumadu et al., 2018).

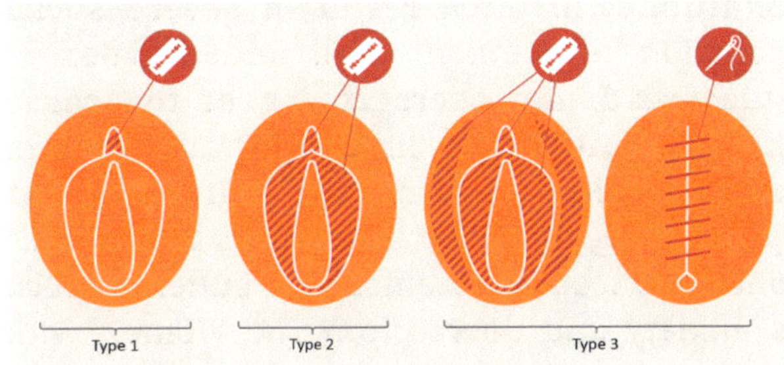

Figure 5.8. Female genital mutilation.

Source: https://codeblue.galencentre.org/wp-content/uploads/2019/02/FGM_types_.png

In the development of a society in which women's health becomes the central issue, it is important to implement educational activities that redefine cultural attitudes toward women's independence. Mobilization programs among communities for the deconstruction of stigma over fistulae and FGM have been successful in fostering awareness and discussion. By putting women's experiences with fistulae on the public health agenda, organizations can advocate policy that not only minimizes the short-term health impact but also seeks to reverse the sociocultural factors fueling the issues. Secondly, multidisciplinary coalitions between health care providers, community leaders, and legislators need to be implemented in a way that creates an infrastructure that promotes women's reproductive well-being and acts against destructive practices. To this end, change in society requires a multifaceted intervention to bridge the gap between healthcare access and cultural acceptability to comprehensively address the implications of female genital fistulae (Broussard et al., 2008; Emelumadu et al., 2018).

5.3.1. Stigmatization of Affected Women

The stigmatization of women with female genital fistula is an entrenched social issue that transcends individual suffering. The condition will often result in severe social exclusion of women, with added woes of widespread misunderstanding of the cause and implications of fistula. Fistula women often experience internalized stigma and end up believing that they themselves caused this condition, leading to emotional suffering such as anxiety and depression. The women with fistula are further stigmatized as unclean or broken, thus further marginalizing them, and typically resulting in the disintegration of their social networks and support systems. The stigma comes in three forms—enacted stigma, internalized stigma, and structural stigma—that not only extend to the women but also to their families and communities, perpetuating cycles of discrimination and exclusion (Barr-Walker et al., 2025). Also, the implications of such stigmatization are brutally evident in the daily lives of such women. It has been established through studies that a significant percentage of women suffering from fistula are forced to endure divorce or separation, triggered by social rejection and shame following their condition, and with composite prevalence rates for divorce/ separation as high as 35% (Barr-Walker et al., 2025).

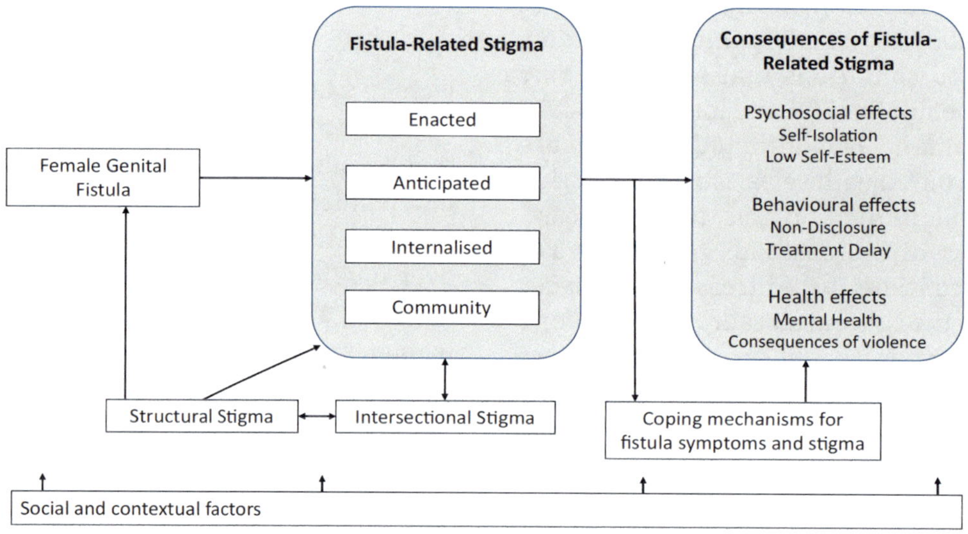

Figure 5.9. Conceptual framework for fistula-related stigma.

Source: https://www.researchgate.net/figure/Conceptual-framework-for-fistula-related-stigma_fig1_332778174

This abandonment not only impacts their psychological condition but also their financial position. Employment opportunities are not exempt, either, as women tend to be ostracized and cannot seek employment due to societal perception of their condition. The isolation that this induces can be a vicious cycle, with less interaction and support serving only to strengthen their isolated position. Awareness and education efforts on fistula issues are critical in dispelling such negative narratives and promoting social support for the women afflicted with fistula. Multifaceted interventions involving clinical and community-based interventions are necessary to eliminate stigma on female genital fistulae. While there is emphasis on effective stigma interventions from the literature, none of them have been systematically rolled out within the clinical practice framework (Barr-Walker et al., 2025). Such interventions would work towards developing a tolerant environment where fistula and the stigma of it are made normal and its psychological impact is worked upon. Community programs may also work towards improving support systems, which research has found to be a buffer against the impact of stigma and also towards greater mental health improvement. By interacting with society's sentiment and provoking honest dialogue in terms of diversity and health, stakeholders can work toward reducing stigma, thus significantly improving the lives of women who have fistula.

5.3.2. Impact on Family and Community Dynamics

The effect of female genital fistulae reaches far beyond the woman, having a strong impact on family and community life. In most cultures, fistula is stigmatized, resulting in the social exclusion of affected women. Social exclusion creates fissures within families, usually ending in the collapse of support systems at the family level. Statistics indicate that up to 35% of women who experience fistulae experience divorce or separation, not only destabilizing family life but also further burdening such women's mental health and economic status. The psychological impacts, besides heightened anxiety and depression, only help to deter women from engaging in familial and communal responsibilities, which ultimately destroys the very fabric of family care that is so crucial during recovery. These disruptions underscore the need for community education and supportive interventions to roll back the stigma surrounding fistulae and reestablish family ties. Community function is also significantly affected by the incidence of female genital fistulae because such a health condition reflects gender attitudes in society and attitudes towards health. Internalization of stigma in society leads to a widespread misconstrual of fistula and affects both the available treatment and the overall support system for fistula patients. Evidence supports the fact that social support has the capacity to buffer against the negative outcomes of stigma, reinforcing the importance of community-based interventions for the treatment of health conditions like fistulae. Furthermore, the intersection of stigma of infertility, disability, gender, and poverty complicates a complex array of social issues that undermine community cohesion. Enhanced comprehension and accommodation can be achieved by using wide-ranging awareness campaigns to address such stigmas. An integrated community strategy is thus imperative in addressing deeply entrenched stigmas and enabling the enhanced quality of life for women with fistulae. Further, the effect of female genital fistulae is not merely socioeconomic or psychological but also demands broader conceptual shifts within society in attitudes to sexual and reproductive health. Again, like the atypical genitalia and disorders of sex development (DSD) conditions, there is a focus on the need for multidisciplinary management, suggesting that specialist referral can assist families with dealing with these issues. The education obtained through effective clinical practices can motivate communities and parents to learn how to co-exist with changing social expectations regarding diversity and tolerance. With the shift in perspectives regarding gender and health, particularly at the local level, the harmonization of data collection for orphan diseases is critically needed. Through the creation of a supra-registry for exchange of clinical data, communities are able to create a stronger evidence-based platform for social services that are built to reduce stigma and improve quality of life for women with fistulae, and ultimately re-integrate these patients into society.

5.3.3. Cultural Beliefs and Misconceptions

Cultural beliefs and misconceptions form the core of the existence and formation of female genital fistulae, particularly in developing nations where traditional practices are more paramount than medical knowledge. For example, social and economic circumstances are major contributory factors to the existence of obstetric vesico-vaginal fistula. In Nigeria, research highlights the relevance of effective communication interventions that engage men in maternal health issues, whose opinions are not thoroughly examined despite playing a decisive role in the health outcomes of the family and community (Ebeze et al., 2015). Without the destruction of misconceptions regarding women's health issues, it fosters cyclical ignorance that deters the development of medical treatment and the well-being of women afflicted with fistulae. Furthermore, cultural traditions such as female circumcision complicate the issue of fistulae and attest to deep beliefs around women's bodies and sexuality. In Somalia, where rates of circumcision are near-universal, challenging health consequences can arise, including increased risks of childbirth complications often leading to fistulae (Tatah et al., 2016). Such practices are usually explained away by social convention and uninformed assumptions about hygiene and fertility, and highlighting the necessity of comprehensive education that discourages such myths. The necessity to correct such myths is essential, as it not only affects the health of individual women but also collective societal attitudes on women's rights and access to healthcare. It is only by dispelling these cultural myths and beliefs that effective prevention and care of female genital fistulae can be obtained. Merging education, advocacy, and community mobilization with a multi-component intervention will decrease harmful practices and cause better habits. Interventions that aim to engage men in maternal health issues can be effective vehicles for change, building acceptance and support from communities (Ebeze et al., 2015). Further, the education of women with accurate information about their bodies and reproductive health can combat the culture of stigma around conditions like fistulae and prompt cultural attitude shifts. Only through a nuanced recognition of the intersection of culture, health, and rights can we hope to bring an end to the suffering of victims of fistulae and such conditions.

Test Your Knowledge

1. What impact can female genital fistulae have on family and community dynamics?
2. How do cultural beliefs and misconceptions influence the perception and treatment of female genital fistulae?

5.4. Treatment Options

Learning Outcome

1. Understand the surgical Interventions and non-surgical Management
2. Describe the role of rehabilitation and support services

Proper management of female genital fistulae is predominantly symbolized by surgery, which plays a central role in the maintenance of normal anatomy and function. Surgical closure is often the definitive treatment, aiming to close the fistula while maintaining covering tissue. Trained surgeons utilize several techniques depending on fistula size and location, with successful closure significantly improving the patient's quality of life. Postoperative recovery is very important because it includes managing complications and healing. Additionally, the importance of a multidisciplinary process cannot be overstated; the healthcare professionals who are involved, including obstetricians, urologists, and wound care specialists, must collaborate to provide integrated care and assistance to the patient. Comprehension of the complexities of surgical treatment serves the interests of healthcare providers in addressing efficiently the unique requirements of patients afflicted by this condition to enhance outcomes and enable women to return to society ultimately. Conservative treatments take on a supporting role in the management of female genital fistulae in addition to surgical intervention. These methods often include the placement of catheters, which may help divert urine from flowing through the fistula so that it can heal spontaneously. Ongoing drainage of the bladder may also be employed to prevent urine from always flowing, thereby reducing inflammation and allowing tissues to heal. Finally, psychological and social support are integral components of the treatment. Fistula women are often isolated and stigmatized, which adds to their physical as well as psychological morbidity. Through engaging the services of community health workers and peer support groups, their social burden is minimized because both forms of help foster psychosocial support and practical care. Physical and psychological care is emphasized as crucial because it optimizes general recovery and rehabilitation in women with fistula. Cultural sensitivity is critical when managing female genital fistulae. Healthcare providers must be aware of the patient's ethnically diverse background since it has a significant role in influencing beliefs regarding health and treatment options. As an illustration, migrant women and minority groups are likely to have unique difficulties tied to cultural practices that can complicate healthcare access. Inadequate cultural competence can result in miscommunication, which compromises patient care and the trust of medical professionals. Inability to understand and appreciate differences in cultures, such as beliefs surrounding childbirth and social impacts of fistula, can impede effective treatment and recovery. According to Clark et al. (2019), women's health providers are required to be culturally aware so that they can deliver efficient and meaningful care. Embedding cultural competency within treatment plans not only enhances patient interactions but also diversifies the healthcare environment, which in turn results in an improved health outcome for all at-risk or afflicted women with fistulae.

5.4.1. Surgical Interventions

Surgical treatment remains the mainline therapy for female genital fistulae, most commonly a complication of obstructed labor and leading to disabling physical and psychological sequelae. Restorative surgery for the restoration of normal anatomical function is essential to provide relief from the associated urinary incontinence and ongoing leakage. Optimal time for surgery is generally during the first few months following fistula formation, as long-standing conditions can complicate healing and result in higher risks of bad outcomes. Surgeons employ procedures that involve closing the fistula and restoring the surrounding tissue. Successful repairs not only restore physical health but also are pivotal in reinstating the social identity and self-concept of women so involved, who are exposed to stigma surrounding the condition, as indicated in Barr-Walker et al. (2025). Besides, the use of surgical techniques should be supplemented with extensive pre- and post-surgical management. This entails patient education and counseling of the psychological kind in order to equip women with skills through which they can recover and re-enter society. The response should be multidisciplinary because it facilitates addressing psychosocial problems that correlate with the physical healing of fistula. Evidence indicates that the psychological effects of fistula, such as anxiety and depression, are prevalent among patients and tend to affect their overall well-being (Barr-Walker et al., 2025).

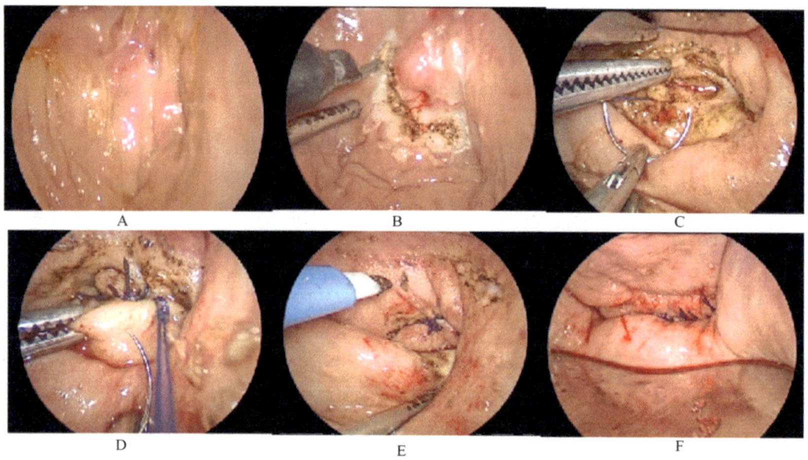

Figure 5.10. Procedure for Transvaginal Repair of Apical Vesicovaginal Fistula via Notes. (A).A high vesicovaginal fistula(VVF) in our surgical field; (B). On the outside of the fistula, a circular incision is made at the normal mucosa. Then free the flap to the outside, but the scar and sinus tract on the inside of the incision are not necessary to cut; (C). Use 3 – 0 Monocryl suture to close the fistula; (D). Use 3 – 0 Monocryl again to close the incision for 2 ~ 3 layers; (E,F). Finally, close the vaginal mucosa with a 3 – 0 Monocryl suture.

Source: https://www.nature.com/articles/s41598-024-82366-y

Follow-up after surgery on a long-term basis is critical, as it can detect potential complications and aid prevention programs that reduce the incidence of fistulae in subsequent pregnancies. Women's health clinics have the potential to ensure such continuity of services and facilities.

Finally, the broader implications of surgery extend beyond individual cases into community health and socio-economic factors. Repairing female genital fistulas through medical means not only reduces personal suffering but also allows for societal change that erodes stigmas around the condition. With the outcome of surgery creating windows of opportunity for women to regain their livelihoods and social status, massive improvements in community well-being are possible. However, access to surgical care, particularly in poorer hospitals, continues to remain restricted, necessitating increased systemic provision. Furthermore, as documented in research, respect for the cultural contexts of fistulae can promote greater acceptance and success of surgical programs. Surgical treatment is hence both a health imperative and the basis for empowerment of gender equity and health justice among affected populations.

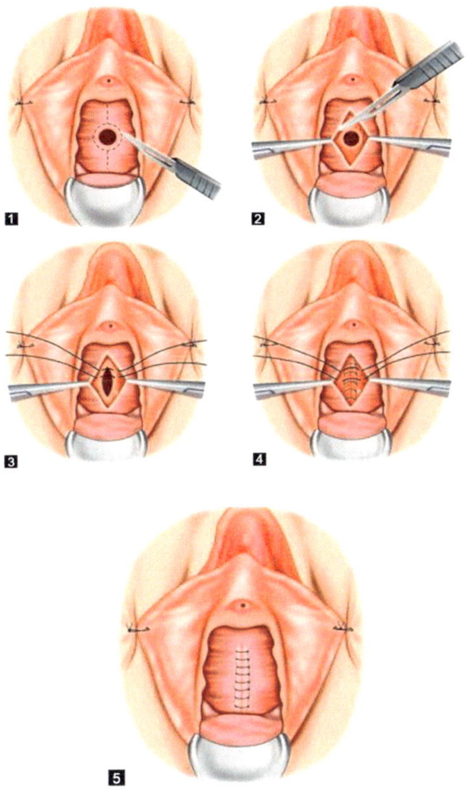

Figure 5.11. Principal steps of repair of old VVF by flap method. 1. Line of incision. 2. Separation of the vaginal wall from the bladder. To excise the fibrous tissues around the margin of fistula. 3. Closure of the bladder opening by interrupted sutures taking bites through the muscle wall excluding the bladder mucosa. 4. Reinforcing interrupted sutures taking superficial muscle and bladder fascia. 5. Look of the suture line after final repair.

Source: https://oshimu.com/wp-content/uploads/2021/07/Gynaecology-DC-Dutta.pdf

5.4.2. Non-Surgical Management

Treatment of female genital fistulae needs a holistic approach, particularly when talking of non-surgical management. Non-surgical management can be extremely effective as an adjunct to surgical closure or when surgery is not on the immediate horizon. It alleviates symptoms and promotes healing before any surgery. An emphasis is laid on nutritional therapy, as nutrition is essential to support the healing of the tissue, especially in those patients who may have been malnourished due to chronic leakage from the fistula. Psychological counseling is equally crucial, as the patients of fistulae tend to be stigmatized and emotionally traumatized. With the physical and psychological treatment, non-surgical management offers a holistic care environment, ultimately improving surgical outcomes. Besides, treatment can be non-surgical and given through urinary catheter use or vaginal packing, thereby controlling incontinence and reducing infection risk. The use of absorbent pads can also prove useful with a more dignified experience for the women affected, but they are short-term measures. In cases where surgery is not possible or where patients are not willing to undergo surgery, these non-surgical measures do help alleviate the situation and help patients cope with daily activities. Proper and constant education on pelvic floor exercises may also be essential in making the bordering muscles strong, helping with overall pelvic function. Such treatment not only provides immediate relief but also empowers women with the ability to manage their health in a more proactive manner, enhancing their independence. Finally, support groups in the community and health education constitute part of the non-surgical management of female genital fistulae. Raising awareness through outreach activities can assist in breaking the stigma around fistulae, making it easier for more women to seek earlier presentation. Educational interventions ought to work towards understanding the etiology of fistula development, improve reproductive health education, and promote preventive interventions.

Specialized interventions assist women in gaining an understanding of their conditions, being empowered in their experiences, and acquiring knowledge on management options. Generally, these non-surgical practices emphasize a care-focused, patient-centered practice in which women are not only cured comprehensively but also empowered to own their health processes confidently (Pigot et al., 2021; Ngarambe et al., 2017).

5.4.3. Role of Rehabilitation and Support Services

Rehabilitation and support services play a core role in addressing the complex needs of women suffering from female genital fistulae. The services encompass, besides surgery, holistic psychosocial, physical, and economic rehabilitation that seeks to reintegrate them back into society. Women suffering from obstetric fistula experience a range of challenges that may hinder the quality of their lives, including stigma and limited access to treatment. The importance of understanding such multi-dimensional outcomes is emphasized in the literature, which pushes for a holistic health care system considering both medical and emotional healing (Hayter et al., 2017). Furthermore, without proper support, women may be discriminated against even after corrective surgery, making their process of reintegration even more complicated. This emphasizes the need for thoroughgoing rehabilitation services that address these social determinants in a manner that promotes self-esteem and community integration. Psychosocial counseling is an important component of postoperative care for women who have undergone genital fistula repair. There is evidence to suggest that women receiving counseling and psychosocial therapy rate their mental health and satisfaction with rehabilitation more positively. A trial evaluating a multi-component reintegration intervention revealed that women who were given health education and psychosocial counseling experienced improvement in physical and psychosocial quality of life after surgery (Akori et al., 2024). Such would imply that support services given due to the immediate physical aftermath of surgery not only address the physical aftermath of the operation but also help women regain their self-sufficiency and social standing. The provision of economic support, among other types of rehabilitation services, also enhances their chances for successful reintegration, symbolizing the inextricable bond between health and socio-economic factors in the healing process. Nor is the role of community-based support services exaggerated in the rehabilitation of female genital fistula. The local organizations have a tendency to move as central connections connecting women with the resources they need, creating support systems that promote empathy and acceptance among their home communities. Certain of these services might include reproductive health education, stigma reduction programs, and peer support groups that provide mutual experiences and emotional healing. Such involvement by the community not only provides a supportive environment but also facilitates cultural shifts towards improved perceptions of women with fistulae, which are necessary for long-term change (Hayter et al., 2017). Lastly, increasing the availability and access of support and rehabilitation services will not just improve the individual health statuses of women with fistula, but also support further public health goals as well as women's empowerment in poor communities.

Test Your Knowledge

1. What are common surgical interventions used to treat female genital fistulae?
2. What non-surgical management options are available for female genital fistulae?

5.5. Prevention Strategies

Learning Outcome

1. Define education and awareness programs
2. Discuss the access to quality maternal healthcare
3. Explain the advocacy for women's rights

Preventive strategies against female genital fistulae are predominantly focused on stemming the causes of this debilitating condition. A fundamental approach in this direction is to increase access to good prenatal and obstetric care. Women who experience prolonged labor, something that in most instances happens in ill-equipped facilities, stand most at risk of acquiring fistulae. By making sure that skilled birth attendants conduct the delivery and by offering comprehensive maternal health care services, obstetric fistulae can be significantly prevented. In addition, training programs that promote the value of early medical interventions during childbirth can empower women and their families to receive the treatment they need, which may avert physical and mental damage associated with fistulae. According to the literature, strengthening maternal health services is a precious component in effective prevention measures designed to reverse the condition's prevalence among vulnerable communities (Blanchfield et al., 2011). Another key prevention strategy is focused on increasing awareness and altering social attitudes towards violence against women (VAW). Research has proven that cultural normalization of VAW, including early and forced marriage, is a dominant factor in the predisposition towards fistulae occurrence among women. By implementing large-scale education programs that challenge harmful gender norms and emphasize women's rights, communities can dismantle the stigma of obstetric complications and compounded discrimination. Furthermore, integrating anti-VAW components into general health programs can lead to a more cohesive approach that is centered on prevention so that women can receive medical care without fear of violence or exclusion. As highlighted by recent research, these measures are crucial to enable women to access timely assistance and care through their reproductive health cycle to ultimately realize a decline in the incidence of fistulae (Blanchfield et al., 2011).

Finally, supportive networks and community programs are essential for prevention and campaigns against female genital fistulae. They ought to incorporate psychosocial counseling of the women afflicted by obstetric fistula, as well as education of men and leaders in the community on the impacts of fistulae and the importance of maternal health. They can foster an environment conducive to change, diminishing stigma on both fistulae and the affected women. In addition, the successful reintegration of women upon treatment also demands continued support mechanisms addressing their particular needs. Empowering women through education and their involvement in communities can contribute to ending the cycle of discrimination and marginalization. Greater awareness and advocacy can subsequently open doors to a successful system of using preventive measures, thus addressing the multifaceted nature of female genital fistulae (Hayter et al., 2017).

5.5.1. Education and Awareness Programs

Education and awareness campaigns are essential components of the control of female genital fistulae because they play the central function of prevention as well as early treatment. Through educating communities about the causes, consequences, and treatment of fistulae, these campaigns can greatly improve maternal health outcomes. Providing information on the dangers of giving birth, particularly where skilled birth attendants are lacking, is necessary.

Most women are unaware that prolonged labor can lead to obstetric fistula, and therefore, extensive education for childbearing age women as well as for healthcare providers is necessary. Such programs can also address traditions that lead to the prevalence of this condition towards a cultural transition of having healthier reproductive health practices, as in the case of challenges brought by some cultures, such as female genital mutilation. Furthermore, social-inclined programs addressing the socio-economic determinants leading to fistula prevalence highlight the interconnected relationship between poverty alleviation and health education. Studies are indicative of low levels of education and limited healthcare access exacerbating risk factors for childbirth and eventual fistula development. According to research, poverty elimination, improving maternal health, and increasing access to health care are all important steps that can be integrated into education. Awareness should not only be offered through the programs but also educate women and provide them with economic opportunities. As societies learn of the value of good maternal care and engage in health-promoting customs, the prevalence of obstetric fistula can be significantly reduced, emphasizing the necessity to overcome disparities in education and improve overall health care. In the end, the impacts of good educational and awareness interventions are long-term beyond specific direct health effects, influencing long-term societal attitudes toward women's health. By providing education on fistula prevention and treatment at the community level, these programs can provide a conducive environment where women can access medical intervention without fear of being stigmatized. Furthermore, educating health workers on how to identify and handle cases of fistula can lead to early intervention, thereby improving maternal health outcomes. The findings from research indicate that continuous education of the patients as well as providers is essential to avoid fistula formation. With changing educational strategies, they must correlate with the new social environment to make awareness and advocacy peak concerns in healthcare matters and thus contribute to a future where obstetric fistulae are preventable on a large scale and are properly managed, as through the successful strategies established in community health programs.

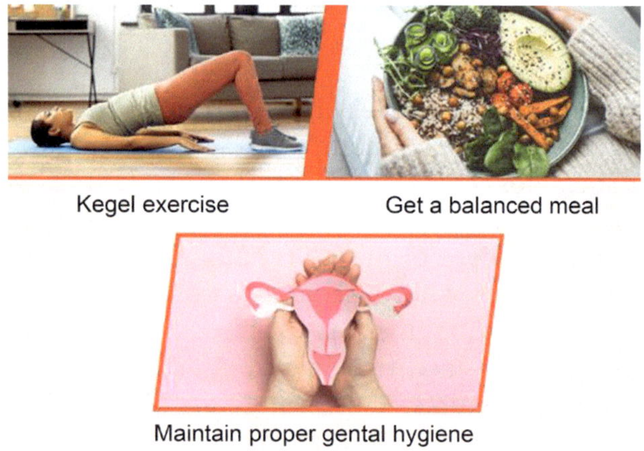

Source: https://www.medindia.net/health/conditions/obstetric-fistula.htm

5.5.2. Access To Quality Maternal Healthcare

Access to quality maternal health care is a central determinant of the outcome of maternal health, particularly in poor-resource settings where conditions such as female genital fistulae are prevalent. The intersection of poor health care services and culture-based stigmatization maintains a system of neglect that causes the high rate of obstetric complications. Improved pre- and postnatal care can significantly reduce the risk of acquiring complications like fistula, which in most cases result from obstructed labor without access to healthcare. Consistent with evidence compiled in the field, there is a direct knowledge gap that lies beneath women's access to healthcare in developing countries, suggesting that reforms must not only accommodate the quantity of resources but also the needs and attitudes of individual women towards their own health (Rizvi et al.,

2006). Therefore, improving access to quality maternal care requires a paradigm change that places supreme attention on women's voices and experiences. The impact of poor maternal care extends to physical health, with adverse effects on the mental and social well-being of women as well. Female genital fistula, a disabling injury occurring from obstructed labor or poorly performed medical treatment, tends to cause extreme stigmatization, leading to isolation, depression, and compromised quality of life. This stigma is not only gendered but also disability-affiliated and poverty-related, which makes it challenging for women to access reproductive health care in time (Barr-Walker et al., 2025). To solve these problems, there must be an integrated health system that, in addition to offering surgery for fistula repair, encourages the whole community environment to be supportive. These programs can facilitate conversation about stigma and social reintegration, which are crucial to enhancing the quality of life for infected women. The medical response to maternal conditions like female genital fistula should also be integrated and collective, incorporating a number of different stakeholders such as healthcare providers, policymakers, and local citizens. Enhancing maternal health care is not only a call for prioritization of clinical care, but also a need to acknowledge socio-economic barriers to women's access to health care. Public sector investment must be enhanced to develop efficient reproductive care services tailored to the needs of women, particularly in developing regions where resources are scarce (Rizvi et al., 2006). Moreover, encouraging community responsibility for women's health can lead to opening avenues for the mobilization of support services and advocating for health equity. The holistic strategy is central to unearthing the composite dimensions of maternal access to healthcare and ultimately reducing the prevalence of afflictions such as female genital fistulae.

5.5.3. Advocacy For Women's Rights

The struggle for women's rights has increasingly become a cry for attention to urgent health issues such as female genital fistulae, the situation that is most often founded on gender inequalities. Governments, non-governmental organizations, and local civil society groups are increasing the response levels to this public health problem, particularly in regions where women cannot get good maternal health care. The social shame of fistula patients tends to compound their misery, closing off their possibilities for social rehabilitation and psychological healing. Thus, advocacy campaigns seek not merely to increase awareness of fistulae but to inform communities about prevention and cure as well. By placing women's health at the forefront and emphasizing access to care, such advocacy initiatives seek to shatter the cultural customs underpinning discrimination and muzzling of women's voices regarding reproductive health. Legislative measures are also significant in the advocacy for women's rights, particularly maternal health care and an end to female genital mutilation/cutting, closely linked to fistulae prevalence. Aids such as the Africa Coordinating Centre for the Abandonment of Female Genital Mutilation/Cutting work hard to consolidate best practices and develop comprehensive training guidelines for medical professionals. This is essential, given that medical professionals trained on these matters are typically the last line of defense against the ramifications of such practices that disregard women's health and agency (Kimani et al., 2016).

5.5.4. Effective Advocacy

Effective advocacy has to be multi-dimensional and involve policymakers, health professionals, and community members to all work together to treat the issue of fistulae in women and to fund forward-thinking interventions to prevent their formation in the first place. In addition to health interventions, advocacy needs to respond to social and cultural determinants that hinder women's rights and access to care. For instance, educational interventions for the destigmatization of female genital fistulae have the potential to empower women, create supportive settings, and raise community awareness about this condition. Facilitating open discussions around female health concerns is essential in the fight against norms that devalue women and their health experiences. Further, as is highlighted by the reference to current legislative changes concerning adolescent sexual rights, there is also a clear need for policies that address the realities of young women (Chirkut et al., 2016). Advocacy for women's rights here not just addresses short-term health requirements but also strives to achieve long-term social change that supports gender equality and pushes women towards reclaiming their rights to health and dignity.

Test Your Knowledge

1. How do education and awareness programs help in preventing female genital fistulae?
2. Why is access to quality maternal healthcare crucial for reducing obstetric complications?

SUMMARY

In short, therapy for female genital fistulae has to be an interdisciplinary approach with a focus on both medical interventions and de-stigmatizing. Women with fistulae often experience severe psychological and social repercussions in the form of depression, anxiety, and severe social exclusion. Research reveals that approximately 35% of infected women experience divorce, and approximately 65% experience depression, which is an indicator of the significant impact of stigmatization on the quality of life (Barr-Walker et al., 2025). Hence, health interventions should target not just surgical repair but also treatment with full mental health care and education in the community to transform public attitudes toward individuals afflicted by fistulae. Effective interventions must also consider the cultural contexts in which female genital fistulae are formed. Many of them are rooted in practices that are causes of prolonged obstructed labor in settings with limited medical facilities. In addition, the interplay of gender, poverty, and social expectations is the cause of obstetric fistula. Since women from 41 countries have demonstrated, the problems related to fistulae cannot be left to clinical resolution (Barr-Walker et al., 2025). Instead, action should involve community-based interventions promoting understanding and compassion as well as efforts to eliminate prevailing myths about the disease. Moreover, the extensive prevalence of female genital mutilation (FGM) presents an urgent necessity for ongoing change in society. Despite efforts to eradicate the practice, cultural and traditional beliefs remain very entrenched, which leads to both FGM and its resultant complications, including fistulae. The challenge lies in developing educational awareness and participation at the grassroots level to alter attitudes and practices in the long term. In working toward a holistic improvement of women's reproductive health, an interlinking of legal measures, education, and outreach at the community level has the most promising chances for changing lives and maintaining the dignity and well-being of women with fistulae. Intersecting these problems calls for ongoing commitment and collaboration across levels.

Information about female genital fistulae addresses a variety of key issues, beginning from their aetiology to impacts on women's health and social standing. Fistulae in the first place are most often the result of prolonged obstructed labor, particularly where there is inadequate access to healthcare. The process results in an abnormal connection between the vaginal tract and urinary or intestinal tracts and has devastating physical and psychological consequences for the involved females. The stigma of fistulae also worsens such effects, causing social stigmatization, psychological trauma, and economic hardship. The systematic scoping review once again confirms that 35% of women with fistula experience divorce or separation from marriage, and approximately 65% become depressed, illustrating the far-reaching interdependency between fistula and stigma and how much it negatively affects the overall quality of life for the majority (Barr-Walker et al., 2025). In addition, the study on stigma for female genital fistulae demonstrates different aspects of social disrespect as enacted, internalized, and expected stigma. These stigmas overlap with a variety of other forms of discrimination like gender, disability, and poverty stigma, while demonstrating a complex web of oppression affecting women's everyday lives. Interestingly, social support has been identified as a buffer factor that can counter the effect of stigmas on mental well-being, mobilizing communities to promote resilience among victims. Examining the psychosocial context of fistulae, the causative link between stigma and mental health problems is paramount in formulating successful interventions. Painfully few interventions have been documented within the literature, and there is a large gap in support mechanisms specifically developed that are able to enhance the quality of life for women with fistula (Barr-Walker et al., 2025).

Female genital fistulae must be tackled in an integrated manner that includes healthcare reforms and community participation to enhance women's health outcomes. Emergency responses need to focus on training frontline providers in fistula women's care management, allowing for prevention and treatment interventions at the community level. Synthesis of evidence about the health effects of female genital mutilation/cutting (FGM/C) is useful for training guideline development that can inform healthcare policy and practice. These evidence-based guidelines provide a firm foundation for understanding and managing the problems of fistula care. Future research should penetrate deeper into the health implications of fistulae, designing well-organized interventions to reduce the burden on women and promote change at the community level towards abandonment of harmful practices.

KEY TERMS FROM THIS CHAPTER

- Female genital cutting (FGC)
- Fistula formation
- Genital schistosomiasis
- Comorbidities
- Disorders of sex development (DSD) conditions,
- Maternal health
- Obstetric complications
- Obstetric fistulae
- Obstructed labor
- Sexual violence
- Surgical interventions
- Female genital fistulae
- Fistula prevalence
- Health education
- Conservative treatments
- Healthcare strategies
- Obstetric care
- Obstetric fistula
- Obstetric injuries
- Reproductive health education
- Social isolation
- Violence against women (VAW)

CRITICAL THINKING QUESTIONS

1. **What is a female genital fistula?**
   a. A benign tumor in the female reproductive tract
   b. An abnormal connection between the genital tract and another organ
   c. A cyst found in the ovaries
   d. A hormonal imbalance affecting menstruation
2. **The most common cause of obstetric genital fistula is:**
   a. Bacterial infection during menstruation
   b. Prolonged obstructed labor causing tissue necrosis
   c. Congenital malformation of the uterus
   d. Endometriosis
3. **Which organs are most commonly involved in female genital fistulae?**
   a. Uterus and fallopian tubes
   b. Bladder and vagina
   c. Ovaries and cervix
   d. Rectum and uterus
4. **A key symptom of vesicovaginal fistula (VVF) is:**
   a. Painful menstruation
   b. Continuous leakage of urine from the vagina
   c. Severe abdominal cramps
   d. Irregular vaginal bleeding
5. **The primary treatment for female genital fistula is:**
   a. Antibiotic therapy
   b. Hormonal therapy
   c. Surgical repair of the fistula
   d. Chemotherapy

Short Answer Questions

1. What are the common causes of female genital fistulae?
2. What symptoms typically indicate the presence of a genital fistula?
3. How is female genital fistula diagnosed?
4. What are some societal and cultural implications of female genital fistulae?
5. What treatment options are available for female genital fistulae?
6. What prevention strategies can help reduce the incidence of female genital fistulae?

Answer to Critical Thinking Questions

1. (b) 2. (b) 3. (b) 4. (b) 5. (c)

REFERENCES

1. Ahmed, S. F., & Markosyan, R. (2017). Sex assignment in conditions affecting sex development. https://core.ac.uk/download/150597685.pdf (accessed on 15th June 2025).
2. Akori, S., Ali, S., Barageine, J., Byamugisha, J., et al. (2024). Development and pilot test of a multi-component intervention to support women's recovery from female genital fistula. https://core.ac.uk/download/617035268.pdf (accessed on 15th June 2025).
3. Al-Riyami, A., Browning, A., Bulut, A., Holme, A., Adler, A. J., Karateke, A., Prual, A., et al. (2013). Estimating the prevalence of obstetric fistula: A systematic review and meta-analysis. https://core.ac.uk/download/42631348.pdf (accessed on 15th June 2025).
4. Alves, I., Di Giovanni, E., Duarte, L., Cunha, A. M., et al. (2016). Tuberculosis endometrial simulant um carcinoma do ovaria. https://core.ac.uk/download/62707676.pdf (accessed on 15th June 2025).
5. Barageine, J., Byamugisha, J., El Ayadi, A. M., Kakaire, O., et al. (2019). Trajectories of women's physical and psychosocial health following obstetric fistula repair in Uganda: A longitudinal study. https://core.ac.uk/download/323082515.pdf (accessed on 15th June 2025).
6. Barr-Walker, J., Conway, A., El Ayadi, A. M., Kennerly, H., et al. (2025). A comprehensive understanding of global female genital fistula and stigma: A systematic scoping review and meta-analysis. https://core.ac.uk/download/649473132.pdf (accessed on 15th June 2025).
7. Barry, T. H., Beavogui, A. H., Bouedouno, P., Camara, M., et al. (2017). Fistula recurrence, pregnancy, and childbirth following successful closure of female genital fistula in Guinea: A longitudinal study. https://core.ac.uk/download/153399435.pdf (accessed on 15th June 2025).
8. Bergström, A., Boene, H., CLIP working group, Hanson, C., et al. (2017). Obstetric fistulae in southern Mozambique: Incidence, obstetric characteristics and treatment. https://core.ac.uk/download/141439339.pdf (accessed on 15th June 2025).
9. Blanchfield, L., Margesson, R., Salaam-Blyther, T., Serafino, P., et al. (2011). International violence against women: U.S. response and policy issues. https://core.ac.uk/download/5131183.pdf (accessed on 15th June 2025).
10. Broussard, P. A. (2008). Female genital mutilation: Exploring strategies for ending ritualized torture; Shaming, blaming, and utilizing the Convention Against Torture. https://core.ac.uk/download/62547998.pdf (accessed on 15th June 2025).
11. Chirkut, S. (2016). Ethico-legal concerns in relation to adolescent sexual intercourse. https://core.ac.uk/download/188775680.pdf (accessed on 15th June 2025).
12. Christinet, V., Lazdins-Helds, J. K., Reinhard-Rupp, J., Stothard, J. R., et al. (2016). Female genital schistosomiasis (FGS): From case reports to a call for concerted action against this neglected gynecological disease. https://core.ac.uk/download/pdf/82099896.pdf (accessed on 15th June 2025).
13. Clark, V. (2019). An analysis of major issues for culturally-minded professionals in women's health care. https://core.ac.uk/download/213463629.pdf (accessed on 15th June 2025).
14. De Pessemier, B., Grine, L., Debaere, M., Maes, A., Paetzold, B., & Callewaert, C. (2021). Gut–skin axis: Current knowledge of the interrelationship between microbial dysbiosis and skin conditions. *Microorganisms, 9*, 353–353. https://doi.org/10.3390/microorganisms9020353 (accessed on 15th June 2025).

15. Ebeze, U. V., & Odoemelam, C. C. (2015). Patterns of exposure to communication interventions on obstetric fistula among men in Ebonyi State, Nigeria. https://core.ac.uk/download/234652659.pdf (accessed on 15th June 2025).

16. Emelumadu, O. F., Epundu, U. U., Ibeh, C. C., Ilika, A., et al. (2018). The epidemiology of female genital mutilation in Nigeria–A twelve-year review. https://core.ac.uk/download/478449068.pdf (accessed on 15th June 2025).

17. Gumodoka, B., Lilungulu, A., Nassoro, M., Soka, D., et al. (2018). Obstetric fistulae, birth outcomes, and surgical repair outcomes: A retrospective analysis of hospital-based data in Dodoma, Tanzania. https://core.ac.uk/download/478462746.pdf (accessed on 15th June 2025).

18. Hayter, M., Laurenson, M., & Mafo Degge, H. (2017). An integrative review on women living with obstetric fistula and after treatment experiences. https://core.ac.uk/download/151161489.pdf (accessed on 15th June 2025).

19. Heller, A. (2015). Interrogating the superlative sufferer: Experiencing obstetric fistula and treatment seeking in Niger. https://core.ac.uk/download/233212176.pdf (accessed on 15th June 2025).

20. Hilton, P. (2019). Urogenital fistula: Studies on epidemiology and treatment outcomes in high-income and low-and middle-income countries. https://core.ac.uk/download/334997530.pdf (accessed on 15th June 2025).

21. Ingram, J. R., Collier, F., Brown, D., Burton, T., Burton, J., Chin, M. F., Desai, N., et al. (2018). British Association of Dermatologists guidelines for the management of hidradenitis suppurativa (acne inverse) 2018. *British Journal of Dermatology, 180*, 1009–1017. https://doi.org/10.1111/bjd.17537 (accessed on 15th June 2025).

22. Kimani, S., Muteshi-Strachan, J., & Njue, C. (2016). Health impacts of female genital mutilation/cutting: A synthesis of the evidence. https://core.ac.uk/download/229808562.pdf (accessed on 15th June 2025).

23. Magoha, G. A. O., & Magoha, O. B. (2009). Current global status of female genital mutilation: A review. https://core.ac.uk/download/478296343.pdf (accessed on 15th June 2025).

24. Ministry of Health Kenya. (2015). *Kenya Adolescent Sexual and Reproductive Health Policy*. https://core.ac.uk/download/229801675.pdf (accessed on 15th June 2025).

25. Ngarambe, C., & Peng, D. (2017). Female urinary incontinence: A systematic overview and non-surgical treatment. https://core.ac.uk/download/539901161.pdf (accessed on 15th June 2025).

26. Ngoma, J. (2011). Prevention of vesicovaginal fistula: A literature review and experience from Zambia. https://core.ac.uk/download/38026955.pdf (accessed on 15th June 2025).

27. Pigot, G. L. S. (2021). Gender urology: Outcomes of urological care in gender affirming process: Gender urology. https://core.ac.uk/download/387936561.pdf (accessed on 15th June 2025).

28. Richens, J. (2004). Genital manifestations of tropical diseases. https://core.ac.uk/download/1669842.pdf (accessed on 15th June 2025).

29. Rizvi, J., & Zuberi, N. F. (2006). Women's health in developing countries. https://core.ac.uk/download/84855120.pdf (accessed on 15th June 2025).

GENITAL MALIGNANCY

6

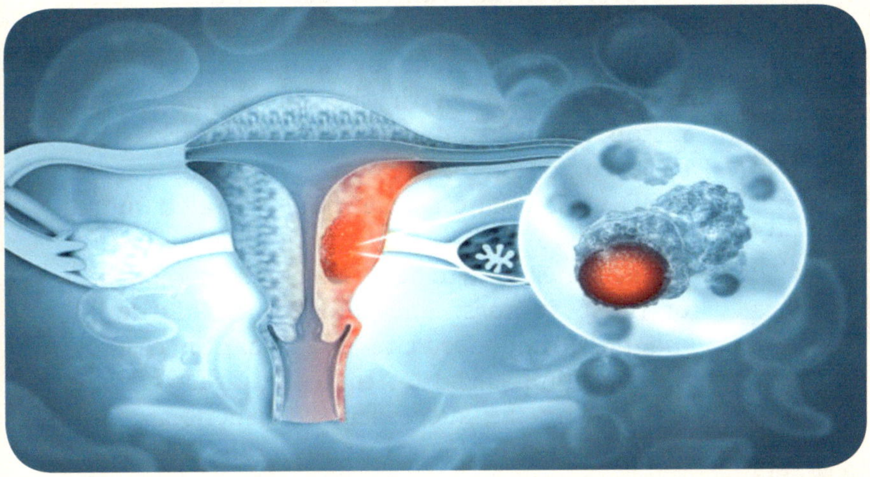

LEARNING OBJECTIVES

After studying this chapter, you will be able to:

1. Describe the different types of genital malignancies
2. Identify the risk factors associated with genital malignancies
3. Recognize the symptoms and diagnostic methods for genital malignancies
4. Evaluate the treatment options available for genital malignancies
5. Discuss the psychological impact of genital malignancies on patients

Introduction

Genital cancer is a field of research covering a variety of tumors targeting the reproductive system, and which calls for profound studies in clinical practice and medical science. Understanding of these cancers is at the forefront not only of developing diagnostic techniques but also of constructing therapeutic modalities. The multifactorial pathogenesis of these diseases reflects the interaction between genetic determinants, environmental factors, and lifestyle parameters that all equally contribute to cancer causation. With increased awareness of genital cancers, there is a corresponding challenge to professionals in diagnosing symptoms and early intervention, ultimately placing them in a position to enhance patient prognosis. The use of advanced imaging technology, along with new forms of therapy, relies on ongoing research and clinical trials to advance the treatment regimens further, which explains the need for ongoing education among practitioners as society strives to grasp the character of the disease. Recent developments in imaging modalities and diagnostic techniques have radically modified the profile of genital cancer detection and therapy. Out of all these modalities, ultrasound (US) has been found to be a very valuable tool in the evaluation of anatomical abnormality and estimation of risk of malignancy from specific features noted on imaging. It serves as a cost-effective, painless initial evaluation, allowing the clinicians to choose patients who need intervention, i.e., FNA biopsy. Through coded classification systems, phrased in report language and interpretation of the ultrasound findings, the greatest importance is placed on optimizing the pathways of care for patients. All these advances are based on a literature foundation enabling imaging to be applied in correlating presentation with risk of malignancy, hence active management interventions to maximize survival and quality of life for the involved (David et al., 2024). Also, the genital malignancy is not merely a complicated presentation, but it also mirrors in psychological, social, and other patient experience and outcome determinants to a very great extent. Conditions such as chronic genital arousal disorder/genitopelvic dysesthesia (PGAD/GPD) are a complicated state of genital health wherein drug treatments can have a paradoxical effect to aggravate or ameliorate the symptoms. Evidence suggests that although certain drugs can be relieving, they also have the potential to exacerbate symptoms in some individuals, showing just how fine the line is that a clinician has to tread when prescribing drugs for genital-based illnesses (Kruger et al., 2024). Heightened appreciation of such conditions underlines the necessity for an integrated policy in treatment planning, including patient-centered care that encompasses the physiological as well as the psychological. The presentation of malignancy of the genitals is not only utilized here as an introduction to the subject for purposes of discussion of clinical interest but also to underline the necessity for an integrated, multidisciplinary treatment and management plan.

Definition of Genital Malignancy

The term genital malignancy is a synonym for a wide range of malignant neoplasms that develop mostly in the genital organs, including the male and female reproductive systems. Such a definition encompasses various kinds of tumors, including squamous cell carcinoma, adenocarcinoma, and testicular germ cell tumors, with their own distinctive pathophysiological characteristics and corresponding risk factors. Genital tumors are clinically and epidemiologically significant, usually needing careful management by diagnosis, staging, and treatment. With the developments in histopathologic and molecular characterization, as documented in the latest revisions of the WHO classification, attention is drawn more strongly to utilizing both morphologic and molecular criteria to benefit from the complexity of these tumors. The importance of timely diagnosis and accurate classification cannot be overemphasized, as they are direct factors influencing the success of treatment as well as patient prognosis (Moch et al., 2022). In female genital cancers such as cervical and ovarian cancer, there has been a strong focus on preventive approaches and early detection regimens. The human papillomavirus (HPV) vaccine has also become a bedrock of primary prevention for cervical cancer, a malignancy with a strong association with infection with HPV. Through mass screening programs like Pap smears, the detection of precancerous lesions at an early stage has significantly raised survival, thereby indicating the central role of public health interventions to tackle these cancers. Also, in male genital cancer, particularly in testicular cancer, early awareness campaigns and self-examination result in early treatment and diagnosis. As research develops to include molecular markers in the classification of these tumors, their etiology, risk factors, and pathogenesis need to be known (Garbe et al., 2022).

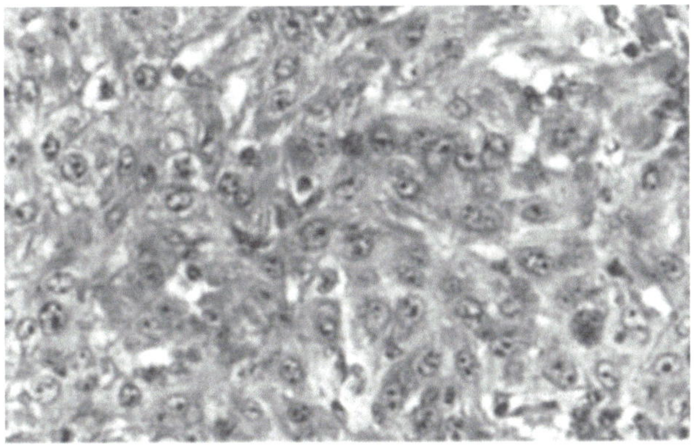

Figure 6.1. Histologic picture of vulval squamous cell carcinoma.

Source: https://oshimu.com/wp-content/uploads/2021/07/Gynaecology-DC-Dutta.pdf

Apart from this, treatments for genital cancers have progressed from traditional surgery to more advanced therapies, including immunotherapy and targeted therapy. These therapies are based on new developments in tumor genomics, which allow for the identification of exact genetic changes and the initiation of specifically formulated therapeutic regimens. For instance, advances in subclassification of penile and renal tumors allow us to differentiate between HPV-positive and HPV-negative malignancies, which can have significant treatment implications. Tumors such as testicular neuroendocrine tumors provide a demonstration of the heterogeneity of this category, necessitating a complex understanding of each tumor's individual biology to treat it effectively. With progress in the area, it is essential to pursue research and clinical trials to refine treatment protocols and maximize patient outcomes in the diverse scenario of genital malignancies (Moch et al., 2022).

Importance of Studying Genital Malignancies

The significance of the study of genital cancer cannot be overstressed because such cancers represent a spectrum of tumor types which have the potential to greatly influence physical and mental health. Through study of the etiology and progress of such malignancies, research scientists can devise targeted prevention strategies, early detection, and treatment protocols. For example, the study of correlations between previous cancers and the development of secondary malignancies is of great significance. Research has established that any underlying malignancy has a greater risk of secondary acute lymphoblastic leukemia development, and most importantly, there are critical implications for overall survival in young patients. The correlation illustrates the ripple effects of malignancies of the genital organs, not only in terms of the immediate health consequences but also for patient management and long-term health follow-up (Brunson et al., 2017). Given such intricacies, the study of genital malignancies is important to improve patient outcomes and reduce death rates of this group of cancers. Also, examination of surgical interventions, such as hysterectomy, offers more refined details in risk factors that affect ovarian cancer incidence.

Fresh evidence refutes the assumption that hysterectomy in the absence of oophorectomy is universally protective of ovarian malignancies. Instead, the connection is understood to be rooted in large part on some patient characteristics, such as the occurrence of conditions like fibroids or endometriosis, which can drastically alter risk profiles. The evidence shows that hysterectomy among women with these co-existing conditions has the potential to significantly reduce the risk of ovarian cancer, implicating a convergence of cardinal significance among surgical decision-making and cancer prevention measures (Dixon-Suen et al., 2019). This awareness supports the significance of integrating a thorough understanding of genital malignancies into clinical practice, as it will likely lead to more effective and tailored healthcare measures.

Lastly, the application of learning about genital malignancies is relevant on the sociocultural level of women's health problems. Learning and awareness regarding these malignancies contribute significantly towards guaranteeing early diagnosis, stigma elimination, and inspiring women to seek early medical intervention. Sex and reproductive health issues are stigmatized in most societies, leading to late diagnoses and unfavorable prognoses. Through open discussion and public awareness, women can be empowered by clinicians and researchers to raise their voice for their health issues and identify the importance of frequent screening. Further, with increasing health disparities globally, social determinants of such cancers should be thoroughly researched to create interventions among various populations. Positioning genital cancers in the center of inquiry can thus initiate serious public health transformation, enhancing treatment and awareness for vulnerable groups with higher vulnerability.

6.1. Types of Genital Malignancies

Learning Outcome

1. Define male genital malignancies and female genital malignancies
2. Discuss rare types of genital cancers

Of all the several forms of genital cancer, cervical cancer is most prevalent among females worldwide. It is usually associated with persistent infection by certain high-risk forms of human papillomavirus (HPV), which plays a significant role in the progression from benign lesions to invasive carcinoma. Cervical cancer pathology can be divided into adenocarcinomas and squamous cell carcinomas, both with varied histological patterns as well as risk factors. Pap smear screening and HPV immunization have decreased the incidence of cervical cancer in most industrialized countries tremendously. Persistent disparities in mortality rates continue to exist, particularly in low-resource populations where preventive services are not accessible. The fact that cervical cancer is a women's health concern works to underscore the necessity of continued public health intervention and inquiry into prevention and early detection. Endometrial cancer, whose association is largely with the lining of the uterus, is also a leading type of genital cancer. Although most prevalent in postmenopausal women, other risk factors such as obesity, diabetes, and estrogen exposure elevate rates of occurrence even in young women. Endometrial carcinoma is typically subdivided into type I and type II, type I being linked with endometrial hyperplasia and typically a good prognosis, but more aggressive and typically later diagnosed than type II. Clinical presentation is most commonly abnormal vaginal bleeding, but it can be utilized as an early warning. With the rising incidence of obesity and its associated metabolic disease, knowledge of endometrial carcinoma pathophysiology and lifestyle influences becomes increasingly important to prevent risk and optimize patient outcomes. Less common but no less significant are the primary fallopian tube carcinomas (PFTC), an uncommon female genital tract malignancy. Most common in postmenopausal patients, PFTC is likely to be misinterpreted as ovarian cancer based on the collective clinical presentation and imaging characteristics. Characterized by sensitive pelvic abdomen and paraovarian discharge, it is frequently diagnosed coincidentally during an operation for unrelated pathology, and hence, early diagnosis may be challenging. The prognosis for PFTC is generally poorer compared to such ovarian cancers, despite presenting at an earlier stage. Research suggests PFTC management is similar to ovarian cancer, agreeing that there is a need for greater awareness on the clinical level as well as research in this rare disease with respect to women's health, as established by studies calling for multidimensional management strategies (Bafna et al., 2011). In addition, synchronous cancers of the female genital tract, such as concomitant endometrial and ovarian cancer, introduce yet another level of treatment and management complexity to which there have been calls for personalized therapeutic approaches by specific histological type and stage (Arsenijevic et al., 2013).

6.1.1. Male Genital Malignancies

Male genital cancer geography has been strongly linked to a variety of risk factors that can influence prevalence as well as prognosis. Among the risk factors, age, ethnicity, and HIV status have been strongly linked with cancer incidence. For instance, the studies indicate that HIV-infected men are at risk for the development of Kaposi sarcoma and lymphoma, among other cancers, and these are manifested in these patients as a second malignancy. Male cancer incidence rates, age adjusted, reveal disparities that are to be addressed specially. More specifically, the evidence necessitates more aggressive screening and treatment protocols specific to treat the specific vulnerabilities of men, particularly in the case of immunocompromised cases or chronic disease such as HIV (Detels et al., 2019).

The presentations of male genital cancers are enormously variable, with penile cancer and testicular cancer being the most pertinent. Testicular cancer is not as prevalent as other cancers, but the fact that it is very prevalent among young men, usually in late teens to early thirties, makes it special. Alternatively, penile cancer would be more likely to appear in older populations and has risk factors of hygiene and human papillomavirus infection (HPV). Current research draws attention to the significance of HPV vaccination in the prevention of penile cancer and recognizes prevention measures as a component of public health strategies. Both cancers emphasize the need for education and awareness campaigns to reduce stigma and promote early detection in men, and this can significantly enhance survival rates and quality of life (Brunson et al., 2017). Moreover, the outcome of male genital cancers also largely depends on when they are diagnosed, in addition to how well the subsequent treatment goes. Early diagnosis tends to work better, but the majority of patients with these cancers have a poor understanding of symptoms and signs of genital cancers, which results in delays in visiting the physician. Specifically, the personal shame surrounding learning about genital health dissuades men from making themselves available for preventive care. By promoting open discussion of male genital problems and requiring regular check-ups, medical providers can help turn these trends around. There has to be coordination among clinicians, public health practitioners, and community leaders to guarantee an environment that awakens men's health interest and enables early interventions (Detels et al., 2019; Brunson et al., 2017).

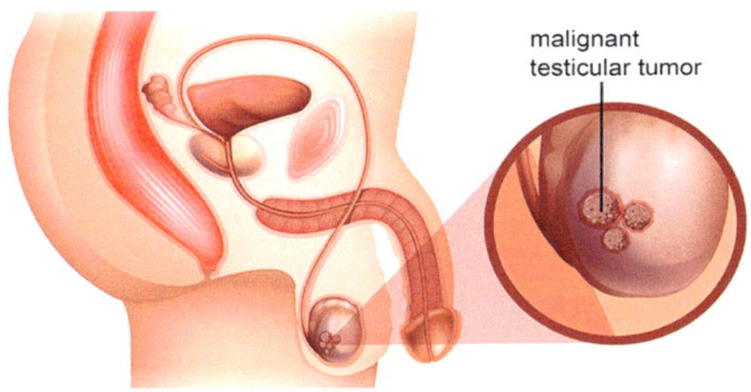

Figure 6.2. Testicular Cancer.

Source: https://www.metromaleclinic.com/wp-content/uploads/2020/07/testicular-cancer-metromale-clinic-fertilty-center-treatment-web.jpg

6.1.2. Female Genital Malignancies

The clinical picture of female genital malignancy is varied and rich with a range of types, each with its own characteristic features, risk factors, and presentation. Of the malignancies, embryonal rhabdomyosarcoma (RMS) is a remarkably rare condition, particularly in adult females. Although this malignant neoplasm is more frequent in the pediatric and adolescent populations, incidences in adults are extraordinarily rare, with the incidence rates estimated to be between 0.4% to 1%. In adults, RMS occurs in a non-typical manner, most commonly being diagnosed when patients complain of dyspareunia and post-coital bleeding. The necessity for aggressive therapy with radical surgery and chemoradiation points to the aggressiveness of this malignancy. The case of the anaplastic variant RMS diagnosis of a 36-year-old female is a haunting reminder that uncommon cancers can present in patients who are at presumably lower risk, and this is a reminder of awareness and identification of unusual symptoms pertaining to female genital cancer (Jadhav et al., 2023).

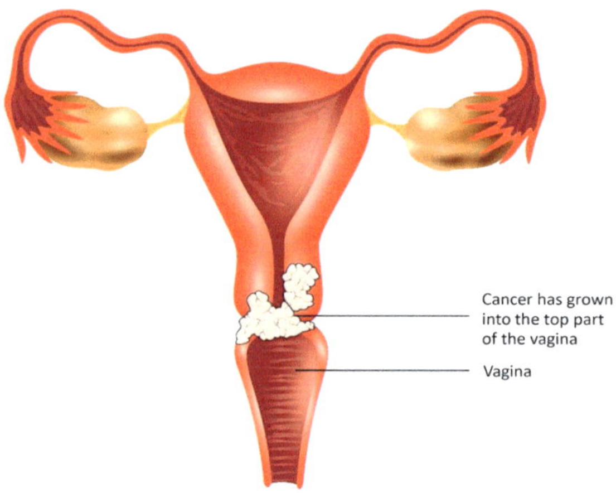

Figure 6.3. Vaginal Cancer Stage I.

Source: https://www.frontiersin.org/files/Articles/883805/fonc-12-883805-HTML-r1/image_m/fonc-12-883805-g005.jpg

The second salient aspect of female genital cancers is the impact of chronic infection, in this case, schistosomiasis, on cervical well-being. Female genital schistosomiasis, caused predominantly by Schistosoma haematobium, is a primary juncture for infectious disease and gynecologic oncology. Most endemic throughout sub-Saharan Africa, the disease places special stress upon women's health, as the genital form is best related to sequelae like increased HIV transmission and malignancy.

The cervix is particularly vulnerable, with the lesions frequently misdiagnosed as cervical intraepithelial neoplasia due to analogous clinical presentations. This diagnostic dilemma calls for a high index of suspicion on the part of health workers, particularly in hyperendemic regions. The diagnosis of schistosomiasis as a potential precursor to cervical cancer validates the relevance of combined screening policies in gynecological practice, in effect merging efforts towards addressing both infectious and malignant concerns (Gk et al., 2022).

Understanding the intricacies of infections and cancer in women's genital health sheds light on broader implications for public health interventions. As concern grows that some infections potentially cause women to be at risk of developing cancers, particularly in disease-endemic regions like schistosomiasis, the imperative need for particular preventive interventions cannot be overstated. One highly significant step is to implement rigorous screening programs that are responsive to the individual epidemiologic settings of different populations in order to allow early detection and intervention. In addition to that, promoting awareness among medical practitioners on the potential for unusual presentations of malignancies, such as RMS and schistosomiasis-related lesions, can promote diagnosis and eventually save patient lives. In learning these issues, it is clear that the management of female genital cancers is more than clinical care; it is a many-faceted learning that involves prevention, education, and access to healthcare services that are tailor-made to the requirements of women of different backgrounds and geographies.

6.1.3. Rare Types of Genital Cancers

Of the cancers of the genitals, the uncommon cancers present unique diagnostic and treatment challenges that must be addressed through formal clinical assessment. These cancers, though less common than some of their more prevalent relatives, for example, prostate or cervical carcinoma, have a significant impact on patients' quality of life and prognosis. Most notable among these rare entities are penile and vulvar cancers, which, although making up a minority of all genital cancers, when they do occur, can manifest with atypical presentation like severe pain and alteration of body function. Additionally, their rarity normally causes clinical unawareness, and consequently, diagnoses are delayed, resulting in more extensive disease at presentation. These rare cancers should be understood with subtlety in their characteristics by medical personnel so that they may be treated early and correctly. These are representative rare genital cancers with disproportionate burden in some populations, such as those with compromised immunity, such as patients with HIV.

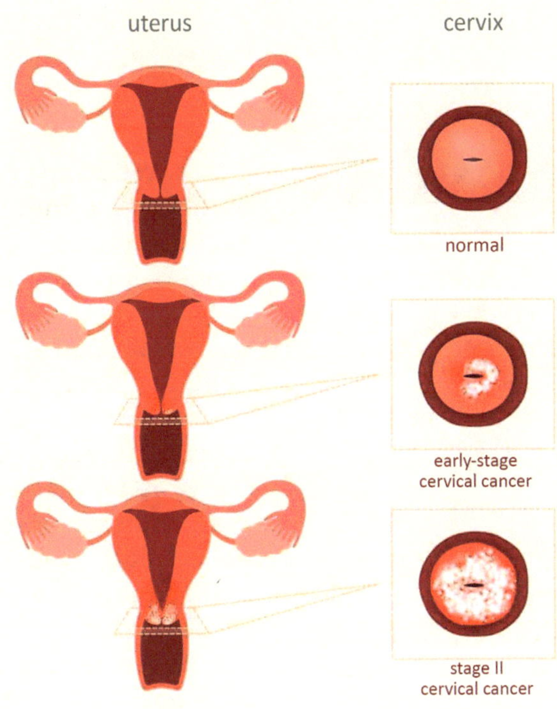

Figure 6.4. Cervical Cancer.

Source: https://rsphealth.org/wp-content/uploads/2021/07/Cervical-Cancer-1.jpg

According to the data available, age-standardized rates of malignancy incidence in this category show a stark contrast, with less common cancers like Kaposi sarcoma having a standardized incidence rate of 2,639.8 in males, reflecting a high rate of malignancies in this category. The presentation of these cancers is not merely linked with the direct pathophysiology of the cancer but also with overall health issues such as access to healthcare resources and screening services, which in low-resource settings may be limited. These weaknesses must be tackled to maximize outcomes and reduce the overall burden of genital cancer. Besides Kaposi sarcoma, other rare malignancies such as some sarcomas and neuroendocrine tumors are also found in the genital area, making the clinician's diagnostic challenge. The rarity of the tumors necessitates an extremely high index of suspicion and expertise in their management. In addition, geographic variability has its effect; e.g., research indicates that cervical cancers continue to be more common in some localities despite heightened screening modalities, proving that the topography of pathogens is different around the world. It is important that ongoing research identifies the epidemiological patterns of these rare cancers, as understanding their incidence is a clue to furthering early detection, prevention, and treatment methods, particularly in populations at greatest risk (Detels et al., 2019; Kumar et al., 2018).

Test Your Knowledge

1. What are the common types of male genital malignancies?
2. Which malignancies are most frequently found in the female genital tract?

6.2. Risk Factors

Learning Outcome

1. Explain the role of genetic predisposition in the development of genital malignancies
2. Analyze how environmental influences contribute to genital malignancies
3. Assess the impact of lifestyle choices on the risk of genital malignancies.

In the risk factors for genital malignancy, the genetic predisposition also has a crucial role. Certain inherited syndromes, including Lynch syndrome and familial breast-ovarian cancer syndrome, are predisposed to a higher incidence of genital tract cancers. Individuals harboring gene mutations BRCA1 and BRCA2 have a high risk of developing malignancies of the type of ovarian and breast cancer, which are typically related to secondary malignancies of the genitalia. These genetic processes facilitate tumor development by disrupting normal cellular regulatory processes. With increasing advances in genetic testing, identification of individuals at higher risk becomes feasible, allowing targeted surveillance and prevention, eventually with the goal of reducing genital malignancy occurrence in high-risk individuals. The integration of genetic counseling into patient care is a vital element of this preventive strategy, stressing the significance of inherited risk factors to oncologic medicine. Infection, in addition to genetic susceptibility, is also a significant risk factor for the development of genital cancers. Infection with Human Papillomavirus (HPV) is noteworthy; it is solely the etiologic agent detected in cervical carcinoma, directly incriminating viral pathogens as a cause of malignancy. The existence of high-risk types of HPV can potentially initiate oncogenic processes through integration of viral DNA into host genomes and thus disrupt normal cellular functions and provide a contribution to malignant transformations. Moreover, long-term infections, such as herpes simplex virus and *Chlamydia trachomatis*, may also contribute to elevated risks. Public health interventions aimed at the vaccination of HPV and promotion of safe sex are therefore imperative in minimizing such infections. These interventions not only lower the risk of genital malignancies from HPV but also improve overall reproductive health.

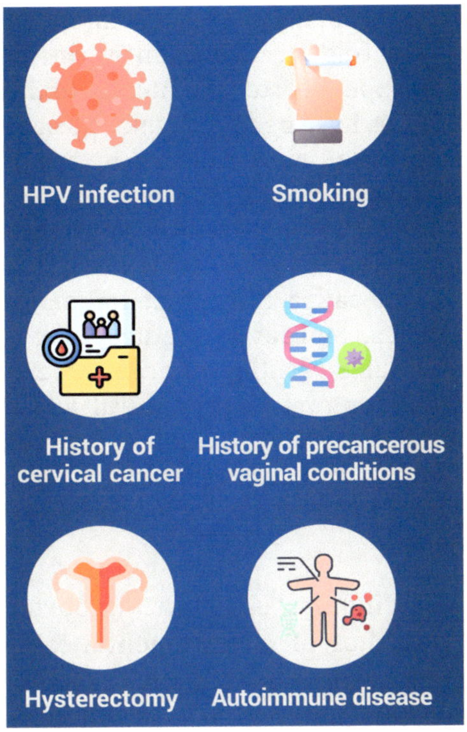

Figure 6.5. Risk Factors for vaginal cancer.

Source: https://actchealth.com/images/can-vaginal-cancer-be-prevented/02.png

Environmental and lifestyle exposures contribute to the risk factor profile of genital malignancy. Tobacco smoking, for example, has been implicated in the development of numerous types of cancer, including cancers of the genital tract, on the basis of its ability to cause carcinogenically altered changes in epithelial tissues. Diet and obesity contribute to a heightened risk profile, potentially through mechanisms that involve chronic inflammation and hormonal imbalance. The combination of these environmental exposures with infections and genetic susceptibility in an individual creates a multidimensional risk profile. Modulation of the modifiable risk factors by lifestyle interventions has a direct effect on public health outcomes. Education about the impact of environmental exposure, as well as prevention strategies for lifestyle modification, is essential to reducing the prevalence of genital malignancies and overall health in populations.

6.2.1. Genetic Predisposition

Genital cancer and genetic susceptibility, in particular, underscore the necessity to uncover inherent risk factors of the majority of cancers, particularly human papillomavirus (HPV) infection. Genetic diversity plays an important role in determining the susceptibility of an individual to particular malignancies, including disease-causing mutations in the GATA Binding Protein 2 (GATA2). Such patients tend to manifest HPV-associated anogenital cancer at much younger ages compared to their counterparts in the normal population, which speaks of a high element of genetic predisposition. This underscores the need for enhanced vigilance and prophylactic measures in already established genetic risk patients due to the fact that awareness of such predispositions can guide early intervention capable of blunting the effect of genital cancers. In addition to that, technological advances in genetic susceptibility determination have the potential for targeted interventions for cancer prevention and management. The development of risk scores based on environmental and genetic factors, for instance, allows clinicians to risk-stratify individuals for the risk of developing specific neoplasms of the genitals. Such stratification is particularly important in groups affected by conditions such as GATA2 haploinsufficiency, where risk for HPV disease is significantly higher prior to the typical age of onset. This, therefore, means that diagnosis can be performed early enough through meticulous monitoring of such high-risk individuals, hence enhancing therapeutic outcomes. With increasing advances in the field of medicine, including the inclusion of genetic susceptibility in practice, it is highly essential that patient prevention is maximized in the treatment of genital cancers. In addition, identification of the role played by genetic susceptibility in genital cancers is not only a risk measure but also an element in treating and follow-up too. Genetically at-risk patients will manifest more advanced disease, as indicated by the higher prevalence of HSIL in women who have GATA2 haploinsufficiency.

The need for multiple operations in these patients indicates that genetic susceptibility not only contributes to initial cancer development but also to rendering subsequent treatment difficult. Formulating tailored treatment strategies that target such genetic vulnerabilities can enhance patient outcomes and lower recurrence rates. Finally, addressing concerns of the complexity level of genetic predisposition is essential in simplifying prevention and treatment approaches of genital cancers, which emphasizes the complicated interaction between oncological services and genetics.

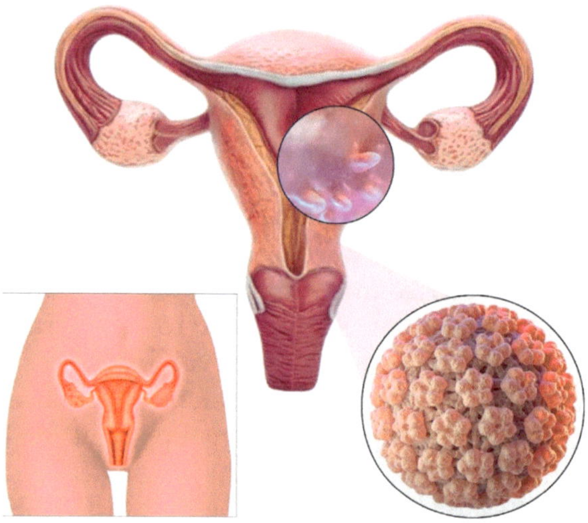

Figure 6.6. Human papillomavirus (HPV).

Source: https://nycgyne.com/wp-content/uploads/2025/01/human-papillomavirus-treatment-in-midtown-manhattan.jpg.webp

6.2.2. Environmental Influences

Environmental influences significantly influence the causation and occurrence of malignancies in the genitals, which indicates the interaction between external influences and an individual's health. Various environmental influences, including exposure to chemicals, toxins, and ways of living, have been recognized as causative factors for acquiring cancers in the genital tract. For instance, prolonged exposure to endocrine-disrupting agents such as phthalates and bisphenol A (BPA), which are found in plastics, can cause hormonal imbalance and malignancies. Moreover, studies have shown that individuals residing in areas where there is heavy industry or agricultural application of pesticides develop a higher frequency of reproductive cancers, revealing a causative association between environmental toxicity and cancer.

These findings show the importance of ongoing studies of environmental factors on cancer risk profiles and suggest the importance of regulatory policy aimed at reducing toxic exposures to the advantage of public health. Furthermore, lifestyle behaviors exert important influences on the environmental environment of genital cancers.

Cigarette smoking, excessive alcohol consumption, and diet can add to the risk of environmental hazards. For instance, smoking has already been conclusively linked to a number of cancers found in the genital area, given the numerous carcinogens involved with the ingestion of tobacco products. Similarly, consumption of a high quantity of processed foods but low in vegetables and fruits can weaken the ability of the body's detoxification mechanisms against carcinogenic substances, further raising the risk of cancer.

In addition, the epidemic of obesity driven by poor diet and physical inactivity has also been associated with increasing trends in particular cancers, including endometrial and prostate cancer. The self-reinforcing factors of lifestyle underscore the multifactorial patterns of environmental exposure to genital cancers and the necessity for a comprehensive strategy of cancer control that includes lifestyle intervention combined with environmental health programs.

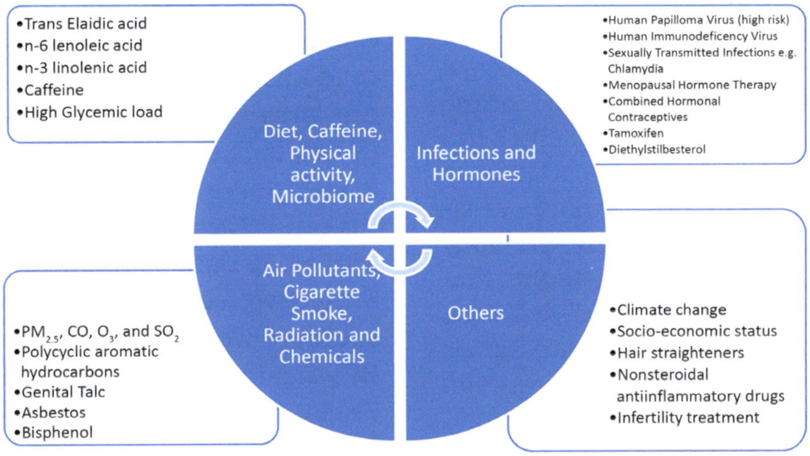

Figure 6.7. Environmental determinants of gynaecologic cancers.

Source: https://www.frontiersin.org/files/Articles/1430532/or-18-1430532-HTML-r1/image_m/or-18-1430532-g001.jpg

Finally, the socioeconomic determinants need to be recognized as a central component of the environmental determinants of genital cancers, which can lead to extreme differences in outcomes of cancer across various populations depending on the variation in access to health care, education, and health knowledge. Populations from a lower socioeconomic category may reside in areas with high exposure to environmental toxins and limited access to healthcare centers, resulting in delayed diagnosis and poor prognostics. Furthermore, educational disparities can affect an individual's ability to make healthy choices, like awareness of the dangers of certain environmental toxins. There has been evidence that the groups affected by socioeconomic disparities have more aggressive cancer types at higher rates, like the trends observed in recent survival rate epidemiological research among various demographic populations. This evidence points to the importance of public health initiatives towards addressing such discrepancies and towards bringing about a fairer environment where all individuals can achieve the highest possible outcomes in terms of health, particularly for genital cancers.

6.2.3. Lifestyle Choices

Lifestyle is a pivotal aspect of determining the risk of contracting genital cancers and therefore reflects the importance of people leading a better lifestyle. Within all these lifestyles, smoking has been found to be one of the largest risk factors for various cancers, including penile cancers. Cigarette smoke contains a number of carcinogens that compromise the immune system of the body and raise the rate of cell mutations. Additionally, poor hygiene is especially relevant to genital cancers because improper hygiene will lead to conditions of chronic inflammation that enhance cancer-promoting factors. By controlling for these behavioral factors proactively, individuals are able to reduce their chances of getting genital malignancies and contribute towards overall public health. Research into the crossover of lifestyle habits and cancer prevention is a vital aspect of enhancing individual health and reducing the occurrence of such debilitating diseases. Further, dietary habits play a vital role in determining whether or not an individual contracts genital cancers. Diets that are high in processed foods and low in fruits and vegetables can make one prone to cancer, meaning diet directly affects general health outcomes. Wholesome foods, particularly those containing antioxidants and anti-inflammatory substances, can fortify the body against carcinogenesis. Research highlights that men who consume vegetable and fruit-rich diets possess a decreased incidence of prostate cancer, further solidifying the connection between diet and risk for malignancy. Such data prove that healthy consumption of food can be an effective preventive measure for genital cancers.

Therefore, public health measures aimed at improving food choices are an essential aspect of cancer prevention programs, substantiating the fact that educated lifestyle decisions can be quantifiably beneficial. Finally, sexual health practices are also a significant part of lifestyle choices that dictate the development of genital cancers. Safe sex practices, such as the use of condoms and reducing the number of partners, can prevent sexually transmitted infections (STIs), including human papillomavirus (HPV), a well-proven risk factor for certain genital cancers. The prevalence of HPV in sexually active populations reaffirms the imperative for protective factor education and awareness. In addition, prevention through vaccination against HPV significantly lowers rates of related cancers. Programs designed to enhance public awareness of safe sex can go a long way in reducing the number of genital cancers. Therefore, including sexual health education in lifestyle change programs is necessary in managing the multifaceted risks of genital cancers, thereby improving the health outcome for heterogeneous populations.

Test Your Knowledge

1. What are the common risk factors associated with the development of genital malignancies?
2. How do lifestyle, genetic, and infectious factors contribute to the risk of genital cancers?

6.3. Symptoms and Diagnosis

Learning Outcome

1. Identify the common symptoms associated with genital malignancies
2. Describe diagnostic procedures and tests used for genital malignancies.
3. Explain the importance of early detection in the management of genital malignancies.

Early symptoms of genital malignancies are often subtle and nonspecific and lead to delayed diagnosis. Common presentations are abnormal vaginal bleeding or discharge, pelvic pain, and changes in urinary or bowel function. Importantly, these symptoms are usually caused by a range of benign disease processes and may not be diagnostic of underlying malignancies. This can be seen in cervical cancer, for example, in which late presentation is typical, particularly where access to healthcare is poor (Majinge et al., 2011). This highlights the importance of education and awareness about what constitutes atypical symptoms. Active symptom recognition may allow earlier intervention, with a dramatic impact on treatment outcome and survival rates. Diagnosis of genital cancers is frequently a combination of clinical examination, imaging studies, and histopathological tests. In cervical cancer, for example, Pap smears and

HPV tests play a pivotal role in early detection and screening (Majinge et al., 2011). Patients with abnormal results are typically referred to colposcopy, which allows direct visualization of the cervix and targeted biopsies. Additionally, in the case of sex disorders or ambiguous genitalia, thorough genital examinations are important to establish an unequivocal diagnosis. These thorough diagnostic tests also underscore the importance of multidisciplinary approaches in accurately diagnosing malignancies and implementing suitable treatment regimens. Apart from the initial diagnosis, the challenges in diagnosing genital malignancies also continue, as the majority of patients experience hindrances that complicate their long-term care. These barriers could include socio-economic causes, anxiety over diagnosis, and lack of access to follow-up treatment. For instance, studies show that patients in low-resource settings present with late stages of cancer, and these correlate with poor prognosis (Majinge et al., 2011). In addition, patients' reluctance to present themselves for treatment of symptoms can also be a contributing factor in late presentation, as it lowers the efficacy of available treatment. Enabling a healthcare environment with emphasis on education and accessibility can avoid such challenges and facilitate early diagnosis, ultimately improving the fate of the victims of genital cancers.

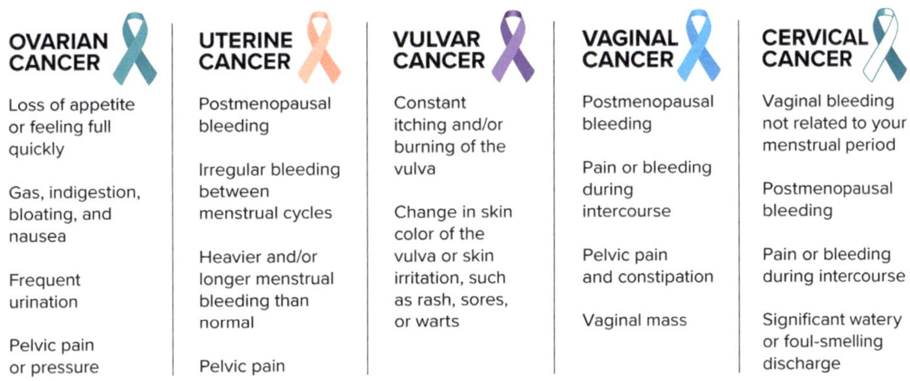

Figure 6.8. Signs and symptoms of gynecologic cancers.

Source: https://www.onealcanceruab.org/wp-content/uploads/sites/2/2022/12/gyn_cancers.jpg

6.3.1. Common Symptoms Associated With Genital Malignancies

Genital cancers have a myriad of symptoms that are frequently nonspecific or misinterpreted, thus delaying treatment and diagnosis. Abnormal bleeding is usually one of the initial signs, but this appears in varying ways in varying cancers. For instance, postmenopausal bleeding (PMB) is a useful symptom in deciding on endometrial cancer because it occurs 12 months or later from the woman's last menstrual period and can occur with or without concomitant underlying pathology. The irregular bleeding needs to be fully assessed clinically since it is a common clinical presentation that is associated with genital malignancies, prompting histopathological evaluation to determine its etiology. Recognition of these symptoms is necessary to facilitate on-time intervention, as timely diagnosis tremendously improves the prognosis in malignancies (Talwar et al., 2024). In addition to irregular bleeding, patients may experience urinary or bowel habits that must be evaluated.

These symptoms can be an increased frequency of urination, urgency, or pain while urinating, and may indicate cancers of the cervix or vagina. Conversely, gastrointestinal symptoms such as spontaneous changes in bowel habit can point to anal cancers. The patients would also feel pressure or pain in the pelvic area, which can easily be underappreciated and misattributed to benign processes such as fibroids or dysmenorrhea. This symptom, particularly if chronic and alongside other presentations such as abnormal discharge, should raise suspicion for potential malignancy, highlighting the significance of careful investigations in patients who present with such a common symptom encountered in genital malignancies (Talwar et al., 2024).

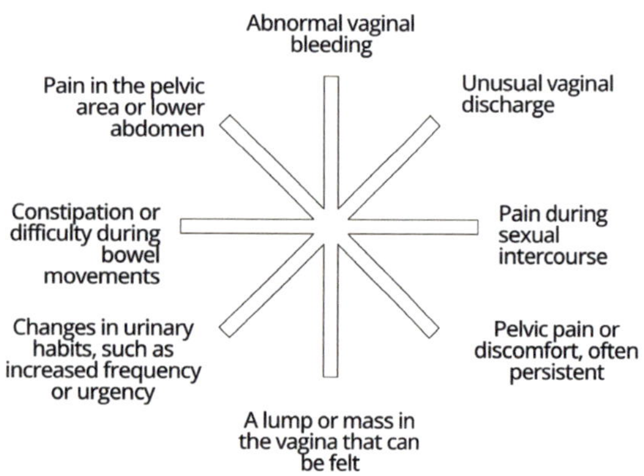

Figure 6.9. Symptoms of vaginal cancer.

Source: https://continentalhospitals.com/uploads/mceu_57892447121700202872037.jpg

Notably, genital cancer symptoms are also accompanied by more diffuse signs of advanced disease. Loss of appetite, weight loss, and fatigue are most often observed in advanced genital cancers such as vulvar or ovarian cancers. These systemic presentations can lead to misdiagnosis since they are attributed to other conditions of an illness, thereby necessitating the inclusion of malignancy in differential diagnoses while presenting such nonspecific symptoms in patients. Secondly, infertility as an outcome can be a devastating effect of female genital malignancies, particularly in young women presenting with such diagnoses. This is a more sophisticated description of the symptoms that will necessitate increased awareness and education regarding genital malignancies, which would allow for earlier diagnosis and prognosis in such affected persons (Roy et al., 2025).

6.3.2. Diagnostic Procedures and Tests

In the diagnosis of genital cancers, an accurate understanding of diagnostic tests and examination is critical. Initial evaluations typically involve physical examination that includes visual inspection and palpation of genitalia to identify any abnormality from normal. Subsequently, practitioners normally employ imaging devices such as ultrasound, MRI, or CT scans to further image a potential malignancy. These imaging modalities play a significant role in determining the extent of disease and aiding in planning the treatment. Moreover, serum tumor markers, such as CA-125 or alphafetoprotein, are taken; these markers may prove to be very useful in detecting the presence and status of some genital cancers. Accurate diagnosis at this point is of paramount importance, as it forms the platform for subsequent therapeutic maneuvers and is a vital determinant of patient prognoses. Biopsy remains the gold standard of diagnostic methods for the diagnosis of genital malignancies after initial screening and imaging. Punch, excisional, and fine-needle aspiration biopsy are various techniques of biopsy done to enable histopathological analysis of suspicious lesions. The choice of the biopsy type can be informed by the nature and accessibility of the lesions. Histological examination by a pathologist gives clinicians critical information regarding the grade, type, and invasive nature of cancer, hence informing treatment. For instance, the diagnosis of lichen sclerosus, a subacute inflammatory process sometimes associated with squamous cell carcinoma, is significantly enhanced with the addition of serum autoantibody measurement, as seen by recent advances in diagnostic approaches (Alarcon-Segovia et al., 2004).

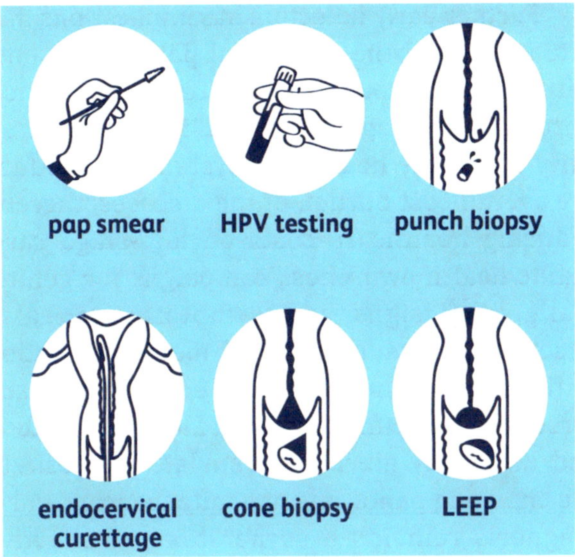

Figure 6.10. Cervical cancer diagnosis.

Source: https://www.verywellhealth.com/thmb/vj9VrorZubf3a-oNCPZvX2a518o=/1500x0/filters:no_upscale():max_bytes(150000):strip_icc()/cervical-cancer-diagnosis-5b647ce246e0fb0025341fff.png

This indicates the way the evolving context of diagnostic practice, focusing on timely and accurate diagnosis, is central to improving patient outcomes in the case of genital malignancies. As a means to enhance diagnostic precision, standardized assessment tools such as the Quality Assessment of Diagnostic Accuracy Studies 2 (QUADAS-2) have been developed to measure the quality of cancer-screening and treatment-related studies. With cervical cancer-specific modifications, these instruments ensure comprehensive assessments of the quality of diagnostic test findings. For instance, based on a recent study, the majority of post-treatment studies had significant risks of bias, predominantly in patient selection. They can create significant discrepancies in the efficacy of diagnostic tests utilized among various populations (Clarke et al., 2020). Therefore, by the utilization of systematic assessment tools, not only is a deeper understanding of the diagnostic picture obtained, but also a setting where there is constant enhancement of diagnostic methods. The modification of these quality tools is needed in future studies because it is used directly in clinical practice, ensuring that patients are given the best and evidence-based care for genital malignancies.

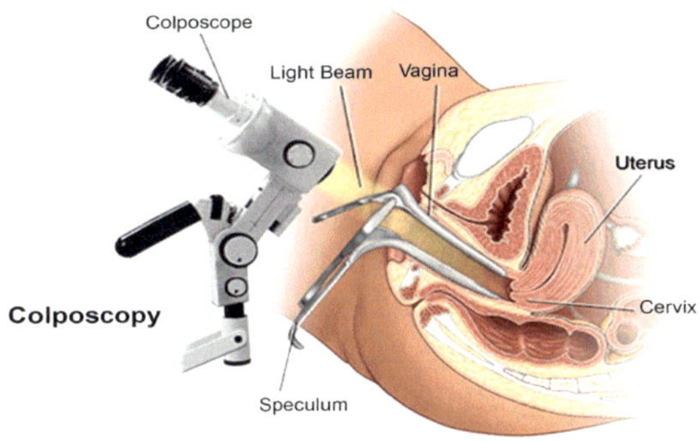

Figure 6.11. Colposcope is a magnifying instrument used to find out whether there are abnormal areas in the cervix or vagina.

Source: https://www.medifee.com/blog/cervical-cancer-testing-symptoms-risk-factors-diagnosis-prevention/

6.3.3. Importance of Early Detection

The significance of detection in genital malignancies cannot be overstressed, as it plays a central role in increased patient outcomes and survival. Unlike most cancers, genital malignancies often present with nonspecific and vague symptoms, consequently leading to delayed diagnosis. For instance, primary lymphoma of the female genital tract may present with symptoms like abdominal pain and vaginal bleeding that are typical of benign gynecological conditions. As indicated by the literature, patients are more likely to present in gynecological departments where nonspecific symptoms may precipitate misdiagnosis or undue delay in treatment. Early detection through intensive screening and education among medical professionals is essential since early treatment has the potential to completely alter the character of the disease and optimize therapeutic outcomes (Wang et al., 2025). The intricacies introduced by genital cancers underscore the need for specially tailored screening protocols properly matched to varied populations and risk groups. For instance, while squamous cell carcinoma of the lower lip is relatively rare, the absence of conventional risk factors in certain patients may render attempts to identify such early onerous, underlining the need for clinical vigilance. As is evident in the case of malignancies presented by patients with no conventional risk factors, medical staff must be extra cautious and resort to differential diagnoses. Effective early detection techniques can include regular testing and patient education of potential symptoms, thereby enabling early intervention. Early detection can ultimately result in the provision of a multidisciplinary treatment protocol comprising gynecologists, oncologists, and pathologists working in collaboration to optimize patient outcome (Rageh et al., 2025).

Further, early detection has implications that extend beyond the individual patient outcome because it has broader public health significance. Through the diagnosis of malignancies at an early stage, the healthcare systems can reduce the overall cost burden of the diseases, thereby reducing healthcare costs on late-stage care. Public health awareness campaigns for genital malignancy signs and symptoms can also encourage individuals to seek medical attention in time. Such schemes would ensure increased screening rates, improved risk factor awareness, and, ultimately, morbidity from late diagnosis. In the changing panorama of genital cancers, early diagnosis remains a cornerstone of effective health measures, playing a major role in survival and quality of life in affected patients (Wang et al., 2025).

Test Your Knowledge

1. Which diagnostic procedures and tests are typically used to confirm genital malignancies?
2. Why is early detection crucial in the management of genital malignancies?

6.4. Treatment Options

Learning Outcome

1. Describe surgical interventions used in the treatment of genital malignancies
2. Explain the roles of chemotherapy and radiation therapy in managing genital malignancies
3. Discuss emerging treatments and the significance of clinical trials in genital malignancy care

The therapy for genital cancers is generally multidisciplinary and needs a multi-treatment approach tailored to the individual patient. The therapy often consists of surgery, radiation, and chemotherapy, each appropriate to the given histological type and degree of cancer. Extirpation by surgery remains the cornerstone of therapy for the majority of genital cancers, especially localized cancers. For example, radical vulvectomy is being commonly employed in the therapy of vulvar cancers because it is capable of removing the tumors completely and yielding curative outcomes. However, such a brutal surgical procedure can lead to catastrophic morbidity, so less invasive treatments and adjuvants have been explored to avoid complications without sacrificing efficacy. When surgery in advanced cases is not curative enough by itself, multimodal therapy is indicated. Chemotherapy and radiation therapy are also commonly employed to supplement surgical resection, particularly in cases of regional lymph nodes or distant metastasis. Chemotherapy can be with a regimen that is a mixture of drugs that are targeted against proliferating tumor cells, while radiation can be either the major treatment modality or administered as an adjunct to surgery. Both can reduce tumors, palliate symptoms, and increase survival rates. Despite such improvements, the result of treatment can vary greatly based on the nature of the tumor and the patient, necessitating a personalized treatment approach for each case (Ciofalo et al., 2017). Involvement of a multidisciplinary team is important in the management of genital cancers to maximize results and deliver comprehensive treatment. Interdisciplinary coordination among oncologists, surgeons, radiologists, and supportive care providers becomes feasible to ensure a more synchronized regimen of treatment that addresses the physical, psychological, and psychosocial requirements of the patient. For instance, conditions such as paraneoplastic pemphigus that have been known to occur in relation to cancers of the genital tract require careful planning of oncological and dermatological therapies (Ciofalo et al., 2017). Prompt diagnosis and early interventions, in conjunction with patient education and counseling, are key elements of effective management since they can have the maximum influence on recovery and overall quality of life for patients faced with such colossal threats.

6.4.1. Surgical Interventions

Surgical interventions play a pivotal role in the management of genital malignancies, influencing both the success of treatment and patients' quality of life. Surgical interventions tend to remove malignant growths, reconstructively restore anatomical deformity, and prevent relapse of the disease. Radical operations, such as partial or entire resection of affected tissues, are required for effective management of advanced genital malignancies. Where there are malignancies as a secondary complication of the treatment of another disease, such as hematopoietic stem cell transplantation (HSCT), the need for surgical intervention is higher. Complications of hormone replacement therapy and chronic genital graft-versus-host disease create a demand for surgical intervention to restore normal function and improve general well-being in patients, demonstrating the intricate interdependence of surgery and quality of life in the context of genital malignancy (Kamada et al.,

2021). In the context of atypical genitalia from disorders of sex development (DSD), surgery must be mature and multidimensional. Surgeons, endocrinologists, and psychologists must collaborate to create individualized treatment plans in light of the individual challenges presented by each patient. The improvement in medical knowledge and technology has aided medical experts to gain a clearer understanding of the implications of various DSDs, thus facilitating better surgical decision-making. Early surgical exploration in cases where malignancies are suspected based on atypical presentations is essential. Such interventions not only address oncological requirements but also take away the psychosocial burdens from congenital genital conditions. With altered attitudes within society towards diversity and openness regarding gender identity, surgical management of genital conditions requires a wise balance between medical necessity and ethics, once again underlining the complexities of surgical intervention here (Ahmed et al., 2017).

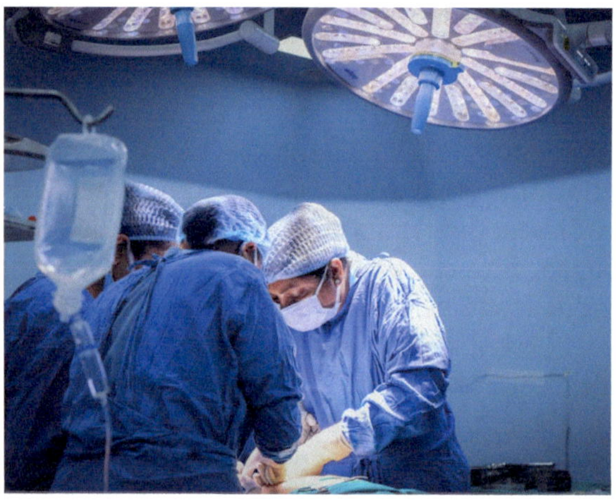

Source: https://www.mgmch.org/images/gynoclogy-about.jpg

Lastly, surgical interventions within the field of genital cancer need to not only aim at the physical removal of cancerous tissue but also global patient management. These include psychological care, rehabilitation, and ongoing hormonal treatments following surgery. Proficient surgical interventions can significantly enhance the comfort of recovery, reduce the possibility of complications, and achieve a better quality of life through effective reconstructive techniques. The effects of these interventions can have a strong influence on the psychological and social quality of life of a patient as they progress with cancer. With improvements in the studies of this field, the importance of individualized surgical methods taking into account unique cases and patient preferences cannot be overstressed. Surgical procedures are therefore an important component of successful genital malignancy management, such as clinical efficacy and patient-centered care (Kamada et al., 2021).

6.4.2. Chemotherapy and Radiation Therapy

The therapeutic situation for cancers of the genitals is dominated by the two modalities of radiation therapy and chemotherapy, both with their roles and actions. Chemotherapy employs cytotoxic drugs aimed at killing cancer cells by disrupting their ability to divide and multiply. This systemic modality is particularly effective for cancers such as cervical cancer, where the treatment can involve targeting metastases in a remote site. Investigations have revealed that chemotherapy, when combined with radiation therapy, can enhance the efficacy of treatment and survival rates, particularly in advanced disease. The use of such treatments together is thus crucial in designing efficient treatment schemes that take into account the biological behavior of the tumors and the health status of the patient, thereby revolutionizing a multidimensional method in treating genital malignancies. Radiation therapy in the form of external beam radiation and brachytherapy is a significant modality of treatment for most genital cancers, such as cervical and endometrial cancer. For instance, large groups of patients with advanced cervical carcinoma were treated with teletherapy as a first-line treatment at the Ocean Road Cancer Institute. The findings indicate that while the external beam radiation works, its work also greatly relies on the stage of the illness and the dosage of radiation given.

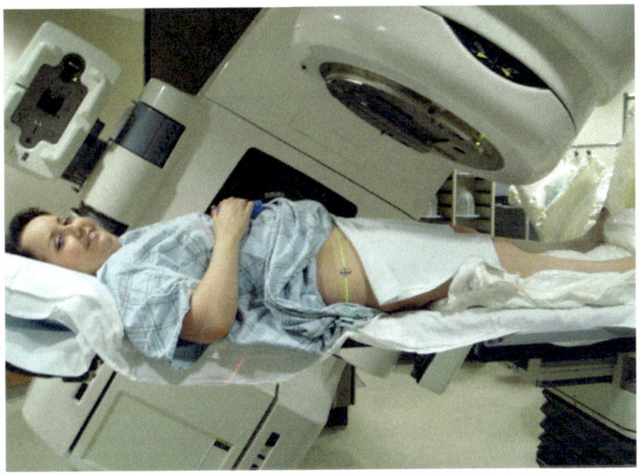

Figure 6.12. Radiation therapy

Source: https://upload.wikimedia.org/wikipedia/commons/d/d5/Radiation_therapy.jpg

Moreover, patient follow-up and compliance difficulty contribute to the challenge in treatment planning outcome evaluation, which further requires creative solutions to care delivery. These points highlight the intrinsic interrelationship between radiation dosing, therapy planning, and outcome prediction among genital malignancies and the need for tailored solutions. In even more precise cases, such as embryonal rhabdomyosarcoma, particularly the botryoid type that involves the female genital tract, the treatment regimen often requires a subtlety of management to balance effective management with the preservation of future fertility. The cancer, although very uncommon, has been found to be very responsive to a combination of local surgery and adjuvant chemotherapy, thereby circumventing the use of radiation exposure that could adversely affect reproductive capacity. A personalized treatment plan is called for, especially with respect to how virulent this cancer is. Notably, studies show that having a multi-disciplinary approach can lead to favorable outcomes, e.g., better disease-free survival if early diagnosis and personalized therapy are employed. The advancing information in treatment protocols underscores the need to continue researching so as to develop innovative therapeutic protocols for difficult genital cancers (Majinge et al., 2011; Almperis et al., 2023).

6.4.3. Emerging Treatments and Clinical Trials

The treatment environment for genital cancers is continually evolving, with the push of innovative research and clinical trials aimed at improving patient outcomes. Newer therapies, namely immunotherapies, have come into focus due to their capacity to make the immune system recognize and destroy cancer cells more efficiently. Research on the effectiveness of checkpoint inhibitors, including PD-1 and PD-L1 inhibitors, has been encouraging, particularly when used in combination with traditional therapies such as chemotherapy. For instance, the use of immunotherapy in conjunction with chemotherapy regimens has the ability to improve response rates for certain tumour types, as seen in observations pointing towards specific protein markers mediating potential responses to chemotherapy, such as ERCC1 and TOP2A. Such findings are supportive of the concept that an approach to precision oncology, founded on biomarker analysis, can enable the development of individualized treatment strategies, hence optimizing the treatment of genital cancers (Arguello et al., 2020). Clinical trials of penile squamous cell carcinoma (PeSCC) and germ-cell tumors (GCT) are pivotal advancements in the topic. While they are uncommon, both of these cancers are significant due to their prevalence among young people and risk for poor prognoses if they are not treated according to set guidelines. Current clinical trials are exploring the use of new chemotherapeutic agents in combination with the standard of care, and promising findings indicate that a high rate of compliance with prescribed treatment protocols can greatly increase survival (Gauler et al., 2019).

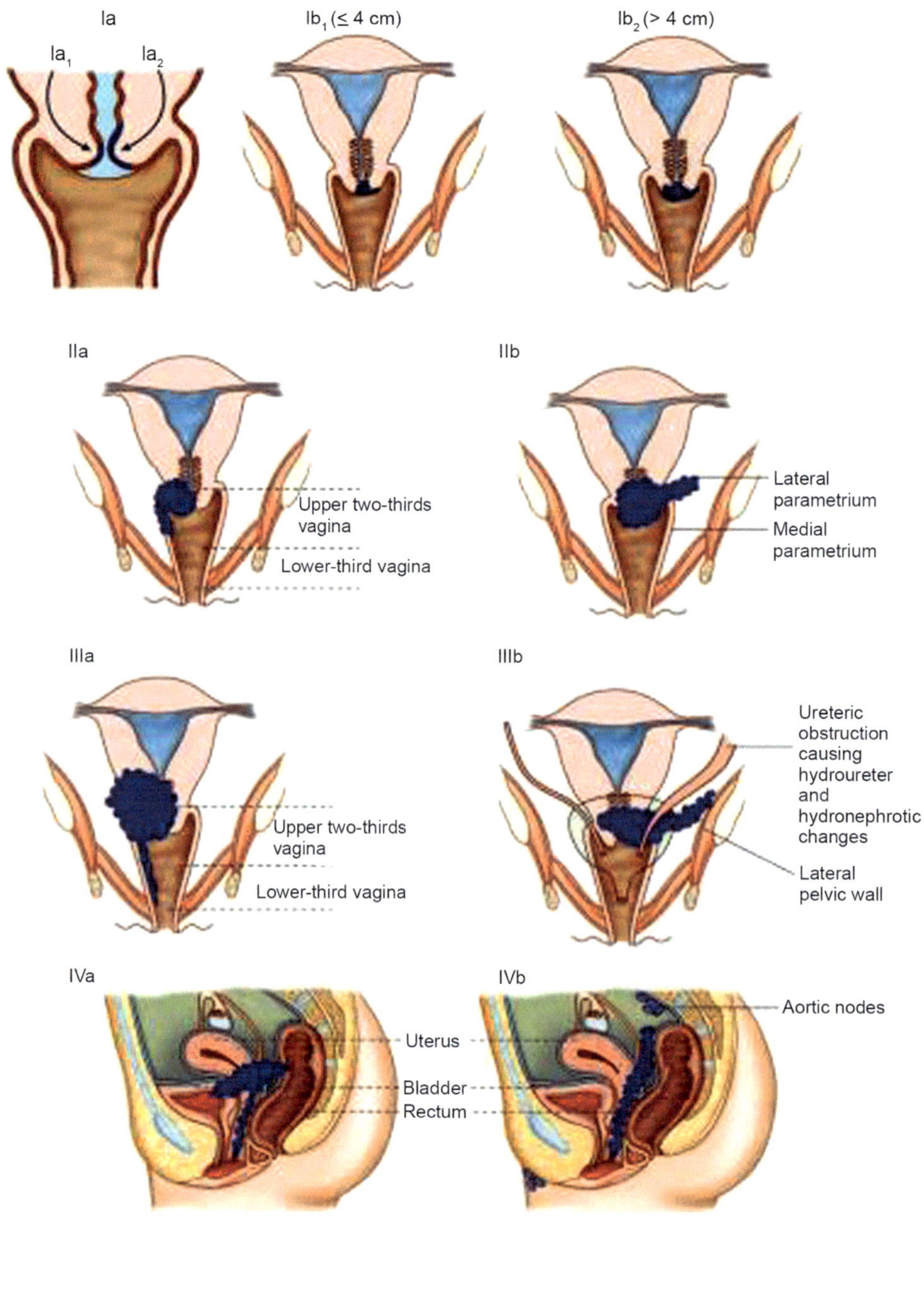

Figure 6.13. Diagrammatic representation of staging of carcinoma cervix according to FIGO.

Source: https://oshimu.com/wp-content/uploads/2021/07/Gynaecology-DC-Dutta.pdf

In addition, clinical networks such as the ERN EURACAN identify the benefit of being treated in centers of excellence so that the patient can receive state-of-the-art therapies and multidisciplinary therapy (Almar et al., 2019). The cooperative nature of such trials has the potential to produce more optimal management plans and eventually better patient prognosis. With ongoing research, it will be crucial to sustain surveillance of novel combinatorial therapies. The use of next-generation sequencing and biomarker discovery is critical in guiding the clinical application of new therapies. For example, microsatellite instability or high tumor mutational burden identification has been linked to improved responses to immunotherapy, providing a rationale for personalized treatment regimens. Ongoing clinical trials are exploring the delineation of the efficacy of these therapies in heterogeneous patient populations, allowing for broader generalizability of successful strategies. The importance of accurate data collection and analysis in these trials cannot be overstated because they have the mission of illuminating the paths to effective therapies and eventually advancing genital malignancy therapy (Arguello et al., 2020).

Test Your Knowledge

1. How are chemotherapy and radiation therapy utilized in managing genital cancers?
2. What emerging treatments and clinical trials are currently being explored for genital malignancies?

6.5. Psychological Impact

Learning Outcome

1. Understand the emotional effects on patients
2. Define support systems and counseling
3. Discuss coping strategies for patients and families

Diagnosis of genital cancer can have profound psychological effects on the affected individuals, as well as their families. The first reaction to the receipt of such a diagnosis is usually a range of feelings from shock, denial, and fear of the unknown. These emotional disturbances are added to by societal attitudes towards genital health and sexuality, and these may result in feelings of shame or isolation. Patients may become preoccupied with issues of their identity, body image, and future relationships. Emotional suffering due to a malignancy in such a private area can be paralyzing, complementing the physical challenges posed by the disease itself. Moreover, support systems fail to effectively meet the emotional and psychological needs of patients because they lack the necessary resources or expertise to provide adequate support in such cases. Moreover, treating genital malignancy at times involves not only medical interventions but also profound psychological adjustments. Patients may undergo surgical operations that alter their physical appearance and function, and thus make their emotional response even more complex. For example, operative alterations can lead to loss or feelings of incompleteness, impacting sexual identity and self-esteem. As was reported in recent studies, psychological support throughout therapy has become very necessary, necessitating an integrated approach to patient care that will address both the physical and psychological effects of diagnosis and treatment. It is essential that health practitioners offer open communication so that patients can express their concerns and anxieties during their treatment process, thereby offering a conducive environment that recognizes and touches on the psychological nature of their care. Multidisciplinary interventions are highly prized as essential in addressing the psychological impact of genital cancers. Having mental health specialists be part of the care team can significantly enhance patients' overall quality of life, allowing them to cope with the nuances of their condition more effectively. Interprofessional collaboration is particularly important in addressing the psychological implications of diseases such as disorders of sex development (DSD), where issues of personal identity and societal stigma intersect. As demonstrated in current research, those with abnormal genitalia are likely to bear psychological burdens that emanate from their medical conditions, especially when combined with weak support structures. By way of application of methods including counseling, supporting peers, and educational content, medical professionals can curtail the psychological impact of genital cancers and improve quality of life for those afflicted while fostering increased resilience through the recovery process (Eugster et al., 2017; Ahmed et al., 2017).

6.5.1. Emotional Effects on Patients

The psychological state of genital cancer patients is greatly affected by the complicated issues they face. The diagnosis will trigger a snowball of psychological responses, which comprise anxiety and depression, and can greatly undermine the quality of life of a patient. Isolation is an emotion that could set in as the patients deal with the social stigma of genital cancers, which heightens their emotional distress. As cancer progresses and treatment cycles start, the physical side effects of fatigue and loss of sex function further exacerbate these emotional effects, most often leading to hopelessness. Awareness of the extent of such emotional reactions not only informs clinicians of the psychological needs of their patients but also emphasizes palliative care throughout the course of cancer. Anemia is among the most prevalent complications in cancer patients and carries major emotional implications, particularly in genital cancer. Approximately 68% of patients with newly diagnosed solid tumors, i.e., gynecologic cancers, are anemic, with clinically evident symptoms presenting as fatigue, reduced appetite, and impairment of cognitive function. Apart from causing physical disability, these symptoms diminish emotional resilience, causing increased anxiety and a lower quality of life. The coexistence of anemia and emotional distress necessitates that medical practitioners closely monitor and manage both these issues. Active management of anemia enables medical practitioners to alleviate some of the emotional load for patients and thus enhance their capacity to cope with the psychological effects of cancer treatment and other illnesses (Dandavate et al., 2023).

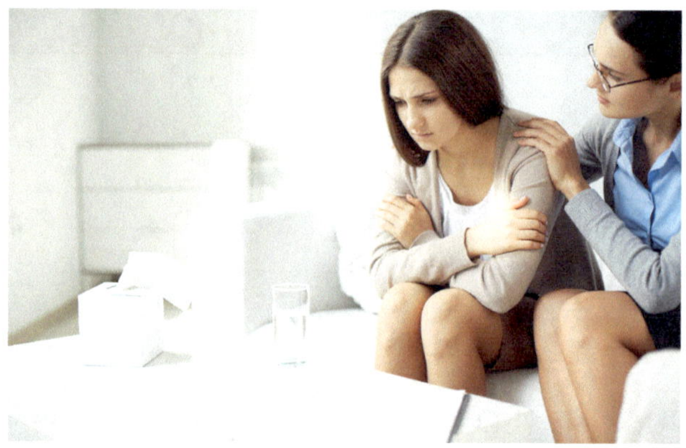

Source: https://uat.medpsychmd.com/wp-content/uploads/2021/09/psychologist-with-patient-pressfoto-smaller.jpg

Of note, advances in therapeutic modalities such as peptide receptor radionuclide therapy (PRRT) have also demonstrated beneficial impacts on health-related quality of life (HRQoL) in neuroendocrine neoplasm patients. Although studies indicate that interventions significantly improve overall HRQoL, including emotional function, they indicate a deficit in studies addressing their effect on sexual function—an important aspect of genital cancer patients' well-being. Since cancer treatments often cause extreme changes in body autonomy and sexual health, the psychological effect of these changes can be extremely distressing. Subsequent research must explore these dimensions further, as addressing emotional impact in relation to sexual function can help break the door open for more holistic care methods that have respect for the complexity of the experiences and emotional demands of the patients during cancer treatment (Malandrino et al., 2022).

6.5.2. Support Systems and Counseling

Support systems play a critical role in the management of patients with genital cancers. Those complex and often extensive health conditions have a tendency to cause considerable emotional and psychological distress that needs a strong support system. Family and friends, doctors, and professionally established specialized support groups for patients who have gone through similar conditions are typically part of support systems.

These supportive relationships can significantly reduce distressing feelings of loneliness and anxiety and increase patients' resilience. Secondly, collaborative care programs that include mental health professionals such as psychologists and counselors ensure emotional wellness alongside physical care. Being able to discuss with others, access shared knowledge, and receive emotional support from peers navigating the same vulnerabilities creates a holistic approach to coping with their diagnosis and treatment. Counseling for the diagnosis of genital malignancy is more than just psychological counseling; it is an integral component in the overall treatment protocol. Trained counselors have the ability to apply various therapeutic techniques to address such issues as depression, anxiety, and body image problems, which are typically exhibited upon learning of the malignancy diagnosis. Cognitive-behavioral therapy (CBT), as one example, has been found to be helpful in helping patients reframe negative thinking and cope with the uncertainty of their condition. Aside from individual counseling, group therapy is also a powerful tool for collective experience and support. In these group therapy sessions, patients gain coping mechanisms and emotional resources that are so badly needed in addressing the psychological effects of their disease.

These multi-dimensional counseling interventions are essential in building psychological resilience and enhancing the overall well-being of patients with genital malignancies. The role of the multidisciplinary care systems cannot be overstressed, particularly in the case of patients with disorders of sex development (DSD) who have common challenges in surmounting their health conditions. Research emphasizes that an integrated care model involving endocrinologists, urologists, and mental health professionals is necessary while keeping in view medical as well as psychosocial requirements.

As noticed through a review, early diagnosis and treatment minimize life-threatening complications and psychosocial distress associated with DSD (Asikin et al., 2024). Secondly, the review points out that collaborative decision-making involving the patient and their family for care planning is crucial. An inclusive process in this way empowers individuals, making them learn and strengthening their coping strategies, thus promoting an environment that is supportively healthy to heal. Therefore, integrating holistic support systems with evidence-based counseling is crucial for improving long-term results for victims of genital cancers and related conditions (Ahmed et al., 2012).

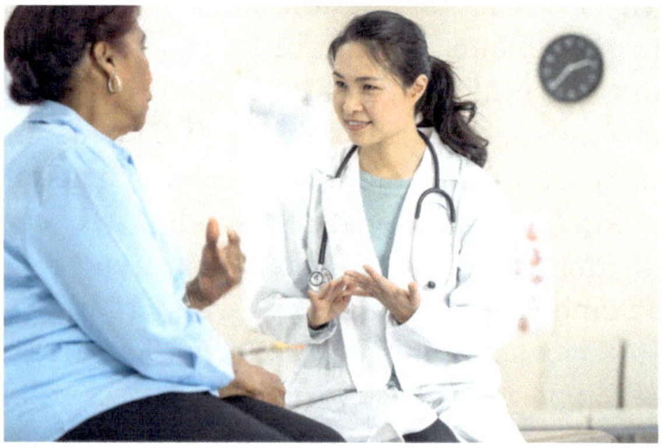

Source: https://uamshealth.com/wp-content/uploads/2024/08/dr-and-patient-1024x683.jpg

6.5.3. Coping Strategies For Patients and Families

Genital cancer diagnosis permanently alters the equation for the patients and their families, necessitating effective coping methods to weather the resulting emotional and psychological distress. Notably, families play a very important role in the support system of the patient, and it follows that communications between family members need to be open. A supportive environment allows the family to process collectively, issues, feelings, and information, ultimately ensuring resilience.

This engagement not only includes receptiveness to the treatment process but also information about the disease itself that can reduce the feeling of isolation and confusion that occurs at diagnosis. It is a multidisciplinary intervention in which the health care providers offer counseling, teaching, and support that can aid the coping of the family so that issues practical and emotional are addressed appropriately as they are capable of coping with the complexity of coping with genital malignancy (Achermann et al., 2010). In addition to support from the family, coping mechanisms on an individual level are also crucial in the psychological adaptation of victims of genital malignancy. Patients may be assisted by structured psychological therapies such as cognitive-behavioral therapy (CBT), which can significantly reduce symptoms of anxiety and depression. CBT results in patients restructuring unhelpful thinking and acquiring helpful coping skills, thus enhancing emotional regulation throughout treatment.

Support groups may prove to be a valuable resource since they provide a discussion forum for experiences and acquiring knowledge from other individuals with the same problem for both patients and families. Mindfulness practice, such as meditation and yoga, has also been found to be beneficial in achieving emotional stability as well as decreasing stress levels. As much as patients and their families attempt to rediscover normalcy amid uncertainty, these interventions can support their resilience when they attempt to foster hope against hope with genital malignancy (Ediati et al., 2021). Besides, it is an extremely difficult issue to navigate the health system, which has the tendency to exacerbate stress among patients and their families.

Therefore, knowledge of their rights and what they are entitled to is the only means of evading the helpless feeling that one gets most frequently during treatment. Families and patients must become active with healthcare staff, posing questions and inquiring about treatment procedures, potential results, and the nature of follow-up care. Financial planning is also an essential part of adaptation, as medical treatment can result in additional expenses.

Patients can benefit by exploring financial assistance programs, coverage, or government programs for patients with medical challenges. Educating families on the ins and outs of patient care, such as navigating visits and arranging support services, allows for a more effective coping model. By developing an informed, engaged response, families and patients are actually able to contribute significantly to their capability to cope with the myriad of problems created by genital malignancy (Achermann et al., 2010).

Test Your Knowledge

1. How do support systems and counseling benefit patients dealing with genital cancers?
2. What coping strategies can patients and their families use to manage the challenges of genital malignancies?

SUMMARY

The pathogenesis of genital cancers presents a complex interaction of environmental and genetic determinants of their onset and prognosis. Insight into the pathogenetic principles of malignancies such as Müllerian clear cell carcinoma can enhance clinical outcomes. The presented case is associated with a rare mutation in RAD54L, making genetic profiling the crucial component of therapy for malignancies. This information gives clinicians insight that dictates unique therapeutic strategies and, in the process, could increase survival rates. The findings underscore the necessity for ongoing studies to decipher the molecular biology of these rare cancers, as the information will eventually be used to guide treatment regimens and maximize patient care in the future (Deng et al., 2024). Also of note is the role played by human papillomavirus (HPV) in genital cancer epidemiology, primarily within the younger population.

As is clear from the results of the systematic review, infection with HPV is highly variable in line with demographic factors, including age and abuse history. The high incidence of low-risk HPV types in children underscores the need for aggressive public health measures to teach families and clinicians about prevention and management. The rarity of HPV in girls under 12, especially in instances of sexual abuse, necessitates caution in carrying out research on malignancy within them. Thus, attending to such matters through particularized research can unravel strands of early intervention as well as enhanced health outcomes (Bispo et al., 2024). Advancement of the science of genital malignancy is crucial for the facilitation of detection, treatment, and prevention protocols. Integration of genetic knowledge, including that relating to RAD54L mutations, with an insightful comprehension of HPV dynamics provides a means for the redefinition of clinical practices. The results gleaned from recent studies highlight the urgent need for a collaborative approach to fill the gaps in existing knowledge on these disorders, in a bid to improve patient management. Through research and study of these complex interdependencies, the medical community can develop more effective ways of dealing with genital cancers and ultimately see to the well-being of affected individuals (Deng et al., 2024; Bispo et al., 2024).

In genital malignancy, some relevant factors are important in understanding its nature and significance. Such malignancies may be challenging due to the varied anatomical and physiological characteristics of the genitalia. Particularly in ambiguous genitalia and DSD, management by more than one specialty is necessary for accurate diagnosis and appropriate treatment. Multidisciplinary teams enable thorough assessments and personalized treatment plans, not just addressing medical needs but also psychological and sociocultural implications of genital cancer. Prompt treatment and scheduled follow-up are significant in guaranteeing positive health outcomes and all-around care to affected individuals, particularly when such conditions arise early in life. The very character of these conditions underscores the necessity of specialist care by seasoned practitioners within a tertiary care setting, which shall result in enhanced prognostic outcomes. The key advancements in screening techniques have also become pivotal for early diagnosis of genital cancer. Just like standard cancer screening protocols, effective early detection remains paramount for reducing levels of advanced disease stages. Dermoscopy has proven to be valuable in the diagnosis of skin-related cancers with increased accuracy compared to normal examinations. Some features of genital lesions can identify malignant lesions from benign lesions, enhancing the chances of early treatment initiation. In addition, identifying the features of melanoma that are specific to the genital area assists medical practitioners in identifying abnormalities with greater ease and in modifying screening guidelines accordingly. Thus, the integration of advanced diagnostic technologies into established clinical procedures ultimately serves to enhance patient outcomes for patients with these cancers.

Finally, follow-up and long-term support are required facets of genital malignancy care. The psychological and emotional toll of such diagnoses necessitates ongoing counseling and support services, which need to be incorporated into treatment protocols. In addition, regular follow-up of patients following therapy is necessary to monitor for recurrence and to manage any subsequent complications or side effects of therapy. This need for comprehensive care emphasizes the importance of an interdisciplinary approach, which synergistically blends medical management with psychosocial care. An entire understanding of the genital cancers includes not only the clinical aspect but also the need for a comprehensive response that addresses the physical, emotional, and social dimensions of the care for the patients with the ultimate aim of improving the quality of life of the affected.

KEY TERMS FROM THIS CHAPTER

- Abdominal pain
- Anogenital cancer
- Cancer prevention measures
- Colposcopy
- GATA2 haploinsufficiency
- Genital cancer
- Genital tract cancers
- Human papillomavirus (HPV) vaccine
- Male genital cancer
- Pap smears
- Vaginal bleeding
- Alphafetoprotein
- Cancer detection
- Cognitive-behavioral therapy (CBT)
- Endometrial cancer
- Genetic predisposition
- Genital malignancy
- HIV transmission
- Lymphoma
- Malignant neoplasms
- Unequivocal diagnosis

CRITICAL THINKING QUESTIONS

1. **Which of the following is the most common type of cervical cancer?**
   a. Squamous cell carcinoma
   b. Adenocarcinoma
   c. Small cell carcinoma
   d. Melanoma
2. **Which human papillomavirus (HPV) types are most strongly associated with genital malignancies?**
   a. HPV 6 and 11
   b. HPV 16 and 18
   c. HPV 1 and 2
   d. HPV 31 and 33
3. **Which of the following is a major risk factor for ovarian cancer?**
   a. Early menopause
   b. Nulliparity (never having given birth)
   c. Use of oral contraceptives
   d. Regular exercise
4. **The common presenting symptom of vulvar cancer is:**
   a. Vaginal bleeding
   b. Vulvar itching and ulceration
   c. Pelvic pain
   d. Abdominal swelling
5. **The Pap smear test is primarily used to screen for which genital malignancy?**
   a. Endometrial cancer
   b. Cervical cancer
   c. Ovarian cancer
   d. Vaginal cancer

Short Answer Questions

1. What are the common types of genital malignancies in females?
2. List major risk factors associated with genital malignancies.
3. What symptoms typically suggest the presence of a genital malignancy?
4. Which diagnostic methods are used to detect genital malignancies?
5. What are the common treatment options for genital malignancies?
6. How can genital malignancies impact a patient's psychological well-being?

Answer to Critical Thinking Questions

1. (a) 2. (b) 3. (b) 4. (b) 5. (b)

REFERENCES

1. Achermann, J. C., Barnicoat, A., Brain, C. E., Carmichael, P. A., et al. (2010). Holistic management of DSD. https://core.ac.uk/download/1854753.pdf (accessed on 15th June 2025).
2. Ahmed, A., American Academy of Pediatrics, American Academy of Pediatrics Council on Children with Disabilities, Baskin, L. S., Blackless, M., Byne, W., et al. (2012). Disorders of sex development. https://core.ac.uk/download/pdf/8678248.pdf (accessed on 15th June 2025).
3. Ahmed, S. F., & Markosyan, R. (2017). Sex assignment in conditions affecting sex development. https://core.ac.uk/download/150597685.pdf (accessed on 15th June 2025).
4. Alarcon-Segovia, D., South, A. P., Bhogal, B. S., Bousema, T., Bushkell, L., D'Cruz, D., et al. (2004). Development of antigen-specific ELISA for circulating autoantibodies to extracellular matrix protein 1 in lichen sclerosus. https://core.ac.uk/download/20448727.pdf (accessed on 15th June 2025).
5. Almar, E., Arveux, P., Autelitano, M., Baldi, I., Bara, S., Barchielli, A., Benfatto, L., et al. (2019). Testicular germ-cell tumours and penile squamous cell carcinoma: Appropriate management makes the difference. https://core.ac.uk/download/287859186.pdf (accessed on 15th June 2025).
6. Almperis, A., Dinas, K., Kourti, M., Laganà, A. S., et al. (2023). Sarcoma botryoides: Optimal therapeutic management and prognosis of an unfavorable malignant neoplasm of female children. https://core.ac.uk/download/559262112.pdf (accessed on 15th June 2025).
7. Amicuzi, U., Balsamo, R., Barone, B., Coppola, M., et al. (2024). Exploring the multifactorial landscape of penile cancer: A comprehensive analysis of risk factors. https://core.ac.uk/download/636827512.pdf (accessed on 15th June 2025).
8. Argenziano, G., Chester, J., Cinotti, E., Longo, C., et al. (2023). Dermoscopy of melanoma according to different body sites: Head and neck, trunk, limbs, nail, mucosal and acral. https://core.ac.uk/download/577489483.pdf (accessed on 15th June 2025).
9. Arguello, D., Barkauskas, D. A., Gatalica, Z., Kurzrock, R., et al. (2020). Relationship between protein biomarkers of chemotherapy response and microsatellite status, tumor mutational burden and PD-L1 expression in cancer patients. https://core.ac.uk/download/323065796.pdf (accessed on 15th June 2025).
10. Arsenijevic, P., Arsenijevic, S., Djuric, J., Milosavljevic, T., et al. (2013). Synchronous primary ovarian endometrioid carcinoma and poorly differentiated endometrial stromal sarcoma. https://core.ac.uk/download/551558443.pdf (accessed on 15th June 2025).
11. Asikin, H. G., Saktini, F., Sarjana, A. S., Widodo, U., et al. (2024). Disorders of sex development: A review of medical and psychosocial aspects. https://core.ac.uk/download/639997267.pdf (accessed on 15th June 2025).
12. Bafna, U. D., Balaiah, S., Prakash, G., Shetty, S., et al. (2011). Primary fallopian tube carcinoma. https://core.ac.uk/download/pdf/14745.pdf (accessed on 15th June 2025).
13. Bahrami, M., Sheikhpour, E., Karami, M., & Mehrabani, S. (2024). Risk factors of second malignant neoplasms in childhood cancer survivors. *Iranian Journal of Pediatric Hematology & Oncology*. https://www.semanticscholar.org/paper/593da17fd40f5d091cd58cdf495210763aefe43b (accessed on 15th June 2025).

14. Bispo, R. K. A. de, Fonseca, M. C. M., & Speck, N. M. de G. (2024). Prevalence and type of HPV genital infection in girls: A systematic review and meta-analysis. *Journal of Lower Genital Tract Disease.* https://www.semanticscholar.org/paper/cc293e5aa54adc74a2dc6e1b761cd1e1b44e2591 (accessed on 15th June 2025).
15. Brunson, A., Jonas, B. A., Keegan, T. H. M., Paulus, J. K., et al. (2017). Secondary acute lymphoblastic leukemia is a distinct clinical entity with prognostic significance. https://core.ac.uk/download/323071816.pdf (accessed on 15th June 2025).
16. Ciofalo, A., Didona, B., Bialy-Golan, A., Didona, D., Moliterni, E., Iannella, G., Paolino, G., et al. (2017). Paraneoplastic pemphigus: Insight into the autoimmune pathogenesis, clinical features and therapy. https://core.ac.uk/download/141696210.pdf (accessed on 15th June 2025).
17. Clarke, M. A., Cremer, M., Darragh, T. M., Einstein, M. H., et al. (2020). Reporting and assessing the quality of diagnostic accuracy studies for cervical cancer screening and management. https://core.ac.uk/download/323064986.pdf (accessed on 15th June 2025).
18. Dancy, E., Stratton, P., Pichard, D., Marciano, B. E., Cowen, E. W., McBride, A. A., Van Doorslaer, K., et al. (2024). Human papillomavirus disease in GATA2 deficiency: A genetic predisposition to HPV-associated female anogenital malignancy. *Frontiers in Immunology, 15.* https://www.semanticscholar.org/paper/9be027afa4e0b4de8e434ce8695dc07c9632c78d (accessed on 15th June 2025).
19. Dandavate, N., Gadkari, N., Rajbhoj, A., Patil, M., Gaikwad, N., & Bankar, A. (2023). Study of anemia in non-luminal solid tumors. *International Journal of Advances in Medicine.* https://www.semanticscholar.org/paper/1fff721c07c7fa8b732fee62c0afa22f321a200a (accessed on 15th June 2025).
20. David, E., Grazhdani, H., Tattaresu, G., Pittari, A., Foti, P., Palmucci, S., Spatola, C., et al. (2024). Thyroid nodule characterization: Overview and state of the art of diagnosis with recent developments, from imaging to molecular diagnosis and artificial intelligence. *Biomedicines, 12.* https://www.semanticscholar.org/paper/631652d6b5dbf034b27c920e5bb39ea558d38f31 (accessed on 15th June 2025).
21. Deng, H., Ding, Y., Yin, D., Jia, Y., Wang, Z., Liang, X., & Liu, Y. (2024). Novel association of RAD54L mutation with Müllerian clear cell carcinoma of the male urethra: New insights regarding the molecular mechanisms of a rare tumor. *Current Cancer Drug Targets.* https://www.semanticscholar.org/paper/cdb83dd0af1874ede7fff9cabdea1ab6524c8a8c (accessed on 15th June 2025).
22. Detels, R., He, N., Mao, Y., McGoogan, J., et al. (2019). Spectrum of malignancies among the population of adults living with HIV infection in China: A nationwide follow-up study, 2008–2011. https://core.ac.uk/download/323078520.pdf (accessed on 15th June 2025).
23. Dixon-Suen, S. C., Jordan, S. J., Stewart, L. M., Tuesley, R., et al. (2019). The association between hysterectomy and ovarian cancer risk: A population-based record-linkage study. https://core.ac.uk/download/213608144.pdf (accessed on 15th June 2025).
24. Ediati, A., Faradz, S. M. H., Fitrianingrum, I., Winarni, T. I., et al. (2021). The evaluation of parental acceptance towards children with sex chromosomal disorders of sex development using a mixed-method. https://core.ac.uk/download/426938102.pdf (accessed on 15th June 2025).

25. Eugster, E. A., & Tica, S. S. (2017). How often are clinicians performing genital exams in children with disorders of sex development? https://core.ac.uk/download/160755303.pdf (accessed on 15th June 2025).

26. Garbe, C., Amaral, T., Peris, K., Hauschild, A., Arenberger, P., Basset-Séguin, N., Bastholt, L., et al. (2022). European consensus-based interdisciplinary guideline for melanoma. Part 1: Diagnostics: Update 2022. *European Journal of Cancer, 170*, 236–255. https://doi.org/10.1016/j.ejca.2022.03.008 (accessed on 15th June 2025).

27. Grover, I. S., Kaur, I., Pannu, J. S., Randhawa, S., et al. (2019). Retrospective study of enormity of cancer in a tertiary care center in Punjab, India. https://core.ac.uk/download/539896297.pdf (accessed on 15th June 2025).

28. Jadhav, T., Madakshira, M. G., & Garud, S. (2023). Embryonal rhabdomyosarcoma of the uterine cervix in an adult female. *Autopsy & Case Reports, 13*. https://www.semanticscholar.org/paper/4c3890495333f530c3f95efaf613ce19b9171a20 (accessed on 15th June 2025).

29. Kaizilege, G. K., Kiritta, R., Chuma, C., Ndaboine, E., Ottoman, O. E. E., Zinga, M. M., et al. (2022). Female genital schistosomiasis, a neglected differential of cervical precancerous and cancerous lesion: A wakeup calls for on-job training for healthcare workers in endemic areas. *Austin Journal of Clinical Case Reports*. https://www.semanticscholar.org/paper/281fa234724f6d096db1133ce04d3fcf73cbffe8 (accessed on 15th June 2025).

30. Kamada, Y., Kashino, C., Kubo, K., Kusumoto, T., et al. (2021). Surgically treated genital chronic graft-versus-host disease in women: A report of three cases. https://core.ac.uk/download/482298387.pdf (accessed on 15th June 2025).

31. Khalid, S., Arshad, S., Aqeel, M., Ameer, R., Shaukat, A., Ghous, M., Khaliq, H., et al. (2024). Epidemiology and risk factors of breast cancer: A global perspective on incidence, mortality, and prevention strategies. *Biological and Clinical Sciences Research Journal*. https://www.semanticscholar.org/paper/f49ce2febe19670778d4dc1343106ea0d58a5a85 (accessed on 15th June 2025).

32. Kruger, T. H. C., Köhne, S., & Kümpers, F. (2024). Pharmacotherapy of persistent genital arousal disorder/genito-pelvic dysesthesia: An updated review and data from a registry. *Expert Opinion on Pharmacotherapy, 25*, 2005–2013. https://www.semanticscholar.org/paper/b301e9633c2ea824e9b679e8d02c61041e3b562e (accessed on 15th June 2025).

33. Kumar, R. (2018). Prevalence of female reproductive tract cancer in a teaching hospital of Rohtas District, Bihar, India. https://core.ac.uk/download/539912694.pdf (accessed on 15th June 2025).

34. Majinge, P. M. C. (2011). Treatment outcome of cervical cancer patients at Ocean Road Cancer Institute, Dar es Salaam. https://core.ac.uk/download/pdf/11307434.pdf (accessed on 15th June 2025).

35. Malandrino, P., Mazzilli, R., Puliani, G., Di Molfetta, S., Pugliese, G., Olana, S., Colao, A., et al. (2022). The effects of radioligand therapy on quality of life and sexual function in patients with neuroendocrine neoplasms. *Cancers, 15*. https://www.semanticscholar.org/paper/cf365f55f9361b1704b9c4235f0b98cefdca1f80 (accessed on 15th June 2025).

36. Moch, H., Amin, M. B., Berney, D. M., Compérat, É., Gill, A. J., Hartmann, A., Menon, S., et al. (2022). The 2022 World Health Organization classification of tumors of the urinary system and male genital organs—Part A: Renal, penile, and testicular tumors. *European Urology,*

82, 458–468. https://doi.org/10.1016/j.eururo.2022.06.016 (accessed on 15th June 2025).

37. Nahar, K., & Nahar, N. (2021). Radical vulvectomy for a rare case of squamous cell carcinoma vulva: A case report. https://core.ac.uk/download/539902592.pdf (accessed on 15th June 2025).

38. Preudhomme, C., Steward, C. G., Pilz, D. T., Dafou, D., Tsai, F. Y., Connell, F. C., Brice, G., et al. (2011). Mutations in GATA2 cause primary lymphedema associated with a predisposition to acute myeloid leukemia (Emberger syndrome). https://core.ac.uk/download/10674800.pdf (accessed on 15th June 2025).

39. Rageh, O. A., Elmadhoun, W., Alshameeri, M. M. M., & Farag, A. (2025). Well-differentiated squamous cell carcinoma of the lower lip in Aden, Yemen: A case report highlighting importance of early detection. *Yemeni Journal for Medical Sciences*. https://www.semanticscholar.org/paper/0e5d0939ecb859ce88b814a0355bbda37a20df5f (accessed on 15th June 2025).

40. Roy, R., Chandanwale, S., Raj, A., Singh, M., & Tambile, A. (2025). Primary ovarian tuberculosis: A case report with unusual clinical presentation. *The International Journal of Mycobacteriology*. https://www.semanticscholar.org/paper/b0ecc898a9eb40e88bf7d63c0a64086af13c88dd (accessed on 15th June 2025).

41. Talwar, S., Kaur, H., Tapasvi, I., Nibhoria, S., & Tapasvi, C. (2024). Clinical and histopathological characteristics in women with postmenopausal bleeding: A study of 120 women in a tertiary care hospital in Punjab. *Cureus, 16*. https://www.semanticscholar.org/paper/c8c015b20b6abb0ca80c05320848b8707761eb76 (accessed on 15th June 2025).

42. Wang, B., Lu, Y., Zhao, J., Li, L., Qiu, L., Qian, Z., Zhou, S. Y., et al. (2025). Early detection and central nervous system prophylaxis in patients with high-risk features of primary lymphoma of the female genital tract: The key to improved prognosis. *Hematological Oncology, 43*. https://www.semanticscholar.org/paper/0daeef09bb03548749e6591cfdf8d82e4faca975 (accessed on 15th June 2025).

43. Wunderlich, K., Suppa, M., Gandini, S., Lipski, J., White, J., & del Marmol, V. (2024). Risk factors and innovations in risk assessment for melanoma, basal cell carcinoma, and squamous cell carcinoma. *Cancers, 16*. https://www.semanticscholar.org/paper/410338a6baf5385210a0bc6330e6ccfcb8b1a9ca (accessed on 15th June 2025).

FIBROIDS (LEIOMYOMA)

7

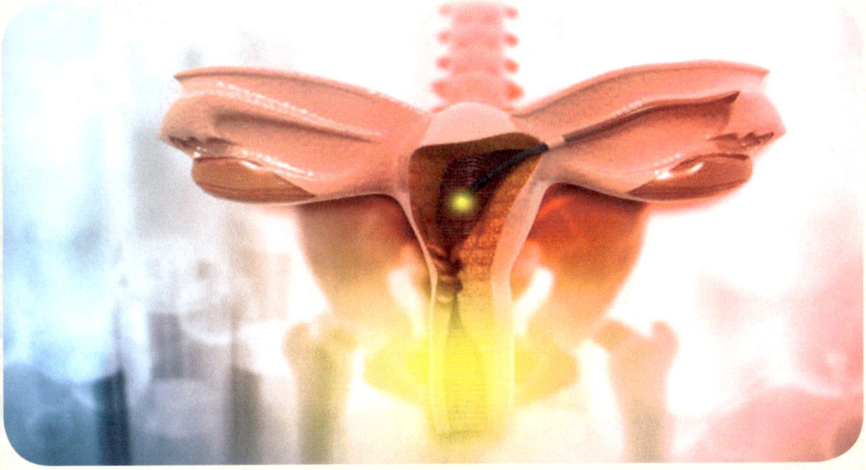

LEARNING OBJECTIVES

After studying this chapter, you will be able to:

1. Identify the different types of fibroids
2. Explain the causes and risk factors associated with fibroids
3. Recognize common symptoms of fibroids
4. Describe diagnostic methods used for fibroids
5. Discuss treatment options available for managing fibroids

Introduction

Fibroids, or leiomyomas and myomas, are benign uterine tumors that develop from the smooth muscle of the uterus. They are the most common type of pelvic tumor found in women of childbearing age. When discussing fibroids, or leiomyomas, the need arises to define the significance of the benign tumors, particularly in regard to women's reproductive health. While as prevalent as they are, found in an estimated 20-80% of women by age 50, fibroids often take on a complex pattern of symptoms, including abnormal bleeding, pain, and pressure, which can significantly impact their quality of life. An understanding of the nuances of fibroids is crucial to ensuring proper treatment plans and improving outcomes in patients. This fundamental knowledge forms the foundation for more comprehensive research into uterine leiomyoma pathological processes, demographics, and treatment options, and ultimately to the broader gynecological health discussion. The pathogenesis of uterine leiomyomas is a subject that remains under investigation, with many factors having been implicated in their development and growth. Notably, the function of the hormonal effects, particularly estrogen, emerges heavily throughout the literature. Epidemiologic observations demonstrate that estrogen receptors, ER and ER types, are of critical significance in the pathobiology of these malignancies, in influencing their course and responsiveness to treatment. Demographics similarly provide disparities in incidence and response to treatment, most strikingly in African American women, among whom more prevalent rates and more crippling symptomatology are found. The monetary expense of treatment for fibroids also underscores their significance as a public health concern, prompting research into prevention and therapeutic discovery. This investigation of these factors provides a deeper understanding of the multifaceted character of uterine leiomyomas worthy of attention. Based on an examination of existing treatments of fibroids, there is a range of alternatives, ranging from conservative management to surgery. Therapy is typically determined by symptom severity, fibroid size, and patient preference, and leads to a broad array of approaches that range from drug therapy to minimally invasive surgery to hysterectomy. Emerging data provide promise for the role of selective estrogen receptor modulators, which target estrogenic activity with the aim of shrinking fibroids without the loss of uterine integrity. As the medical community continues to advance treatment models and explore further new horizons of therapy, debate about the value of patient-centered care becomes increasingly relevant. A reasoned appreciation of fibroids by contemporary research enables healthcare providers to offer targeted interventions to maximize the health of women who carry leiomyomas.

Definition of Fibroids (Leiomyoma)

Fibroids, also referred to as leiomyomas in the medical field, are benign growths that occur in the uterine muscular wall. They develop from smooth muscle cells and can be of different sizes, numbers, and positions in the uterus. Most women would live their lives without ever realizing they have symptoms of fibroids, yet they can also lead to serious health issues, such as profuse menstrual bleeding, pelvic pain, and complications during pregnancy. The prevalence of fibroids is high, especially among women of reproductive age, and they are the leading cause of hysterectomy. Understanding the character of fibroids is crucial not only in the diagnosis and treatment of the disease but also in realizing their impact on women's reproductive health and quality of life, as abnormal uterine bleeding can disrupt daily functioning and quality of life (+11 more authors et al., 2020).

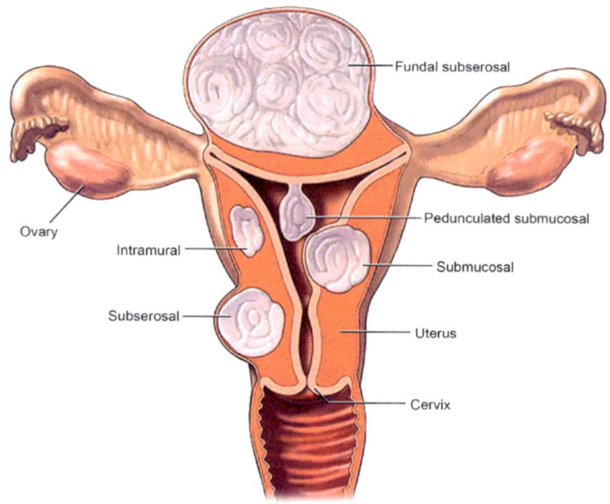

Figure 7.1. Uterine fibroids.

Source: https://www.mayoclinic.org/-/media/kcms/gbs/patient-consumer/images/2013/11/15/17/38/ds00078_-my00501_im01586_hdg7_fibroidlocationthu_jpg.jpg

The size and location of the fibroids are typically employed to categorize them. Intramural fibroids are the ones that grow within the uterine wall. Submucosal fibroids protrude into the uterine cavity. Subserosal fibroids extend out from the uterus. Surprisingly, fibroid size correlates with complication risk, i.e., greater fibroids, particularly those >4 cm, have a progressively greater risk of women undergoing major uterine surgery, such as hysterectomy (Baird et al., 2015).This perception points towards the importance of regular monitoring and diagnostic imaging to assess fibroid burden in women, especially those with symptoms. The continued research in this area is critical to develop individualized management programs considering medical and surgical approaches. While fibroids are largely benign in origin, their ability to cause pain and lead to considerable reproductive health issues increases their intrinsic mechanisms' importance to research. Recent studies highlight the significance of further research into menstruation and fibroids in efforts to alleviate knowledge deficits that affect millions of women globally. Clinicians and scientists endeavoring to create more effective treatment regimens are reliant upon the understanding of the basic biology of fibroids, their role in menstrual health, and how they interact with variables such as hormonal fluctuations. Disruptions in this sensitive balance can lead to disease states such as abnormal uterine bleeding, so research and clinical attention are essential to improving outcomes for women managing disorders of fibroids (+11 other authors et al., 2020).

Prevalence and Demographics

The prevalence of fibroids, or leiomyomas, varies widely between demographic groups and geographic regions. Previous studies have established that benign tumors are particularly common among women of childbearing age, with worldwide prevalence varying from 20% to 80%. Variations in estimated prevalence could be attributed to factors such as ethnicity, age, and environmental exposure. As an illustration, there is evidence that African American women have a greater incidence of fibroids compared to their Caucasian counterparts, which attests to the role of genetic and possibly socio-economic factors in the susceptibility of the disease. Further, the dramatic impact of lifestyle determinants, such as diet and exercise, illustrates how recent changes in society could influence fibroid development in certain populations. Age is a significant demographic factor that affects the incidence and clinical presentation of fibroids. Statistics show that the risk of getting fibroids is greatly heightened in women aged 31 to 50 years, pointing to a clear age-risk correlation. It was found in a research in Uganda that the prevalence of uterine fibroids in reproductive-aged women was 28.2%, and most of these had symptoms such as pelvic pain and menorrhagia. This is reflective of a broader pattern where women commonly have fibroids when they are at their most productive reproductive age, indicating that endocrine changes through aging can play a key role in fibroid development. In addition, the symptomatology experienced by these patients highlights the importance of higher sensitization of fibroids among health providers caring for women in this age bracket. The interaction between population and fibroids also exists in the landscape of infertility, which is often exacerbated by such tumors. Among infertile women, a study recognizes uterine abnormalities, including fibroids, as one of the leading causes of female infertility. A significant result from a separate study indicates that women between 21 and 30 years have the highest rate of infertility, leading one to infer that even younger women may be subject to barriers due to the existence of fibroids. Since fibroids may be responsible for complications like pelvic pain and menorrhagia, their effect on fertility is such that it calls for a close examination of women's reproductive health. These results highlight the imperative of continued research into the demographic disparities in fibroid occurrence and their significant impacts on women's health outcomes, especially on fertility and general wellbeing.

Importance of Understanding Fibroids

A basic part of reproductive health is understanding uterine fibroids, or leiomyomas, which significantly impact many women. Benign growths made up of smooth muscle and connective tissue within the uterus have symptoms that differ and detract from quality of life. Understanding fibroids is crucial because they can lead to problems such as heavy menstrual bleeding, pelvic discomfort, and urinary obstruction. Also, patients may experience emotional distress due to the unpredictability and severity of symptoms. The recognition of such issues highlights the necessity for medical practitioners to receive proper education on fibroids to enable them to make correct diagnoses and treatment protocols as required in individual cases. Greater knowledge among providers can also enable early detection, which can further relieve potential complications pertaining to fibroids that have not been diagnosed and enable patients to become more proactive in taking care of their own reproductive wellness. In addition to increasing the awareness of health professionals, awareness of the etiology and risk factors of fibroids plays a vital role in prevention and intervention. Current evidence indicates a multifactorial etiology in leiomyoma development with genetic susceptibility and hormonal factors, particularly the effect of estrogen. Such knowledge can be applied in developing specific medical therapies, such as selective estrogen receptor modulators, which can effectively treat fibroid symptoms. Understanding these inherent mechanisms not only helps healthcare professionals with the creation of personalized treatment protocols but also helps patients to be in the position to make informed lifestyle choices that reduce their risk factors. Such an understanding of the biological processes and causative factors of uterine fibroids is also important for improving the overall reproductive health of the affected as well as educational public health initiatives on women's health issues. Additionally, the socio-economic background of being aware of fibroids cannot be downplayed. The observation that uterine fibroids are highly prevalent in certain groups, such as African American women, justifies intervention through public health means. These can help deal with the prohibitive health costs of fibroid management as well as the potential loss of productivity due to the presence of these comorbid conditions. A thorough understanding of fibroids enables researchers to spur better access to care, greater research dollars for fibroids, and education initiatives to raise awareness. In addition, educating women with information regarding fibroids enables them to advocate for themselves within the healthcare environment, fostering a better working alliance between healthcare providers and women. Lastly, understanding fibroids is not only important for individual health but also has broader societal significance in terms of ensuring overall well-being for communities affected by this very common condition, as seen in existing controversies in Koomson et al. (2017) and Nasiriddinovna et al. (2023).

7.1. Types of Fibroids

Learning Outcome

1. Discuss intramural fibroids
2. Define subserosal fibroids and submucosal fibroids

The typing of fibroids, or leiomyomas, typically relies on where they are located in the uterus and effectively decides the presenting signs and treatments that can be given to the patients. Fibroids within the uterus are categorized into three general classes: submucosal, intramural, and subserosal. Submucosal fibroids arise just beneath the endometrial lining and can grow into the uterine cavity, potentially causing profuse menstrual bleeding and infertility. Similarly, intramural fibroids develop in the muscular walls of the uterus and can lead to a whole range of complications, from discomfort or pressure-type symptoms. Subserosal fibroids, however, develop on the outer surface of the uterus and are less likely to result in symptoms. However, depending on their size, they also exert pressure on nearby organs, generating other types of complications that need to be handled with care and necessitate specifically adapted care mechanisms. The impact of fibroids on menstrual health is considerable, affecting a vast number of women across the world. Heavy menstrual bleeding (HMB) is amongst the most common symptoms of fibroids and has become a significant problem, disrupting the quality of life in afflicted individuals. The biological processes of menstruation intertwined with fibroid pathology point to the importance of fibroids in the larger context of menstrual well-being. Critical research here identifies that abnormal uterine bleeding, such as presenting symptoms of fibroids, occurs in an estimated one in four women of reproductive age. Extensive studies attempt to partition the mechanisms of menstruation and abnormal uterine bleeding to facilitate effective diagnostic and therapeutic interventions. Knowledge of the relation of fibroids to menstruation will even shed more light on the complexity of uterine physiology, emphasizing the need for personalized treatment modalities based on individual physiological responses (Critchley et al., 2020 (a); Critchley et al., 2020 (b)).

Even though the presence of fibroids causes issues, advancements in medical science provide an arena for a way forward in handling these issues. Treatment ranges from conservative, such as drug treatment to manage the symptoms, to more aggressive approaches such as myomectomy or hysterectomy to remove the fibroids. With the progress being made in the biology of fibroids, targeted therapy such as selective progesterone receptor modulators (SPRMs) is in the pipeline to offer specific treatment choices. Developments of this type are critical to meet the unmet needs of patients with heavy menstrual bleeding as a consequence of fibroids. In addition, the recognition that many women delay pregnancy or choose uterine-sparing procedures only serves to further assert the necessity for investigations attempting to define the whole range of fibroid pathology. By facilitating greater insight into the etiologic causes for fibroids and how they present clinically, health practitioners can optimize patient outcomes along with minimizing society's impact of fibroid illness (Critchley et al., 2020; Critchley et al., 2020).

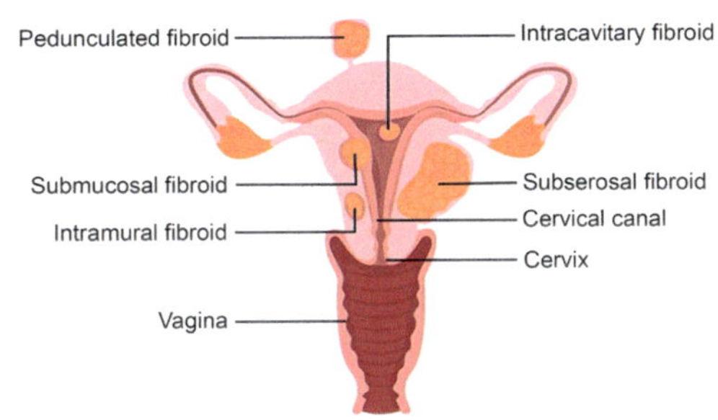

Figure 7.2. Types of Uterine fibroids.

Source: https://www.astraveinvascular.com/wp-content/uploads/2021/11/types-of-uterine-fibroids.jpg

7.1.1. Intramural Fibroids

Intramural fibroids, a type of uterine leiomyoma, develop in the muscular uterine wall and, therefore, manifest with a wide array of clinical symptoms. Intramural fibroids are usually reported in relation to location, as they occur within the myometrium and therefore disrupt the uterine architecture. While the majority of women with intramural fibroids remain asymptomatic, some other women may experience severe health complications, such as abnormal uterine bleeding, pelvic pain, and increased abdominal pressure. The aetiology of such fibroids is not yet fully understood, though factors like hormonal and genetic influences have been suggested to contribute towards their pathogenesis. Diagnosis is typically made by clinical history, examination of the pelvis, and by imaging techniques like ultrasound or MRI, which give accurate localisation and measurement of size and thus useful information for management planning (N/A, 2021). Intramural fibroids' symptomatology can profoundly impact the woman's quality of life, to the extent that an appreciation of treatment must be achieved. Although the majority are asymptomatic, intramural fibroids may produce debilitating symptoms of dysmenorrhea, frequency, and even infertility. The plan of treatment should be individualized to address unique needs such as symptomatology, fibroid size, and the desired fertility of the patient. Pharmacologic therapies, including hormone therapy and selective progesterone receptor modulators, are usually used as first-line treatments to manage symptoms. In severe cases, however, surgical intervention such as myomectomy or hysterectomy may be necessary when quality of life or fertility is compromised by high fibroid burden (Zaher et al., 2010).

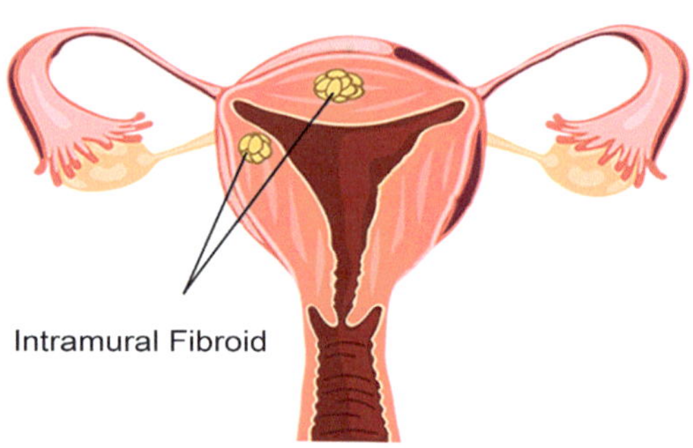

Figure 7.3. Intramural Fibroids

Source: https://drranjanadhanu.com/wp-content/uploads/2024/02/Intramural-Fibroid.jpg

Recognition of the complex presentation of intramural fibroids plays a pivotal role in the choice of the most appropriate intervention. The latest development of minimally invasive treatments presents promising prospects in the management of intramural fibroids. Procedures such as uterine artery embolization and Magnetic Resonance guided Focused Ultrasound Surgery (MRgFUS) have emerged as alternative choices, yielding symptom relief without sacrificing the uterus and loss of reproductive function. MRgFUS, in particular, is a leading example of the shift towards less invasive procedures, allowing women the opportunity to stay away from the physical and emotional burden of traditional surgical procedures. Not only do such new technologies provide assurance of shorter recovery times, but they also facilitate providing improved overall patient satisfaction. With ongoing research providing further insight into the long-term effectiveness and safety of such therapies, hope for a revolutionary shift in the treatment of intramural fibroids within gynecological practice to better women's health outcomes is presented (Zaher et al., 2010).

7.1.2. Subserosal Fibroids

Subserosal fibroids, a specific type of uterine leiomyoma, are characterized by their growth pattern, that is, from the outer uterus wall in an outward direction towards the pelvis. Their exophytic nature is capable of creating a variety of clinical presentations, which are able to obscure the initial diagnosis. Unlike their submucous counterparts, which present clearly with prominent major menstrual abnormalities, subserosal fibroids are capable of progressing to being asymptomatic for decades. They are, in some instances, discovered only incidentally on imaging tests to diagnose other illnesses. Their manifestations depend upon their size and position and can range from mild in the case of large fibroids, where they may cause abdominal pain or press on nearby organs. It is important to know their clinical profile to manage them accordingly and to decide on the appropriate line of treatment, ranging from watchful waiting to operative procedures, based on symptom severity and growth potential. The impact of subserosal fibroids on fertility health cannot be overlooked. Even though the majority of women with these fibroids do not experience severe issues, others are at risk of undergoing pregnancy complications or giving birth. Since the fibroids cause the uterine cavity to become distorted in shape or compress surrounding organs, they will most likely present with issues such as fetal malpresentation or increased chances of cesarean section. Further, their impact on complicating conditions like placental abruption is of concern, as can be seen from certain research. For instance, volume reduction in leiomyoma after uterine artery embolization is considerable, with submucosal and subserosal fibroids showing a substantial decrease in size, hence potentially reversing their adverse effects on pregnancy outcomes (Affonso et al., 2014). Clinicians must scrutinize patients with subserosal fibroids carefully, weighing against one another the risks and benefits of treatment and conservative management, especially in women of reproductive age. With advances in the surgical management of fibroids, more minimally invasive methods are being used increasingly to control symptomatic subserosal fibroids. Methods such as uterine artery embolization have been found to be highly effective in reducing the size of fibroids while preserving uterine function. Studies have shown that the average shrinkage in leiomyoma dimensions is significant, with extremely large effects being observed at the subserosal locations when quantified by means of magnetic resonance imaging. A high reduction of over 50% in the size of the fibroids achieves symptomatic relief and improved quality of life in the involved women (Affonso et al., 2014). Further, identification of fibroid characteristics, such as the node-to-muscle ratio, can identify the outcomes. Therefore, integrating imaging technology in the therapeutic regimens of subserosal fibroids enables personalized therapy, allowing patients to receive the most effective treatment based on their specific situation.

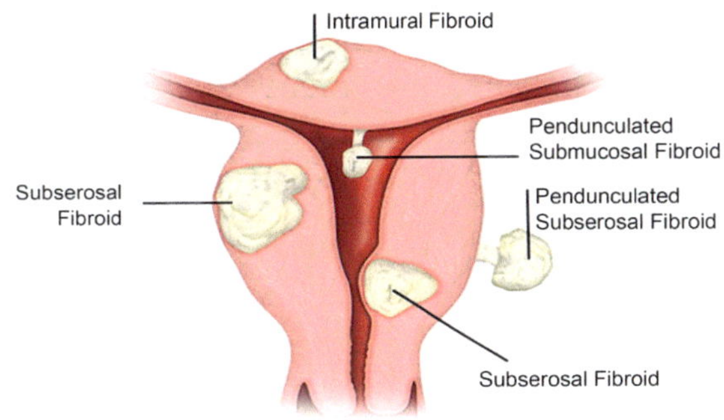

Figure 7.4. Subserosal Fibroids.

Source: https://www.astraveinvascular.com/wp-content/uploads/2021/11/Subserosal-Fibroids.jpg

7.1.3. Submucosal Fibroids

Submucosal fibroids represent a unique type of uterine leiomyomas that develop just beneath the endometrial lining, the innermost layer of the uterus. The site of growth is of particular relevance since it is more likely to create typical symptoms in conjunction with the uterus's functional activities. Submucosal fibroids are commonly reported by women who complain of increased menstrual flow, both regular and irregular, and experience pain or pressure in the pelvis. In the process, they can interfere with normal reproduction processes to make conception and pregnancy difficult. Since fibroid development has hormonal dependences, their treatment tends to require a careful balance of care to address these symptoms effectively while considering the patient's health and reproductive plans (N/A, 2021). It is necessary to comprehend the clinical presentation and implications of submucosal fibroids to diagnose and prepare for treatments. The advancement of imaging technologies has significantly enhanced the diagnosis of submucosal fibroids, making it possible to identify the lesions and their respective influence on reproductive health. Magnetic resonance imaging (MRI) has emerged as a leading technique, with good images of uterine morphology and localized fibroid attributes. Research shows that the size and precise location of submucosal fibroids are treatment outcome prognostic factors, especially when undergoing minimally invasive treatments such as uterine artery embolization. MRI findings demonstrate a significant reduction in fibroid size following treatment, especially those that are submucosal and possess a greater node-to-muscle ratio, evidenced by T2-weighted images (Affonso et al., 2014).

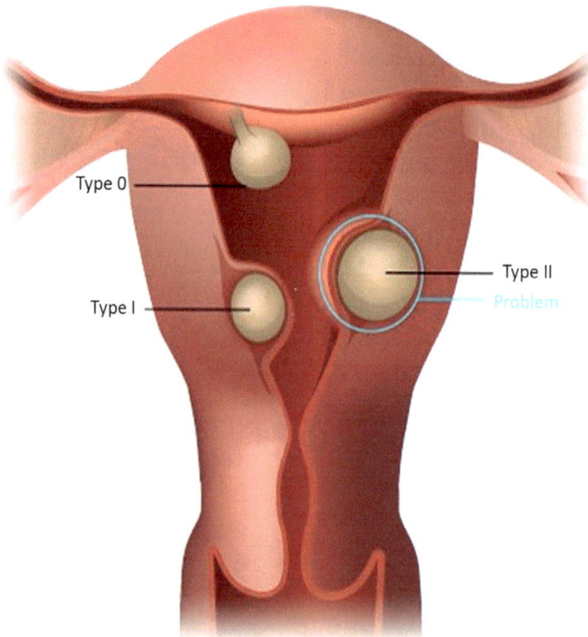

Figure 7.5. Submucosal fibroids.

Source: https://kjkhospital.com/submucosal-fibroids/

Therefore, the interface between imaging results and clinical presentation remains a field of utmost investigation, with a sharp emphasis on accurate diagnosis to be able to effectively manage. Submucosal fibroids are managed around the clock with a variety of treatment alternatives to alleviate the diverse range of symptoms for these affected women. Medical treatment can include hormonal therapy that regulates the menstrual cycle and offers symptom control, and surgery can be considered in more severe cases.

Uterine artery embolization has become very prominent as a less invasive treatment, facilitating substantial shrinkage of fibroids—particularly beneficial for submucosal types. Evidence indicates that this treatment has an effectiveness in volume loss of over 50% and enhances the quality of life in women with symptoms as a result of these fibroids (Affonso et al., 2014).

Thus, a comprehensive approach considering both the physiological and psychosocial aspects of management is required to provide optimum long-term management of submucosal fibroids, enhancing reproductive outcomes and overall well-being.

Test Your Knowledge

1. What defines an intramural fibroid, and where is it located in the uterus?
2. How do subserosal fibroids differ in location and symptoms compared to other types?

7.2. Causes and Risk Factors

Learning Outcome

1. Discuss the hormonal influences
2. Explain the genetic predisposition

The pathogenesis of fibroids, or leiomyomas, is still not clearly understood, with a multifactorial interplay of genetic, hormonal, and environmental influences. Of particular note, estrogen and progesterone are documented to promote the growth of fibroids, and thus researchers have been studying the role of the menstrual cycle in the formation of fibroids. Women between reproductive ages have cyclically varying levels of hormones, and this may be a factor in the prevalence and growth of fibroids. Further, studies indicate that fibroids are more common in women of childbearing age, and most importantly, in African descendants, pointing towards racial and ethnic disparities as main risk factors. Such a population distinction is critical in understanding susceptibility due to potential genetic predisposition or variability in hormonal responses, hence necessitating greater scrutiny of differentiated risk assessment and targeted interventions. In addition to the influence of hormones, the risk of fibroids has also been implicated with lifestyle components such as obesity and diet. Observations from healthcare epidemiology have shown that elevated body mass index (BMI) has been linked with increased incidence and size of fibroids. Greater adipose tissue can lead to greater levels of estrogens in the body because adipocytes convert androgens to estrogens, hence promoting the formation of fibroids. Nutrition is also to blame, with red meat consumption and low fruit and vegetable intake associated with a greater risk of fibroids.

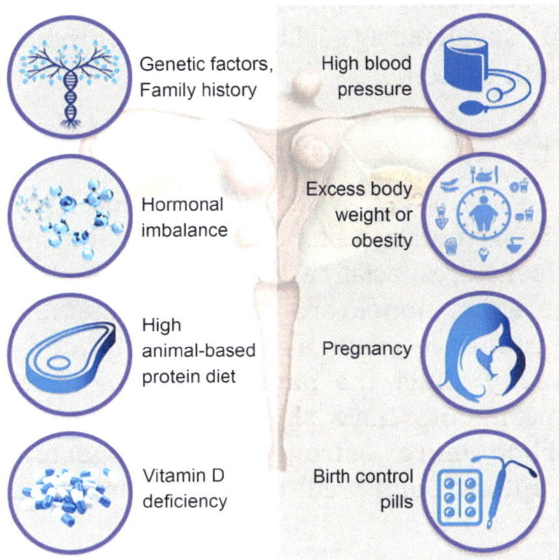

Figure 7.6. Major causes of uterine fibroids.

Source: https://www.astraveinvascular.com/wp-content/uploads/2021/11/Major-causes-of-uterine-fibroids.jpg

Determination of these modifiable risk factors is crucial for the development of prevention programs as well as guiding life habits in at-risk populations, demonstrating the need for nutrition and weight control education. Chronic conditions such as diabetes and hypertension can also predispose women to the development of fibroids. More evidence suggests that metabolic diseases influence the equilibrium of hormones and growth in connective tissue, thereby promoting fibroid formation. Specifically, elevated blood pressure has been associated with an increased incidence of fibroids, most probably due to the fact that chronic inflammation and vascular lesions exert a deleterious influence on uterine tissue. Moreover, hormonal imbalances brought about by health conditions can stimulate the development of fibroids. These observations underscore the importance of comprehensive health screening among women with regard to risk-contributing underlying health conditions and subjecting them to an overall management plan for enhancing quality of life and reproductive health outcomes.

7.2.1. Hormonal Influences

The growth and evolution of uterine fibroids, or leiomyomas, are largely driven by hormonal influences, especially estrogen and progesterone. These hormones are crucial in the female reproductive cycle, and their variations can directly affect the pathogenesis of fibroids. Experiments have shown that leiomyomas harbor more estrogen and progesterone receptors compared to normal myometrial tissue, a fact that would suggest that the tumors will respond differently to fluctuating hormones as the life cycle of a woman continues. Given that estrogen levels are higher during the reproductive years of a woman's life, so too is the size and quantity of fibroids, which in turn normally is accompanied by symptomatology endured by women, including heavy menstrual loss and pelvic discomfort. Explaining hormonal factors is of prime importance in developing targeted therapeutic approaches to managing fibroids and minimizing the accompanying complications (Nasiriddinovna et al., 2023). Apart from the immediate effect of estrogen and progesterone, interaction among other growth factors and hormones merely enhances the dynamics of forces behind leiomyoma growth. Insulin-like growth factors (IGFs), for instance, can be demonstrated to facilitate the effects of estrogens on fibroids toward growth. Furthermore, studies indicate that fibroids can also be controlled by local growth factors such as transforming growth factor-beta (TGF-β) that aid in the overproduction of extracellular matrix and tumor formation.

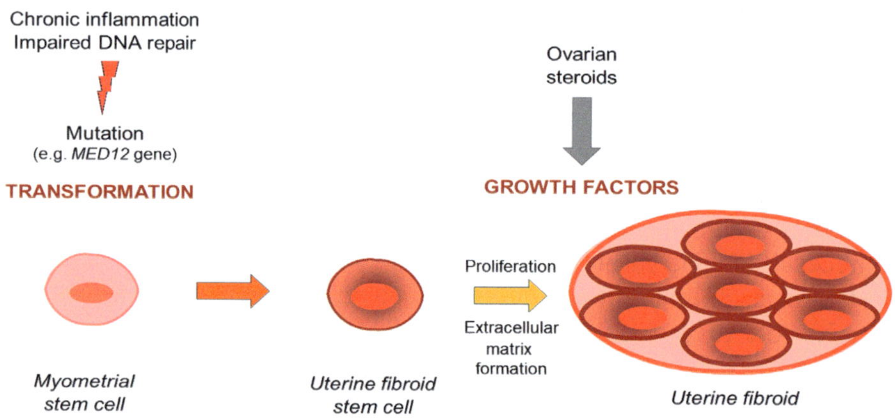

Figure 7.7. Development and growth of uterine fibroid—simplified scheme. Importance of mutation-derived transformation and stimulation of hormones and growth factors.

Source: https://www.researchgate.net/figure/Development-and-growth-of-uterine-fibroid-simplified-scheme-Importance-of_fig1_341391656

These interactions with hormones and growth factors are what illustrate the intricacy of the hormonal environment that is involved in fibroid development and the potential of multiple treatment avenues. By unraveling these complex relationships, researchers are optimistic about finding novel therapeutic methods for hormone-mediated fibroid development (Koomson et al., 2017). The identification of selective estrogen receptor modulators (SERMs) is a promising research direction to therapeutically target uterine fibroids, as they will be capable of specifically modulating hormonal action and minimizing side effects associated with systemic hormone therapy. The varied roles of estrogen receptor subtypes ER and ER introduce yet another layer to fibroid biology: both receptors exert varied actions, which promote or inhibit fibroid growth. Thus, future research aims to elaborate on the individual roles of these receptors and their interactions in fibroid pathogenesis. With the utilization of developments in pharmacology and molecular biology, there is not only innovative but also necessary potential to design receptor-specific therapies, which have the possibility of delivering more effective, targeted treatments for women afflicted with the conditions of uterine fibroids (Koomson et al., 2017).

7.2.2. Genetic Predisposition

The mechanism of genetic susceptibility plays a dominant role in the development of uterine fibroids, clinically also known as leiomyomas. Research has established that certain genetic factors may predispose an individual to the growth of these benign tumors. For instance, genome-wide association studies (GWAS) have identified various loci that are associated with increased risk for developing leiomyomas. These findings suggest that genetic variations could lead to alterations in cellular function behind tumor growth, thereby highlighting the hereditary component of fibroid growth. Identification of the genetic cause not only tells us why some women are more likely to develop fibroids than others, but also challenges the utility of family history in the clinical assessment of patients presenting with fibroid symptoms.

The genetic intricacy of leiomyomas has been highlighted in current studies through the discovery of specific genetic loci implicated in their pathogenesis. Interestingly, nine major loci were identified in one study through a large GWAS of more than a thousand cases and controls, which demonstrated significant association of genetic variants with the risk of fibroids. One of them, a novel locus at 12q23.2, was discovered to have a significant role in gene regulation and tumorigenesis. Furthermore, subgroup analysis also identified certain loci as having high impact across different categories of leiomyomas, such as submucous fibroids, and hence emphasizing the importance of personalized strategies in research as well as treatment protocols. These findings provide insights into the complex interaction of genes with the pathogenesis of uterine fibroids, further indicating the need for the characterization of genetic susceptibility in the overall frame of gynecological health (Aoki et al., 2020).

The effects of genetic susceptibility transcend the simple understanding of leiomyoma formation; they influence clinical management and patient outcomes as well. Knowledge of specific genetic markers in fibroids can enable clinicians to screen candidates based on family history assessment and genetic testing. Early intervention strategies can be implemented, potentially preventing the physical and emotional burdens of fibroid-associated symptoms. In addition, identification of the genetic underpinnings of fibroids allows clinicians to tailor management plans based on genetic characteristics, enhancing personalized medicine in gynecologic care. In addition, advancing knowledge of the genetic foundation of leiomyomas has the potential to lay the groundwork for new therapies, targeted toward molecular pathways implicated in tumor growth and proliferation. By integrating genetic considerations into treatment models, clinicians can significantly enhance outcomes among women with fibroids (Adamo et al., 2017).

7.2.3. Lifestyle Factors

Habitual Physical activities are a significant etiologic factor in the causation and management of fibroids (leiomyoma), with some habits causing the causation or the enhancement of such benign growths in the uterus. Obesity has been shown in research to be among the most significant risk factors; women with a higher body mass index (BMI) have higher rates of fibroids. This is partly because of excess estrogen levels, because the adipose tissue has the ability to produce estrogen, and this will promote the growth of fibroids. In addition, sedentary lifestyles that result in obesity may also be linked with hormonal imbalances that will cause the development of fibroids. Education on lifestyle risks and fibroid development is critical for at-risk women, since the acceptance of an improved diet and the incorporation of exercise on a regular basis can lower these risks.

Lifestyle also has a significant impact on the risk of uterine fibroids, where certain eating patterns have a protective or adverse effect. Consumption of a high dietary intake of fruits, vegetables, and whole grains is associated with lower rates of fibroids, while excessive consumption of red meat and processed foods is associated with increased rates. Also, adequate intake of vitamin D is relevant; research indicates that lack of vitamin D may be linked to an increased risk for fibroid formation, with an odds ratio of about 2.4, ranking its relevance relative to other risk factors like age and family history (Jaiyeola et al., 2023). Consequently, women are recommended to look into their intake of micronutrients, particularly vitamin D, as it can have a central role in the maintenance of reproductive health as well as in fibroid prevention.

Finally, socioeconomic status and overall maintenance of health cannot be overlooked regarding fibroids. Healthcare availability, reproductive health education, and resources all influence a woman's access to early diagnosis and treatment of fibroids. Additionally, changes in lifestyle like stress-reduction techniques, including physical exercise and mindfulness, have been linked to improved general health and hormonal balance, which can influence fibroid pathology. Women's appreciation of the way their lifestyle choices are intertwined—everything from eating and exercise to stress and access to healthcare—needs to exist. Through the use of preventive steps to deal with these things, women are able to not only enhance their health but also overcome fibroid' issues in a proactive way (Nasiriddinovna et al., 2023).

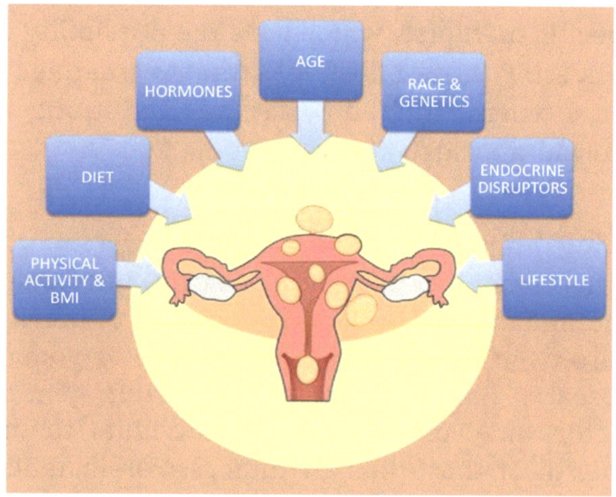

Figure 7.8. Uterine fibroids risk factors.

Source: https://ars.els-cdn.com/content/image/1-s2.0-S1521693417301372-gr1.jpg

Test Your Knowledge

1. How do hormonal influences contribute to the development of fibroids?
2. What role does genetic predisposition play in the occurrence of fibroids?

7.3. Symptoms of Fibroids

Learning Outcome

1. Discuss the heavy menstrual bleeding
2. Define pelvic pain and pressure
3. Identify the urinary and bowel issues

The presentation of fibroids can be extremely varied among women, primarily on the basis of leiomyoma size, number, and location within the uterus. The majority of women remain asymptomatic and only discover they have them incidentally from routine surveillance. Some symptomatic women, however, may experience physical or psychological manifestations. Common complaints include heavy menstrual bleeding (menorrhagia), prolonged menstrual periods, and increased menstrual cramping, which can impede daily activities. The psychological impact of fibroids should not be underestimated; the stress caused by chronic pain and menstrual irregularities can affect mental health and quality of life. Detection of these symptoms is essential, as they tend to push women suffering from them towards seeking medical care and can serve as a point of origin for further diagnostic tests. In addition to the primary symptoms, fibroids can lead to various complications that further worsen a woman's condition. As fibroids grow larger, they have the ability to press against surrounding organs such as the bladder or rectum and cause additional symptoms such as a frequent need to urinate, constipation, and pelvic pressure or pain. Large fibroids in severe cases can cause swelling of the abdomen, which can be mistaken for weight gain or other illnesses. Some women also develop reproductive issues such as infertility, which is typically caused by the size and site of fibroids.

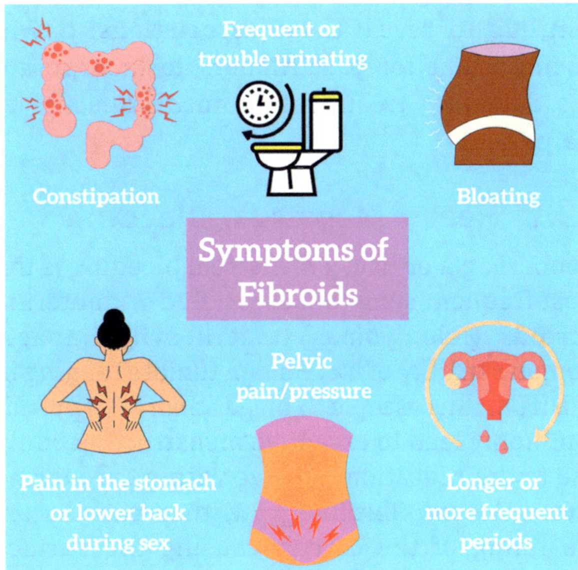

Figure 7.9. Symptoms of fibroids.

Source: https://www.hotteamama.com/cdn/shop/articles/Symptoms_of_Fibroids_1.png?v=1720004409

The connectivity of these symptoms establishes the importance of vigilant observation and assessment. For those needing more respite, a range of remedies is available, from hormonal therapy to surgery, tailored to their specific symptoms and level of health. Contemporary studies have also explored the potential connections between symptoms of fibroids and other influences on well-being, such as diet. A study indicates that there is a link between low concentrations of vitamin D and the incidence and growth of uterine leiomyomas. Subjects who had fibroids had lower serum vitamin D levels than women without fibroids, and it is argued that vitamin D may have a role in tumor regulation. The implication is that supplementation with vitamin D may be a useful adjunct to symptom relief and fibroid shrinkage. It becomes evident that an integrated approach, considering hormonal, nutritional, and lifestyle factors, is essential to the broader understanding of fibroid symptoms. As studies continue to reveal these associations, it will be important for practitioners to incorporate this data into treatment protocols specific to the patient.

7.3.1. Heavy Menstrual Bleeding

Menorrhagia or heavy menstrual bleeding is the most frequent symptom associated with uterine fibroids (leiomyomas) that heavily impacts women's quality of life. Benign tumors ranging in size from microscopic to bigger than a grapefruit commonly lead to excessive menstrual bleeding due to their location and size within the uterine cavity. As the fibroids grow, they can distort the lining of the uterus, causing the surface area across which the endometrial tissue sheds during menses to expand. Therefore, women may experience extended bleeding or excess blood loss, typically resulting in debilitating fatigue or anemia. The correlation between fibroids and menorrhagia highlights the importance of proper diagnosis and assessment, particularly since these symptoms may be inappropriately attributed to normal cyclic changes alone instead of pathologies like leiomyomas (N/A, 2021).

In the treatment of heavy menstrual bleeding secondary to fibroids, clinicians must carefully weigh the treatment against the needs and desires of patients, particularly preservation of fertility. While hysterectomy remains an effective surgical procedure in the case of symptomatic fibroids, sometimes it is incompatible with the desires of women who wish to preserve their reproductive capabilities (N/A, 2021).

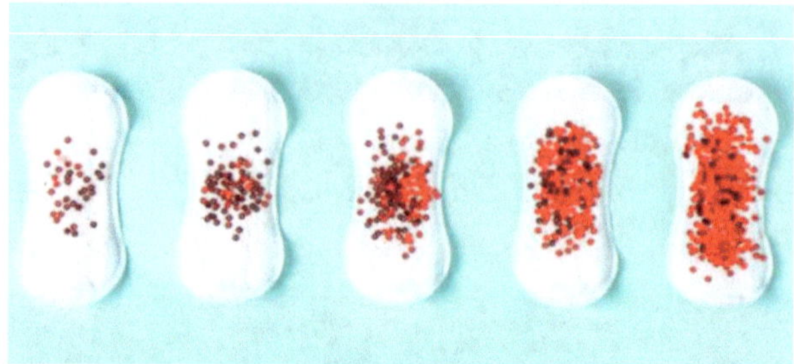

Source: https://static.wixstatic.com/media/dc8b7e_09e9b6ce45764498a9021a58c40ca2dc~mv2.jpg/v1/fill/w_720,h_480,al_c,lg_1,q_80/dc8b7e_09e9b6ce45764498a9021a58c40ca2dc~mv2.jpg

Some of the medical treatments could be initiated to manage symptoms, such as hormone therapy or non-steroidal anti-inflammatory drugs (NSAIDs) that could regulate menstrual cycles and restrict bleeding. Alternatively, less invasive procedures such as uterine artery embolization or myomectomy could be considered, which preserves fertility but involves a massive improvement in quality of life through reduction of heavy menstrual bleeding (Allaire et al., 2015). Research has shown that the prevalence of uterine fibroids and associated heavy menstrual bleeding is significant in reproductive-age women, particularly those who are older than 30 years (N/A, 2021). Considering that a significant proportion of the affected women have severe symptoms, clinical impacts extend beyond physical well-being, with the causative stress from heavy menstrual bleeding finding equivalency in mental and emotional well-being, leading to restriction of lifestyle and decreased productivity. It becomes crucial for clinicians to know the pathophysiology of fibroids and the resulting symptomatology to provide customized care. This is only possible with full guidelines to aid in the decision-making process for optimal interventions based on the safety as well as efficacy of dominant treatment processes, along with a woman's unique health history and preference (Allaire et al., 2015).

7.3.2. Pelvic Pain and Pressure

Pressure and pelvic pain are common complaints of uterine fibroids (leiomyoma), a significant source of morbidity in women. They are benign tumors, but they can compress overlying pelvic structures and cause pain that is variable in terms of duration and intensity. The size and position of the fibroids will dictate the extent of symptoms. For instance, the larger the fibroids or if they are in the intramural or subserosal sites, the more likely they are to have noticeable pressure effects with an acute or chronic pelvic pain as one of the most common results. Thus, patients experience not just physical discomfort but also psychological suffering arising from the impact of these signs on work and interpersonal relationships. Treatment of such symptoms is essential to improving overall health and well-being in women with fibroids. Beyond this, the management of pelvic pain due to fibroids has become more sophisticated, including both conservative and surgical options. Pain may be alleviated by medication such as nonsteroidal anti-inflammatory drugs (NSAIDs); however, they are not equally effective in different individuals. Hormonal treatment, including the use of ulipristal acetate, has, in some cases, been examined for its impact on symptom relief and quality of life in symptomatic women with fibroids. Current analysis indicates that ulipristal acetate can lead to increased relief from pelvic pressure and menorrhagia, which makes it a promising non-conservative treatment option (Cornejo et al., 2023). Conversely, surgical treatment for severe cases is indicated, especially when pain impairs routine function, so an evaluation of the status of the patients and their preference for treatment is appropriate. Clinically, pelvic pressure and pain resulting from fibroids can also mimic other gynecologic disorders, thus complicating the diagnosis. Differential diagnoses like endometriosis, ovarian cysts, or pelvic inflammatory disease must be carefully considered in order to prevent misdiagnosis and treatment. Lymphoma Correct Evaluation with imaging modalities such as ultrasound or MRI can assist clinicians in differentiating fibroids from other pain-producing causes. Because pain may be multifactorial in origin, the inclusion of psychosocial assessment, along with physical examination, can further clarify the patient's experience with fibroids. With the complications of symptomatology unfolding, treatment modalities can be tailor-made for each patient, offering the optimal care for fibroid patients and associated pelvic pain and pressure (Besharat et al., 2012).

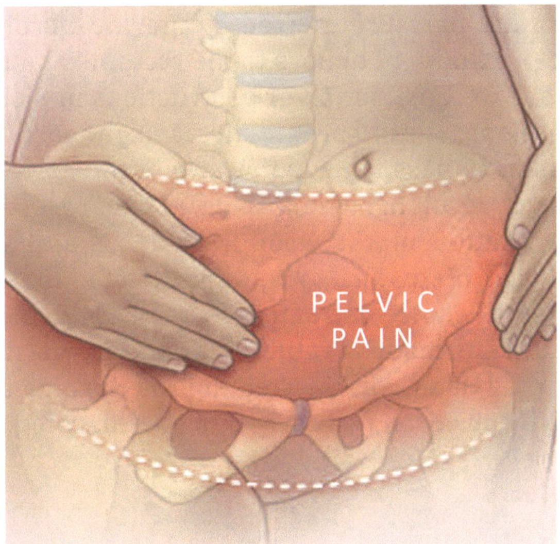

Source: https://lh7-us.googleusercontent.com/Tc6W37c_-AeHecGR0YCgWr-NJEHF5j4FX-uO5smcSTJjFDXFC8hH_vIyN8hEPiLjrPr5T-Kaq7ZVz1l_WxD5rlBb0xaEDZmLGf5KHADMI-jF6tbBX2S0UJfHFIB6uYD3SKbmV7ecJf9_jh-8gcTETVZ1BCs

7.3.3. Urinary and Bowel Issues

The development of uterine fibroids (leiomyomas) has significant implications for bowel and urinary function in women. Benign neoplasms have the capability of compressing adjacent organs, most significantly the bladder and rectum, and developing a range of symptoms. For instance, the majority of women have urinary frequency or urgency as the fibroids compress the bladder and decrease urination capacity. In addition, the pressure may lead to incomplete emptying of the bladder, which frequently causes urinary tract infections. The discomfort of such a symptom can significantly affect a woman's quality of life. Thus, treatment of urinary symptoms associated with fibroids is essential because such disturbances may cause general problems concerning physical and mental well-being, particularly in women of childbearing age who may have multiple tasks to accomplish simultaneously (Zaher et al., 2010). Bowel abnormalities can also result from the pressure exerted by uterine fibroids. The proximity of tumors to the rectum is bound to lead to constipation or obstructions in worse situations. It can become increasingly hard for women to pass regular bowel movements, and this can result in bloating, pain, and more issues. The relationship between fibroid size and site and gastrointestinal symptoms dictates that, in making a choice of treatment, a full assessment should be made. Problems of the bowel are not only dealt with by treating the fibroids but also by performing dietary and pharmacological maneuvers to improve gastrointestinal function and transit. This emphasizes the need for health practitioners to assess symptoms holistically, considering the impact fibroids can have on both bowel and urinary functioning (Zaher et al., 2010). While therapeutic management of fibroids will generally focus on symptom relief from menstruation, alleviation of urinary and bowel symptoms is equally significant. Treatment options range from pharmacologic therapy to surgical interventions like myomectomy or hysterectomy. Of special interest are emerging advances in non-surgical treatments, specifically Magnetic Resonance guided Focused Ultrasound Surgery (MRgFUS). The therapy holds the promise of decreasing risks associated with traditional surgery while effectively shrinking fibroid size and related symptoms, such as urinary and bowel function impairments. Having the preferred treatment be compatible with a woman's reproductive goals and overall well-being remains most essential. The breakthrough of minimally invasive treatments brings relief to those who wish to be free from the debilitating effects of fibroids on a daily basis, indicating a shifting trend in treating fibroids.

Test Your Knowledge

1. How can fibroids lead to heavy menstrual bleeding in affected individuals?
2. What causes pelvic pain and pressure in patients with fibroids?

7.4. Diagnosis of Fibroids

Learning Outcome

1. Define pelvic examination
2. Understand the imaging techniques (ultrasound, MRI)
3. Explain the hysteroscopy

Diagnosis of leiomyomas or fibroids involves more than one step and encompasses clinical evaluation, imaging studies, and in selected cases, laboratory tests. Clinicians will first use a complete patient history and physical examination, where irregularities in shape and size of the uterus often result in additional testing. Of interest, transabdominal or transvaginal ultrasound remains the preferred imaging modality since it is readily available, noninvasive, and effective for detecting the presence and size of fibroids. These methods can precisely demonstrate the quantity and size of fibroids and thus be helpful in assessing the likelihood of any association with symptoms such as menorrhagia or pelvic pain. Although used in combination with ultrasound, magnetic resonance imaging (MRI) gives clearer images of fibroids and surrounding tissue with accurate information regarding their characteristics. MRI is particularly valuable in the planning of treatment as it can differentiate between various forms of fibroids, i.e., submucosal or intramural fibroids, and establish any possible complications. Additionally, recent advances in Doppler imaging techniques, as highlighted by recent literature, improve accuracy in diagnosing leiomyomas based on vascular characteristics. For instance, a study indicates that Dopplerometry can elucidate differences in blood supply between malignant and benign tumors, enabling differential diagnosis and ultimately guiding patients' management plans (Sukhin et al., 2018). On rare occasions, fibroids can lead to life-threatening situations such as hypovolemic shock resulting from acute hemorrhage from a ruptured fibroid. Diagnosing it is challenging since initial diagnoses may reveal nonspecific abdominal symptoms. Use of computed tomography (CT) can provide rapid confirmation of hemoperitoneum secondary to avulsion of a pedunculated leiomyoma, facilitating early surgery. As case reports clearly show, imaging with CT clarity can be life-saving and emphasizes the importance of early and accurate diagnosis in avoiding serious outcomes. Hence, the integration of multiple imaging modalities with clinical assessment remains key to achieving effective diagnosis and treatment planning for fibroid patients (Adamo et al., 2017).

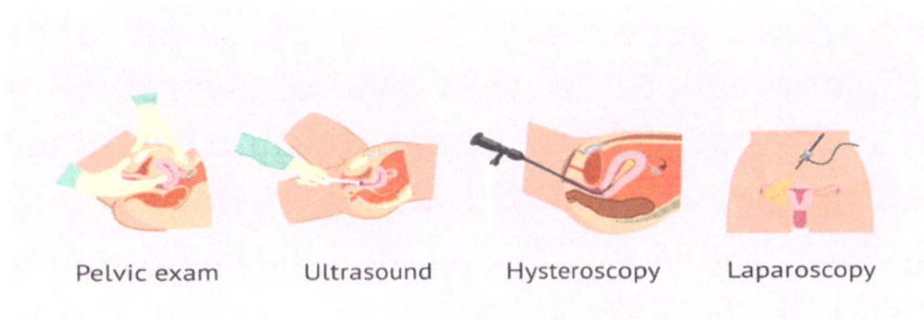

Figure 7.10. Most used techniques in fibroid diagnosis.

Source: https://www.invitra.com/en/wp-content/uploads/2019/12/diagnosis-fibroids.png

7.4.1. Pelvic Examination

The pelvic examination is a routine part of diagnosing and treating many gynecological conditions, such as uterine fibroids. With a complete examination, health practitioners are able to detect the physical characteristics of masses present, if any, such as size, location, and tenderness. Such an examination is typically performed under both visual and bimanual palpation, such that the practitioner is able to check the uterus's position (anteverted, retroverted, or midline) and check for adnexal pathology. For instance, an enlarged uterus can suggest the presence of fibroids, which may be misinterpreted as other conditions. This physical examination offers a window for other diagnostic tests, such as ultrasound or CT scans, to make the diagnosis, and therefore it is a crucial first step in the clinical management of fibroids and their associated symptoms. For fibroids, the pelvic exam can make visible several symptoms that the patients may present, which can indeed impact their quality of life. The majority of women with fibroids have symptoms like abnormal vaginal bleeding, pelvic discomfort, and pressure symptoms from larger masses. The pelvic examination assists in elucidating these symptoms because medical providers are able to detect abnormalities within the size and shape of the uterus. Furthermore, an excellent pelvic examination can reveal additional fibroid complications, like urinary or gastrointestinal symptoms secondary to compression upon adjacent structures. This level of awareness is critical to identifying the appropriate treatment pathways, be it medical management, surgery, or observation, thus correlating the examination with optimal care directly.

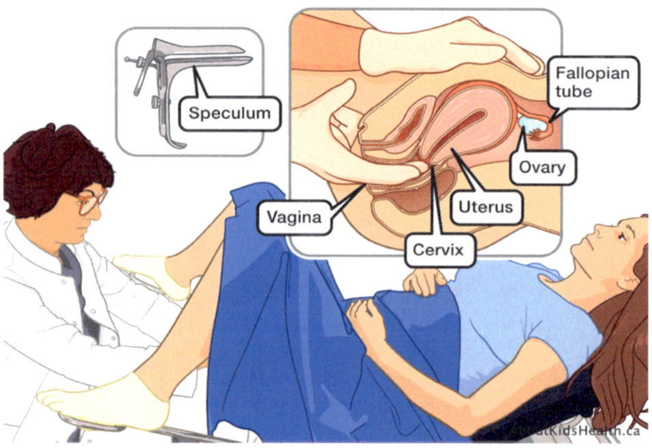

Figure 7.11. Pelvic examination.

Source: https://teens.aboutkidshealth.ca/globalassets/assets/pelvic_exam.jpg

One of the important considerations in a pelvic exam is the emergent situation among fibroid patients. Although the majority of them are stable, there are cases that develop severe complications such as hemoperitoneum with an expanding or bleeding leiomyoma, which necessitates immediate treatment. For example, a case such as this was documented in the literature where a patient presented a case of hypovolemic shock due to hemorrhage from a pedunculated fibroid, identified through both imaging and pelvic exam (Adamo et al., 2017). Such a case reminds us how clinicians must remain aware of the presence of acute complications during routine exams. This vigilance not only ensures timely intervention but also encourages a preventive approach towards management of the myriad symptoms of fibroids, so that women are offered safe and effective treatment as part of reproductive health care (N/A, 2021).

7.4.2. Imaging Techniques (Ultrasound, MRI)

Familiarity with imaging tests utilized to diagnose fibroids (leiomyomas) is warranted in light of the prevalence of these benign tumors in women of childbearing age. Ultrasound remains one of the most common imaging methods, primarily due to its availability, low cost, and ability to provide immediate information. Transabdominal and transvaginal ultrasound can easily identify fibroids, measuring their diameter, number, and location in the uterus. This non-invasive method not only allows early diagnosis but also settles clinical decision-making based on treatment options and plans. However, while ultrasound is proficient at identifying the presence of fibroids, it may be deficient in terms of needed accuracy concerning precise characterization of tissues and, therefore, may lead to misdiagnosis or failure to detect other pathologies. Thus, further imaging modalities may be warranted to confirm diagnosis and assess properties of fibroids comprehensively (Zaher et al., 2010). Magnetic Resonance Imaging (MRI) is a technologically more advanced and high-resolution imaging technique with specific advantages in the evaluation of uterine fibroids. MRI gives high-resolution images that enable accurate assessment of fibroid dimensions and pinpoint localization, thereby adding to surgical planning and possible intervention plans. Moreover, MRI is better at differentiating between fibroid types and other masses of the pelvis and providing helpful information that dictates management. Research has established that Magnetic resonance-guided high-intensity focused ultrasound (MRgFUS) uses the imaging features of MRIs to enhance the outcome of treatment in symptomatic patients. MRgFUS is a non-surgical procedure for treating fibroids, which not only reduces symptoms such as menorrhagia and dysmenorrhea but leaves uterine anatomy intact. The growing body of evidence supporting the efficacy and safety of MRgFUS underscores the role of MRI in the management of uterine fibroids and enhances patients' clinical pathways (Baracat et al., 2017).

The integration of ultrasound and MRI in managing uterine fibroids not only improves diagnostic accuracy but also informs treatment options. Fibroid-related symptoms can significantly impact the quality of life, prompting the need for targeted interventions. MRIs' advanced imaging capabilities enable the measurement of treatment effectiveness over time, so clinicians can monitor changes in fibroid size and symptomatic expressions after treatments like MRgFUS or standard surgical interventions. Longitudinal evaluation is most crucial for developing patient-specific treatment regimens that maximize outcomes the most. Moreover, applications of these imaging modalities have led to an increase in minimally invasive methods in gynecology as an indication of a cultural shift towards patient safety and fertility conservation. By facilitating a comprehensive understanding of fibroids through advanced imaging technologies, the medical community has the potential to facilitate better control of this prevalent condition and improve the quality of care for affected women (Zaher et al., 2010)..

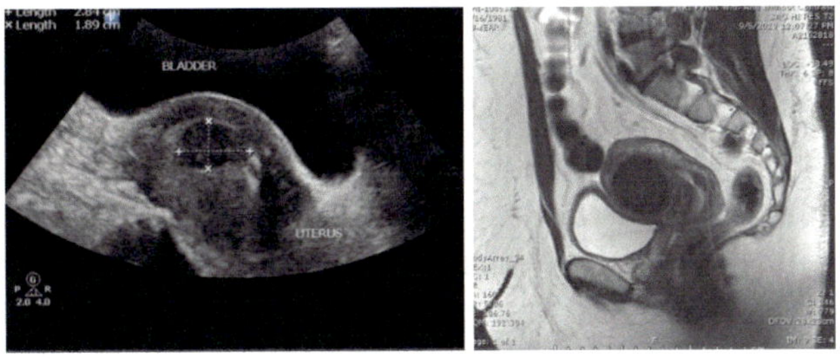

Figure 7.12. Pelvic MRI.

Source: https://freefromfibroids.org/wp-content/uploads/2021/08/mri-vs-ultrasound-e1629207102571.jpg

7.4.3. Hysteroscopy

Use of hysteroscopy for the management of uterine fibroids, particularly submucous fibroids, has been a topic of great interest among clinicians. Application of hysteroscopy as a minimally invasive surgical procedure allows direct visualization of the uterine cavity and intervention without exposing women to extensive abdominal surgery. The ability to excise submucous fibroids by hysteroscopy can enhance reproductive outcomes in women presenting with unexplained infertility or with complications related to these fibroids. In addition, studies reveal that when performed prior to assisted reproductive therapies, i.e., intrauterine insemination (IUI) or in vitro fertilization (IVF), hysteroscopic surgery can improve the chances of successful pregnancy by curing uterine cavity anatomical abnormalities, therefore optimising embryo implantation and pregnancy conditions (Bosteels et al., 2015). The prevalence of uterine fibroids, or leiomyomas, is very common, and hence, effective treatment modalities are required. Leiomyomas are often asymptomatic but can cause a host of problems, including abnormal uterine bleeding, pelvic pain, and infertility (N/A, 2021). Hysteroscopic myomectomy, particularly in submucous fibroids, has been found to be an effective treatment, which may increase the likelihood of achieving clinical pregnancy rates in cases of women with fertility issues. Evidence indicates that hysteroscopic removal yields better outcomes compared to other conservative treatments, offering a targeted approach to eliminating the blockage created by fibroids. This approach is thus more and more regarded as a potential intervention in the therapeutic strategy, particularly given its minimally invasive nature and minimal recovery time compared to traditional techniques. Despite its advantages, the use of hysteroscopy in managing submucous fibroids is still under research regarding its efficacy and safety. While some studies have demonstrated promising results, other studies reveal that rates of clinical pregnancy after hysteroscopic myomectomy may be variable. For instance, even though increased clinical pregnancy rates have been shown, firm proof is limited and additional randomized controlled trials are required to confirm these and to ascertain long-term effects of hysteroscopic procedures on fertility outcomes. The subtle appreciation of the way in which hysteroscopic methods can be most optimally applied for fibroid patients is essential in fine-tuning treatment models and providing optimal management for women encountering the threat of fibroids and associated infertility (Bosteels et al., 2015).

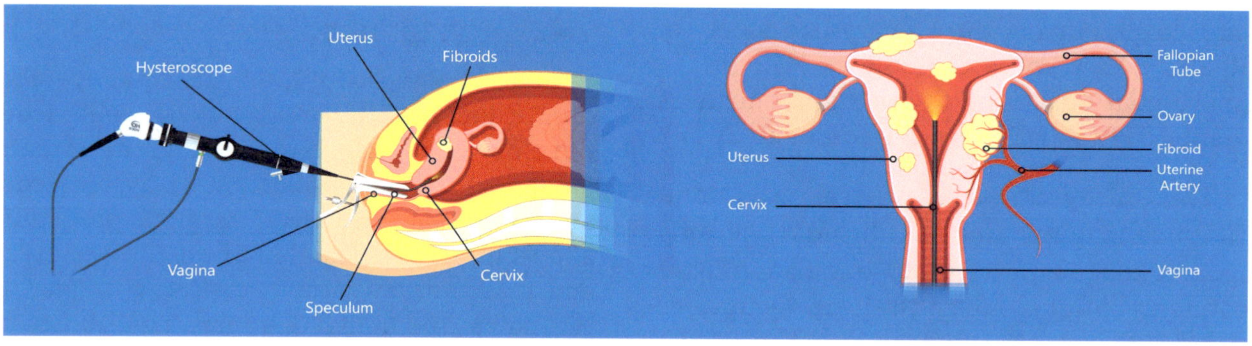

Figure 7.13. Hysteroscopic Resection of Fibroids.

Source: https://images.squarespace-cdn.com/content/v1/5bd10d14523958814df7900c/1540791940134-ZUQCYHEH5ANGJ7GEM9XY/shutterstock_1194708523.jpg

Test Your Knowledge

1. Demonstrate the ability to perform and interpret findings from a pelvic examination.
2. Explain the role and application of imaging techniques such as ultrasound and MRI in diagnosing gynecological conditions.

7.5. Treatment Options

Learning Outcome

1. Discuss the medication management of treating uterine fibroids
2. Explain the surgical interventions
3. Define non-invasive procedures

Treatment of uterine fibroids, or leiomyomas, is diverse and tailored to the individual requirements of each patient. For patients in whom fibroids are an incidental discovery and asymptomatic, active surveillance is generally the optimal approach, as the majority of patients have negligible effects on their lifestyle. Treatment, however, is warranted when fibroids are symptomatic, such as heavy menstrual bleeding or pelvic pressure. Common treatments include hormone therapy aimed at normalizing menstrual outflow and symptoms. Specific interest has been shown in selective estrogen receptor modulators that bind to estrogen receptors and may reduce the size of fibroids while managing associated symptoms. However, treatment choice should take into account the patient's desire for future fertility, overall health, and risk-to-benefit ratio of the alternatives, with emphasis placed on the demand for individualized care in the management of leiomyomas (Allaire et al., 2015).

Surgical procedures also take center stage in treating symptomatic fibroids. Myomectomy, where the removal of the fibroids is done, sparing the uterus, is normally the option of choice for women who would prefer to preserve reproductive function.

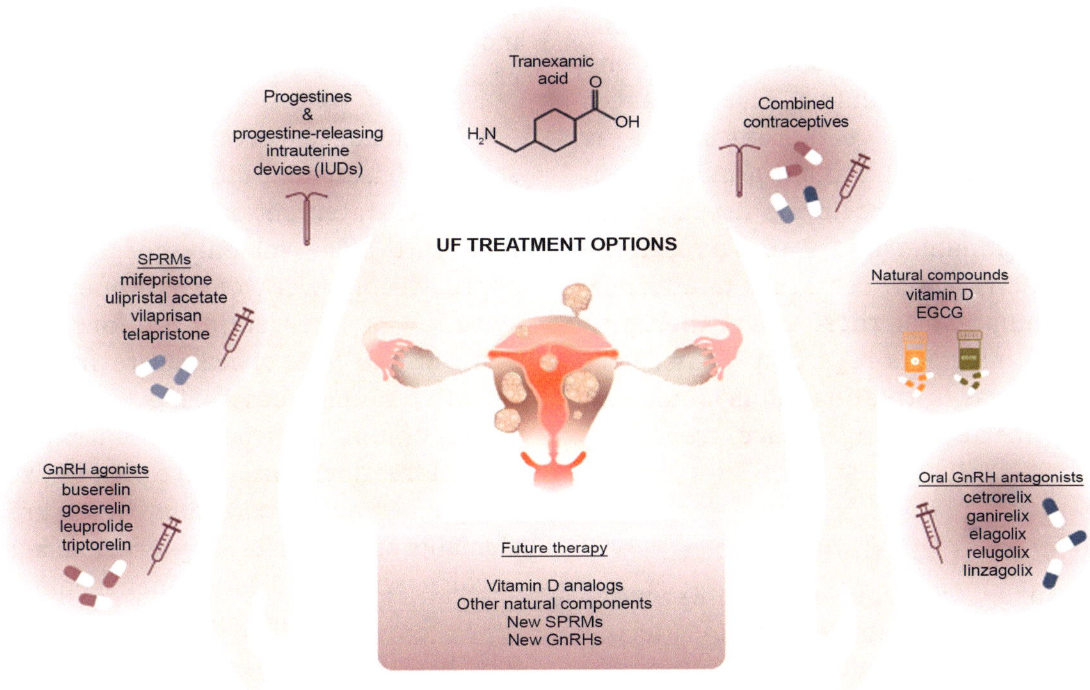

Figure 7.14. Current and emerging treatment options for uterine fibroids.

Source: https://media.springernature.com/lw685/springer-static/image/art%3A10.1007%2Fs40265-023-01958-6/MediaObjects/40265_2023_1958_Fig1_HTML.png

This procedure can alleviate symptoms and also allow for a later pregnancy. Alternatively, hysterectomy, or the excision of the uterus, is seen as an ultimate option, particularly for individuals with intense symptoms or no longer wishing to preserve fertility. Selection of these procedures depends not only on symptom severity but also on the patient's long-term reproductive goals. Significantly, each procedure has its risks as well as benefits, and hence, detailed consultation between the patient and the doctor is necessary while choosing surgical treatment (Allaire et al., 2015).

Aside from surgery and medicine, there are other non-surgical procedures that can treat fibroids. One of them is uterine artery embolization (UAE), in which the blood supply to fibroids is cut off, and hence fibroids shrink and symptoms disappear. It is a less invasive technique, which is appealing for women who do not wish for a traditional surgery since this procedure requires less time for recovery and less postoperative discomfort. Also, advances in technology of ablative therapies such as MRI-guided focused ultrasound provide novel treatment options, where fibroid tissue can be ablated with minimal injury to surrounding structures. As research continues to advance, ongoing evaluation of these novel therapies continues to inform us regarding their safety and effectiveness in treating leiomyomas and assists us in developing future treatment paradigms.

7.5.1. Medication Management

Effective drug control is an important component in the management of uterine fibroids (leiomyoma), particularly in those who need non-surgical measures. Medical therapy, including hormonal treatment with oral contraceptives and gonadotropin-releasing hormone (GnRH) agonists, may be useful in significantly alleviating symptoms of fibroids, including menorrhagia and pelvic pain. These drugs work by altering the hormonal environment, which may also lead to fibroid shrinkage and symptomatic relief. Of particular importance, patient education on drug use and the side effects of drugs is essential because adherence would be strongly promoted by a patient's awareness of their treatment regimen. Also, careful monitoring is essential in order to evaluate medication management effectiveness and implement any necessary adjustments so that patients can maintain optimal control of symptoms with consideration to their overall reproductive health. Complementary and alternative treatments have emerged as significant adjuncts to standard medication therapy among women with uterine fibroids. Many patients attempt such things as changes in diet, herbal supplements, exercise, and acupuncture alongside medication. Research has indicated that these complementary treatments lead to great symptom relief without surgery or more invasive procedure side effects (Gregorich et al., 2014).

For instance, participants of recent studies showed considerable quality-of-life improvement after such intervention was incorporated into their care plan. Not only does this combined approach empower women by offering a greater selection of intervention options, but it also reaffirms the value of healthcare providers being sensitive to and recognizing varying symptom management approaches. Emphasizing a unified treatment program can optimize patient compliance and satisfaction, which are critical elements of successful long-term management of fibroids. While medication management is often the first step in managing symptomatic fibroids, patients should be informed about the potential need for surgery in cases where pharmacologic therapies are insufficient. Uterus-preserving procedures, such as myomectomy and uterine artery embolization, are viable alternatives for women seeking symptom relief while maintaining fertility. Decision-making should involve explicit discussion of the benefits and complications of all treatments, the implications of potential surgery (Zaher et al., 2010). An individualized treatment plan combining medication management, complementary care, and surgery can help guide women in making informed healthcare decisions. Lastly, the solution calls for an interdisciplinary strategy with ongoing communication between patients and health practitioners to achieve the maximum therapeutic benefit and tackle the extremely complicated issues that uterine fibroids present.

7.5.2. Surgical Interventions

Surgical procedures are an important avenue for treating uterine fibroids when conservative management is unsuccessful in reducing symptoms. Myomectomy is one of the mainstay surgical modalities that has found favor due to its advantage of removing fibroids without compromising uterine function, thereby being the modality of choice for those desiring preservation of fertility. It is particularly suited for symptomatic fibroids with menorrhagia, pelvic pain, and pressure symptoms. Surgery can be done by various techniques—abdominal, laparoscopic, or hysteroscopic—and each has its own advantages depending on the size and location of the fibroids and the patient's preference.

But deciding to go for myomectomy should weigh rigorously against the risk of complication and recovery time and in favor of symptom relief and improvement in quality of life, emphasizing the need for individualized treatment planning (Koomson et al., 2017). In certain cases, hysterectomy presents itself as a complete cure for symptomatic fibroids, especially in women who have completed childbearing or whose symptoms have a drastic impact on their quality of life. Hysterectomy is the process of removing the uterus and is most often advised in women with severe symptoms that fail to respond to other ways, such as incapacitating pain or heavy bleeding leading to anemia. While this intervention is a definitive remedy for the fibroid problem, it impacts a woman's fertility, and hence, thorough counseling prior to surgery becomes essential. In addition, the cost-effectiveness of hysterectomy must be considered in that procedure, and associated healthcare costs could be significantly high. The necessity to deal with fibroid symptoms is most often of an emergency nature that needs to be weighed against such considerations as the relative benefits of possible long-term relief of symptoms (Koomson et al., 2017).

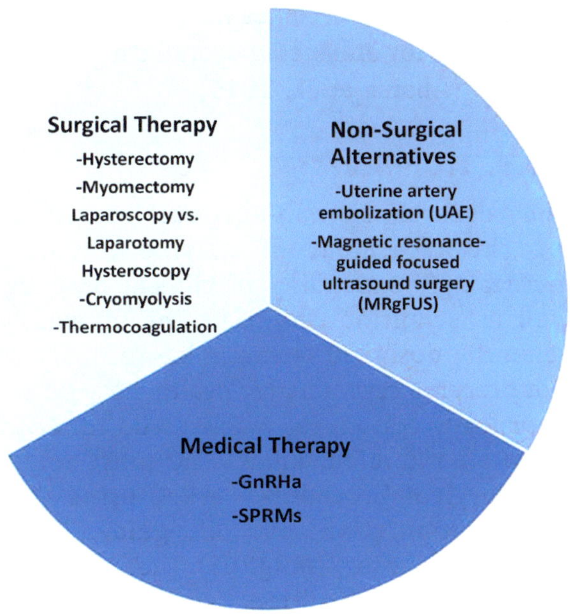

Figure 7.15. Surgical, non-surgical and medical therapy for the management of fibroids.

Source: https://www.researchgate.net/figure/Surgical-non-surgical-and-medical-therapy-for-the-management-of-fibroids-the-current_fig7_305697512

There are also novel minimally invasive techniques that have significantly impacted surgery for fibroids and offer more choices for patients. Of these therapies, uterine artery embolization (UAE) has been given attention because of its ability to reduce the size of fibroids by cutting off their blood supply. This procedure generally results in a shorter recuperation time and less post-operative pain compared to traditional operations. And another one that minimizes scarring and recuperation time is laparoscopic myolysis, which coagulates and thus kills fibroids through the application of thermal or laser heat. It is most important for healthcare professionals to remain current with such evolving techniques, as they not only expand the surgical arsenal but also respond to mounting pressure for less invasive therapy. With the ongoing evolution of surgical procedures, ongoing research becomes necessary for optimal results and for enhancing overall care of uterine fibroids (Allaire et al., 2015).

7.5.3. Non-Invasive Procedures

The research on non-surgical interventions for the treatment of uterine fibroids is increasingly expanding in clinical practice as well as scientific research. The alternatives, generally designed to minimize recovery time and preserve reproductive health, have emerged as primary options for women who suffer from symptomatic leiomyomas. The most common non-surgical procedures are Uterine Artery Embolization (UAE) and MRI-guided focused ultrasound surgery (MRgFUS). These techniques offer options to traditional surgical techniques like hysterectomy, particularly for women who would like to maintain fertility or do not want extended convalescence periods after surgical interventions. Both procedures have also been proven to be effective in controlling heavy menstrual bleeding and pelvic pain symptoms, thus enhancing the quality of life and well-being of affected women (Allaire et al., 2015). UAE specifically involves the selective interruption of blood flow to the fibroids, causing their shrinking and subsequent relief of symptoms. This in-office procedure will frequently require minimal sedation, and patients can go home the same day. Clinical experience suggests that UAE can be associated with substantial improvement in symptoms, with many patients experiencing reduced menstrual bleeding and pain within months. At the same time, MRgFUS employs high-frequency ultrasound waves to ablate and destroy fibroid tissue, thereby offering a non-surgical method of treating fibroid symptoms with no cuts involved. Evidence indicates that MRgFUS also enhances patients' quality of life in that women can avoid surgical risks while efficiently tackling their fibroid-related problems (College A of Obstetricians and Gynecologists et al., 2020). While there is potential in these non-surgical techniques, keep in mind that they are not suited to all patients. Further one-on-one assessment of fibroid size and location, as well as patient preference, is part of determining the suitability of these techniques. Further, while seemingly with fewer complications, they may not fully resolve the requirement for future intervention. Women must engage in well-informed discussions with their doctors to weigh the potential benefits against the risks of each treatment. Ultimately, the development of guidelines that encompass non-surgical interventions in addition to guidelines for standard operating procedures for surgery is envisioned to provide a complete approach in managing fibroids in order to enhance decision-making among women who suffer from uterine leiomyomas (Allaire et al., 2015).

Test Your Knowledge

1. Explain the pharmacological options available for the management of uterine fibroids and their mechanisms of action.
2. Describe the indications, techniques, and outcomes of surgical interventions used to treat uterine fibroids.

SUMMARY

In summarizing the complexity of the management of fibroids (leiomyoma), patient-specific treatment clearly comes first. The range of symptoms that fibroids are capable of inducing, from severe abdominal pain to infertility, demands a patient-specific therapeutic strategy. Despite established alternatives such as hysterectomy and myomectomy, newer non-invasive treatments such as Magnetic Resonance guided Focused Ultrasound Surgery (MRgFUS) have been in vogue due to their benefits of minimizing surgery risk and the loss of the uterus. The evidence that is coming in indicates a significant relief in symptoms and success for women who could otherwise undergo invasive intervention. Thus, the choice of treatment should specifically consider patient preference, fertility desire, and symptom severity to ensure informed decisions are made that represent individual circumstances (Zaher et al., 2010). Also, if UAE is considered as an option other than myomectomy, several questions regarding future pregnancy ensue. Although the UAE seems to be less invasive with the additional advantage of relief of symptoms and reduced recovery periods, how it affects future pregnancy outcomes is unclear. The literature available to date reveals an association with risks of adverse maternal outcomes, including spontaneous abortion and abnormal placentation. Until more robust and large-scale studies bring attention to this treatment's long-term consequences, myomectomy will likely remain the gold standard of care for women who wish to maintain fertility. Therefore, the clinical fraternity must embrace a high priority for ongoing research and patient education regarding adapting to the evolving environment of fibroid treatment modalities (Wimber et al.). Overall, the conclusion arrived at from current evidence emphasizes an integrated approach towards managing fibroids. The synergy of innovative therapeutic methods, appropriate patient selection, and astute understanding of each option's risks will significantly enhance patient quality of life. The growing body of evidence supporting MRgFUS and the careful balancing of UAE paved the way for less invasive and more successful treatments for women plagued with fibroid-related problems. With progressive clinical practice, the continuously pressing need for patient-specific treatment pathways becomes more and more obvious, ensuring that women are treated in line with their own unique health needs and context (Zaher et al., 2010).

Uterine fibroids, or leiomyomas, are frequent benign neoplasms arising from smooth muscle tissues of the uterus that affect a high percentage of women worldwide. The tumors often manifest with various symptoms, from menorrhagia to pelvic discomfort and pressure manifestations on adjacent organs. The presentation of fibroids may significantly affect a woman's quality of life, and therefore, a variety of treatment modalities ranging from medication to surgery are undertaken. Specifically, myomectomy and hysterectomy have been characterized as effective surgical interventions for fibroid management that allow women to maintain their reproductive function in conjunction with relief of bothersome symptoms. With a complete understanding of the effect of fibroids and their management, healthcare providers can deliver personalized treatment plans tailored to the specific requirements of each patient that optimize quality and outcome of care in individuals with this common condition. Recent studies emphasize the potential benefits of surgical procedures like hysteroscopic myomectomy, stating that they can maximize pregnancy rates in women who are experiencing subfertility after fibroids. For instance, the removal of submucous fibroids has been found to be related to an increased probability of successful pregnancies either naturally or following assisted reproductive techniques like in vitro fertilization (IVF). Specifically, research indicates that women undergoing hysteroscopic removal of fibroids have greater clinical rates of pregnancy compared to those who do not undergo it, and as such, it is an important alternative for women undergoing unexplained subfertility (Bosteels et al., 2015). Nevertheless, the success of the interventions can be tempered by the general health status and reproductive goals of the woman, and as such, personal assessments are required in treatment approaches. Furthermore, advancements in techniques such as in-bag morcellation have enhanced the safety profile of laparoscopic myomectomy, reducing concerns of complications with older power morcellation. The in-bag method allows for safe fibroid removal without disseminating tissue within the abdominal cavity and thus decreasing the risk of spreading malignant cells if present. This guideline of safety is especially important in the context of the rare but problematic risk of leiomyosarcoma being confused with benign fibroids during surgical procedures (Raffone et al., 2020). Ongoing evaluation of these techniques is significant, as large studies must be conducted in order to provide us with ultimate evidence of their impact on outcomes and complications. Systematic reviews of these strategies will ultimately result in maximizing treatment regimens and patient safety in fibroid management.

KEY TERMS FROM THIS CHAPTER

- Abnormal uterine bleeding
- Computed tomography (CT)
- Dopplerometry
- Endometrial tissue
- Estrogenic activity
- Fibroid pathogenesis
- Hysterectomy
- Insulin-like growth factors (IGFs)
- Leiomyomas
- Muscle cells
- Reproductive health education
- Body mass index (BMI)
- Diagnostic accuracy
- Dysmenorrhea
- Estrogen
- Fetal malpresentation
- Heavy menstrual bleeding (HMB)
- Hysteroscopy
- Intrauterine insemination (IUI)
- Menorrhagia
- Receptor-specific therapies
- Submucosal types

CRITICAL THINKING QUESTIONS

1. **What are uterine fibroids (leiomyomas)?**
   a. Malignant tumors of the uterus
   b. Benign smooth muscle tumors of the uterus
   c. Cysts filled with fluid in the uterus
   d. Infections of the uterine lining
2. **Which symptom is most commonly associated with uterine fibroids?**
   a. Heavy menstrual bleeding (menorrhagia)
   b. Sudden weight loss
   c. Frequent urination due to infection
   d. Irregular heartbeat
3. **Which of the following factors is believed to promote the growth of fibroids?**
   a. Low estrogen levels
   b. High progesterone levels
   c. High estrogen levels
   d. Low progesterone levels
4. **The most common diagnostic tool used to detect uterine fibroids is:**
   a. Pelvic ultrasound
   b. CT scan of the abdomen
   c. Mammography
   d. Colonoscopy
5. **Which of the following is NOT a typical treatment option for uterine fibroids?**
   a. Myomectomy
   b. Hysterectomy
   c. Antibiotics
   d. Uterine artery embolization

Short Answer Questions

1. What are the different types of uterine fibroids?
2. What are the common causes and risk factors for developing fibroids?
3. What symptoms are typically associated with uterine fibroids?
4. Which diagnostic methods are used to detect fibroids?
5. What treatment options are available for managing fibroids?
6. How do fibroids affect a woman's reproductive health?

Answer to Critical Thinking Questions

1. (b) 2. (a) 3. (c) 4. (a) 5. (c)

References

1. Adamo, R., Kaushik, C., & Mizrahi, D. J. (2017). Hypovolemic shock and hemoperitoneum from spontaneous avulsion of a large pedunculated uterine leiomyoma. https://core.ac.uk/download/83049907.pdf (accessed on 15th June 2025).
2. Affonso, B. B., Baracat, E. C., Baroni, R. H., de Lorenzo Messina, M., et al. (2014). Predictive factors for pelvic magnetic resonance in response to arterial embolization of a uterine leiomyoma. https://core.ac.uk/download/268269394.pdf (accessed on 15th June 2025).
3. Allaire, C., Chen, I., Laberge, P. Y., Leyland, C., et al. (2015). The management of uterine leiomyomas. https://core.ac.uk/download/534389307.pdf (accessed on 15th June 2025).
4. American College of Obstetricians and Gynecologists, Bhave Chittawar, P., Gupta, J. K., Lethaby, A., Low, M. S. Y., Murji, A., et al. (2020). Epidemiology and management of uterine fibroids. http://deepblue.lib.umich.edu/bitstream/2027.42/154526/1/ijgo13102.pdf (accessed on 15th June 2025).
5. Anitha, A., Fathima, H., Nousheen, S., Parunandi, Y., et al. (2024). An observational study on causes of female infertility. https://core.ac.uk/download/620836115.pdf (accessed on 15th June 2025).
6. Aoki, D., Arisawa, K., Chiyoda, T., Fukushima, A., et al. (2020). Identification of a novel uterine leiomyoma GWAS locus in a Japanese population. https://core.ac.uk/download/347090797.pdf (accessed on 15th June 2025).
7. Armstrong, A., Daniels, A., Golan, A., Lethaby, A., Lieto, A., Zimmermann, A., Audebert, A. J., et al. (2016). Medical therapies for uterine fibroids–A systematic review and network meta-analysis of randomized controlled trials. https://core.ac.uk/download/79500438.pdf (accessed on 15th June 2025).
8. Baird, D. D., Hill, M. C., Saldana, T. M., Schectman, J. M., et al. (2015). A single baseline ultrasound assessment of fibroid presence and size is strongly predictive of future uterine procedure: 8-year follow-up of randomly sampled premenopausal women aged 35–49 years. https://core.ac.uk/download/230764903.pdf (accessed on 15th June 2025).
9. Bajunirwe, F., Kanyesigye, H., Ngonzi, J., Adawe, M., Sezalio, M., Kajabwangu, R., & Okello, S. (2022). Prevalence, clinical presentation and factors associated with uterine fibroids among women attending the Gynecology Outpatient Department at a large referral hospital in Southwestern Uganda. https://core.ac.uk/download/524771448.pdf (accessed on 15th June 2025).
10. Baracat, E. C., de Lorenzo Messina, M., dos Santos Simões, R., Peregrino, C., et al. (2017). Review of magnetic resonance-guided focused ultrasound in the treatment of uterine fibroids. https://core.ac.uk/download/268270024.pdf (accessed on 15th June 2025).
11. Besharat, M., & Tabandeh, A. (2012). Successful myomectomy during pregnancy. https://core.ac.uk/download/86410577.pdf (accessed on 15th June 2025).
12. Bosteels, J., Broekmans, F. J., D'Hooghe, T. M., Kasius, J. C., et al. (2015). Hysteroscopy for treating subfertility associated with suspected major uterine cavity abnormalities. https://core.ac.uk/download/55847628.pdf (accessed on 15th June 2025).
13. Cornejo, M. Y. L., García, A. G. G., Palacios, A. A. M., Vespero, E., et al. (2023). Shifting paradigms in uterine fibroids treatment: Insights from current therapeutic approaches. https://core.ac.uk/download/579951690.pdf (accessed on 15th June 2025).

14. Critchley, H., Babayev, E., Bulun, S. E., Clark, S., Garcia-Grau, I., Gregersen, P. K., Kilcoyne, A., et al. (2020). Menstruation: Science and society. *American Journal of Obstetrics and Gynecology, 223*, 624–664. https://doi.org/10.1016/j.ajog.2020.06.004 (accessed on 15th June 2025).

15. Critchley, H., Maybin, J. A., Armstrong, G. M., & Williams, A. (2020). Physiology of the endometrium and regulation of menstruation. *Physiological Reviews, 100*, 1149–1179. https://doi.org/10.1152/physrev.00031.2019 (accessed on 15th June 2025).

16. da Silva, A. P. F., Cavalcanti, C. L. B., dos Santos, E. R. R., de Albuquerque Mello, L., de Melo-Junior, M. R., & Paz, S. T. (2016). Histopathological and digital morphometrical evaluation of uterine leiomyoma in Brazilian women. https://core.ac.uk/download/207207515.pdf (accessed on 15th June 2025).

17. Egeonu, R. O., Eleje, G. U., Enechukwu, C. I., Ezeama, C., et al. (2024). Association between serum vitamin D status and uterine leiomyomas: A case-control study. https://core.ac.uk/download/619411146.pdf (accessed on 15th June 2025).

18. Engman, M. (2011). Mifepristone for preoperative treatment of uterine leiomyoma. https://core.ac.uk/download/70339764.pdf (accessed on 15th June 2025).

19. Gregorich, S. E., Jackson, R., Jacoby, A., et al. (2014). Use of medical, surgical and complementary treatments among women with fibroids. https://core.ac.uk/download/46964821.pdf (accessed on 15th June 2025).

20. Guleria, S., Pathania, K., & Thakur, S. (2021). Huge fibroid uterus mimicking an ovarian malignancy. https://core.ac.uk/download/544390322.pdf (accessed on 15th June 2025).

21. Jaiyeola, O. O. (2023). Modeling the incidence of uterine fibroids among women in the US. https://core.ac.uk/download/573334490.pdf (accessed on 15th June 2025).

22. Koomson, J. N. (2017). The role of estrogen receptors alpha and beta in the development of uterine leiomyomas. https://open.bu.edu/bitstream/2144/23835/5/Koomson_bu_0017N_12892.pdf (accessed on 15th June 2025).

23. Mahmadiyeva, D. N., & Mahmadiyorova, Z. S. (2023). Uterine fibroids. https://core.ac.uk/download/587416894.pdf (accessed on 15th June 2025).

24. Raffone, A., Saccone, G., Venturella, R., Zullo, F., et al. (2020). In-bag manual versus uncontained power morcellation for laparoscopic myomectomy. https://core.ac.uk/download/541658918.pdf (accessed on 15th June 2025).

25. Sukhin, V., Tamm, T., Yakovenko, E., et al. (2018). The importance of the study of the hemodynamics of the uterine tumors by the method of Dopplerometry in the two- and three-dimensional echography modes for differential diagnostics of simple, proliferating leiomyomas and uterine sarcomas. https://core.ac.uk/download/322516352.pdf (accessed on 15th June 2025).

26. Wimber, C. (2025). Preservation of fertility after uterine artery embolization: A review of pregnancy following non-surgical intervention for leiomyoma. https://core.ac.uk/download/pdf/48843764.pdf (accessed on 15th June 2025).

27. Zaher, S. S. (2010). Magnetic resonance guided focused ultrasound surgery–A novel treatment for uterine fibroids. https://core.ac.uk/download/pdf/48843764.pdf (accessed on 15th June 2025).

SEXUALLY TRANSMITTED INFECTIONS (STIS) AND HIV IN FEMALES

8

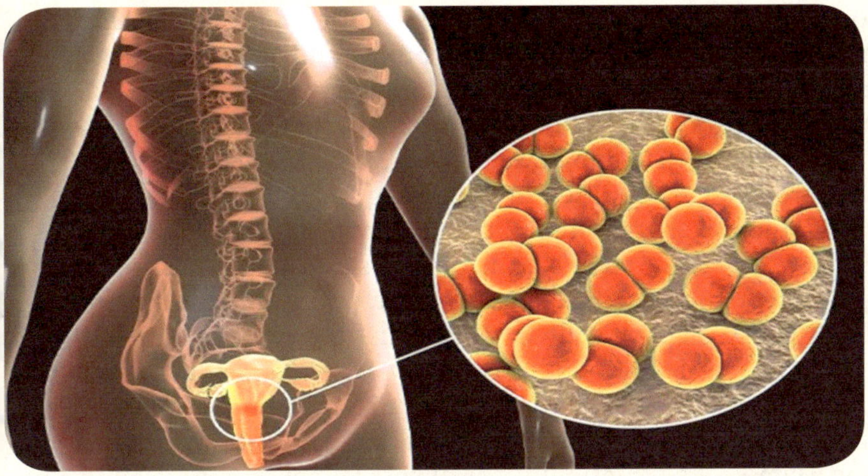

LEARNING OBJECTIVES

After studying this chapter, you will be able to:

1. Describe the prevalence of STIs and HIV among females
2. Identify the risk factors contributing to STIs and HIV infection in females
3. Recognize the common symptoms and diagnostic methods for STIs and HIV
4. Analyze the impact of STIs and HIV on female health
5. Evaluate effective prevention strategies for STIs and HIV in females
6. Discuss treatment and management approaches for STIs and HIV

Introduction

The increasing incidence of sexually transmitted illnesses (STIs) among women highlights a significant matter of public health that requires an extensive inquiry. STIs have been found to take a heavy toll on women's reproductive health and are even likely to lead to severe illnesses such as infertility, chronic pain, and increased susceptibility to HIV. Social stigma of STIs also adds to treatment delays, further compounding health effects among infected individuals. From a recent scoping review for developing diagnostic technologies, there has been a growing need for the improvement of point-of-care testing. This would enable timely diagnosis and improved treatment outcomes for women who have STIs, ultimately reducing the resulting health burdens within communities (Osipenko et al.). With the intersectionality of sexual health, gender, and ability to access health care, a knowledge of the STI and HIV sensitivities among women is essential to facilitate appropriate health responses. The need for patient involvement in STI testing in this context cannot be overstated. One qualitative study indicated that the perceived interaction with medical staff directly influences women's decisions regarding where to have STI testing. Patients preferred genitourinary medicine services over general practice because there was higher specialization and a greater range of tests available. This is a huge failure within the healthcare system in that general practitioners cannot provide adequate STI screening and treatment modalities. Other determinants such as previous experiences, relationships with the health care providers, and the reception of the test results further complicate decisions around STI testing (Cairns et al., 2012). Evidently, STI testing cannot be addressed in a one-size-fits-all fashion; thus, certain measures must be taken to address the differing needs of women across various health care settings. Additionally, the inclusion of effective public health education and campaign programs is of paramount significance in reducing the transmission rates of HIV and STIs among women. These need to focus on increasing awareness and knowledge about STIs, the removal of the stigma attached to diagnosis, and the promotion of regular screening as a vital aspect of sexual health. Innovative solutions using digital platforms and community outreach can help women put their sexual health at the forefront of their agenda without fear or embarrassment. By putting information out there and addressing the specific concerns of women, health authorities can significantly enhance the preventive and curative measures. Finally, STIs and HIV are best addressed through a multi-component method that engages collaboration between medical care providers, policymakers, and community resources aimed at generating an environment that is supportive of women's health and well-being.

Definition of STIs and HIV

Sexually transmitted diseases (STDs) refer to the diseases that are largely spread by sexual intercourse, i.e., vaginal, anal, and oral intercourse. Both men and women can be infected by these diseases, but they typically have certain repercussions on women's health. Women are more susceptible to the ill effects of STIs because of anatomical and physiological factors like the female genital structure, through which the infective agent spreads easily. Also, the clinical presentation of STIs among women is usually insidious, and this would thus entail delayed diagnosis as well as treatment. Unmanaged STIs would thus complicate and lead to complicated reproductive health issues such as pelvic inflammatory disease, infertility, and chronic pain. It is necessary to gain adequate knowledge about STIs for prevention and control, particularly among at-risk populations like women who might face difficulties in accessing health care services. Human Immunodeficiency Virus (HIV) is among the most significant STIs because it has a life-changing effect. HIV attacks the immune system, specifically the CD4 cells, and compromises the body's ability to fight disease and infection. Women's risk for HIV acquisition is influenced by a range of factors, including biological susceptibility, social determinants, and systemic inequities in health care. Women constitute a considerable group among individuals with HIV infection, particularly in high-prevalence countries, where they are also subjected to stigma and discrimination that undermine their health care. Other STIs co-infection could also help spread HIV, forming a vicious circle that enhances the vulnerability of the parties involved. Suitable education and prevention measures, such as pre-exposure prophylaxis (PrEP) and regular testing, are fundamental in reducing the prevalence of HIV among females. With the prevalence of STIs and HIV worldwide, particularly among females, awareness and education are fundamental. Global Burden of Diseases, Injuries, and Risk Factors Study 2017 brings forth significant information regarding the prevalence and incidence of STIs with high gender disparity in morbidity and health impacts of the disease (James et al., 2018). Knowledge of transmission modes, risk factors, and the cost of

STIs and HIV at a societal level can also inform public health policy and interventions tailored to the needs of women. Health education of health activity should also aim to eliminate stigma towards STIs and HIV, promote open dialogue about sexual health, and promote preventive options. By addressing all these areas, healthcare professionals can promote women's well-being and reduce the spread of STIs and HIV among women, therefore improving their quality of life and health.

Importance of Studying STIs and HIV in Females

The role of education in sexually transmitted infections (STIs) and HIV among women is central to public health programs that have the ability to reduce rates of infections as well as improve health outcomes. Women are more adversely affected by STIs and HIV due to a number of issues related to biology, society, and the economy. For instance, differences in anatomy can exaggerate vulnerabilities to STIs, particularly with intercourse. Additionally, cultural norms and expectations will regularly limit women's autonomy, controlling women's control over negotiating safe sex. The effects of these problems extend into education and access to healthcare, where women's access to early STI and HIV treatment and testing is potentially halted. With an enhanced comprehension of these dynamics, we can undertake specially tailored education interventions and prevention efforts that are both clinically efficacious and culturally palatable. The disease infection epidemiology also highlights the need for focused research among women for HIV and STIs. Adolescent girls are a most vulnerable subgroup, and existing data have uncovered these stark trends in infection even among sexually inactive women. For example, studies indicate that among certain populations, a greater percentage of HIV infection among adolescent girls was found in those who said that they were virgins, suggesting misreport or other transmission processes (Deuchert et al.). The divergence requires careful scrutiny of population and behavioral dynamics influencing the sexual health of adolescent girls. Identification of such determinants informs STI and HIV studies to educate outreach and prevention activities that address underlying causes, including peer pressure and parent communication, which are also core in adolescent sexual behavior formation (Mmbaga et al., 2012). Finally, STI and HIV studies in women inform comprehensive sexual health education strategies that influence overall society's health. The blending of demographic information and psychological issues enables more effective public health communication to teen girls and their households. Under the circumstances where teen girls are being increasingly exposed to premature initiation of sexual experience as it relates to peer pressure and cultural beliefs, education programs need to cover more than the biology; they need to address the youth sexuality complex social environment (Mmbaga et al., 2012). By focusing on women's STI and HIV research, we are not only ensuring better health for individuals but also contributing to the development of a knowledgeable society that is capable of overcoming the stigma and myths surrounding these infections as a group. That is fundamental to preventing the transmission of STIs and HIV among women and, hence, healthier populations in the long run.

8.1. Prevalence of STIs and HIV among Females

Learning Outcome

1. Define statistical data on STIs and HIV rates in females
2. Describe the demographic factors influencing prevalence
3. Explain the geographic variations in infection rates

The incidence of sexually transmitted infections (STDs) and HIV among women is a complex issue, one that is best illustrated in the instance of certain groups, like young African-American women. It has beenproven that youth are more informed concerning STDs and the implications thereof, which should normally lead to risk-decreasing sexual habits. Nevertheless, this knowledge does not necessarily translate to safe sexuality. A study among first-year college students who were African-American discovered that even though the participants were highly knowledgeable about STIs, there were participants who practiced riskier sex, which leads to high-risk behavior for infection. This is a reminder of the necessity for intervention to be at an individual level that not only addresses the behavior but also the perceptions and beliefs that are behind sexual health decisions (Annang et al., 2012). Therefore, it is important that the socio-cultural context of such conduct be made a reality in order to significantly reduce the prevalence of STIs among this population. Risk epidemiology of STIs and HIV is also complicated further by a combination of the accessibility of health, socio-economic status, and level of education. The evidence suggests that women living in STI-endemic settings are likely to be faced with decreased accessibility to prevention interventions and education. This reduction in resources will likely leave a gap in the knowledge of women regarding transmission and prevention practices. For instance, it was established in research done on Dar Es Salaam that it exhibited high percentages of young women who are HIV infected, either practiced unprotected sex or had multiple partners, mainly due to the lack of proper information regarding the transmission of STIs (Leyna et al., 2013). These revelations bring to the fore the necessity for such comprehensive sexual education programs that cater to such knowledge lacuna, aimed at educating women with such information in order to empower them to protect themselves. Secondly, the function of health systems in bringing solutions to these cannot be overemphasized. These ignorant women who do not know their partners' HIV status or are ill-educated about STIs stand to get infected easily. The prevalence of unprotected intercourse among young women who are HIV positive is a textbook case of this public health problem, in which structural circumstances actually place them at increased risk. Specifically, studies have ascertained that being on antiretroviral drug treatment is not necessarily an indicator of safe sex, particularly for individuals who lack the information or support (Leyna et al., 2013). Strengthening health systems and promoting education programs in the community are the key steps towards reducing HIV and STIs among women. Developing a system by which women are able to access preventive and therapeutic services, public health programs are capable of combating infection in the group effectively.

8.1.1. Statistical Data on STIs and HIV Rates in Females

Sexually transmitted diseases (STDs) and the prevalence of human immunodeficiency virus (HIV) in women constitute a major public health problem, highlighted by a number of studies tracking these rates in recent years. An understanding of the demographic and medical profile of women with STIs can direct interventions to be more specific. For example, a retrospective survey in India at the Surakhra Clinic found 1.74% of female attendees HIV positive, showing a major health risk to be addressed straight away, and with needed resources to counteract. Secondly, as rates of prevalence for other STIs such as gonorrhea and chlamydia are 3.36% and 11.78%, respectively, these underscore that mass sexual health education and routine screening must be put in place so that detection rates as well as the effectiveness of treatment among these healthcare-access-barred groups must be enhanced (Abu-Hammad et al., 2024).

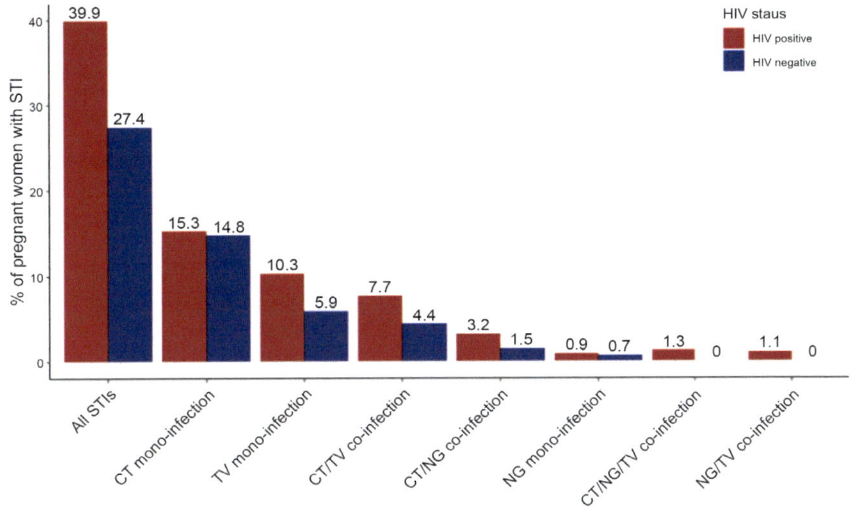

Figure 8.1. STI prevalence by HIV status in pregnant women screened at first antenatal visit in South Africa, 2016-2019.

Source: https://www.researchgate.net/figure/STI-prevalence-by-HIV-status-in-pregnant-women-screened-at-first-antenatal-visit-in-South_fig2_344452631

Statistical data also indicate that the prevalence of HIV and STIs among women varies based on various factors such as age, socioeconomic status, and geographical location. Notably, a meta-analysis of male patients with monkeypox found 40% of them to be co-infected with HIV or other STIs, reflecting cross-cutting exposures that can extend to the women in the same settings whose sexual networks overlap. Understanding these patterns can guide public health policy to make sure that women are not overlooked in health initiatives toward STIs and HIV. Public health administrators must focus on integrating gender-sensitive approaches to the provision of care, considering the social determinants that often place women at an increased risk of such infection. The co-epidemic of high STI prevalence among women also demands more efficient prevention interventions among women, crossing the barriers of health access and facilitating sexual health education (Abu-Hammad et al., 2024). Further, the interconnectedness of STIs and HIV with education, employment, and healthcare factors has a decisive influence on infection among women. The results of the Suraksha Clinic study illustrate the need for more extensive intervention in the community to complement not only medical treatment, but sexual health education among women on a larger scale. Given that over 34% of the female interviewees were referred for HIV testing, this indicates that there exists a large disparity in the knowledge of their sexual health status and the need for active testing and counseling intervention. More interprofessional collaboration among healthcare workers, educators, and health officials can translate to improved health outcomes in women with a higher risk of STIs and HIV. By having effective outreach techniques and a culture that makes discussing sexual health easy, public health programs can better prevent and combat the disease burden of STIs in women (Muralidhar et al., 2024).

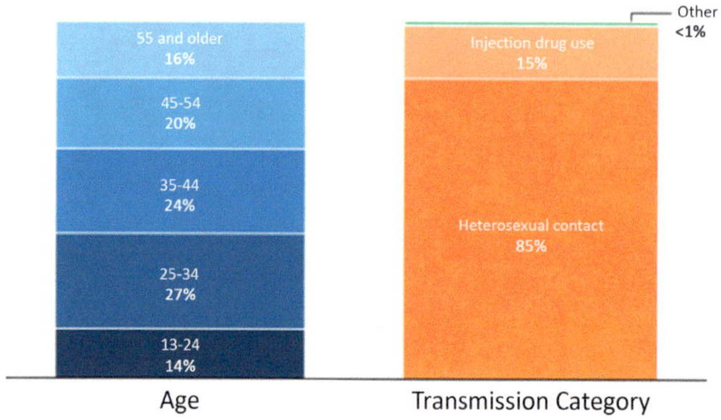

Figure 8.2. HIV Diagnosis among woman and girls, by age and transmission category 2018.

Source: https://artpictures.club/autumn-2023.html

8.1.2. Demographic Factors Influencing Prevalence

Demographic factors are a key factor in understanding the incidence of sexually transmitted diseases (STIs) and HIV among women, both in susceptibility and access to treatment. Geographic location remains a factor, as differing characteristics between nations such as Tanzania and Norway show the large differences in rates of STIs. For example, 33% of Tanzanian patients were found to be HIV antibody positive in a survey, with the prevalence being much higher among females (43%) than among males (26%) (Chalamila et al., 2006). These kinds of findings not only determine the strength of geographical differences in using health care but also show how varying cultural environments lead to varying health outcomes. The existence of cultural stances in relation to sexuality, gender roles, and health-seeking behavior also leads to these discrepancies and needs specially trained public health interventions for various population groups.

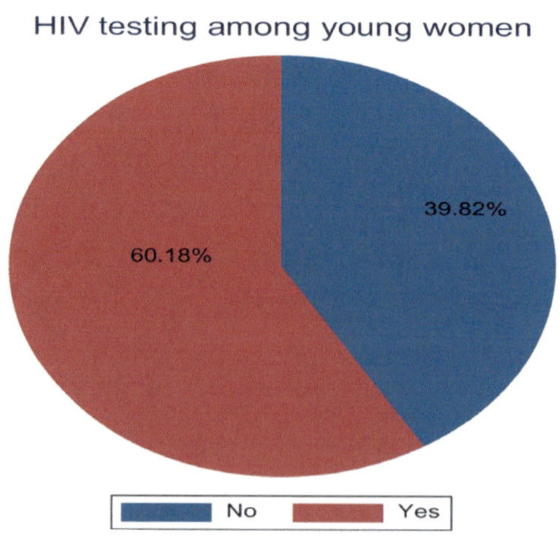

Figure 8.3. Prevalence of HIV testing among young women in Tanzania.

Source: https://www.frontiersin.org/files/Articles/1518314/fpubh-12-1518314-HTML/image_m/fpubh-12-1518314-g002.jpg

The age of the individual also plays an important role in the transmission of STIs and HIV, particularly among young females. As stated by the World Health Organization, a significant number of new cases of HIV infection are seen in individuals aged 15-24 years (Girum et al., 2017). This category of individuals tends to carry out risky sexual behaviors due to a lack of proper sexual health education, peer influence, and a lack of parental guidance. Among secondary school students in Gondar City, high rates of unsafe sex were reported in a study, where 12.8% of the students had ever had unprotected sexual intercourse. Contributing factors to this were alcohol consumption, parental neglect, and lack of sex discussions. These rates suggest that such age groups and socioeconomic aspects must be prioritized in attempts to reduce the rates of STIs and HIV among young women. Socioeconomic status (SES) is also seen to be a significant predictor of STI and HIV infection among women. Poor women are likely to be faced with all types of obstacles to medical care access, including scarce economic resources, lack of insurance, and restricted access to preventive and educational services. These socioeconomic factors tend to leave vulnerable populations in the absence of the means to use safe sex or to receive medical treatment in a timely fashion. In most cases, this population context results in conditions under which STIs will increase due to high rates of unsafe sex and poor information on prevention. As such, understanding how SES and health outcomes interact dictates the proper design of public health efforts in response to specific needs of different demographic populations and, ultimately, enables an integrated response to combating STIs and HIV among women.

8.1.3. Geographic Variations in Infection Rates

Geographic variations in sexual infection (STI) and HIV illness among women reflect significant inequalities, with the underlying social, economic, and cultural determinants. In the UK, over the last decade, paradigm shifts in STI epidemiology have occurred particularly in some groups such as young adults and minority ethnic individuals whose patterns are determined by socioeconomic status and access to health services. Those service delivery and public health gains in STI have not been achieved evenly by all, leading to entrenched sexual health disparities. The emergence of localized endemicity speaks to targeted approaches, which consider the unique population at increased risk within these communities, paralleling the interaction between geography and infection prevalence (Field et al., 2015). Thus, an awareness of such geographic variation is essential to the development of effective public health interventions for addressing the burden of STIs and HIV in women. The epidemiological context of gonorrhoea in England provides a very acute illustration of spatial-temporal variation in infection prevalence. Four endemic regions, which virtually all consisted of urban regions such as London, where over 86% of diagnoses were conducted, were detected in a study making use of Kulldorff's scan statistics. In this instance, men who have sex with men (MSM) had a disproportionately higher likelihood of diagnosis than heterosexual men, pointing to the necessity of disaggregation of data by sexual orientation and gender in order to inform public health interventions. Within these endemic areas, the rate of infections due to heterosexual transmission must also be taken into account, as it demonstrates that women face varying risk profiles based on geographic location. These determinations drive health authorities to strategically allocate resources and scale up interventions specifically designed for those communities with greater infection rates (O'Brien et al., 2018). Moreover, the role of partner notification (PN) as an instrument for gonorrhoea diffusion control is yet another degree of complexity that follows geographic disparities in infection rates. PN intervention effectiveness was extremely heterogeneous in terms of demographic factors, such as a significant difference between urban and less urban settings. In research, 14.5% of gonorrhoea diagnoses were due to PN, revealing both the value of such programs and the need for ongoing efforts at outreach and education to individuals about healthy sexual behavior. Geographically, high-prevalence areas differ in how successful they are in prompting individuals diagnosed by PN to seek out treatment. The heterogeneity lies behind the necessity for region-level public health campaigns, and hence, maximizing the intervention programs to lower STIs and enhance female sexual health outcomes (O'Brien et al., 2018).

Test Your Knowledge

1. What are the current trends in statistical data regarding STI and HIV rates among females?
2. Which demographic factors are known to influence the prevalence of STIs and HIV in females?

8.2. Risk Factors for STIs and HIV in Females

Learning Outcome

1. Discuss the biological susceptibility of females
2 .Explain the behavioral risk factors
3. Identify the socioeconomic factors affecting vulnerability

The prevalence of sexually transmitted diseases (STIs) among women shows a high correlation with some risk factors that increase the susceptibility to HIV. The most suitable factor is sexual partner multiplicity because it is clear that women who have more than one partner are at high risk of STIs and therefore increase the risk of getting HIV. This was further corroborated by research findings from studies carried out in Siaya County, whose results indicated that the rate of STIs among their HIV-positive population was much higher than that of their HIV-negative counterparts, demonstrating the correlation between these illnesses (Awuoche et al., 2024). Furthermore, sexual relationship dynamics and partner choice are most important, as social norms and expectations may encourage women to practice more unsafe sex, leading to an increase in the problem. Another crucial riskdetermining factor for STIs and HIV among women is drug use, that is, psychoactive drugs that affect judgment and decrease sexual health decision-making. Where the prevalence of HIV is high, the risk-taking behaviors that go hand-in-hand with substance abuse can lead to unprotected sex and thereby increase STI rates. This issue was identified in a study demonstrating a strong link between substance abuse and STI prevalence among men and indicating a similar pattern among women, although less studied (Awuoche et al., 2024).

The applicability is critical when it comes to public health interventions since the treatment of substance use in the context of sexual health will possibly have a profound effect on the reduction of the incidence of STIs and HIV infection transmission among women. Prevalence and STI trends among women highlight the importance of targeted health interventions addressing education and prevention strategies. In Chhattisgarh, for example, the gender disparities in STI prevalence warrant an immediate imperative to gender-specific health interventions towards women's health and empowerment. Early diagnosis and treatment of STIs are significant, not only because untreated infection not only threatens HIV acquisition but also sustains the chain of infection in communities. Comprehensive sex health education, enhanced access to care services, and effective screening programs are crucial in avoiding such risks. Public health authorities, through creating settings that permit open sexual health discourse and engaged participation of women in preventive healthcare, can effectively counter the emerging concern of STIs and HIV among women and lead to better outcomes.

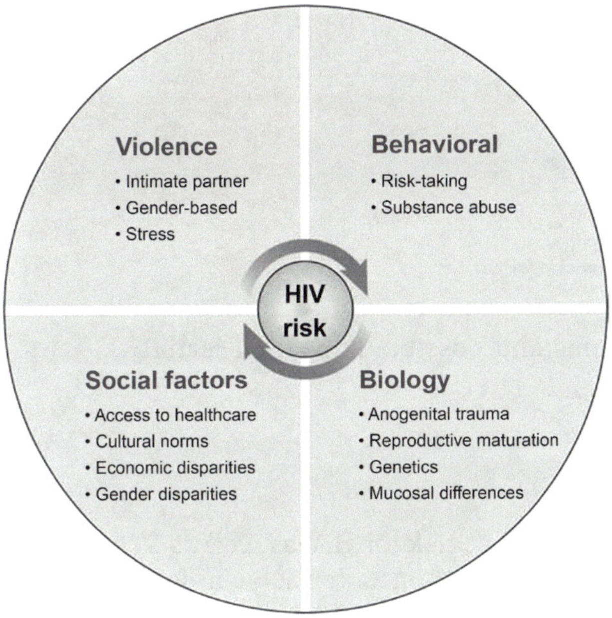

Figure 8.4. The complex spectrum of risk factors affecting HIV susceptibility.

Source: https://www.researchgate.net/figure/The-complex-spectrum-of-risk-factors-affecting-HIV-susceptibility_fig1_309567522

8.2.1. Biological Susceptibility of Females

The vulnerability of women to sexual diseases (STIs) and HIV is a body of research that needs to bring forward the physiological disparity between men and women. The female genital tract's anatomy includes a higher risk of infection due to the increased mucosal area exposed during coitus. This increased exposure would enhance the spread of pathogens, and therefore, young women are at a greater risk for STIs as well as HIV. Furthermore, hormonal alterations demonstrated during menstruation also influence susceptibility as these alterations may modulate mucosal immunity and disrupt vaginal microbiota, creating the niche for infection (Bray et al., 2024). Identification of these biological factors is significant in devising effective prevention strategies targeted specifically for women and removing their risk of acquiring STIs and HIV. Apart from anatomical reasons, immunological disparity between males and females also works to make women more susceptible to STIs, including HIV. Research points out that women produce a stronger inflammatory response to infection, which, at times, rather than resisting it, worsens the condition. The occurrence of certain cytokines may produce an inflammatory environment that can increase infection persistence and severity. Additionally, women with a history of STIs may experience worse outcomes following HIV exposure compared to men with STIs since the inflammation might increase the permeability of mucosal barriers and facilitate virus penetration (Christopher J L Murray et al., 2022).

This immunological response highlights the identification of female biology within disease prevention and epidemiology. Pregnancy also presents other biological challenges that enhance a woman's exposure to STIs and HIV. Pregnancy is characterized by widespread modulation of a woman's immune system for fetal development, which can result in impaired immunity against infection (Bray et al., 2024). This altered immune status renders pregnant women more susceptible to STI infection, with serious complications for both the mother and fetus, including vertical transmission of disease.

Medical interventions need to consider the unique biological vulnerabilities of women at various stages of life, particularly pregnancy. Through the targeting of these most important biological determinants through education and health care access, STI and HIV prevalence among women can be better managed and ultimately lead to improved health for women and their families.

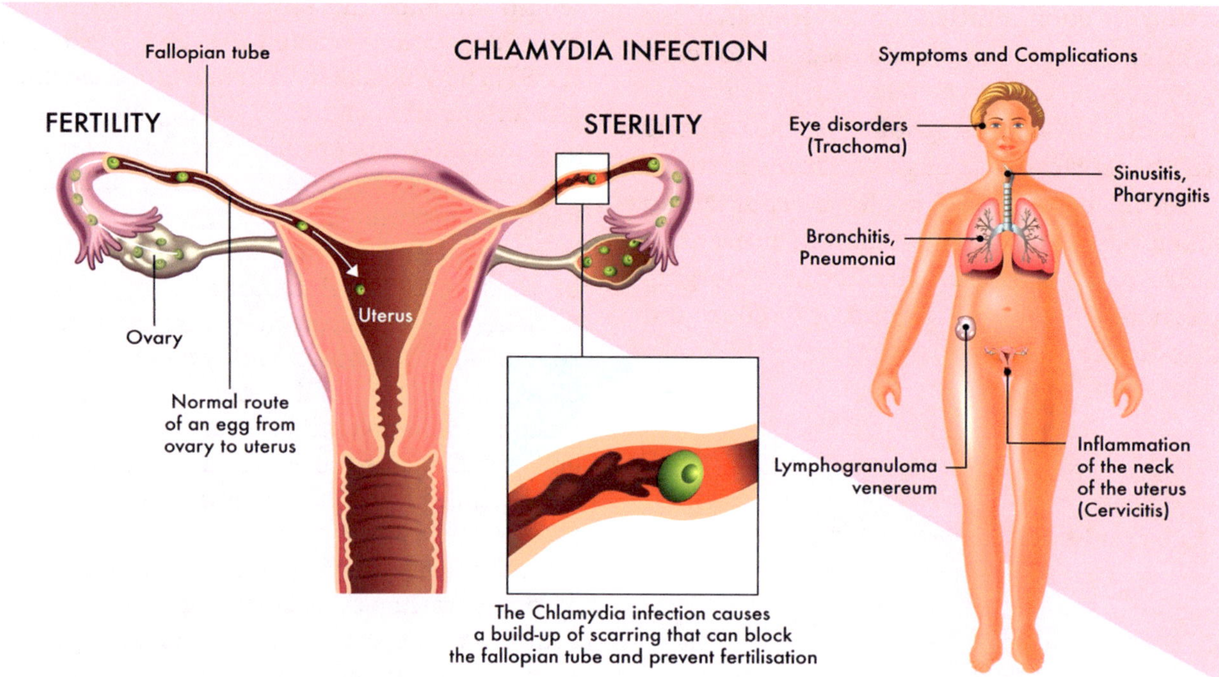

Figure 8.5. *Chlamydia trachomatis* infection. Symptoms and possible impact on fertility.

Source: https://www.mdpi.com/1422-0067/22/4/2170

8.2.2. Behavioral Risk Factors

Behavioral risk factors are the main reason for women to be at risk for HIV as well as STIs. Having unprotected sex with numerous partners raises the risk several times. It has been found through studies that women who have had multiple sexual partners are the most likely to have STIs, primarily due to the intricacies of biological as well as anatomical factors. This is duplicated in one Siaya County study that concluded that independent predictors of STI prevalence were having more than one sexual partner in both men and women, which emphasizes that such behaviors hold the secrets to understanding the dynamics of STIs (Awuoche et al., 2024). Successful sex education targeted at the young women's behavioral choices could be a chief factor in curbing these risks and promoting healthier sex habits. Substance use is also a primary behavioral risk factor for STIs and HIV infection among women. Mixing mind-altering drugs with unsafe sexual behavior can lead to reduced judgment and reduced capacity to negotiate safe sex, thereby making one vulnerable to infections. Research creates a linkage between drug use and rising STI levels, particularly among males in the populations being analyzed; however, its relevance for females is no less pressing as drug addiction diminishes their capacity to make decisions on sexual issues (Awuoche et al., 2024).

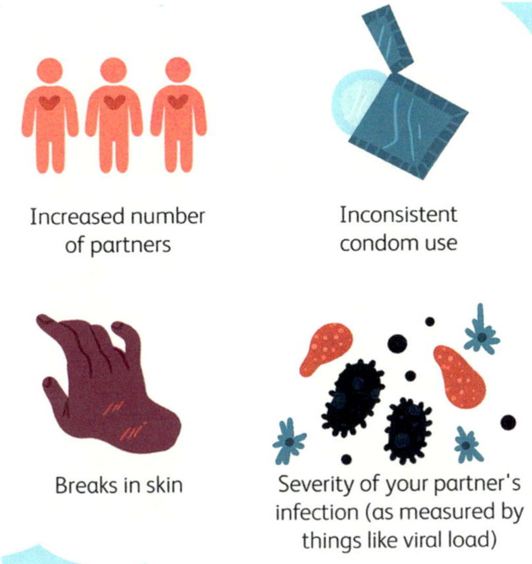

Figure 8.6. Risk factors of STIs.

Source: https://www.verywellhealth.com/thmb/rFnxWDy5OzWTr0B5PoaG5QfkHIQ=/1500x0/filters:no_upscale():max_bytes(150000):strip_icc()/std-causes-3133097-Final-c1cc7e2214db4a22bb86718681dba7cd.png

Thus, medical interventions to inform women about the risks related to substance use and provide them with related resources can balance their impact on sexual health outcomes. Last but not least, socio-cultural forces render women's situation of behavioral risk factors even more complex. Stigma and discrimination against STIs and HIV discourage females from receiving preventative care and testing. A retrospective study highlighted that a number of sociodemographic factors, including education level and sexual orientation, had a strong correlation with the incidence of STIs, reflecting that the social context affects sexual behavior and health-seeking practices. It is crucial that these barriers in society are bridged through targeted community outreach and culturally appropriate education. This serves to empower women to embrace healthy, positive behaviors and consequently decrease the incidence of STIs and HIV among women. Identifying and changing these behavioral risk factors are essential to the continued improvement of public health programs aimed at minimizing the spread of infections.

8.2.3. Socioeconomic Factors Affecting Vulnerability

The interplay of socioeconomic factors and vulnerability to sexually transmitted infections (STIs) and HIV disease in women is a critical topic of research. Economic instability is likely to increase the risk of STIs by limiting access to healthcare, education, and prevention measures. Poor women may lack the means of obtaining proper medical care or engaging in preventive services like regular screening and education for safe sex. Besides, limited access to healthcare services leads to delayed diagnoses and treatment, which increases the likelihood of transmission of STIs and HIV. Thus, economic disadvantage not only determines individual health consequences but also results in broader public health issues through the continuous transmission of infectious diseases. Further, education is an extremely significant factor that determines women's exposure to STIs and HIV. Less educated people lack comprehensive information about sexual health, safe sex, and prevention. Inadequate knowledge is what leads to higher levels of risky sexual behavior, therefore, higher vulnerability to STIs and HIV. Evidence indicates that there exists a correlation between educational interventions and reduced sexual risk behavior, implying that targeted education programs can effectively respond to this vulnerability. For example, interventions aimed at the provision and referral of medical care, particularly those utilizing local community resources, demonstrate higher efficacy in reducing risky behaviors among women, particularly those within disadvantaged socioeconomic strata (Aupont et al., 2012). Providing accessible education and resources is therefore imperative in addressing the intersection of sexual health and education. Moreover, social determinants like discrimination and stigma on the basis of socioeconomic status further enhance the vulnerability of women towards STIs and HIV. Stigma is what discourages the affected from seeking medical care or preventive services, promoting an atmosphere of fear and isolation. In other contexts, for example, Vietnam, where there have been post-industrial social transformations, the processes of HIV and AIDS stigma can encourage discrimination against women in economically poor groups (Nielsen et al., 2009). It generates barriers to healthcare and support systems access, sustaining a pattern of vulnerability. Defeating these social determinants is vital; interventions that reduce stigma, promote inclusiveness, and provide comprehensive health services can imbue women with the power of empowerment to take proactive steps in safeguarding their sexual well-being and health.

Test Your Knowledge

1. What biological factors make females more susceptible to STIs and HIV?
2. How do socioeconomic factors contribute to the vulnerability of females to STIs and HIV?

8.3. Symptoms and Diagnosis of STIs and HIV

Learning Outcome

1. Identify the common symptoms of STIs in females
2. Explain the importance of early diagnosis
3. Define diagnostic methods and testing options

The symptoms of sexually transmitted diseases (STIs) can be extremely variable in patients, with some infections causing little or no apparent symptoms at all. This asymptomatic presentation is particularly concerning in women since, if left untreated, STIs can have severe health consequences like pelvic inflammatory disease, infertility, and vulnerability to HIV. Typical symptoms of STIs like chlamydia and gonorrhea can be vaginal discharge, dysuria, and pelvic pain. But most women might be unaware of their infection status, adding to the problems of delayed diagnosis and treatment. It is necessary that healthcare providers promote frequent screening of STIs, especially in sexually active women under the age of 25 and those who have more than one sexual partner, in order to identify them early and to minimize their long-term health implications. STI diagnosis in females is commonly done by combining clinical evaluation, patient history, and laboratory tests. Healthcare providers can utilize urine, swabs, and blood tests to confirm the identification of specific pathogens. For instance, the availability of molecular tests for Trichomonas vaginalis has revolutionized the diagnosis of this infection to a large extent, elevating the stature of this infection from that of a minor irritant to a significant public health concern. These advances also highlight the importance of diagnosing not only female infections but also emphasizing the importance of co-infections' implications. Most importantly, there is a linkage between T. vaginalis infection and the acquisition of HIV, prompting increased awareness and screening in at-risk populations and high-risk groups, particularly young women and minority groups. The overlap of HIV and STIs warrants a comprehensive sexual health strategy. Public health measures are crucial in increasing awareness and access to HIV and STI testing and treatment. Information from surveillance, as reported by the Health Protection Agency, aids in disseminating data on the occurrence and incidence of these infections and guiding focused interventions and resource allocation. These statistics not only reflect trends in infection rates but also reveal gaps in diagnosis and screening that take place along different groups, particularly in the primary care sectors. These public health indicators help professionals and policymakers organize sexual health services suitably to cater to their population. By filling knowledge gaps and overcoming barriers to care, public health education campaigns have the potential to promote greater awareness and early detection and intervention of STIs and HIV among women, ultimately translating into improved health outcomes and reduced transmission rates across the population as a whole (Cassell et al., 2008).

8.3.1. Common Symptoms of STIs in Females

The occurrence of sexually transmitted diseases (STIs) among women can cause a variety of general symptoms that are most often overlooked because they accumulate slowly. Early detection is vital to avoiding long-term effects on health. Chlamydia, one of the more prevalent infections, typically occurs symptomatically; however, symptoms, when they do emerge, may consist of abnormal discharge in the vagina, burning during urination, and pelvic discomfort. Similarly, gonorrhea may also lead to these symptoms, with females experiencing vaginal discharge and discomfort. The importance of detecting such early signs is brought out through the danger of such complications worsening to develop more severe medical conditions, such as pelvic inflammatory disease, if left untreated. Overall, awareness of such symptoms is paramount for on-time medical assistance as well as for avoiding the spread of STIs in the community at large, especially among women who tend to have more associated health problems with the infection (Rowley et al., 2019).

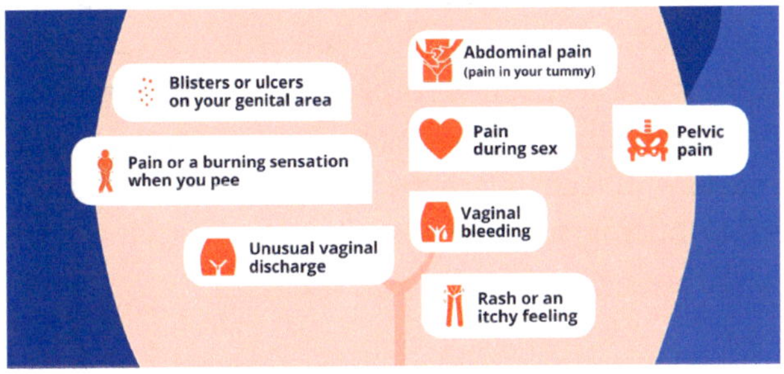

Figure 8.7. Common STI symptoms in women.

Source: https://sukhipariwarclinic.com.np/wp-content/uploads/2024/09/common-symptom-of-STIs-in-women.jpeg

In addition to gonorrhea and chlamydia, trichomoniasis is another significant STI to consider. The infection, caused by a parasite, can lead to frothy, yellow-green discharge from the vagina with a pungent smell. Females will also experience pain during sexual intercourse and vaginitis. Symptoms of trichomoniasis can have a dramatic impact on a woman's quality of life as well as sexual health, and transmission of other STIs, like HIV, is increased if infection with one of these is present. Symptom awareness is particularly important, as most women will confuse them with other vaginal infections' symptoms and hence end up misdiagnosing and getting delayed treatment, further complicating their health and wellbeing (James et al., 2018).

The other very important STI to contend with is syphilis, which occurs both in the primary and secondary stages. In the initial stage, women may present with a painless ulcer, also referred to as a chancre, on the site of infection. If left untreated, syphilis becomes more severe with secondary stages of illness in the form of flu, skin rash, and generalized lymphadenopathy. The unpredictability and even uncertainty of symptoms create difficulty in early diagnosis and treatment, with a high risk for serious illness when the infection is carried untreated. Aside from that, syphilis carries dangerous effects while pregnant, leading to congenital syphilis upon fetal transmission. Overall, awareness of these common symptoms of STIs plays a significant role in educating women about healthy precautionary practices, ultimately contributing to sexual and reproductive health outcomes (Rowley et al., 2019).

8.3.2. Importance of Early Diagnosis

The significance of early detection when sexually transmitted diseases (STIs) and HIV are involved in women cannot be overstated. Early detection not only facilitates early treatment but also plays a key role in the prevention of the transmission of infections to other individuals. For instance, women with STIs, such as gonorrhea and chlamydia, can experience severe reproductive health complications, such as pelvic inflammatory disease or infertility, when left untreated. This emphasizes the significance of early detection and prevention efforts, particularly in high-risk populations. Secondly, active diagnosis methods can significantly reduce long-term health effects and optimize overall public health outcomes. Studies noted that most female gonorrhea cases were diagnosed through partner notification (PN), which effectively managed STIs, and, therefore, early detection is crucial for individual and community health consciousness (O'Brien et al., 2018). Early infection control ultimately results in a better and better-educated society. Another crucial role played by early diagnosis is improving the quality of life of the infected individual. It has been observed that females who test HIV-positive at earlier stages of infection can start treatment on time. This was evident in a Tanzanian research wherein a large proportion of female patients were HIV-positive at an early age, demonstrating the importance of early screening and interventions immediately (Chalamila et al., 2006).

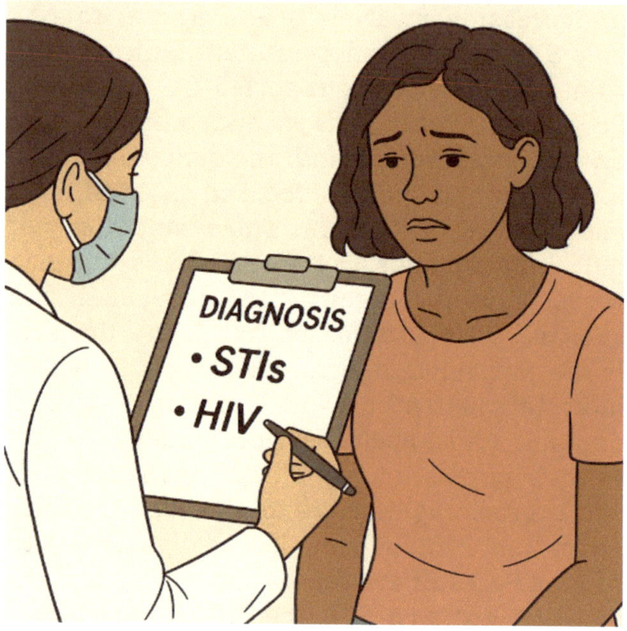

Source: https://sdmntprwestus2.oaiusercontent.com/files/00000000-aba8-61f8-a2a7-fa95d5f315fb/raw?se=2025-05-22T08%3A51%3A14Z&sp=r&sv=2024-08-04&sr=b&scid=65c013f8-f675-5b56-aefb-6e70db75f872&skoid=30ec2761-8f41-44db-b282-7a0f8809659b&sktid=a48cca56-e6da-484e-a814-9c849652bcb3&skt=2025-05-21T20%3A39%3A35Z&ske=2025-05-22T20%3A39%3A35Z&sks=b&skv=2024-08-04&sig=dDZkbcv/GW0upVDfpDAKhmNCwtT5/6ZaMX7yqeSjSNQ%3D

By identifying infections early, healthcare workers can give appropriate treatment regimens, and this decreases rates of morbidity and improves lives. Early detection also empowers women with the power to make independent choices regarding their health and sexual relationships, lessening stigma and facilitating open conversation about sexual health. Thus, making strong campaigns of awareness concerning the importance of frequent testing may urge more women to seek earlier testing, and this will improve reproductive health outcomes. In addition to personal health gain, early diagnosis of STIs and HIV also has a significant role in public health interventions at the community level. Targeted interventions can reduce STI incidence in populations and ease healthcare burdens. Identification of endemic areas and clusters, as in the example of gonorrhea cases in England, assists health agencies in the effective allocation of resources and triggering intervention measures in proportion to respective populations (O'Brien et al., 2018). Further, circumventing healthcare access barriers, particularly for targeted groups, remains essential in facilitating early diagnosis, The difference in STI and HIV prevalence between countries, as inferred from comparisons between Tanzanian and Norwegian populations, mirrors the unequal availability of care and the need for culture-sensitive approaches to education and prevention interventions (Chalamila et al., 2006). Generally, enhancement of early diagnosis mechanisms is not only better for the individuals but also stronger in making society's collective health robust, leading to a healthier public health system.

8.3.3. Diagnostic Methods and Testing Options

Accurate diagnostic testing and diagnostic methods are critical in the treatment of sexually transmitted diseases (STIs) and HIV infection among women. Since most STIs are not symptomatic, screening on a regular basis is important to identify the infections early and minimize complications. Diagnostic methods involve various methods, including serological tests, nucleic acid amplification tests (NAATs), and rapid tests. Serology tests, which detect antibodies or antigens, are particularly helpful in the diagnosis of infections like HIV and syphilis. However, NAATs are highly sensitive and can accurately detect bacterial STIs, such as chlamydia and gonorrhea, which have a disproportionate effect on women's sexual health. The application of point-of-care testing has also improved access and early diagnosis, enabling clinicians to initiate treatment in early stages and avert transmission within populations, and thus promote public health objectives related to STIs and HIV (Palfreeman et al., 2020).

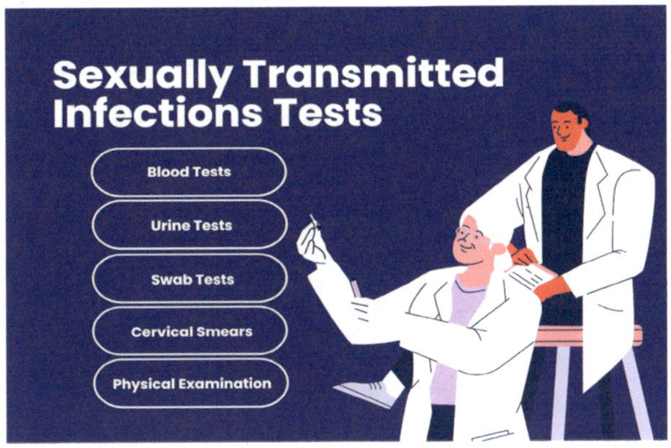

Figure 8.8. Sexually transmitted infections (STIs) Tests.

Source: https://web-assets.elara.care/2023/11/Sexually-Transmitted-Infections-Tests.png

The impact on health from undiagnosed or late-diagnosed STIs and HIV is significant, having a huge impact on women's reproductive health and overall quality of life. Delayed diagnosis greatly increases the risk of complications, including infertility, pelvic inflammatory disease, and susceptibility to HIV. For this reason, testing recommendations emphasize periodic screening, particularly in high-risk groups such as men having sex with men (MSM), sex workers, and those with multiple partners. For the best diagnosis, health workers must implement universal opt-out testing in high-prevalence areas, whereby educational intervention coupled with routine screening can significantly boost rates of testing. Additionally, breaking down barriers such as stigma and access to care is inevitable. Establishing a friendly environment that encourages open sexual health talk, the health systems can maximize early treatment and diagnosis for infected women with STIs and

HIV (Sully et al., 2020). Advancements in testing technology have revolutionized the landscape of STI and HIV testing, with greater facilitation for women. Community-based testing initiatives and self-testing kits are particularly promising, empowering people to be in charge of their health in a comfortable and confidential setting. Self-testing has been found to enable more regular testing in vulnerable populations, encouraging proactive health behavior. In addition, expanding testing services as part of routine healthcare, such as during antenatal care, trivializes the experience and informs women of their sexual health status. These interventions are in line with public health goals of reducing transmission and improving reproductive health. Education of patients and providers is also important to inform individuals of their comfort in going for testing and treatment. In the end, an overall approach that combines innovative testing options with effective health education can significantly enhance outcomes for women with STIs and HIV (Palfreeman et al., 2020).

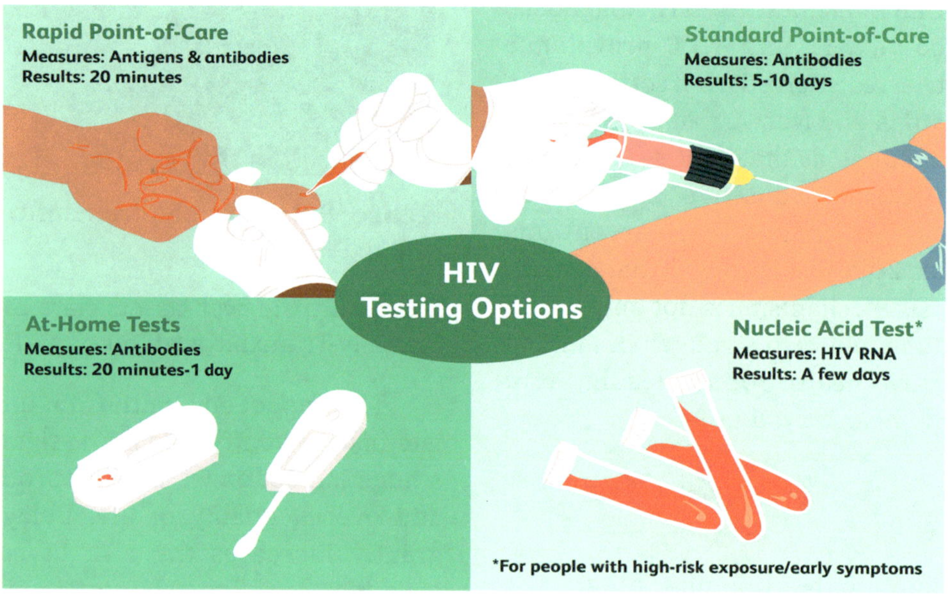

Figure 8.9. HIV testing options.

Source: https://www.verywellhealth.com/thmb/gzUKOyKzYC-YK8rhhoy28npBfWs=/1500x0/filters:no_upscale():max_bytes(150000):strip_icc()/3132731_color2-5ba53e0a46e0fb002594fec7.png

Test Your Knowledge

1. Why is early diagnosis important in the management of STIs in females?
2. What are some commonly used diagnostic methods and testing options for detecting STIs in females?

8.4. Impact of STIs and HIV on Female Health

Learning Outcome

1. Define short-term health consequences and long-term health implications
2. Discuss the mental health effects associated with STIs and HIV

The impact of sexually transmitted diseases (STIs) and HIV infection on women's health transcends direct clinical outcomes, encompassing more socio-economic and psychological factors. Women are over-represented among HIV infections, with approximately 20 million women estimated to be living with HIV in 2022, reflecting a large gender disparity in the prevalence of infection. This imbalance is further compounded by the fact that women are underrepresented in clinical trials of antiretroviral therapies (ART) in the past, limiting our knowledge of how best to optimize such treatment for women. The socio-cultural and biological determinants of women's health necessitate that treatment protocols are optimized individually for their needs. The absence of gender-specific research on HIV management negates the advancement in management strategies as well as possibly perpetuating health inequalities among women fighting this pandemic (Colpani et al., 2024). Moreover, psychosexual implications of STIs and HIV pose tremendous challenges to effective control of health in women. Stigma and discrimination experiences lead to shame or feelings of isolation, culminating in extreme negative impacts on mental health as well as social integration. Women living with STIs or HIV may develop depression, anxiety, and low self-esteem, coupled with the challenge of their interactions with the healthcare system. The psychological burdens are increased where women have to go through care for both their family's health outcomes, putting added pressure on their own well-being. There is a requirement to create supportive environments in order to provide unrestricted sexual health discussion and increase awareness of the effects of STIs and HIV. Assessment of these emotional determinants alongside medical intervention can potentially empower women to take control of their health, ultimately leading to better treatment adherence and quality of life (Skinnes et al., 2023). Aside from mental health determinants, the physical health consequences of STIs and HIV have the potential to drastically impact women's reproductive well-being. STIs such as pelvic inflammatory disease (PID) caused by untreated STIs lead to infertility, chronic pain, and pregnancy complications, worsening the women's health burden. HIV-infected women are also at increased risk for an adverse pregnancy outcome, including vertical transmission of the virus to the fetus and increased morbidity in mother and child.

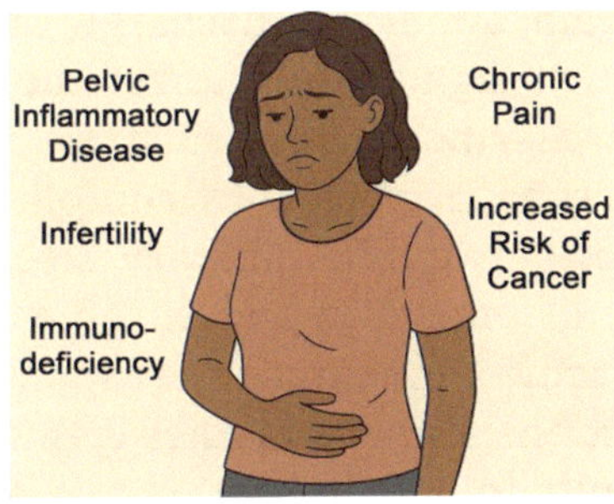

Figure 8.10. Impact of STIs and HIV on Female Health.

Source: https://sdmntprnorthcentralus.oaiusercontent.com/files/00000000-dd8c-622f-9868-14906f6126fe/raw?se=2025-05-23T05%3A26%3A06Z&sp=r&sv=2024-08-04&sr=b&scid=d3398a3d-3173-507b-be93-69cf473976a0&skoid=9ccea605-1409-4478-82eb-9c83b25dc1b0&sktid=a48cca56-e6da-484e-a814-9c849652bcb3&skt=2025-05-22T19%3A41%3A47Z&ske=2025-05-23T19%3A41%3A47Z&sks=b&skv=2024-08-04&sig=4/4SidGtdu0V6IE4WIYGPvC%2B/I9hJzo77LdceRJnCXI%3D

The intersection of STIs and HIV with reproductive health requires integrative models of healthcare to address these converging health imperatives. Public health efforts must address comprehensive sexuality education, access to services for all, and prevention programs targeting women. In doing this, we can significantly alleviate the impact of STIs and HIV on women's health outcomes (Colpani et al., 2024).

8.4.1. Short-Term Health Consequences

The acute physical findings of sexually transmitted infections (STDs) and human immunodeficiency virus (HIV) in women are multifaceted with significant implications for physical and psychological health. During the acquisition of an STI, women can present with a broad spectrum of acute manifestations such as pelvic pain, abnormal discharge, and genital ulcers, which significantly affect their quality of life. Furthermore, STIs such as chlamydia and gonorrhea may lead to complications in the form of pelvic inflammatory disease (PID) with risks of infertility and chronic pain. The resultant acute inflammatory response due to these infections also exacerbates co-morbidities, which results in hospitalization and additional healthcare costs. These immediate health effects necessitate immediate access to health care for effective control and treatment, reminding us of the need for comprehensive sexual health education and preventive measures. Another consideration is heightened susceptibility to secondary infection for women with STIs. The presence of an STI facilitates the transmission of HIV by weakening the mucosal barrier, which increases the susceptibility to infection during unprotected coitus. This risk, coupled with many women's limited access to healthcare services, aggravates the situation, as a significant percentage of them are still unaware of their STI status. It is through research that the acute phase of STIs goes unaddressed due to stigma, fear, and lack of adequate sexual health education, thereby perpetuating the vicious cycle of infection and complexity of public health interventions (Habel et al. ; Maierhofer et al., 2018). The impacts of undiagnosed STIs are far-reaching, characterized by high transmission rates in communities of not just STIs but also of HIV among vulnerable populations, an indication of the requirement for targeted health interventions. Besides, the psychological impact of HIV and STIs is equally debilitating for women. Anxiety and fear of diagnosis, infertility, and stigma regarding STIs are extremely psychologically unsettling. The majority of women feel guilty, ashamed, and depressed when they are diagnosed with an STI, which impacts their social life as well as overall mental well-being. This affective burden can discourage them from seeking further care or treatment, adopting a cycle of neglect in health-seeking behavior (Habel et al.; Maierhofer et al., 2018). Understanding such short-term effects on their health—physical as well as psychological—sets the tone for the need for integrated solutions addressing women's health as a whole. Early intervention, counseling, and education take priority in mitigating such effects and building a healthier and well-informed population of women who cope with the issues of STIs and HIV.

8.4.2. Long-Term Health Implications

The long-term health effects of sexually transmitted diseases (STDs) and HIV infection for women are multifaceted, influenced not only by individual well-being but also by society's health. In young women who have unsafe sex, the odds of acquiring STDs, including HIV infection, are significantly higher. Community health has been shown to influence these behaviors in studies, illustrating the role of neighborhood characteristics in health outcomes related to sexuality. In particular, rates of high-risk sexual behavior in youth vary substantially across regions, and research has shown that community-based interventions can significantly alter such trends (Ugwu et al., 2024). As these infections lead to infertility, pelvic inflammatory disease, or even life-threatening infection, their long-term consequence are dire. Thus, outreach and education among communities must be enhanced to avoid these undesirable health effects in young women, in turn promoting a healthy population. The effects of HIV and STIs go beyond the physical health of women since these diseases severely impact psychological and socioeconomic status. Female teenagers are most likely to experience an increased risk of mental illness due to stigma and social isolation related to HIV and STIs. Adolescent sexual and reproductive health programs that focus on addressing these issues are critical but frequently interrupted by unforeseen events, like the COVID-19 pandemic. The pandemic has further widened existing inequalities, with young women at greater risk of unwanted pregnancies and sexual exploitation from limited access to health services (Murewanhema, 2020).

STD	Symptom				Long term effects / complications
	Discharge	Painful skin lesions	Painless skin lesions	May have no clear symptoms	Without treatment, STD can lead to:
Chlamydia	X			X	Pelvic Inflammatory Disease (PID), which can lead to infertility, scarring, chronic pain
Gonorrhea	X			X	PID
Syphilis			X		Paralysis, personality changes, blindness, damage to joints, etc.
Trichomo-niasis	X			X	Mild to severe inflammation
HSV		X			Recurring symptoms possible
HPV			X	X	Some types of HPV produce genital warts; may lead to cervical or other cancers

Figure 8.11. Long term health implications of sexually transmitted infections (STD).

Source: https://4.bp.blogspot.com/-gj3OkrjN_DQ/WCCeNRxBjdI/AAAAAAAAAcY/9TrNUZeSvdMnjsrgmAyD9568mXhX8pIEwCLcB/s1600/symptoms_effects.png

The long-term health implications, therefore, encompass not only the physical manifestations of STIs but also the emotional and psychological impacts on the victims. This calls for an integrated healthcare strategy to deal with the various impacts of STIs on women's overall wellbeing. Most important, however, are the long-term health implications of STIs and HIV in women that need a multifaceted healthcare intervention plan beyond emergency clinical management. As countries recover from interruptions like the COVID-19 pandemic, sustainable models that ensure continuous access to sexual and reproductive health services are crucial in ensuring that all individuals get the necessary attention they need. Having all the stakeholders, like doctors, teachers, and community leaders, get together is key in having a strong support structure that allows young women to make healthy decisions. Through intervention into the increased dangers of sexual violence and exploitation propagated by social unrest, proactive measures can be directed towards protecting the most vulnerable groups (Murewanhema, 2020). As such, the resolution of the long-term health impacts of STIs and HIV in women requires concerted effort and commitment to improved individual and public health outcomes.

8.4.3. Mental Health Effects Associated With STIs and HIV

The crossroads of mental health and sexually transmitted disease (STD) is a multifaceted issue, most particularly for those women who are disproportionately affected by such diseases. STIs like HIV can bring about severe psychological distress through societal stigma, fear of disease progression, and implications for reproductive health. Women also report more depression and anxiety after receiving an STI diagnosis due to problems with relationship dynamics, fertility, and social acceptance. This psychic burden is added to by the sensation of being singled out or stigmatized by partners and communities harboring negative attitudes towards those infected with STIs. Further, the psychological weight is not only confined to the original diagnosis. However, it is likely to spill over into a continuous struggle with mental health, in which guilt and shame feelings may be profound. This factor of mental health matters in the appreciation of the public health impact of STIs among women at large (Ally et al., 2025).

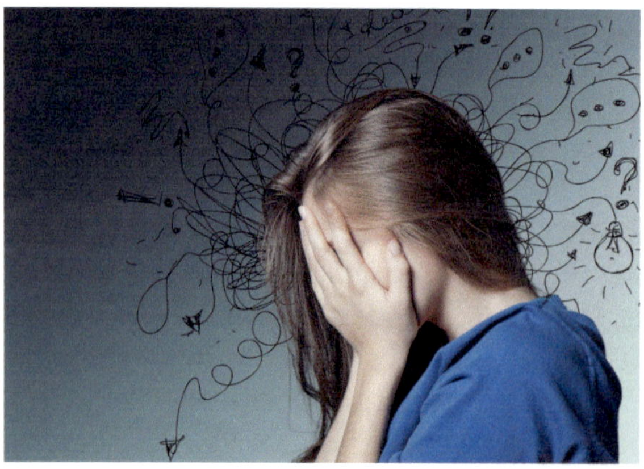

Source: https://www.oglethorpeinc.com/wp-content/uploads/2019/04/anxiety.jpg

Further, the psychological effect of STIs and HIV is powerful in young women who have society's pressures and expectations most likely to overwhelm them. Most societies' young women bear a dual burden of taking care of their sexual health and adhering to stringent social norms of female sexuality. Stigma associated with STIs might lead to feelings of low self-esteem and hopelessness, and even deepen the psychological dilemma they are facing. For instance, symptoms of depression and anxiety have been shown to arise much more often in STI sufferers, particularly those living in unstable socio-economic conditions. Adolescent girls may also experience difficulty accessing proper mental health care for their particular circumstances, further making their recovery and coping harder. Mitigation of such psychological impacts is essential in comprehensive STI and HIV prevention and treatment interventions, so that a multi-dimensional intervention can be provided with psychological counseling (Gitonga et al., 2025). Finally, intervention programs must consider that not only must attention be given to the biological dimensions of STIs and HIV, but also to mental health care focused on meeting the infected women's specific needs. Medical practitioners can also have a crucial role in identifying mental health conditions at the start of the STI treatment and referring women to mental health care where necessary. Moreover, effective educational interventions that reduce STIs can empower women so that they can seek assistance without fearing judgment. A combined model, which addresses the psychological factors of STIs and HIV as well as physical treatment, can provide improved outcomes for women patients. Last but not least, addressing the psychological factors of STIs, in combination with proper treatment guidelines, can contribute towards a more holistic method of managing women's health in sexually transmitted infections (Ally et al., 2025).

Test Your Knowledge

1. What are some common short-term health consequences of STIs and HIV in females?
2. What long-term health implications can result from untreated STIs and HIV?

8.5. Prevention Strategies for STIs and HIV

Learning Outcome

1. Define safe sex practices
2. Discuss the vaccination options (e.g., HPV vaccine)
3. Describe the role of education and awareness programs

Effective prevention of STIs and HIV among women relies heavily on both behavioral and biomedical interventions. Behavioral interventions, such as sexual education, play a crucial role in raising awareness and knowledge levels about STIs and HIV risk factors. Education programs emphasizing the importance of practicing safe sex, including condoms and monogamy, can enable women to make informed choices concerning their sexual health. Secondly, programs encouraging honesty when it comes to sexual history with a partner are essential in averting stigma and illness. Community involvement in these conversations also translates into women not just being educated but empowered to take positive action against STIs and HIV transmission. In addition to behavioral interventions, biomedical interventions have been an essential arsenal of measures against STIs and HIV. The development and promotion of pre-exposure prophylaxis (PrEP) have proven considerably effective in reducing HIV transmission among at-risk women. Also, incorporating routine STI tests in routine health care guarantees early diagnosis and treatment, thus reducing transmission rates considerably. The effects of sex hormones on susceptibility to infection are particularly intriguing; for instance, certain contraceptives have been associated with increased HIV susceptibility (Jocelyn M Wessels et al., 2018).

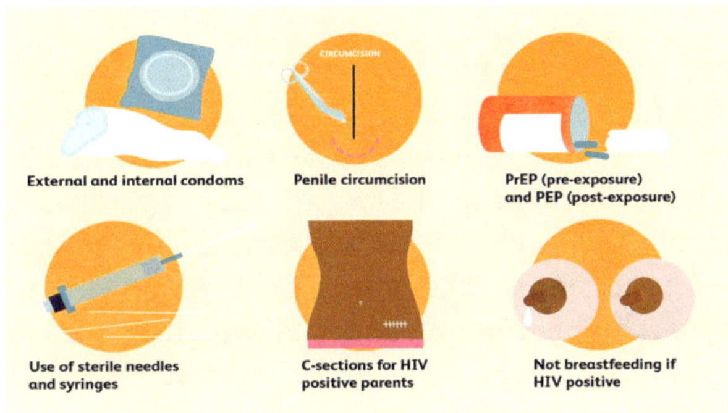

Figure 8.12. Preventions of HIV.

Source: https://www.verywellhealth.com/thmb/D5G3g8GqYWHV6PDrnlxy5KkDYgw=/1500x1000/filters:no_upscale():max_bytes(150000):strip_icc()/Hiv-transmission-rates-5211202_final-984de837f4e54b7ca81c2d21cc4d0f94.jpg

Understanding and management of such hormonal influences can enhance prevention strategies to ensure they address the unique health needs of women. Last but not least, the vaginal microbiome's role in susceptibility to infection has emerged as an important area of research, which might influence prevention against STIs and HIV. A favorable vaginal microbiota dominated by *Lactobacillus spp.* has been found through studies to offer protection. A polymicrobial microbiome can provide protective benefits against infection, whereas a polymicrobial microbiome related to bacterial vaginosis can increase susceptibility to HIV-

1 (Wessels et al., 2018). Therefore, including the health of the microbiome in public health interventions can provide an added layer of prevention in women's health. Additionally, enhancing interventions that strengthen vaginal health, with traditional prevention, can improve overall efficacy against HIV and STIs. With these prevention measures ahead, an integrated strategy combining the behavioral, biomedical, and microbiological information will be required in order to address the STIs and HIV in women.

8.5.1. Safe Sex Practices

Adopting safe sex habits is paramount in the prevention of sexually transmitted illnesses (STIs), including HIV, particularly among females who are more vulnerable. Prevention is anchored in the consistent practice and correct utilization of condoms, which have been identified as among the most effective measures for HIV prevention transmission.

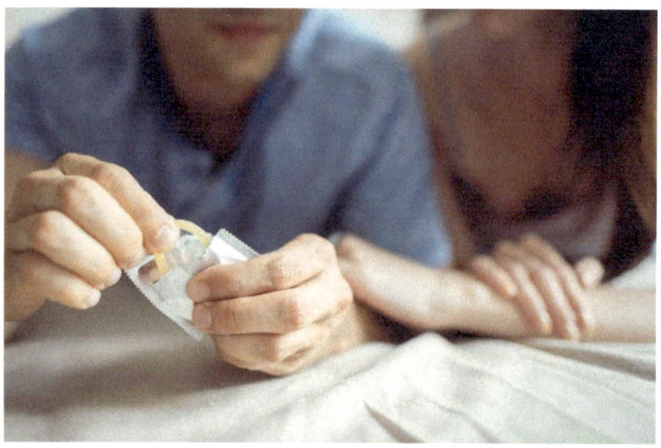

Source: https://novusacs.com/wp-content/uploads/2024/01/1.31-8_11zon.jpg

Despite proof of effectiveness, the gap between practice and knowledge is enormous. For instance, research indicates that while the majority of students possess HIV/AIDS knowledge, few of them use condoms during sex, with some of them prioritizing pregnancy protection over STI protection (Anaetor ISC et al., 2025). This difference in priorities explains why sexual education courses need to focus not only on the biological aspects of disease but on encouraging responsible sex and dispelling common myths regarding STIs and safe practice as well. Moreover, myths about STIs continue to exist, and safe sex is not practiced by young women. A study revealed that many adolescents falsely believed having sex without protection was safe, hence leaving them at risk of infections (Ambaye et al., 2023).

This is coupled with societal stigmas that may deter individuals from undergoing repeated testing or safer sex methods. Hence, education programs must address and surmount such falsehoods and emphasize the importance of identifying one's own and one's/partner's health status. Campaigns promoting not just condom usage but repeated testing can essentially lower HIV and other STIs in the female population. Providing young women with reliable information and testing sites is key to enabling them to make informed choices about their sexual health. It is also essential to examine the sociocultural factors that impede women's practice of safe sex. Such hindrances as limited access to sexual health information, stigmatization of STI testing, and gender inequalities may render best practices second fiddle. The results of low condom use in the majority of studies are a reflection of such hindrances, with the majority of young women indicating that perceived stigma and low risk of infection were among the factors that discouraged them from using protection during sexual activity (Anaetor et al., 2025). Such sociocultural determinants can be overcome by targeted interventions that engage communities and provide supportive milieux that can facilitate the process of moving toward safer sexual practice. By promoting open and honest debate on issues of sexual health and challenging unhelpful gender stereotypes, individuals are better able to make themselves a priority for health, with possibilities of positive impact on the rates of STI and HIV transmission among women.

8.5.2. Vaccination Options (e.g., HPV Vaccine)

The HPV vaccine is a vital measure in the prevention of sexually transmitted illnesses, particularly for young women and other high-risk individuals. Human Papillomavirus is also one of the most widespread STIs, and it has the possibility of causing severe health issues, including cervical and other genital cancers. Not only is vaccination reducing the risk of these cancers, but it is also playing a crucial role in preventing the incidence of genital warts. The vaccination strategy in the majority of countries is targeting girls aged 11 to 12 years, at a time when sexual activity begins. This foresight approach aims at developing immunity before viral exposure, thus making the vaccine work entirely. The public health activities also continue to stress the importance of vaccination receipt, especially in those groups that may experience increases in HPV illness, such as women below the age of 30, with their uptake having been found higher compared to other groups, as illustrated through more recent evidence from STI clinic users in Bologna, Italy (Cleva et al., 2024). The updated Korean Association of Urogenital Tract Infection and Inflammation guidelines make vaccination strategies contingent upon adaptation based on epidemiological trends and evidence. The guidelines recommend the use of various HPV vaccines like bivalent, quadrivalent, and 9-valent vaccines, which are seen to provide effective coverage for various strains of HPV involved in STIs as well as cancers. Vaccination schedules are also defined, including age groups and dosing regimens, which are critical in order to maximize coverage and optimize immunogenicity. Significantly, immunocompromised persons, for example, HIV-infected persons, are also urged to be given three doses of the vaccine to provide adequate protection. This recommendation emphasizes the need for healthcare providers' awareness and active participation in the vaccination process among vulnerable populations, offering personalized counseling and facilitating access to vaccination services (Choi et al., 2024).

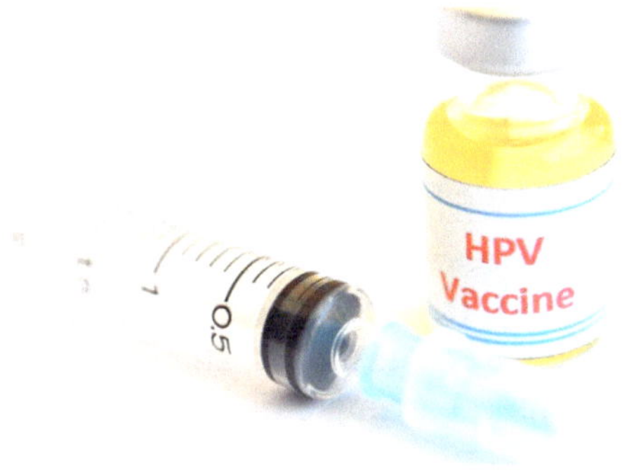

Figure 8.13. HPV vaccine.

Source: https://ichef.bbci.co.uk/news/976/cpsprodpb/1337F/production/_107791787_gettyimages-994979234.jpg

Despite the proven advantages and systematic recommendations for HPV vaccination, inequities in vaccination coverage continue as a major concern. Research indicates that groups such as transgender individuals and men who have sex with men have reduced rates of vaccination coverage, and this addresses the problem caused by sociocultural barriers and access to services. Program interventions for these groups, such as health education campaigns that counteract myths on vaccine safety and effectiveness, play a central role in increasing vaccination coverage among such groups. Identification of the specific concerns of specific demographic populations aids in creating more effective public health interventions. In addition, the availability of the HPV vaccine in STI clinics and other similar outlets is pivotal in increasing awareness among the high-risk population, hence enhancing prevention strategies against sexually transmitted diseases and their associated health complications (Cleva et al., 2024).

8.5.3. Role of Education and Awareness Programs

Educational and awareness schemes are instrumental in tackling sexually transmitted diseases (STIs) and HIV among women, promoting preventive strategies as well as attitudinal change. By providing citizens with correct information, the programs seek to demystify myths and misconceptions that usually blur sexual well-being. For instance, a study of students from historically black colleges and universities revealed widespread knowledge gaps regarding HIV, and overall awareness of the disease (Hardnett et al., 2014). High misperceptions regarding safe sex can enhance the risk of transmission in high-risk groups.

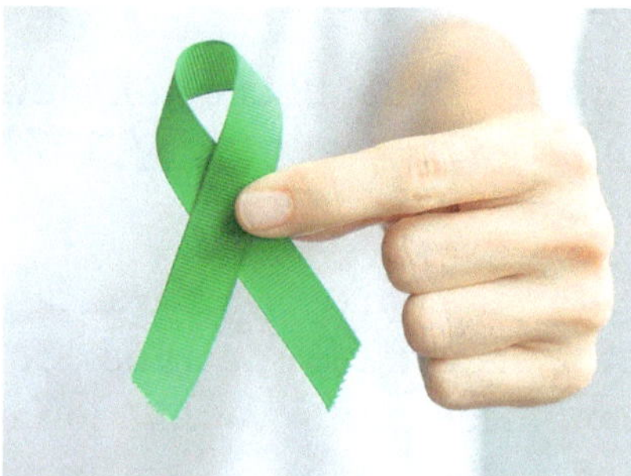

Source: https://nationaltoday.com/wp-content/uploads/2022/08/16-Sexually-Transmitted-Diseases-STD-Education-and-Awareness-1200x834.jpg

Therefore, targeted educational interventions are significant in resolving these misconceptions and enhancing knowledge regarding safe sex, thereby contributing to a considerable decrease in new infections among women. Incorporating comprehensive sexual education in school curricula as well as community outreach programs is essential in empowering women with information regarding STIs and HIV. These programs should not only cover the biological aspects of such infections but also prioritize the importance of double protection strategies, including female condoms. Female condoms are said to give women an important option for protection against unplanned pregnancy as well as STIs in those situations when male condoms may not be available (N/A, 2014).

Through promotion of awareness and availability of female condoms, educational programs can facilitate an enabling environment for women to assume an active role in reproductive health decisions. Empowerment is essential for controlling the incidence of STIs and HIV among women, especially among groups that are disproportionately affected by the infections. More critically, the efficacy of education and awareness efforts depends on culturally appropriate strategies that resonate with the target audiences. Tailoring messages to speak to the unique experience and challenges of women raises motivation and involvement in more safety-enhancing practices. For instance, interventions targeting adolescent African American women need to consider the social networks that organize sexual behavior and decision-making within their community. In this manner, they can lead to higher appropriateness and acceptability of health messages, subsequently constructing protective behavior. Engaging community leaders and opinion leaders can also go a long way in broadening the reach and impact of these interventions, influencing healthier behavior in young women and playing significant roles towards the larger goal of STI and HIV prevention among women groups.

Test Your Knowledge

1. What are some common safe sex practices that help prevent STIs?
2. Which vaccinations are available to protect against certain sexually transmitted infections, such as HPV?

8.6. Treatment and Management of STIs and HIV

Learning Outcome

1. Define available treatment options for STIs
2. Discuss antiretroviral therapy for HIV
3. Explain the importance of regular medical follow-up

Effective management and treatment of sexually transmitted infections (STIs) and HIV require a multi-dimensional approach with early diagnosis, appropriate treatment regimens, and patient counseling. Advances in technology in the field of diagnosis have facilitated rapid and effective detection of STIs, which is vital for effective management. One good example of a significant innovation here is the creation of point-of-care (POC) tests, where one is able to test and see results right away in clinics, consequently raising the prospects for prompt intervention. In the UK, a concerted drive by the Technology Strategy Board (TSB) and Department of Health (DH) highlights the importance of developing new diagnostics tailored to the unique needs of STIs in order to maximize health gain for women while getting the best value from reductions in infection and treatment costs (Osipenko et al.).

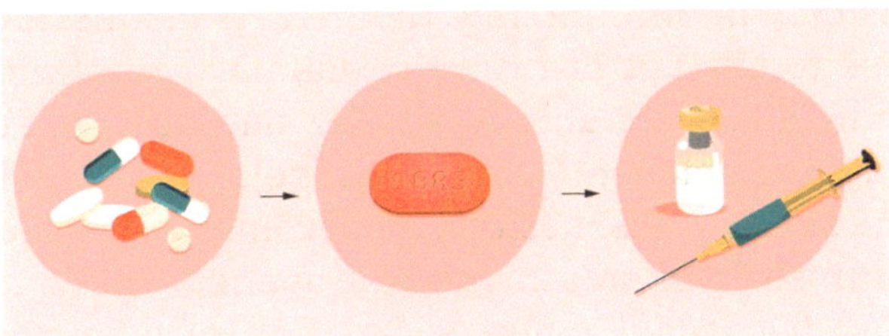

Figure 8.14. The evolution of HIV treatment.

Source: https://post.healthline.com/wp-content/uploads/2022/10/2551537-How-Science-Has-Changed-What-It-Means-to-Have-HIV-1296x728-Body-2.jpg

Moreover, the financial burden of new treatment strategies should not be overlooked, particularly in low-resource environments. Cost-effectiveness assessments hint at the advantages of using POC tests, particularly for frequent STIs like chlamydia, which is most prevalent among women and has severe consequences when left untreated. A study in Botswana concluded that the application of POC tests in antenatal care not only increases the number of cases cured but also reduces overtreatment and improves partner management practices. This integral approach demonstrates how combining POC testing with efficient treatment procedures will render greater health benefits than traditional syndromic management, especially in high-prevalence settings (Hjortdahl et al.). To enhance the impact of STI and HIV treatment programs, education becomes a key driver. Information and knowledge acquisition among patients regarding STIs, modes of transmission, and seeking care cannot be overstated. The process of education should not be confined to the clinical setup but extended through community outreach programs to reverse stigma and empower women in managing their sexual health. Furthermore, ongoing care and counseling following diagnosis are central to compliance with treatment and overall health. Integrating innovative testing, impactful therapies, and robust educational initiatives, health systems can enhance STI and HIV control in women, in the long run resulting in healthier communities and improved public health outcomes.

8.6.1. Available Treatment Options For STIs

The range of the drugs available for the treatment of sexually transmitted diseases (STIs) varies considerably depending on the pathogen involved. The effective cure of bacterial etiologies, e.g., chlamydia, is mainly antibiotic therapy. Azithromycin and doxycycline are utilized most frequently because both agents are extremely effective and have relatively low frequencies of side effects. As researchers have observed, azithromycin is more economical than other antibiotics in certain populations, thereby augmenting the use and availability of treatment among the affected groups (Hjortdahl et al.). Also, the application of point-of-care (POC) testing for chlamydia and other sexually transmitted infections may enhance diagnosis and accelerate treatment, thereby minimizing complications such as pelvic inflammatory disease, especially in young women whose prevalence is greatly high.

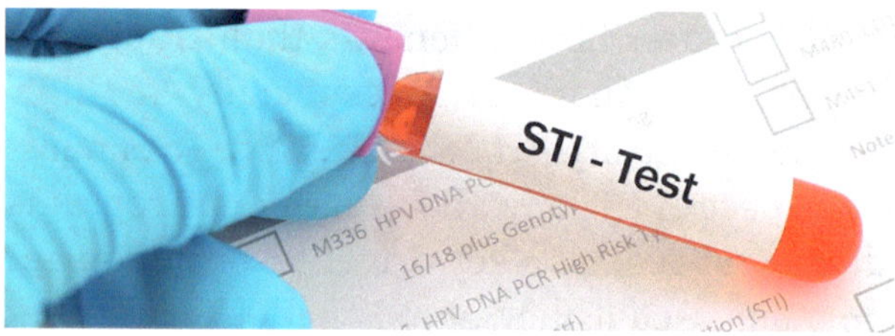

Source: https://external-content.duckduckgo.com/iu/?u=https%3A%2F%2Falergiayalimentos.com%2Fwp-content%2Fuploads%2F2019%2F11%2Fc-5.jpg&f=1&nofb=1&ipt=2422b9ba42edb1704a8e1d6941e01720d1da557ebc352d2ebed0448cdb020fe6

With bacterial STIs, treatment of parasitic diseases such as trichomoniasis has also experienced a new turn with newer diagnostic technologies. Trichomonas vaginalis infections that often go undetected can play a key role in perpetuating reproductive illness and might increase susceptibility to HIV acquisition. Newly established molecular tests have been found to be beneficial in enhancing the detection of T. vaginalis, not only making the treatment process easier but also helping in epidemiological studies to target high-risk populations more effectively (Munson et al., 2016). Previously viewed as a benign infection, the recognition of the severity of untreated trichomoniasis necessitates a re-evaluation of clinical practice to include screening tests, especially among women in high-prevalence areas. Treatment of viral STIs is more in the nature of long-term management strategies rather than cures, especially with respect to human immunodeficiency virus (HIV). Antiretroviral therapies (ART) have transformed HIV from a death sentence to an opportunistic chronic condition that has significantly improved the quality of life of infected individuals. Continued treatment not only keeps the viral level under control but also avoids transmission of HIV by others, particularly crucial for sexual partners' health. In addition, routine STIs, such as HIV, screening promoted by STI programs within clinical environments can facilitate early diagnosis and adherence to treatment. As healthcare policies continue to evolve with the necessity to integrate inclusive STI management processes that comprise prevention, education, and treatment as the optimal solutions addressing the problems of females with STIs and HIV.

8.6.2. Antiretroviral Therapy For HIV

Antiretroviral therapy (ART) has revolutionized HIV treatment, reducing the viral load of individuals infected with the virus significantly and improving their overall health. For females, particularly when it comes to sexually transmitted infections (STIs), effective ART is crucial in minimizing the HIV transmission risk to current or future sexual partners. Once individuals are able to sustain and achieve an undetectable viral load with regular use of ART, the sexual transmission risk becomes negligible. This shift in treatment has opened doors to serodiscordant couples, i.e., one of whom is HIV-positive and the other HIV-negative, who wish to have children without the risk of HIV transmission. As highlighted in recent studies, viral suppression is crucial not just for the health of the HIV-positive individual but also for public health initiatives to curtail the spread of the virus (María Begoña Baza et al., 2019). Adherence to antiretroviral medication is a primary concern, particularly for women, who are likely to face extra sociocultural as well as economic challenges. Knowledge of the determinants of adherence is critical in the case of STIs and HIV among women. Literature has shown that single-tablet regimens are easier to treat and have better rates of adherence. Additionally, men and women in stable, supportive partnerships might show greater adherence, which has a causative relationship with maintaining undetectable viral load. The existence of co-occurring STIs has the potential to complicate the treatment adherence terrain in that these infections can affect the effectiveness of ART. Note that even women with undetectable serum viral loads can still have detectable HIV in genital secretions, creating concerns regarding possible transmission risks during sexual contact, especially in serodiscordant relationships (Gon Mçalves de Melo et al., 2019).

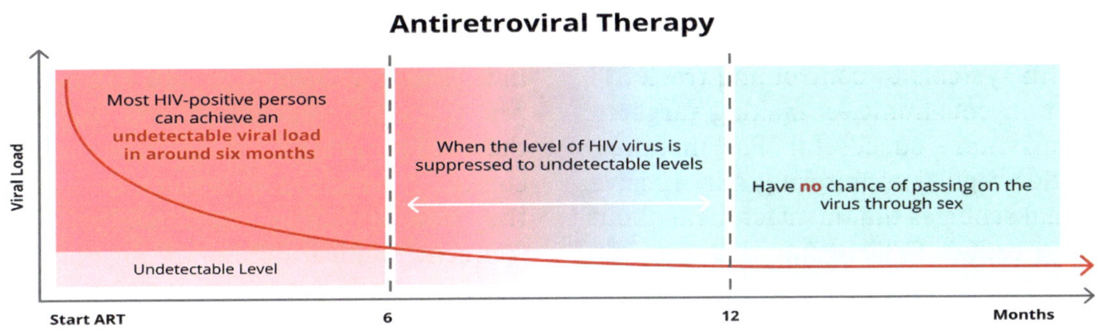

Figure 8.15. Antiretroviral therapy for HIV infection.

Source: https://www.hivtest.gov.hk/en/hiv_treatment_and_care/antiretroviral_therapy.html

In reproductive health contexts, ART facilitates safer conception among serodiscordant couples, highlighting reproductive counseling. According to research, through proper management and adherence to ART, natural conception is achieved by couples without transmitting HIV to their children or the uninfected partner. Reproductive success is brought about by factors like age, absence of fertility disorders, and specific treatment regimens. The accessibility of complete reproductive health care, including the availability of ART, is essential in ensuring women's health and the prevention of sexually transmitted diseases. By enhancing awareness and access to ART, healthcare providers can empower women, particularly those in serodiscordant relationships, to make wise decisions regarding their reproduction while minimizing risks for STIs and HIV transmission (Baza et al., 2019).

8.6.3. Importance of Regular Medical Follow-Up

Continued follow-up medical treatment is of great importance in health outcome management of women exposed to sexually transmitted diseases (STIs) and HIV. Continued monitoring allows healthcare providers to identify potential infections as early as possible, ultimately preventing serious complications and providing appropriate interventions in a timely manner. In particular, this intervention allows for the identification of asymptomatic STIs that are prevalent among women. Without regular check-ups, the infections can progress undetected, leading to severe health complications such as infertility and increased susceptibility to HIV. Studies indicate that regular visits increase women's knowledge regarding their sexual health, thereby promoting an active response towards prevention and treatment interventions that can ultimately improve quality of life and reproductive outcome (Appleton et al., 2006). In addition, not only is the frequency of medical follow-up important on an individual health level, but it also plays a vital role in public health programs. Routine testing and treatment enable health systems to control and track STI rates better in communities, making targeted interventions more successful. For instance, women under regular monitoring may receive informational schemes that instruct them about safe sex and reduce STI stigma. This not only makes individuals stronger but also causes overall transmission rates to decrease within populations. Research shows that when medical care services optimize access and continuity of care, they produce an impressive impact on community health through the dissemination of knowledge and infection prevention (Berman et al., 2002). Lastly, adherence to a program of periodic follow-ups by physicians fosters a trust relationship between patients and providers. This rapport is particularly vital for women because it facilitates open discussions about sexual health issues, including anxiety, stigma, and risk perception concerning STIs and HIV. Under trust, there is a greater probability that patients will present relevant information and concerns, allowing for tailored care that is individually designed to suit them. Also, once providers prioritize follow-ups, they can clarify the need for preventive measures, such as using condoms, which most women do not do when they are in stable relationships. Ultimately, frequent medical follow-up not only enhances patient health outcomes but also allows for a population-level focus on STI and HIV prevention and thereby emphasizes its vital necessity (Appleton et al., 2006; Berman et al., 2002).

Test Your Knowledge

1. What are common treatment options available for bacterial and viral STIs in females?
2. What is the role of antiretroviral therapy (ART) in managing HIV?

SUMMARY

The question of sexually transmitted diseases (STs) and HIV among women is worth noting the different aspects of the challenge posed by this category. Prevalence of STs among women is not so much a health issue, but rather an expression of more profound sociocultural and educational deficiencies. There is proof that comprehensive sexual and reproductive health (SRH) education is a key contribution towards assisting individuals in gaining the knowledge and skills required for them to make accurate decisions regarding their sex life. Just as the qualitative study delineating late adolescents' experiences did, participants who were exposed to SRH education reported better decision-making when it comes to risk behavior, highlighting the significance of existing and applicable education tailored to their interests (Leekuan et al., 2022). Promoting SRH education, then, should be the immediate action towards reducing STI rates and making healthy living achievable among women. In addition, the sociocultural conditions that differentially affect particular groups, such as Black women in the United States of America, illustrate the multifaceted nature involved in understanding STI risks. Such circumstances encompass all of the interrelated conditions affecting sexual behavior and attitudes, such as socioeconomic status, educational level, and support within a community. Research has indicated that these sociocultural contexts may appear in divergent sexual paths, with some women reaching higher-risk conduct due to a variety of pressures and settings (Crooks et al., 2022). By recognizing these complexities, interventions in public health can be designed to address not only the medical aspects of STIs but also the social determinants influencing women's health outcomes. Hence, there is a critical need to develop context-appropriate interventions that account for such realities to serve vulnerable populations more effectively. Because of the stark statistics for STIs and HIV among women, particularly in vulnerable populations, an appeal to action is called for. Public health policy needs to be strengthened to ensure equal access to sexual health services, including testing, treatment, and education. Multilateral action among health care providers, trainers, and policy makers is the most crucial to create an environment in which women feel comfortable without any constraint or stigma. Additionally, the enforcement of the right to informed choice on sexual and reproductive health must be the priority, as observed in the studies above (Leekuan et al., 2022; Crooks et al., 2022). Lastly, a concerted effort to overcome both educational and sociocultural barriers will be the thrust for an imperative drop in STIs and HIV in women and securing a healthier future for generations to come.

The interaction between HIV and sexually transmitted infections (STIs) presents substantial health problems, especially among women. Elaborate comprehension of such interaction is imperative in creating sound prevention measures. For example, STIs have been shown to enhance vulnerability to HIV acquisition, and HIV infection may complicate STI management. Current research has highlighted that women, overall, particularly vulnerable subgroups of women, are more likely to be at risk of STIs due to biological, social, and care access factors. Resolving these issues requires comprehensive sexual health education, better access to preventive interventions, and purposeful intervention in all female groups. Prevention of the incidence of STIs must therefore be integrated into HIV prevention in general. Notably, the epidemiological data on STIs and HIV among women are marked by striking disparities in prevalence and outcome that are influenced by a range of socio-demographic factors. Synthesis of available evidence illustrates that young women and those residing in communities with lower health care access disproportionately carry the disease burden. Programs adopting the know your epidemic (KYE) approach can provide specific information on trends, and they will also define high-risk groups as well as tailor interventions for their needs. This evidence-based system, based on comprehensive reviews of accessible biological, behavioral, and demographic data, ensures that interventions become locally relevant. These focused interventions are critical in the successful mobilization of resources and addressing the unique needs of women in diverse environments (Chikwava et al., 2011). Furthermore, the overlap of STIs and HIV in women is a necessity for integrated public health interventions focusing on prevention and education. While medical breakthroughs have improved treatment for HIV and STIs, these are typically absent if social determinants are not addressed. Other vulnerable groups are usually hindered by inhibitions such as economic insecurity, discrimination, and weak health access, which further heighten their risk of infection. Interventions in public health must thus engage communities, make safe behaviors visible, and make frequent STI and HIV testing accessible. Strengthening the coordination among government and non-governmental organizations has the potential to enable better outreach and support programs for women, eventually to reduce the overall burden of HIV and STIs among this group (Appleton et al., 2006).

KEY TERMS FROM THIS CHAPTER

- Antiretroviral therapies (ART)
- Biological susceptibility
- Emotional determinants
- Genital structure
- HIV infection
- HIV susceptibility
- Mental illness
- Partner notification (PN)
- Point-of-care (POC) tests
- Reproductive health services
- Sexual health decisions
- Asymptomatic presentation
- Chlamydia
- Female population
- Gonorrhea
- HIV management
- Human immunodeficiency virus (HIV)
- Nucleic acid amplification tests (NAATs)
- Pelvic inflammatory disease (PID)
- Public health programs
- Reproductive outcome
- Sexually transmitted illnesses (STIs)

CRITICAL THINKING QUESTIONS

1. **Which of the following is the most common bacterial STI in women worldwide?**
   a. Gonorrhea
   b. Chlamydia
   c. Syphilis
   d. Trichomoniasis
2. **Which STI significantly increases a woman's risk of acquiring HIV?**
   a. Genital warts
   b. Bacterial vaginosis
   c. Herpes simplex virus type 2 (HSV-2)
   d. Candidiasis
3. **One of the early symptoms of HIV infection in women may include:**
   a. Excessive menstrual bleeding
   b. Painless genital ulcers
   c. Flu-like symptoms such as fever and fatigue
   d. Yellowing of the eyes and skin
4. **Which of the following STIs can lead to pelvic inflammatory disease (PID) if left untreated?**
   a. Syphilis
   b. Chlamydia
   c. Candidiasis
   d. Genital herpes
5. **The most effective method to reduce the risk of both STIs and HIV in sexually active women is:**
   a. Use of oral contraceptive pills
   b. Regular douching
   c. Consistent and correct use of condoms
   d. HPV vaccination

Short Answer Questions

1. What is the current prevalence of STIs and HIV among females globally?
2. List two major risk factors for STIs and HIV in females.
3. What are common symptoms of STIs and HIV in women?
4. How do STIs and HIV affect female reproductive and overall health?
5. What are effective prevention strategies for reducing STIs and HIV transmission in females?
6. What treatment and management options are available for females with STIs and HIV?

Answer to Critical Thinking Questions

1. (b) 2. (c) 3. (c) 4. (b) 5. (c)

REFERENCES

1. Abu-Hammad, O., Arabiat, D., Althagafi, N., Eshky, R., Abu-Hammad, A., Jaber, A. R., Jaber, A. R., et al. (2024). Sexually transmitted diseases and HIV co-infection among adult male patients in the 2022 monkeypox outbreak: A systematic review and meta-analysis. *Dermatology Reports, 16*. https://www.semanticscholar.org/paper/4a88cf9f8c4544a68c1c4cef36bb258ccb9d72e0 (accessed on 15th June 2025).
2. Ally, Z. M., Moshi, L., Musoke, R., Mbwana, M. S., Bakari, H. M., Salim, S. M., Karia, L. F., et al. (2025). Trend of genital ulcers and discharge and associated factors among survey respondents in Tanzania, 2004–2022: Analysis of demographic health surveys. *PLOS ONE, 20*. https://www.semanticscholar.org/paper/1905c95b7725f4d7290f47897aa390b4b36b1fa4 (accessed on 15th June 2025).
3. Ambaye, E., Ormago, M. D., & Ali, M. (2023). Sero-prevalence and associated factors of sexually transmitted infections among youth-friendly services attendees. *PLOS ONE, 18*. https://www.semanticscholar.org/paper/bf19170b276de202cf44d8fe4e3b97cd70368a26 (accessed on 15th June 2025).
4. Anaetor, I. S. C., Ikwuka, A. O., & Udeh, F. C. (2025). HIV/AIDS: Safe sex practices, condom use and knowledge among students attending selected tertiary institutions in the Gambia. *World Journal of Advanced Research and Reviews*. https://www.semanticscholar.org/paper/6355ca8b2e5d247c5e12356261b2f0c9d69595ef (accessed on 15th June 2025).
5. Annang, L., Johnson, S. D., & Pepper-Washington, M. A. (2012). The context of sexual risk among African-American female college students. https://digitalscholarship.unlv.edu/cgi/viewcontent.cgi?article=1072&context=jhdrp (accessed on 15th June 2025).
6. Appleton, J., Brooks, F., Bunn, F., & Magnusson, J. (2006). Contraception advice and provision for the prevention of under 18 conceptions and STIs: A rapid review. https://core.ac.uk/download/29841254.pdf (accessed on 15th June 2025).
7. Aupont, L. W., Charania, M. R., Crepaz, N., Henny, K. D., et al. (2012). Efficacy of HIV/STI behavioral interventions for heterosexual African American men in the United States: A meta-analysis. https://core.ac.uk/download/227054367.pdf (accessed on 15th June 2025).
8. Awuoche, H. C., Joseph, R. H., Magut, F., Khagayi, S., Odongo, F., Otieno, M., Appolonia, A., et al. (2024). Prevalence and risk factors of sexually transmitted infections in the setting of a generalized HIV epidemic—a population-based study, western Kenya. *International Journal of STD & AIDS, 35*, 418–429. https://www.semanticscholar.org/paper/4fb17b109a5cd6ddd9c4699e434c59bdd3bf73c1 (accessed on 15th June 2025).
9. Baza, M. B., Jerónimo, A., Río, I., Rodríguez, C., Vera, M., Hernando, V., Castilla, J., et al. (2019). Natural conception is safe for HIV-Sero discordant couples with persistent suppressive antiretroviral therapy for the infected partner. *Journal of Women's Health*. https://www.semanticscholar.org/paper/6f0800e6ce258d33590d9aef0f0a60b6a1093a76 (accessed on 15th June 2025).
10. Berman, J., Longfield, K., & Klein, M. (2002). Multi-country study on trusted partners among youth: Eritrea, Tanzania, Zambia, and Zimbabwe. https://core.ac.uk/download/71342543.pdf (accessed on 15th June 2025).

11. Bray, F., Laversanne, M., Sung, H., Ferlay, J., Siegel, R. L., Soerjomataram, I., & Jemal, A. (2024). Global cancer statistics 2022: GLOBOCAN estimates of incidence and mortality worldwide for 36 cancers in 185 countries. *CA: A Cancer Journal for Clinicians, 74*, 229–263. https://doi.org/10.3322/caac.21834 (accessed on 15th June 2025).

12. Cairns, J., Fisher, M., Llewellyn, C., Miners, A., et al. (2012). Understanding patient choices for attending sexually transmitted infection testing services: A qualitative study. https://core.ac.uk/download/9427630.pdf (accessed on 15th June 2025).

13. Cassell, J., Johnson, S., & Tatem, B. (2008). 2008 sexual health in the South East: A collaborative report by Health Protection Agency South East and the South East Public Health Observatory. https://core.ac.uk/download/2709800.pdf (accessed on 15th June 2025).

14. Chalamila, G., Haarr, L., Langeland, N., & Matre, R. (2006). Demographic and behavioral factors in Tanzanian and Norwegian patients with sexually transmitted infections. https://core.ac.uk/download/pdf/18547605.pdf (accessed on 15th June 2025).

15. Chikwava, F., Fraser-Hurt, N., Gorgens, M., & Hosegood, V. (2011). Know your HIV epidemic (KYE) report: Review of the HIV epidemic in South Africa.

16. Choi, C., Lee, S. J., Choi, J. B., Kim, T. H., Lee, J. W., Kim, J. M., & Bae, S. (2024). 2023 Korean sexually transmitted infections guidelines by the Korean Association of Urogenital Tract Infection and Inflammation: Human papillomavirus vaccination. *Investigative and Clinical Urology, 65*, 108–114. https://www.semanticscholar.org/paper/21b1d1de9f4eb956be63b263198de96d3d3ba39a (accessed on 15th June 2025).

17. Cleva, M., Gaspari, V., Ceccarelli, A., Pianese, G., Griffa, D., Orioni, G., Cintori, C., et al. (2024). HPV vaccine awareness and uptake among sexually transmitted infections clinic users: A cross-sectional study in Bologna, Italy. *International Journal of Environmental Research and Public Health, 21*. https://www.semanticscholar.org/paper/702056efc283b11419bfba431f6769171a2bfa11 (accessed on 15th June 2025).

18. Colpani, A., De Vito, A., Marino, A., Ceccarelli, M., Celesia, B., Conti, G., Spampinato, S., et al. (2024). Viro-immunological efficacy and safety of bictegravir/emtricitabine/tenofovir alafenamide among women living with HIV: A 96-week post-switch analysis from the real-life SHiNe-SHiC cohort. *Biomedicines, 12*. https://www.semanticscholar.org/paper/2d54040c980a2ff73c584ae66f6a8ce42be1677d (accessed on 15th June 2025).

19. Crooks, N., King, B., & Tluczek, A. (2022). Being fast or cautious? Sociocultural conditions influencing the sexual pathways of Black females in the United States. *BMC Women's Health, 22*. https://doi.org/10.1186/s12905-022-01644-x (accessed on 15th June 2025).

20. de Melo, M. G., Varella, I. S., Gorbach, P., Sprinz, E., Santos, B., Rocha, T. M., Simon, M., et al. (2019). Antiretroviral adherence and virologic suppression in partnered and unpartnered HIV-positive individuals in southern Brazil. *PLoS ONE, 14*. https://www.semanticscholar.org/paper/c9dee5b06f04567f7d2b3131ecd525cc94582743 (accessed on 15th June 2025).

21. Deuchert, E. (2025). The Virgin HIV Puzzle: Can misreporting account for the high proportion of HIV cases in self-reported virgins? https://core.ac.uk/download/pdf/6493841.pdf (accessed on 15th June 2025).

22. Field, N. M., & Hughes, G. (2015). The epidemiology of sexually transmitted infections in the United Kingdom: Impact of behavior, services and interventions. https://core.ac.uk/download/29410608.pdf (accessed on 15th June 2025).

23. Girum, T., Kasahun, A. W., Mohammed, B., Yitayal, M., et al. (2017). Risky sexual behavior and associated factors among high school students in Gondar City, Northwest Ethiopia. https://core.ac.uk/download/480549677.pdf (accessed on 15th June 2025).

24. Gitonga, A., King'ang'i, J., Nyawira, J., & Withera, H. (2025). Awareness of contraceptives use among youths aged 18–26 years in Thogoto Market, Kikuyu Constituency–Kenya. *American Journal of Nursing Science*. https://www.semanticscholar.org/paper/2898fb2c97e992a9dc1e16b513fbaa454c0beba2 (accessed on 15th June 2025).

25. Hardnett, F., Huang, M. J., Murray, A., Sutton, M., et al. (2014). Strengthening HIV knowledge and awareness among undergraduate students at historically Black colleges and universities. https://digitalscholarship.unlv.edu/cgi/viewcontent.cgi?article=1236&context=jhdrp (accessed on 15th June 2025).

26. Hjortdahl, P., Hussein, F., Kristiansen, I. S., Romoen, M., et al. (2025). Costs and health consequences of chlamydia management strategies among pregnant women in sub-Saharan Africa. https://core.ac.uk/download/pdf/7107364.pdf (accessed on 15th June 2025).

27. James, S. L., Abate, D., Abate, K. H., Abay, S. M., Abbafati, C., Abbasi, N., Abbastabar, H., et al. (2018). Global, regional, and national incidence, prevalence, and years lived with disability for 354 diseases and injuries for 195 countries and territories, 1990–2017: A systematic analysis for the Global Burden of Disease Study 2017. *The Lancet, 392*, 1789–1858. https://doi.org/10.1016/s0140-6736(18)32279-7 (accessed on 15th June 2025).

28. Leekuan, P., Kane, R., Sukwong, P., & Kulnitichai, W. (2022). Understanding sexual and reproductive health from the perspective of late adolescents in Northern Thailand: A phenomenological study. *Reproductive Health, 19*. https://doi.org/10.1186/s12978-022-01528-1 (accessed on 15th June 2025).

29. Leyna, G. H., Mhalu, A., & Mmbaga, E. J. (2013). Risky behaviors among young people living with HIV attending care and treatment clinics in Dar es Salaam, Tanzania: Implications for prevention with a positive approach. https://core.ac.uk/download/pdf/18410864.pdf (accessed on 15th June 2025).

30. Lidjaja, L. N., Murastami, A., Ellistasari, E. Y., Ivani, & Alia, V. (2024). Prevalence and risk factors of sexually transmitted infections in a tertiary hospital in Surakarta, Indonesia. *Bio Scientia Medicina: Journal of Biomedicine and Translational Research*. https://www.semanticscholar.org/paper/f4fe903cb52d43d6a2c2ae0027fb94fb6ab40ddc (accessed on 15th June 2025).

31. Maierhofer, C., Lancaster, K. E., & Turner, A. N. (2018). Anal sex is more common than having a Twitter account in the United States. *Sexually Transmitted Diseases, 45*, 783–785. https://doi.org/10.1097/olq.0000000000000925 (accessed on 15th June 2025).

32. Mmbaga, E. J., Leonard, F., Leyna, G. H., & Sullivan, P. S. (2012). Incidence and predictors of adolescent's early sexual debut after three decades of HIV interventions in Tanzania: A time to debut analysis. https://core.ac.uk/download/pdf/16666687.pdf (accessed on 15th June 2025).

33. Mohankar, A., & Swain, J. P. (2024). Patterns of sexually transmitted infections: A hospital-based cross-sectional study. *International Journal of Community Medicine and Public Health*. https://www.semanticscholar.org/paper/d9b99c84c21f8f8b2bc4edebf7168acb45fb693b (accessed on 15th June 2025).

34. Munson, E., Munson, K. L., & Napierala, M. (2016). Update on laboratory diagnosis and epidemiology of *Trichomonas vaginalis*: You can teach an "old" dog "new" trichs. https://core.ac.uk/download/213085579.pdf (accessed on 15th June 2025).

35. Muralidhar, S., Gupta, P., Lachyan, A., Singh, S., Rana, R. S., & Khunger, N. (2024). Profile of sexually transmitted infections among attendees of special clinics (Suraksha) at an apex regional sexually transmitted disease center in North India–A five-year study. *Jornal Brasileiro de Doenças Sexualmente Transmissíveis*. https://www.semanticscholar.org/paper/ac48b256d6381a6d5d262fc8e82177c310fe419d (accessed on 15th June 2025).

36. Murewanhema, G. (2020). Adolescent girls, a forgotten population in resource-limited settings in the COVID-19 pandemic: Implications for sexual and reproductive health outcomes. *The Pan African Medical Journal, 37*. https://www.semanticscholar.org/paper/6ac21d9ce4c79a7df2e71c3f9ee6ce416ac004d6 (accessed on 15th June 2025).

37. Murray, C. J. L., Ikuta, K. S., Sharara, F., Swetschinski, L. R., Robles Aguilar, G., Gray, A. P., Han, C., et al. (2022). Global burden of bacterial antimicrobial resistance in 2019: A systematic analysis. *The Lancet, 399*, 629–655. https://doi.org/10.1016/s0140-6736(21)02724-0 (accessed on 15th June 2025).

38. Nielsen, M. H. (2009). From peasant society to manufacturing society. https://core.ac.uk/download/11986270.pdf (accessed on 15th June 2025).

39. O'Brien, A., Sherrard-Smith, E., Sile, B., Simms, I., et al. (2018). Spatial clusters of gonorrhea in England with particular reference to the outcome of partner notification: 2012 and 2013. https://core.ac.uk/download/156739005.pdf (accessed on 15th June 2025).

40. Osipenko, L., & Szczepura, A. (2025). Point of care tests for sexually transmitted infections (STIs). https://core.ac.uk/download/9846212.pdf (accessed on 15th June 2025).

41. Palfreeman, A., Sullivan, A., Rayment, M., Waters, L., Buckley, A., Burns, F., Clutterbuck, D., et al. (2020). British HIV Association/British Association for Sexual Health and HIV/British Infection Association adult HIV testing guidelines 2020. *HIV Medicine, 21*, 1–26. https://doi.org/10.1111/hiv.13015 (accessed on 15th June 2025).

42. Rowley, J., Vander Hoorn, S., Korenromp, E. L., Low, N., Unemo, M., Abu-Raddad, L. J., Chico, R. M., et al. (2019). Chlamydia, gonorrhea, trichomoniasis and syphilis: Global prevalence and incidence estimates, 2016. *Bulletin of the World Health Organization, 97*, 548–562P. https://doi.org/10.2471/blt.18.228486 (accessed on 15th June 2025).

43. Skinnes, M. N., Moe, R., Johansen, T., Lyby, P. S., Dahl, K., Eid, I., Fagertun, T., et al. (2023). Work ability in the year after rehabilitation—Results from the RehabNytte cohort. *Journal of Clinical Medicine, 12*. https://www.semanticscholar.org/paper/e4a46c468f12ccc34ced60706ddf2bf550c939ac (accessed on 15th June 2025).

44. Sully, E., Biddlecom, A., Darroch, J. E., Riley, T., Ashford, L. S., Lince-Deroche, N., Firestein, L., et al. (2020). Adding it up: Investing in sexual and reproductive health 2019. https://doi.org/10.1363/2020.31593 (accessed on 15th June 2025).

45. Thornhill, J., Barkati, S., Walmsley, S., Rockstroh, J., Antinori, A., Harrison, L. B., Palich, R., et al. (2022). Monkeypox virus infection in humans across 16 countries–April–June 2022. *New England Journal of Medicine, 387*, 679–691. https://doi.org/10.1056/nejmoa2207323 (accessed on 15th June 2025).

46. Ugwu, N. H., & Odimegwu, C. (2024). Prevalence and neighborhood determinants of early sexual debut and multiple sexual partnerships among young people in Rwanda, Ghana and South Africa. *African Journal of AIDS Research, 23*, 41–59. https://www.semanticscholar.org/paper/a28ca0cac19b1057a129dcd23415b0b163baa81d (accessed on 15th June 2025).

47. Vos, T., Abajobir, A. A., Abate, K. H., Abbafati, C., Abbas, K., Abd-Allah, F., Abdulkader, R. S., et al. (2017). Global, regional, and national incidence, prevalence, and years lived with disability for 328 diseases and injuries for 195 countries, 1990–2016: A systematic analysis for the Global Burden of Disease Study 2016. *The Lancet, 390*, 1211–1259. https://doi.org/10.1016/s0140-6736(17)32154-2 (accessed on 15th June 2025).

48. Wessels, J. M., Felker, A. M., Dupont, H., & Kaushic, C. (2018). The relationship between sex hormones, the vaginal microbiome and immunity in HIV-1 susceptibility in women. *Disease Models & Mechanisms, 11*. https://doi.org/10.1242/dmm.035147 (accessed on 15th June 2025).

PROLAPSE OF PELVIC ORGANS

9

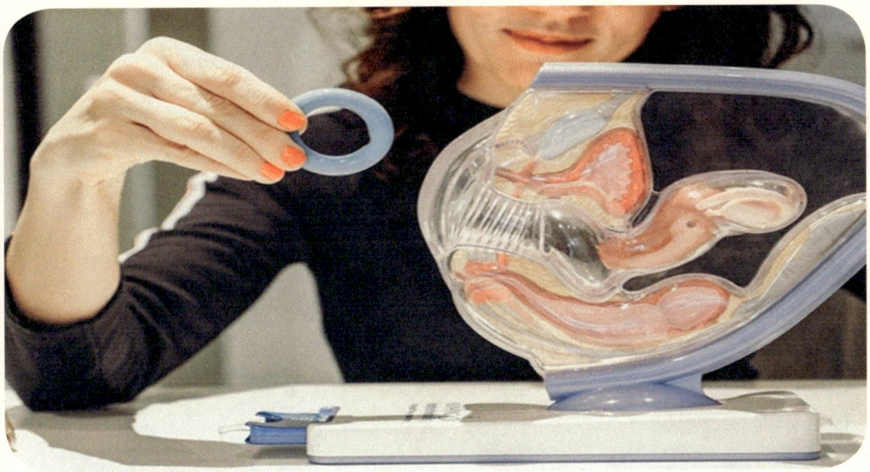

Introduction

Pelvic organ prolapse (POP) a topic of worry in the medical community due to its prevalence and disruption of quality of life in women. POP is a situation in which the pelvic organs, like the bladder, uterus, or rectum, shift from their normal position to cause physical and psychological distress. Understanding of etiology is significant because several factors, such as delivery, age, and heredity, lead to weakening of supporting pelvic tissues. Additionally, understanding the relationship between prolapse and pelvic floor disorders (PFDs) illustrates the complex nature of the condition, requiring a multidisciplinary therapeutic strategy. Treatment of both the physical occurrence and psychological impact is necessary, with new evidence showing a potential causal relationship between PFDs and psychiatric conditions like depression and anxiety, particularly after surgical intervention to cure these conditions (Kalata et al., 2024). Effective surgical treatment for conditions like stress urinary incontinence and pelvic organ prolapse has been a significant research area of interest because

LEARNING OBJECTIVES

After studying this chapter, you will be able to:

1. Discuss the anatomy of the pelvic floor
2. Classify the various types of pelvic organ prolapse
3. Explain the causes and risk factors of pelvic organ
4. Describe the common symptoms and diagnosis of pelvic organ
5. Discuss available treatment options for pelvic organ
6. Examine the psychological and social implications

of its impact on the mental health of women. Recently, various studies have measured the effectiveness of most surgeries, such as native tissue repair and the use of mesh, in alleviating the symptoms of the aforementioned conditions. It has been found that effective surgery can achieve a significant reduction in mental health symptoms, particularly anxiety and insomnia, thus pointing to the interconnectedness of physical and mental health in patients of PFD (Kalata et al., 2024).

This perspective redefines the surgical procedure as much more than anatomical correction but as a life-altering intervention that has the potential to restore overall emotional and psychological equilibrium to the participating individuals. Despite advances in surgery, choosing a surgical technique remains an area for ongoing debate among the medical profession. Numerous studies have compared these different approaches directly, such as native tissue repair, biological xenografts, and polypropylene mesh, in terms of their efficacy and safety profile. Significantly, subsequent studies have shown that while repair surgery can indeed alleviate prolapse symptoms, it does not necessarily result in improvements in long-term pelvic organ prolapse symptom scores, challenging the best practice for treatment. Therefore, additional research is necessary regarding the long-term outcomes of such interventions to determine their applicability to women's physical and psychological well-being. Underpinning this, in essence, is the necessity for comprehensive care mechanisms that not only address anatomical issues but also the psychology of patients to enhance holistic management of pelvic organ prolapse.

Definition of Pelvic Organ Prolapse

Pelvic organ prolapse (POP) is the sliding of any of the organs within the pelvis—such as the bladder, uterus, or rectum—into the vaginal canal due to weakening of the muscles and tissues of the pelvic floor. Prolapse arises when the structures that usually support these organs weaken or are damaged, most often as a result of pregnancy, surgery, aging, or increasing intra-abdominal pressure. POP presentation has the potential to be extremely diverse and range from asymptomatic to highly symptomatic, with a severe impact on quality of life.

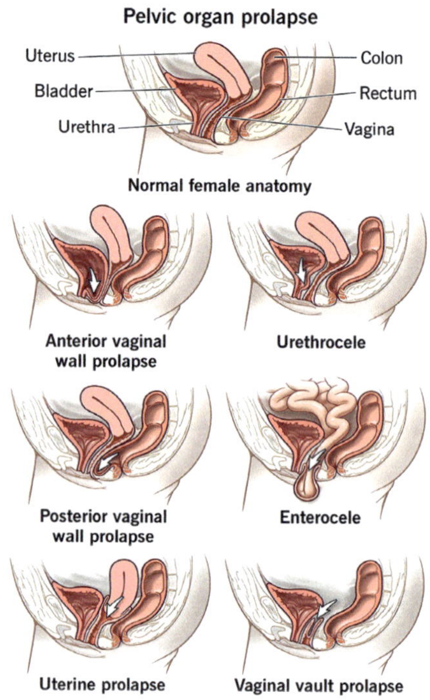

Figure 9.1. Pelvic organ prolapse is when the support in your pelvis weakens, causing one or more organs to sag or bulge into your vagina.

Source: https://my.clevelandclinic.org/health/diseases/24046-pelvic-organ-prolapse

Its clinical significance stems from the relationship between anatomical alteration and loss of function that has the potential for urinary and fecal incontinence or even complete discomfort with exercise, further emphasizing the need for extensive knowledge of this condition. In the past several years, standardization and consistency in the nomenclature of pelvic organ prolapse have also become increasingly important. In a consensus document by the International Urogynecological Association (IUGA) and the International Continence Society (ICS), it has been stated that the development of clear definitions encompassing symptoms, assessment, and classifications of pelvic floor dysfunction, such as prolapse, is designed to make clinical practice easier as well as enhance communication among healthcare practitioners. This multidisciplinary effort emphasizes the importance of terminology precision in the definition of terms that can be used with POP, thereby enhancing effective diagnosis, treatment interventions, and patient education. A well-defined vocabulary not only aids clinicians in management but also research endeavors into pelvic organ prolapse pathophysiology and interventions, providing a foundation for future progress in care and treatment protocols (Abramov et al., 2016).

The diagnosis and delineation of prolapse of the pelvic organs within the scope of general pelvic floor dysfunction are crucial in order to understand its importance on the well-being of women. Research indicates that the incidence of POP can be as high as 50% in women who have delivered, with risk factors for its development including modes of childbirth, integrity of the pelvic tissues, and endocrine changes. The condition itself tends to be underreported since talking about pelvic health is stigmatized, and thus, the barriers to early treatment. Since it is a condition with multifactorial etiology, POP treatment tends to be multidisciplinary. It includes urologists, gynecologists, physical therapists, and other professionals in order to address the individualized needs of the women. Through the convergence of focus on the identification and understanding of pelvic organ prolapse, health disciplines can further fortify preventive strategies and therapeutic interventions (Hamid et al., 2014).

Importance of Understanding the Condition

Both patients and practitioners need to know about the prolapse of pelvic organs. The prevalence of this problem among women, particularly those aged 40 years and older, needs evidence-based management and diagnosis. According to research, 41–50% of women in this category at some point during their lifetime will develop signs of prolapse. However, many women may struggle to access help early enough because they have misconceptions of what constitutes normal or because they feel embarrassed. More knowledge and education can bring down these barriers, enabling early intervention, as well as potentially reducing the severity of symptoms. This knowledge becomes pivotal not only to individual health outcomes but also to planning a patient-focused healthcare environment that prioritizes patient education and empowerment. In addition, treatment of pelvic organ prolapse is evolving, so it is increasingly important that women become more aware of the available options. There is evidence that individualized pelvic floor muscle training does reduce symptoms significantly, demonstrating that conservative management is a valuable alternative to surgery. In one effectiveness study of PFMT, patients who received individualized training reported clinically significant improvement in their symptoms compared to a control group that was offered only lifestyle counseling. This emphasizes the need for women to receive information about treatments for them so that they are empowered to make informed decisions and become participants in their care pathway. As treatment choices expand, understanding the differences between conservative and surgical choices enhances women's ability to speak for themselves. Finally, integrating the voices of women into the discussion about pelvic organ prolapse will assist in progressing care approaches. Women indicate that they often feel disregarded in their own experiences, which tends to lead to dissatisfaction with treatment and encounters with healthcare. Maintenance of active listening to patient experience by healthcare professionals is crucial to the adjustment of interventions to meet the individual's needs and preferences. Research indicates that a multi-professional approach to treatment decision-making, including physiotherapy and patient education, yields more acceptable results. Through setting up an open communication environment and recognizing patients' embodied knowledge as valuable, health systems can adapt their practice to the real-life circumstances of women suffering from pelvic organ prolapse. Through knowledge, consciousness, and advocacy, providers and patients can work together toward more efficient management of the widespread yet often overlooked condition.

9.1. Anatomy of the Pelvic Floor

Learning Outcome

1. Discuss the components of the pelvic floor
2. Explain the functions of pelvic organs
3. Describe the role of connective tissues and muscles

The pelvic floor anatomy is crucial to understanding the dynamics and the potential dysfunctions associated with pelvic organ prolapse. This complex organ consists of muscles, ligaments, fascia, and connective tissues that suspend a number of organs like the bladder, the uterus, and the rectum. The coordination of these structures among themselves is the solution to maintaining the integrity of pelvic organ positioning. Disruption of this anatomical structure, during childbirth, due to hormone shifts, or with aging, can lead to pelvic organ prolapse, in which organs descend into or beyond the vaginal channel. Based on an understanding of pelvic floor functional anatomy, clinicians can make better diagnoses and create successful treatment plans for women with prolapse. Knowledge acquired through anatomy also facilitates the exploration of pathophysiological mechanisms behind these conditions, highlighting the necessity to re-establish support upon prolapse occurrence (Razzak et al., 2018). In addition, improvements in imaging technologies, particularly Magnetic Resonance Imaging (MRI), have improved visualization of the pelvic anatomy in the recent past, and with that, greater diagnostic capability for pelvic floor disorders. From MRI, physicians can dynamically evaluate all the pelvic organs in different planes, thus yielding a more accurate evaluation than with routine physical examination. This is particularly beneficial in the handling of complex cases of multicompartment prolapse or widespread manifestations that may not be determinable by routine clinical evaluation. As the evidence indicates, MRI has proven to have a greater detection rate for abnormalities over physical examination alone, thus enhancing the precision of diagnosis and treatment planning. Through the incorporation of MRI into clinical practice, early intervention measures and customized therapeutic interventions can be made easier, which are essential in the successful management of pelvic organ prolapse (Dave et al., 2017). Moreover, an increased understanding of the support mechanisms of connective tissue in the pelvic floor emphasizes their role in maintaining pelvic organ stability. Consistent with the study that was undertaken by DeLancey, vaginal connective tissue support is classified into three levels, each having a definable role in pelvic stability and function. These are to be understood so that clinical presentations of pelvic organ prolapse can be appreciated and appropriate surgical or nonsurgical corrections may be used. Aging, obesity, and pelvic surgeries are some of the risk factors that could play a notable role in the integrity of such support structures, with a higher incidence of prolapse among such populations. Etiological factors must thus be addressed to enable prevention and effective management of prolapse among such high-risk populations (Razzak et al., 2018).

9.1.1. Components of the Pelvic Floor

The pelvic floor is a muscular and fibrous union of muscles, ligaments, and connective tissue that holds up pelvic organs like the bladder, rectum, and uterus. The pelvic floor is so intricate that it helps support these organs against gravity. Pelvic floor integrity can be lost in childbirth, particularly during vaginal delivery, which is usually the reason for most pelvic floor disorders. Complications such as pelvic organ prolapse (POP) are caused by damage to the pelvic floor, and therefore knowing its components and functions is significant. The pelvic floor's musculature is in charge of urinary and fecal continence management as well as sex function, highlighting its importance to overall well-being and health. This fundamental knowledge is crucial to effective management and prevention of disorders of pelvic floor dysfunction, particularly in the instance of prolapse (RE et al., 2000). The dynamic relationship between the pelvic floor muscles and the organs that it supports accounts for the manner in which compromise of structure leads to functional impairment. When the pelvic floor loses its strength, as happens through childbirth, aging, or other circumstances, the organs it holds are pulled downward from their normal position, resulting in urinary incontinence and POP. It is not a physical illness; it has a huge emotional and psychological impact on individuals afflicted by it. Appropriate evaluation is needed because traditional imaging techniques are incapable of comprehensively evaluating the functional environment of these conditions. The emerging approach that includes advanced imaging technologies, including open MRI, attempts to image the anatomy of the pelvic floor, taking into account the impact of posture and gravity on the movement of pelvic organs to enhance diagnosis and treatment strategies (Abdulaziz et al., 2018).

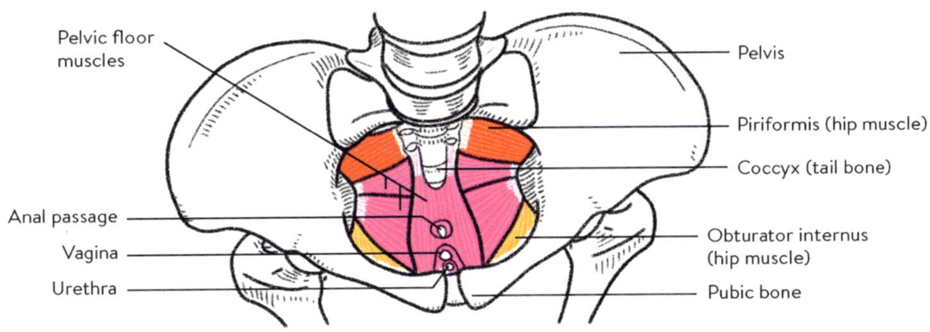

Figure 9.2. The female pelvic floor.

Source: https://images.ctfassets.net/hjcv6wdwxsdz/6e1MD5L55vAoeoPWGDPDL6/fb1ec7c375d6718097b709789be0329a/Pelvic_floor_diagram.png?w=1239&h=523&q=50&fm=png

Also, an extensive understanding of the components of the pelvic floor leads to clinical interventions for the restoration of its integrity. For instance, exercises to the pelvic floor, or Kegel exercises, stimulate the involved musculature, potentially lowering the risk for prolapse. Therapies may also include biofeedback and pelvic floor physical therapy that instruct patients on appropriate contraction and relaxation of pelvic muscles. Risk factor education for the etiology of pelvic floor dysfunction, such as obesity and smoking, directs prevention. With research continuing toward the classification of the complexities that surround the pelvic floor and its relationship to organ placement, it is increasingly important to adopt a multidisciplinary system in the treatment and management of these disorders. This interconnectedness is responsible for the necessity of complete evaluation and treatment to prevent and treat complications like pelvic organ prolapse (RE et al., 2000).

9.1.2. Functions of Pelvic Organs

The pelvic organs play significant roles in a variety of bodily functions, which significantly contribute to the general health and wellness of a person. Such organs encompass organs such as the bladder, uterus, and rectum, which collectively facilitate critical physiological functions such as urination, reproduction, and defecation. The bladder serves as a urine reservoir, allowing for voluntary discharge, while the uterus is focal to reproductive functions, i.e., gestation. Also, the rectum enables the expulsion of waste products, sealing the triad of functions that center within the pelvis. A functional pelvic floor stabilizes all these organs and coordinates their action. Disruption of support in this structure can lead to pelvic organ prolapse, a condition in which organs descend due to weak muscles in the pelvic region, indicating the significance of the organs in maintaining body integrity and normal physiological processes. When pelvic organs are engaged in significant activities, their structural integrity and positional integrity become important. The pelvic floor muscles envelop these organs and house them within a dynamic support system that varies in accordance with physical requirements, i.e., effort or change in posture. These muscles also have functions in sexual function and satisfaction, further emphasizing their multifaceted nature. Moreover, the pelvic organs' wellbeing relies on such factors as body mass index (BMI), age, and childbirth, which can lead to such conditions as pelvic floor dysfunction. In particular, studies indicate that women who undergo vaginal delivery are at a greater risk for pelvic organ prolapse, demonstrating the connection between reproductive health and pelvic organ function. This evidence shows not only the significance of pelvic organs but also the consequences of dysfunction, especially the price of such conditions like prolapse, which can claim a woman's life, as shown in McKinlay et al. (2020).

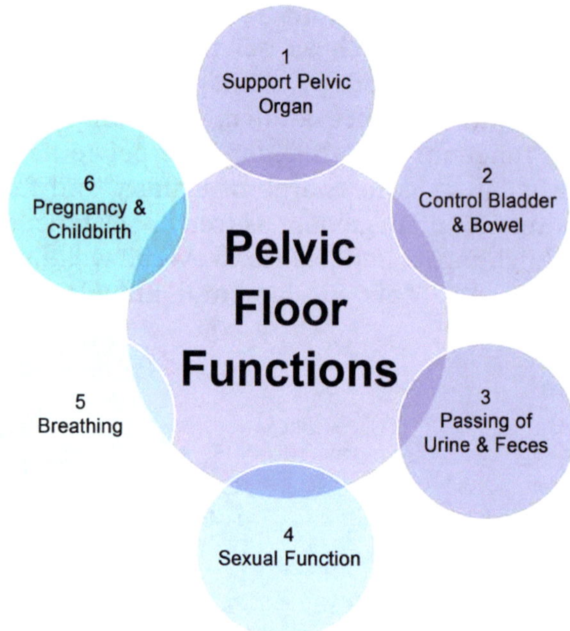

Figure 9.3. The function of the pelvic floor.

Source: https://northwestwellnessgroup.com/the-pelvic-floor/

Knowledge of the function of pelvic organs also necessitates an understanding of their relationships with more significant health outcomes. For instance, the development of pelvic floor disorders like prolapse may impact the psychological well-being of individuals involved, exacerbating anxiety or depression from changing bodies and social disrepute. The biopsychosocial model is a helpful paradigm to consider these interwoven relationships, demonstrating how problems of physical health may spill over into psychological and social arenas. As so prevalent around the globe are pelvic floor disorders, with age, parity, and mode of delivery implicated, knowledge of the whole spectrum of pelvic organ function is needed. Treating these conditions with appropriate medical interventions can significantly improve quality of life, so it is crucial that the research into such surgical procedures, as seen in McKinlay et al. (2020), continues in order to improve healthcare in the future.

9.1.3. Role of Connective Tissues and Muscles

The role of muscles and connective tissues in the pelvis is integral to understanding pelvic organ prolapse mechanisms. Connective tissues like fascia and ligaments serve a critical supportive function to the pelvic organs, maintaining them in position within the pelvic cavity. An explicit comprehension of these tissues is required in prolapse clinicians, as highlighted by studies that emphasize the tension on the interaction between pelvic floor muscles, ligaments, and their supportive tissues. When these supporting tissues fail, various forms of prolapse arise, essentially modifying a patient's quality of life. Increased understanding of the support offered by connective tissue on different anatomical levels, as described by DeLancey, demonstrates how insufficiencies in these tissues can manifest clinically and influence treatment strategy, highlighting the value of thorough anatomical understanding in surgery (Razzak et al., 2018). Intact pelvic organ function is also reliant on muscular support. Pelvic floor muscles, particularly the levator ani, aid in active support and stabilisation of pelvic organs with movement and variations in intra-abdominal pressure. They complement connective tissues in keeping the organs aligned and functioning optimally. When there is muscular weakness or dysfunction, prolapse is very likely, particularly after childbearing or as a result of degeneration with age. The correlation between the quality of the connective tissue and the strength of the muscles comes in the form of patients who have postpartum complications, as the two can lead to an increased risk of having such pathologies as uterine prolapse and cystorectocele. Reversal of the muscular imbalances can then alleviate some of the symptoms that pelvic organ prolapse presents (Braila et al., 2019).

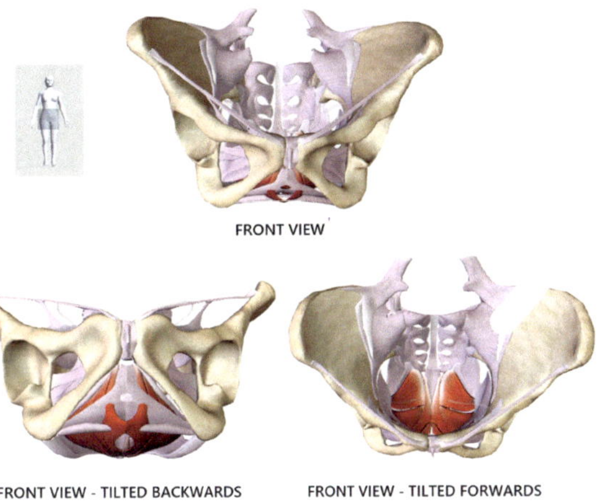

Figure 9.4. Muscles and connective tissue structures.

Source: https://www.baselinehealing.com/images/pelvis-bone-pelvic-floor-CT-female-1.png

In addition, the delicate relationship between muscles and connective tissues is also evidenced in the surgical repair of pelvic organ prolapse. The Manchester operation serves as a good case in point of how an understanding of the anatomical and functional sophistication of the pelvic supports determines the nature of treatment. This method addresses multiple concurrent issues by relocating supportive tissues of the pelvic floor, thereby enhancing both muscle function and connective tissue stability. Via the clinician's role in handling prolapse challenges, an advanced comprehension of the function of these vital tissues guides conservative as well as surgical treatment, such that outcomes are optimized for patients. Lastly, considering the significant functions of muscles and connective tissues in pelvic organ support, the present discourse around effective methods in pelvic organ prolapse prevention and treatment (Razzak et al., 2018).

Test Your Knowledge

1. What are the main components of the pelvic floor?
2. What are the primary functions of the pelvic organs?

9.2. Types of Pelvic Organ Prolapse

Learning Outcome

1. Discuss the cystocele (anterior prolapse)
2. Explain the rectocele (posterior prolapse)
3. Define uterine prolapse

Pelvic organ prolapse (POP) is a state in which prolapse of the pelvic organs occurs due to weakened support structures of the pelvis. POP can be primarily divided into three types: anterior, posterior, and uterine prolapse. Anterior prolapse, or cystocele, is when the bladder bulges into the anterior wall of the vagina, producing urinary symptoms like incontinence or urgency. On the other hand, posterior prolapse, or rectocele, is when the rectum bulges into the back wall of the vagina and causes defecation problems. The third is uterine prolapse, where the uterus drops into the vaginal canal and is most commonly accompanied by pressure and heaviness. Understanding these types helps in diagnosis and proper treatment protocols for such women. Modern treatment for pelvic organ prolapse is varied based on the nature and extent of the condition. Surgical procedures continue to be predominant, with surgery often being classified by the structure involved. For anterior and posterior prolapse, procedures like colporrhaphy are widespread; these reinforce the vaginal walls with sutures or, in some cases, mesh/graft material to provide strength to the pelvic support (Bain et al., 2008). In direct contrast, uterine prolapse can necessitate hysterectomy for marked descent with symptoms. While surgical techniques are effective in restoring anatomical locations, the selection of a procedure will weigh risk, e.g., risk of mesh complications, against benefit, e.g., lower recurrence rate.

This underscores the critical role of practitioners in providing treatment plans based on individual patient circumstances. Specific attention should, in the management of pelvic organ prolapse, also be given to concomitant conditions such as urinary incontinence and dysplasia of the cervix. Those with a prior history of injury from childbirth, such as tears to the perineum, are likely to have accompanying conditions such as cystorectocele and uterine prolapse, as seen in the increased vulnerability of the pelvic floor during labor (Braila et al., 2019). Effective management methods thus require a multi-disciplinary intervention focusing on prolapse and any associated pelvic static disorders. For example, the Manchester operation is a procedure involving several things to be done when there are concurrent lesions treated in one operation, and it provides a convenient solution to prolapse and associated complications. Ultimately, identification of the connection between the prolapse types and associated conditions is vital in optimizing care for patients.

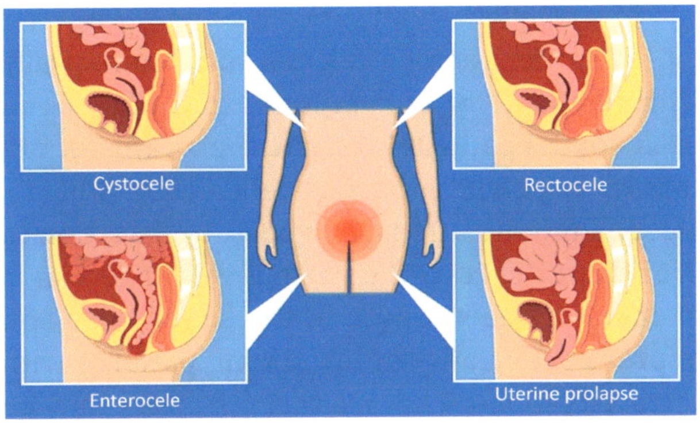

Figure 9.5. Types of pelvic organ prolapse.

Source: https://images.theconversation.com/files/624831/original/file-20241010-17-9ci9d2.jpg?ixlib=rb-4.1.0&q=45&auto=format&w=754&fit=clip

9.2.1. Cystocele (Anterior Prolapse)

Cystocele, or anterior prolapse, refers to bladder bulging into the anterior vaginal wall due to weakened pelvic support structures. Weakening is typically a result of childbirth, age, obesity, or long-standing conditions that apply intra-abdominal pressure to pelvic walls. Cystocele occurs with high frequency; approximately one-third of women are estimated to have pelvic organ prolapse of some level within their lifetime. Symptoms can vary from the feeling of pressure or heaviness in the pelvic region to urination impairment, such as incontinence or increased urination frequency. Due to the holistic nature of the condition, careful understanding of its implications for women's health is crucial to proper handling and treatment.

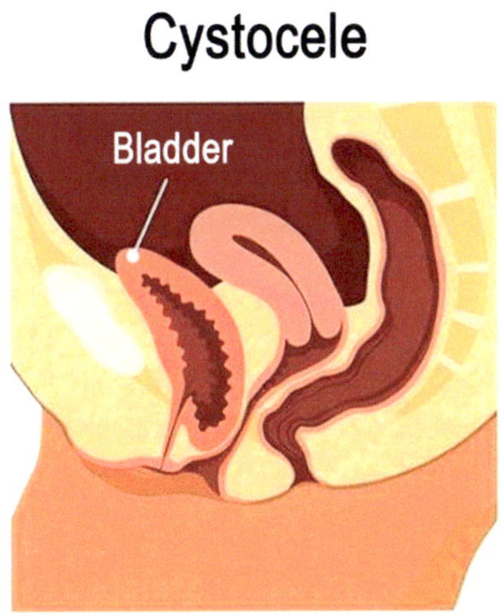

Figure 9.6. Cystocele.

Source: https://nursesrevisionuganda.com/wp-content/uploads/2024/12/Pelvic-Organ-Prolapse-POP-1.jpg

Clinical management of cystocele includes a range of conservative and surgical interventions, in which the choice could be determined by the severity of the disorder and impact on the patient's quality of life. Conservative treatment with the application of pelvic floor muscle training (PFMT) and modification in lifestyle has proved useful in alleviating symptoms. A pilot trial noted that PFMT volunteers experienced considerable improvement in prolapse symptoms and even observed a reduction in the stage of prolapse itself. This finding, which indicates the effectiveness of non-surgical treatment, highlights the need for individually tailored treatment regimens in line with the unique experiences and attitudes of women suffering from this condition (Glazener et al., 2009). Surgical options are normally reserved when conservative management fails, particularly with bad bladder function or major prolapse. The use of mesh or graft materials in surgery has also evoked interest in reducing the rate of recurrence of prolapse. A systematic review indicated that mesh decreased objective recurrence rates significantly over non-mesh methods, though erosion rates are a cause for concern and deserve proper scrutiny (Bain et al., 2008). Such findings have stirred the present debate within the medical practice regarding optimal cystocele management, necessitating strict long-term studies with the purpose of optimizing clinical guidelines and offering the best treatment choice to the affected women.

9.2.2. Rectocele (Posterior Prolapse)

The rectocele, or posterior prolapse condition, is a significant part of pelvic organ prolapse (POP), which occurs in numerous women worldwide. Rectocele refers to the bulge of the rectum into the posterior wall of the vagina through compromised support structures of the pelvis.

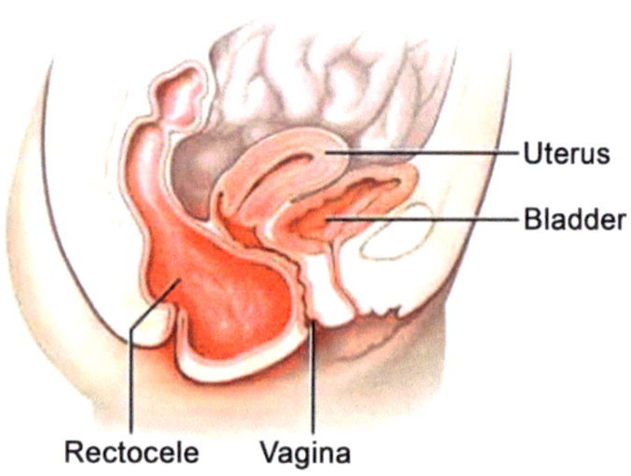

Figure 9.7. Rectocele.

Source: https://www.mayoclinic.org/-/media/kcms/gbs/patient-consumer/images/2013/08/26/10/47/ds00704_im02702_r7_rectocelethu_jpg.jpg

The pathogenesis of this condition is multifactorial, including factors such as childbirth, hormonal changes during menopause, and occupational factors like heavy lifting or long-term constipation. The prevalence of rectocele is high, with studies showing that among women with symptomatic POP, rectocele plays a significant role and impinges on their quality of life. Symptoms such as pain on defecation, sensation of vaginal fullness, and personal hygiene problems may be attributed to rectocele. Detection of such symptoms is vital in the early diagnosis and treatment to minimize suffering due to rectocele among affected women (Zhang et al., 2021).

Treatment of rectocele can vary dramatically with the severity of symptoms and the overall health of the patient. Conservative treatment can consist of pelvic floor muscle training (PFMT), lifestyle modifications, and pessary insertion to provide support to the vaginal wall. The aim is to enhance the strength of the pelvic floor and improve the quality of life among patients with rectocele. In more severe cases, surgery may be performed, with several methods being employed to repair the prolapse. Synthetic mesh and native tissue repair have both been employed, though recent controversy in the application of mesh has been to blame for alarm among healthcare workers and patients alike. The new criticisms highlight the need for care in surgical techniques because the safety and efficacy profile of such procedures is still under development (Petros, 2021). Despite the improvement in treatment options for rectocele, there are still problems with the delivery of optimal outcomes. Surgical treatments, particularly those involving mesh, have come under pressure for high failure rates and complications. These issues have highlighted the importance of developing successful alternatives to current treatment technology. According to recent studies, the emergence of sling techniques holds great future directions in controlling posterior prolapse more successfully. These techniques involve stabilizing the suspensory structures that support pelvic organs, with potential implications for improved patient outcomes. Moreover, ongoing research on the long-term results and success of various treatments makes apparent the complexity of rectocele management and the need once again for new strategies in pelvic health care. Overall, future strategies in the treatment of rectocele must prioritize patient safety, best outcome, and a comprehensive understanding of the multi-sited presentation of pelvic organ prolapse (Zhang et al., 2021).

9.2.3. Uterine Prolapse

Uterine prolapse is a significant part of pelvic organ prolapse, in which there is a downward movement of the uterus into the vaginal canal. Uterine prolapse typically happens as a consequence of conditions such as childbirth, old age, and hormonal changes, leading to weakening of the pelvic supporting structures. It leads to a range of signs that can impact the quality of life of a woman, including pelvic pressure, urine loss, and painful sex.

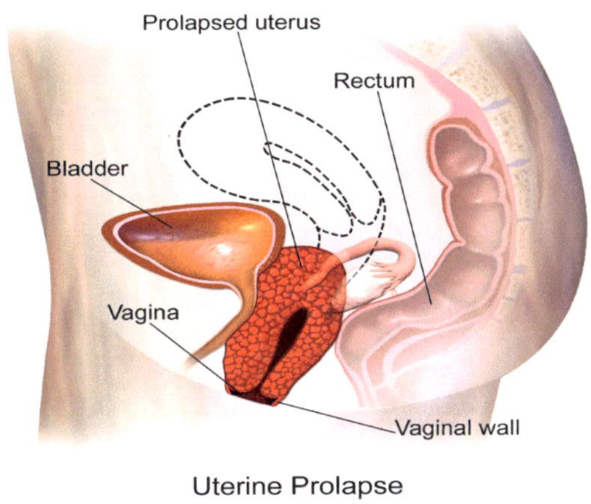

Figure 9.8. Uterine prolapse.

Source: https://en.wikipedia.org/wiki/Uterine_prolapse#/media/File:Uterine_Prolapse.png

The psychosocial impact of uterine prolapse is excellent, and the symptoms render most women ashamed and worried. Because of the taboo surrounding disorders of the pelvic organs, patients may delay treatment, and in so doing, complicate their health and well-being. Understanding the intricate nature of uterine prolapse is crucial for health professionals, as this can inform a more compassionate approach to patient care and point towards the necessity of pelvic health awareness among communities.

In investigating the treatment for uterine prolapse, it has an array of interventions ranging from conservative to surgical. Clinically, it has been demonstrated that surgical interventions are typically offered by individuals who have higher pelvic organ prolapse symptom scores (POP-SS) than those managed conservatively. In particular, the postoperative responsiveness of the POP-SS underscores the possibilities of significant gains following surgery, particularly for women with severe prolapse. For instance, postoperative patients show greater symptom reduction and improved quality of life compared with patients receiving PFMT alone (Abrams et al., 2008).

This evidence is in favor of employing care plans that are specific to the extent of symptoms and the patient's general well-being in the management of uterine prolapse. Despite the utilization of surgery, the decision to perform extensive intervention must be carefully considered, especially in elderly and frail patients. Surgical risk inclines healthcare professionals to be wary, since conditions such as comorbidities and frailty can complicate the recovery process and increase the chances of complications.

A case report on an elderly woman underscored the challenge faced in considering surgical interventions for severe genital prolapse. In her case, a significant restriction in activity in daily life followed, prompting a change of mind in her treatment plan. While surgical procedures can alleviate symptoms, they present inherent risks that will discourage such therapies' prescription in particular populations

(Formosa et al., 2009). These issues necessitate thorough discussions of the risks and benefits of all treatments to allow patients to make informed decisions about their health.

Test Your Knowledge

1. What is a cystocele, and which pelvic structure is involved in anterior prolapse?
2. How does a rectocele differ from a cystocele in terms of anatomical location?

9.3. Causes and Risk Factors

Learning Outcome

1. Define childbirth and its impact
2. Explain the age-related changes
3. Describe the lifestyle factors (obesity, heavy lifting)

The pathology of pelvic organ prolapse is multifactorial, usually caused by factors compromising the supporting structures of the pelvic floor. Among them, the most decisive factor is the trauma of vaginal delivery, causing a pelvic floor injury. Childbirth is most likely to cause conditions such as incontinence of the anus and bladder, alongside pelvic organ prolapse itself, indicating a high correlation between delivery types and pelvic health status. As stressed in the latest literature, the pathophysiology of such disorders points out an urgent need to understand not just the mechanics of childbirth but also its long-term implications on women's health. This background places emphasis on the investigation of preventive approaches and rehabilitation methods that could minimize the occurrence of such complications following delivery, which is in line with the common public health concern in women's health following pregnancy (RE et al., 2000). Aside from being a consequence of childbirth, advancing age is also a significant risk factor for pelvic organ prolapse. Physiological aging—like decreased levels of estrogen and the normal weakening of the strength of tissues—are able to compromise pelvic floor integrity. Elderly women may have widespread prolapse, which may lead to significant disability in activities of daily living. It is therefore a condition faced by the elderly, particularly with regard to mobility and autonomy. As noted in case reports of elderly women who have disabling genital prolapse, the site of surgery raises ethical concerns over their risk-reward ratio. While surgeries, such as vaginal hysterectomy, rectify function, the high likelihood of increased rates of complications among weaker persons necessitates stopping to consider (Formosa et al., 2009).

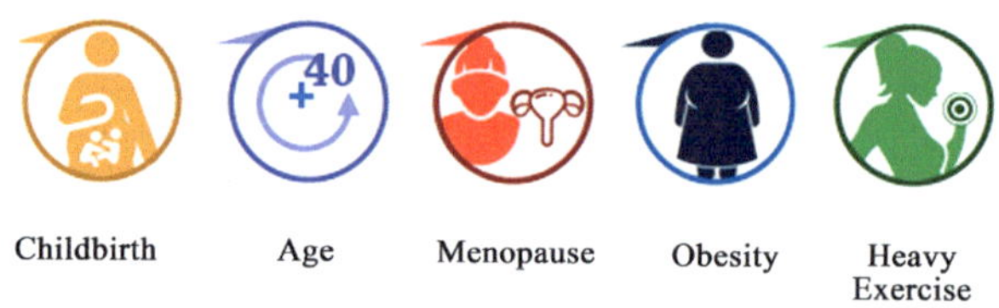

Figure 9.9. Different causes of pelvic organ prolapse.

Source: https://images.medindia.net/patientinfo/450_237/causes-of-pelvic-organ-prolapse.jpg

Other risk factors include obesity, chronic cough, and heredity. Being overweight usually leads to increased intra-abdominal pressure, hence placing additional stress on pelvic support tissues. Disorders such as smoking-related lung diseases that lead to chronic coughing increase pressure on the pelvic tissues, further destabilizing the pelvic floor. Genetic factors also have a notable role to play in the susceptibility of an individual to prolapse, with family history generally indicating a greater risk of developing similar issues. These varied risk factors indicate the multifactorial etiology of pelvic organ prolapse, accepting that it is not always due to lifestyle or physical trauma but an interplay of biological, environmental, and genetic processes determining women's health over their lifetime.

9.3.1. Childbirth and Its Impact

Childbirth itself subjects women to rigorous physical tests, particularly the integrity of the pelvic floor. In vaginal delivery, the pelvic floor, supporting the bladder, uterus, and rectum, is subjected to a significant amount of stress.

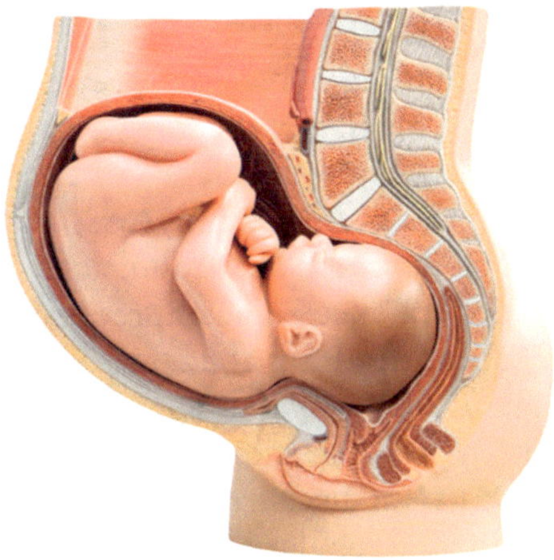

Source: https://media.healthdirect.org.au/images/inline/original/ky3rgb-(1)_c53bbd6a-f309-45f6-b20e-2eb8914f5c67-eeeb18.jpg

Besides physiological changes, childbirth also has radical impacts on a woman's psychological and emotional status. Such an inexplicable lifetime experience of becoming a mother; however, it can be accompanied by anxiety, depression, or loss of identity, particularly for those with adverse health outcomes like prolapse. Fear or threatened pelvic organ prolapse will exacerbate psychological inadequacy or fear of subsequent pregnancy and sexual health. Thus, a woman's psyche is gravely impacted by the corporal sufferings of childbearing. Support networks, including healthcare workers, families, and peer groups, play essential roles in coping with such emotional outcomes, so that women are able to deal with the complexities of motherhood, including any consequent pelvic floor dysfunction (RE et al., 2000). Furthermore, societal attitudes and cultural norms around childbirth will determine how women perceive their experiences and consequent problems, including the risk of pelvic organ prolapse. In all cultures, attention is drawn to an early recovery of pre-pregnancy body shape, which may be unrealistic and cause further psychological upset. Pelvic floor disorder stigma typically keeps women away from approaching healthcare professionals, resulting in chronic suffering and diminished quality of life. Establishing a culture that encourages open dialogue regarding pelvic health and informing women of the realities of postpartum recovery is paramount in reducing stigma and optimizing effective treatment plans. Public education regarding the impact of childbirth on pelvic health can lead to improved health and enable women to take charge of their well-being within the context of their total maternal health (RE et al., 2000).

9.3.2. Age-Related Changes

Aging-related alterations are a dominant factor in the development of pelvic organ prolapse (POP) and influence women's quality of life and health. Throughout life, particularly after childbirth and subsequent pregnancies, the integrity of the structure of the pelvic floor begins to decline. This decline can also be a result of hormonal changes, such as in menopause, that lead to decreased production of collagen and firming up of connective tissues. These biological processes enhance vulnerability to POP, where pelvic organs such as the bladder or uterus shift from their normal positions. The role of age as a risk factor is underscored by studies showing that there is a linear association between increasing age and the state of prolapse, and which requires complex management interventions tailored to older women. Research further elucidates the relationship of age to parity in pelvic organ prolapse etiology.

A study of Indigenous women in Brazil found that age and birth history were important risk factors for the condition, also commenting on the significant impact of birth history on the health of the pelvic floor. Specifically, the study had an odds ratio of 1.03 for age, indicating that with each increasing year, there is a greater likelihood of having POP, while parity had a whopping odds ratio of 9.40, again substantiating that having more than one pregnancy raises the vulnerability to pelvic dysfunction. These results resonate that, in the absence of intervention for other health factors, aging women with vaginal deliveries are particularly vulnerable to prolapse, and therefore need greater awareness regarding preventive strategies. The implications of age-related pelvic floor changes extend beyond physical modifications, having psychological and emotional consequences as well. Women with pelvic organ prolapse often present with urinary incontinence and pain, which, in turn, leads to social restriction and anxiety.

Cumulative effects of childbearing and aging underpin the importance of education and early intervention regarding pelvic floor health. Furthermore, knowledge of changes with age facilitates the formulation of targeted therapies like pelvic floor exercises and lifestyle interventions that can efficiently prevent risks. Thus, the understanding of the interaction between age, childbearing, and pelvic health not only enables clinical management of POP but also fosters a holistic appreciation of women's health across the lifespan.

9.3.3. Lifestyle Factors (Obesity, Heavy Lifting)

The relationship between lifestyle factors and the risk for pelvic organ prolapse (POP) has gained increasing attention in more recent research. Of particular interest, obesity is a significant risk factor, as a higher body mass index (BMI) may put undue stress on the pelvic floor structures. This stress further hastens the risk of pelvic organ descent, with studies indicating that women with higher BMI are more likely to develop symptomatic POP. The epidemiology of obesity in populations is heterogeneous and is usually compounded by socio-economic determinants, making it essential to have focused interventions against this public health issue.

Understanding obesity as a reversible risk factor is crucial in preventive strategies that attempt to lower the incidence of POP among women in their advanced years, especially considering its comorbid conditions such as urinary incontinence and compromised quality of life (Campbell et al., 2022). Heavy lifting is also a significant lifestyle component linked with pelvic organ prolapse and often underestimated in women's health discourse. Every day activities or jobs involving regular heavy lifting have been known to cause increased intra-abdominal pressure, and this could add extra stress on the pelvic floor. Evidence exists to support the fact that women who regularly lift heavy weights are at risk of developing POP, particularly if added to other risk factors such as parity and vaginal delivery.

The heavy lifting body mechanics demand the correct knowledge of body mechanics and pelvic support, as incorrect lifting posture could exacerbate pelvic floor weaknesses. Therefore, education programs for safe lifting are necessary, particularly among women who have job-demanding labor or are caregivers with repetitive lifting needs (Torgbenu et al., 2020). Consequences of lifestyle determinants such as obesity and lifting are greater than mere physical distress, having widespread ramifications for overall quality of life.

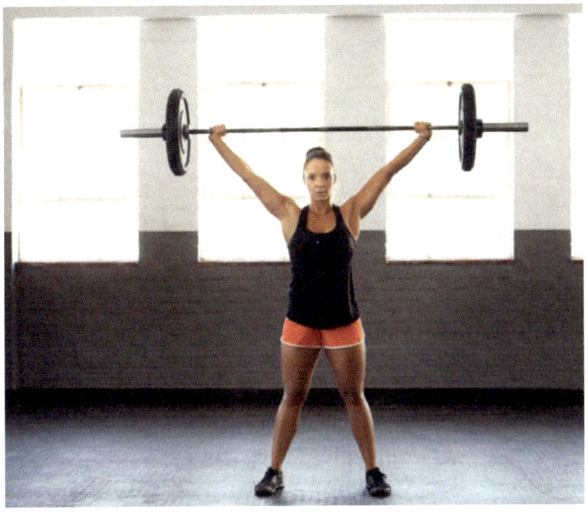

Source: https://d1rig8ldkblbsy.cloudfront.net/app/uploads/2020/01/23121652/getty-weight-heavy-lifting-good-for-women.jpg

Symptomatic POP women are not only likely to experience physical symptoms but also emotional distress, in addition to feeling embarrassed or socially stigmatized regarding urinary leakage and prolapse of the pelvic organs. The combination of obesity with heavy lifting can potentially create a cycle of health disparities, with women susceptible to increased healthcare costs and decreased productivity. Intervention on these lifestyle factors at the population level is indicated, as educating women on the dangers and preventive measures will instill better health outcomes. Lifestyle modifications as a component of routine treatment can increase awareness and support improved habits, and eventually reduce the incidence of pelvic floor disorders among women (Campbell et al., 2022).

Test Your Knowledge

1. How can childbirth contribute to pelvic floor disorders?
2. What age-related changes increase the risk of pelvic floor dysfunction in women?

9.4. Symptoms and Diagnosis

Learning Outcome

1. Identify the common symptoms experienced by patients of pelvic organ
2. Explain the diagnostic procedures (physical exams, imaging)
3. Discuss the importance of early detection

Symptoms of prolapse of the pelvic organs may quite variably vary among women, typically according to the character and severity of the prolapse. Typically reported symptoms are a sense of heaviness or pressure in the pelvis, which most women describe as a sensation of something falling or bulging down. Some experience pain on sexual intercourse, urinary leakage, or the inability to initiate urination and defecation. These symptoms are not only capable of inflicting bodily pain but also emotional distress and social isolation in that individuals are capable of avoiding the things they once loved in order to avoid embarrassment or in order to avoid making their condition worse. Identification of these symptoms is critical not only for the medical well-being of patients but also for encouraging said patients to come forward for appropriate medical evaluation and treatment in a timely manner, and hence the importance of awareness regarding this condition. Diagnosis of pelvic organ prolapse often begins with an adequate clinical assessment, which includes a thorough medical history along with physical examination. Medical practitioners generally employ the pelvic examination in diagnosing the extent of the prolapse as well as the affected organ—bladder, uterus, or rectum. During the process of taking the patient through this examination, the clinician can ask the patient to perform a Valsalva maneuver, which makes it easier to note the prolapse as organs within the pelvis sag with increased intra-abdominal pressure. Further, diagnostic modalities such as transvaginal ultrasound may be employed to visualize the prolapse more clearly and facilitate a more accurate assessment. Current research calls attention to the utilization of proper testing tools to give an accurate measurement of prolapse degree and for ensuing selection of treatment (Bain et al., 2008).

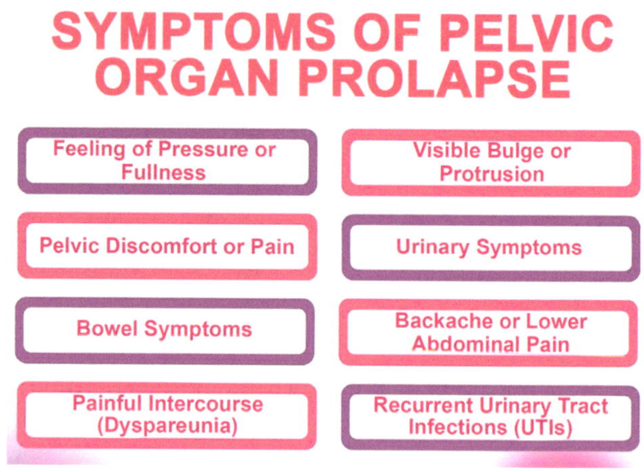

Figure 9.10. Symptoms of Pelvic Organ Prolapse.

Source: https://www.gardenobgyn.com/cdn-cgi/image/format=webp,width=728,height=728/https://www.gardenobgyn.com/sms/dashboard/blog_img/1268867821.png

In addition to diagnostic assessment, standardized grading systems such as the Pelvic Organ Prolapse Quantification (POP-Q) system also play a significant role in diagnosing and grading the severity of pelvic organ prolapse. The system provides an organized approach to grading prolapse, with an unambiguous guideline for clinicians to assess the severity of organ descent and devise appropriate therapeutic interventions. Effective classification not only facilitates tracking of the disease course but also assists in effective communication among patients and providers regarding treatment. Additionally, it is important to understand the effect of prolapse on a patient's health-related quality of life. Systematic reviews have identified the need for the use of both objective and subjective prolapse measurements, with the latter being critical to assessing intervention success in the future (Hamid et al., 2014).

9.4.1. Common Symptoms Experienced By Patients

The prolapse symptom is usually manifested by a variety of symptoms that have a dramatic effect on patients' quality of life. These symptoms include pelvic pressure, either the feeling of heaviness or fullness in the pelvic region. The patients' urinary dysfunction, such as urgency, frequency, or incontinence, can also be described, leading to social embarrassment as well as avoidance of normal activities. Further, others experience painful sexual intercourse, which they associate with the changes in the structure of the pelvic area as a result of prolapse. The pervasiveness of these symptoms establishes the necessity for a critical assessment to determine the precise type of prolapse and complication, which will allow healthcare providers to formulate pertinent interventions and treatment options. Another symptom patients of pelvic organ prolapse often exhibit is rectal dysfunction in the form of constipation, a feeling of incompleteness of bowel evacuation, or fecal incontinence. This is particularly painful because it interlinks with patients' psychosocial well-being, having a tendency to induce anxiety and increase feelings of inadequacy. The symptoms may also be accompanied by more obvious physical symptoms of prolapse, such as palpable bulge upon straining or standing. The multifactorial nature of these symptoms points to the interactive subtleties of the pelvic floor that may engage muscular and connective tissue integrity. High-resolution imaging technologies, such as MRI, have become crucial to accurately defining the degree of prolapse and associated symptoms, elucidating the structural contributions that underlie such complicated clinical presentations (Dave et al., 2017). Moreover, the psychological impact of symptoms of prolapse cannot be undermined. Most patients will complain of a compromised quality of life, namely, embarrassment and isolation from society due to the symptoms. The aforementioned stressed emotional and psychological factors are supplemented by physical restrictions and symptoms perceived, hence creating a cycle of distress. One must remember that symptoms of pelvic organ prolapse, including those related to urinary, rectal, and sexual function, are often quite diverse among patients. Furthermore, the severity of symptoms is not necessarily correlated with the degree of anatomical prolapse, a truth revealing the necessity of careful assessment methods comprised of both clinical examination and advanced imaging modalities. Recognition of the severity of symptoms in patients allows healthcare providers to be more responsive to the complete needs of pelvic organ prolapse patients and enhance the outcomes of treatment (Hamid et al., 2014).

9.4.2. Diagnostic Procedures (Physical Exams, Imaging)

Pelvic organ prolapse (POP) evaluation involves a multidisciplinary diagnostic approach combining physical examination with advanced imaging techniques. Physical examination typically involves a comprehensive medical history and a pelvic examination, allowing clinicians to evaluate severity and prolapse type. During the examination, clinicians can identify bulging of the vaginal wall or other findings consistent with the condition. But to have a better understanding of POP, imaging studies such as three-dimensional endoanal ultrasound (3D EAUS) have emerged as useful tools. Not only does it illuminate the anatomical interrelationships of the pelvic floor, but it also helps in planning surgery by revealing latent defects or dysfunctions of the pelvic musculature. The convergence of these diagnostic methods is critical to getting a reliable diagnosis of POP and subsequently influencing subsequent treatment strategies. Over the last few years, the role of imaging in the diagnosis of pelvic organ prolapse has increased immensely. More advanced imaging modalities supplement standard physical examinations and offer information about dynamic pelvic organ function. For example, 3D EAUS provides meticulous visualization of the pelvic anatomy and can identify occult abnormalities not apparent on physical examination.

Literature has shown that 3D EAUS is particularly helpful in assessing anal and rectal structures and is a must-use tool in patients with pelvic floor dysfunction. Also, it can establish the relation of the pelvic organs to surrounding structures, which is crucial in diagnosing multi-compartmental dysfunction in prolapse conditions. By filling the space between clinical examination and imaging techniques, healthcare providers can better comprehend the complexities of POP, thus enhancing patients' care.

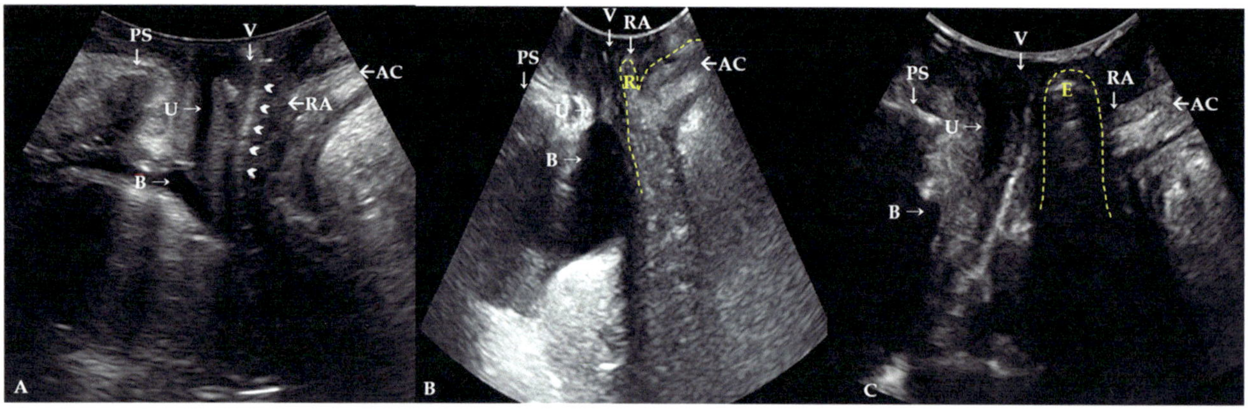

Figure 9.11. Translabial ultrasonography (A) in resting phase. Rectovaginal septum (arrowheads). AC, anal canal; B, bladder; PS, pubis symphysis; RA, rectal ampulla; U, urethra; V, vagina. Translabial ultrasonography in patients with (B) rectocele and (C) enterocele in maximal Valsalva phase. Rectocele filled with stool and air, resulting in hyperechogenicity, and the defect of the rectovaginal septum is observed in the maximal Valsalva maneuver (B). The contents of an enterocele appear generally iso- to hyperechogenic compared with a rectocele and bowel peristalsis is usually observed in the enterocele sac (C). R, rectocele; E, enterocele.

Source: https://www.mdpi.com/2077-0383/10/18/4267

The demand for the right diagnostic procedures is even higher with the prevalence of pelvic organ prolapse among women. It is postulated that approximately 50% of females undergo some degree of POP during their lifetime, influencing their body and psychological status. Despite this reality, the barriers to proper diagnosis and therapy are even greater. The majority of women delay treatment due to incorrect presumptions about the normalcy of their symptoms, and thus get trapped in a cycle of untreated prolapse. Advances in imaging technologies, for example, 3D EAUS, allow quantitation of POP severity and help elucidate interactions between anatomical variations and patients' subjective symptoms. Due to the flaws in current diagnostic procedures, a comprehensive evaluation using both physical assessments and high-tech imaging can develop more effective treatment plans, ultimately improving the overall quality of life of women with POP (de Coura et al., 2018; Sinex et al., 2021).

9.4.3. Importance of Early Detection

Early diagnosis of pelvic organ prolapse is crucial in improving the quality of life for women affected by it. Awareness of the symptoms and perhaps the causes may have a significant impact on the timing of diagnosis and consequent treatment. Most women shy away from seeking help due to social stigma, shame, or their ignorance of normal pelvic health. As the results have shown, it is an infuriating journey to diagnosis for females, with potential dismissal by health care providers. This delay could accelerate the condition to develop into more severe symptoms and make treatment options even more complicated. Consequently, enhancing public sensitization for prolapse symptomology is vital to facilitate an active healthcare strategy, ultimately enabling early diagnosis and more suitable management strategies that are tailored to women's needs and preferences, as emphasized in patient-centered care forums (Adelowo et al., 2019). What is more, ensuring that healthcare personnel are adequately sensitized about pelvic organ prolapse can enable greater rates of early detection. Education courses that train doctors to identify and treat the condition can lead to more precise recommendations and a still more supportive patient environment. In fact, the addition of physiotherapist interventions as first-line management options highlights the importance of a multi-disciplinary model which not only addresses the physical aspects of the condition but actively invokes women's experiences and self-determination in treatment planning. By employing standardized protocols in screening and open patient-practitioner communication, the healthcare system can better deal with women with prolapse symptoms. This would fill the present gaps in awareness and treatments, establishing a healthcare climate in which early intervention becomes standard and effective (Adelowo et al., 2019). Moreover, the therapeutic evolution demands an educational and preventive early diagnosis strategy. The multifactorial character of pelvic organ prolapse, typically associated with other pathologies such as urinary incontinence, demands extensive analyses with the ability to identify more than a single disease at once. As the literature describes, contemporaneous correction of concomitant conditions with prolapse surgery will optimize the outcome, restricting the burden of comorbid diseases such as colpocele and cystorectocele. Patient and doctor education must emphasize the significance of early symptom detection and the collaboration of various pelvic diseases. By creating a climate where awareness translates into timely intervention, we can maximize the effectiveness of treatment and improve women's overall health and well-being considerably.

Test Your Knowledge

1. What are common symptoms experienced by patients with pelvic organ prolapse?
2. Which diagnostic procedures are commonly used to assess pelvic organ prolapse?

9.5. Treatment Options

Learning Outcome

1. Discuss the non-surgical treatments (pelvic floor exercises, pessaries)
2. Explain the surgical interventions (types of surgeries)
- Describe the role of lifestyle modifications in management

Treatment of pelvic organ prolapse (POP) entails many different options, which are modified based on the severity of the condition and the requirements of the patient. Conservative management is typically the first line of treatment. These constitute pelvic floor exercises, also known as Kegel exercises, by which one attempts to strengthen the pelvic floor muscles in an effort to provide greater support to the pelvic organs. Second, the use of pessaries, or the medical device inserted into the vagina to support the pelvic organs, will be helpful to most women, even those who would be bad surgical candidates. The application of these non-surgical techniques will allow for a conservative assessment of how the prolapses are affecting quality of life without the risks of complications that come with surgical procedures. The success or failure of conservative management largely depends on patient motivation and adherence to treatment protocols. When conservative treatments are unsuccessful, surgical intervention is then required. Surgical repair of pelvic organ prolapse is generally aimed at anatomical support and relief of symptoms. Different procedures can be undertaken, from repairs of the anterior and posterior walls specifically to restore function to the bladder or rectum, respectively. In this surgical situation, the use of mesh or graft material has gained much popularity. From studies, it is clear that mesh/graft surgeries in anterior repair are linked with lower rates of prolapse recurrence compared to traditional repair methods, proving to be a strength in management techniques (Bain et al., 2008).

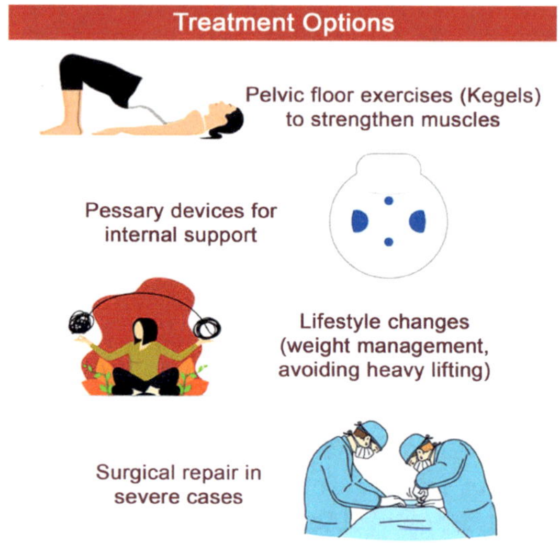

Figure 9.12. Treatment Options of pelvic organ prolapse.

Source: https://www.herobgyn.com/wp-content/uploads/2025/03/pelvic-organ-prolapse-desktop.jpg

However, this procedure is not without risk, since the employment of artificial materials is associated with complications of erosion and infection. Thus, due care must be taken in relation to the general condition of the patient and specific situations prior to the application of surgical intervention. In gynecological malignancies, management of POP involves additional complexities. Females diagnosed with pelvic cancers may have the double load of both malignancy and pelvic floor disorders due to their cancer treatments, such as surgery or radiotherapy (Bodean et al., 2018). The overlap implies the necessity for multidisciplinary therapy; the first priority is still cancer eradication, but the management of pelvic floor disorders is of paramount significance in a bid to enhance the quality of life of survivors. An appreciation of the impact of cancer treatment on the well-being of pelvic organs is necessary since these complications are not always well described by patients or understood by practitioners. Therefore, successful therapeutic interventions for pelvic organ prolapse must have regard not only to the anatomy of the repair but also to the general well-being of the woman when addressing such challenging diagnoses.

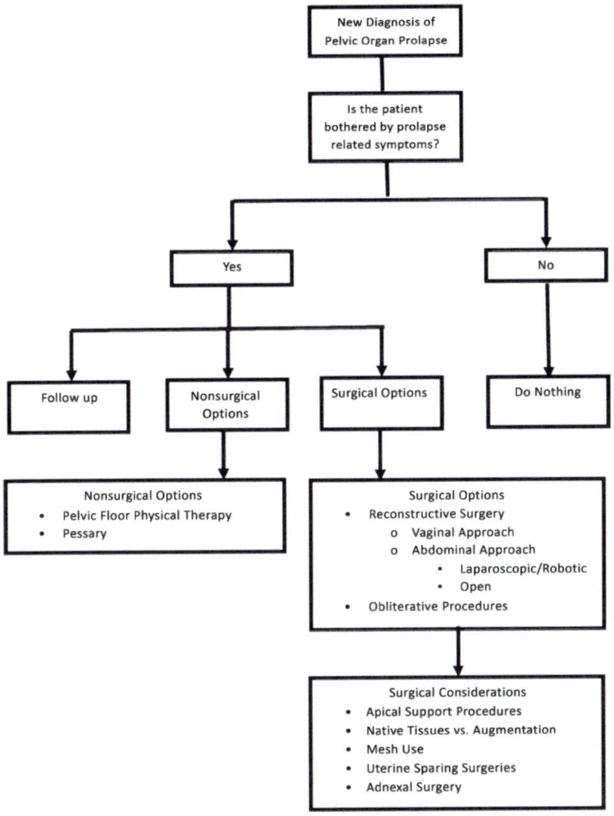

Figure 9.13. Treatment and considerations for pelvic organ prolapse.

Source: https://www.liebertpub.com/cms/10.1089/gyn.2022.0049/asset/images/gyn.2022.0049_figure1.jpg

9.5.1. Non-Surgical Treatments (Pelvic Floor Exercises, Pessaries)

Pelvic organ prolapse (POP) has a number of management strategies, and non-surgical options like pelvic floor exercises and pessaries are increasingly being accepted. Pelvic floor exercises, particularly pelvic floor muscle training (PFMT), are routinely prescribed to strengthen the supportive tissues of pelvic organs. Symptomatic relief in the form of improvement in symptoms of prolapse is possible with such exercises, thereby improving the quality of life of women with prolapse. It has been discovered that individualized PFMT reduces the severity of prolapse symptoms by a significant effect within twelve months. Like in a multicenter randomized controlled trial, individuals who received individualized PFMT experienced a notable relief of pain and a greater opportunity to feel improved from their condition than a control group that received lifestyle advice only (Biskupski et al., 2024). This underlines the importance of individualized interventions in the effective control of POP. Pessaries, another non-surgical procedure, have been with us for centuries in POP control. These devices act by mechanically supporting the pelvic organs and alleviating the associated symptoms from protrusion to urinary incontinence. Pessaries are extremely helpful for women who prefer gradual relief without the need to seek surgical interventions. Their flexibility allows different types to accommodate different stages of prolapse and patient anatomies. There are options for clinicians to offer varied pessary choices, tailoring selection for individual needs and preferences (Biskupski et al., 2024).

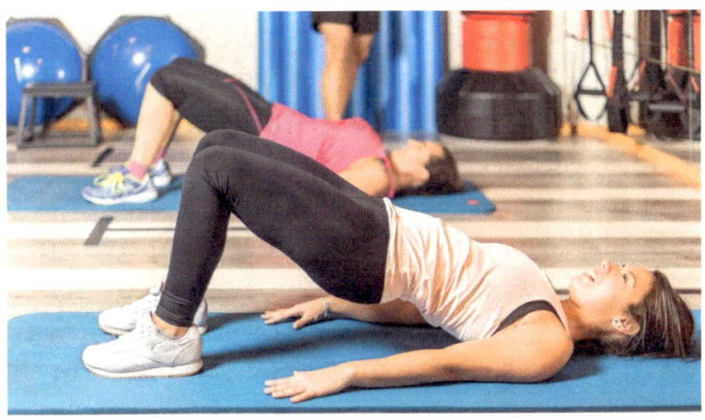

Source: https://myskyn.co.uk/wp-content/uploads/2024/06/Pelvic-floor-exercises-1024x572.jpg

Patient education regarding pessary use and care is most important for comfort and efficacy. Regular follow-up visits are also necessary for monitoring for potential complications or adjustments to changing symptoms. Incorporation of nonoperative management such as pelvic floor exercises and pessaries into overall prolapse care reflects the movement toward conservative treatment. Even if surgery remains an option for them, non-surgical techniques can be effective and empowering, giving women control over treatment. The positive results of PFMT and the versatility of pessaries might contribute toward a radical decrease in the need for surgery. In addition, the fact that they are not invasive, along with them being cost-effective, means they are also well-suited to be used as frontline treatments for POP (Barry et al., 2013). As patient preferences and needs become more understood, integrating these non-surgical interventions into a general care model is also essential to improving overall care of pelvic organ prolapse.

9.5.2. Surgical Interventions (Types of Surgeries)

Understandability of the various surgical procedures employed in pelvic organ prolapse is vital in managing the numerous challenges that the disease poses. Among the common surgical procedures is the use of transvaginal mesh implantation surgery, whose aim is to provide support to the pelvic floor by stabilizing it with synthetic material. This is a more sought-after procedure because it is less invasive and supports rapid recovery. However, the use of mesh has not been without complications, as there have been numerous accounts of complications in the form of long-term pain and infections. These matters culminated in the Parliament of Australia Senate Inquiry, which called for a clear review of the safety and efficacy of such procedures (McKinlay et al., 2020). Thus, while transvaginal mesh surgery is an option for most women, it should be considered with foresight about its long-term consequences. Another type of surgery performed for pelvic organ prolapse is the traditional reconstructive surgery, and this can involve various techniques such as colporrhaphy and hysterectomy. Colporrhaphy itself is the surgical repair of the vaginal wall to maintain anatomical position and function. This procedure is often employed for cases where prolapse involves the anterior or posterior vaginal walls. Hysterectomy may also be performed alongside other procedures if the uterus is a causative agent of the prolapse or if there are other gynecological defects. These procedures are often associated with fewer complications compared to mesh implantations, as reported in recent literature, hence improving patient outcomes (N/A, 2022).

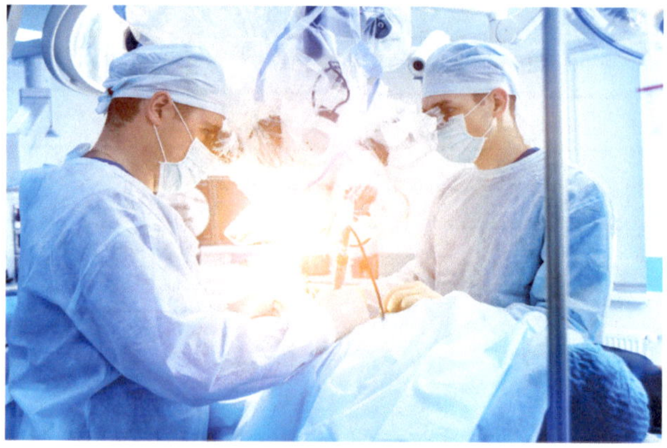

Source: https://www.curianmedical.co.uk/wp-content/uploads/2021/10/surgery-scaled.jpg

While they tend to have longer post-surgery recovery times than mesh surgeries, the procedures are efficient in alleviating symptoms and enhancing the quality of life of the afflicted. It is also essential to consider the general impact surgical procedures have on women's health from a biopsychosocial perspective. Pelvic floor conditions such as pelvic organ prolapse have an enormous effect on women's physical, social, and psychological health, and therefore the necessity of care plans that incorporate more than just surgery. The psychological effects, such as anxiety and depression, due to incontinence or pain, further add to the challenge in treatment and patient satisfaction. Treatment of prolapse with success is therefore commonly interdisciplinary, with physiotherapy and pelvic floor rehabilitation included (N/A, 2022). By dealing with these factors, medical practitioners can more effectively assist women throughout their surgery processes and contribute to better long-term results, which improve their quality of life.

9.5.3. Role of Lifestyle Modifications in Management

Treatment of pelvic organ prolapse (POP) is often multidimensional, with lifestyle change playing a central role. Patients can gain significant advantages from the reduction of risk factors that exacerbate prolapse symptoms. Specifically, dietary modification and exercise can decrease pressure on pelvic tissue and thereby ease discomfort and condition advancement. Moreover, proper fluid intake and dietary changes can alleviate constipation, which has been found to contribute to increased pelvic floor tension. Such a lifestyle adaptation not only boosts general health but can also enhance the effectiveness of conservatively managed treatments, such as pelvic floor muscle training (PFMT), by allowing the associated habits with POP to be addressed effectively (Abrams et al., 2008). Incorporating behavioral changes into the management of pelvic organ prolapse has been found to offer significant clinical benefit. Engaging in frequent exercises that strengthen pelvic floor muscles, including tai chi and yoga, may alleviate POP symptoms. Not lifting heavy objects and avoiding sports with high impact can prevent further deterioration of complications. A clinically grounded consensus report has highlighted the importance of effective communication between physicians and patients regarding lifestyle interventions designed to enhance treatment outcomes for pelvic floor dysfunction (Abramov et al., 2016). As patients adopt more healthy behaviors, they can notice improvement in quality of life, which complements medical or surgical management and is a holistic therapeutic approach to prolapse symptoms. Also to be noted is the incorporation of psychological treatment with lifestyle modifications. Emotional resilience is typically required to deal with the impacts of pelvic organ prolapse, and mental health management can provide a significant input towards the overall prognosis in terms of control. Counseling or support groups that focus on pelvic care can help bolster patients, ensuring adherence to lifestyle modifications and a positive attitude towards their condition. As such, patients will be more motivated to comply with exercise and dietary adjustments required for healing. This lifestyle-based, holistic intervention not only improves physiological health but also emotional well-being, setting the stage for improved pelvic organ prolapse care (Abramov et al., 2016).

Test Your Knowledge

1. What are two common non-surgical treatments for managing pelvic organ prolapse?
2. Name one type of surgical intervention used for pelvic organ prolapse and its purpose.

9.6. Psychological and Social Implications

Learning Outcome

1. Describe the impact on mental health and self-esteem
2. Define social stigma and awareness
3. Understand the importance of support systems

The psychological effect of prolapse is profound, with the majority of women undergoing a significant decrease in a woman's quality of life. Nearly all women with prolapse feel embarrassed, ashamed, and isolated, and these emotions discourage them from seeking assistance. This worsens the emotional burden by society's stigmatization of pelvic health, which minimizes or dismisses pelvic health issues in everyday discourse. As a result, women can endure silently, understanding that they are single-handedly facing their conditions. Moreover, they would normally understand that healthcare providers may not adequately address their problems, and so they experience frustrations and helplessness. These sentiments ought to be understood for the establishment of an enabling environment under which women will feel empowered to report their conditions without reservation and obtain appropriate treatment (Adelowo et al., 2019). Social repercussions also occur notably as a result of the physical impacts of prolapse. Women become less socially active, fearing symptoms manifesting or being judged by their peers. Social withdrawal can thus lead to loss of social support network, increasing feelings of loneliness and depression. Also, the lack of knowledge on pelvic organ prolapse among women and even healthcare professionals contributes to the perpetuation of the stigma and misconception. Literature shows that where women are encouraged to speak about their experience, there is increased overall satisfaction with care given, as well as improved coping strategies (Adelowo et al., 2019). This highlights that not only should interventions enhance awareness, but also debate around prolapse and the impact it has on women's lives. Also, the experience of pelvic organ prolapse can have debilitating impacts on a woman's self-esteem and body image. Along with prolapses, physical symptoms, and functional limitation, many women must struggle with negative self-image and incompetence. Such psychological distress can only make it more probable that treatment will be complicated; patients may avoid treatments or consultations with fear that they will not be able to meet societal expectations of femininity and health. According to studies, an integrated strategy—like psychological counseling and counseling on offered treatments—can effectively enhance women's health outcomes and satisfaction. Hence, addressing these psychosocial effects is not only preferable but also imperative for effective prolapse management in order to enable a recovery process that values and respects patients' emotional landscape.

9.6.1. Impact on Mental Health and Self-Esteem

The mental impacts of pelvic organ prolapse (POP) are a serious experience, primarily in terms of reduced self-esteem and mental illness. Women with POP tend to experience humiliation, anxiety, and depression due to the physical problems and social stigmatization of the condition. It is normal for one to experience a lower sense of self-worth as the body image perception gets intertwined with the physical conditions they possess. Studies identify that POP's psychosocial components affect women's emotional states significantly, influencing their quality of life and sense of self. They may struggle with inferior feelings that may continue even after treatment has been medically achieved, which points towards the necessity of an integrated approach in care that considers psychological management alongside physical cures. Moreover, self-esteem is complex and bound up with body image, particularly in women with POP. A significant majority report a significant shift in the way they view themselves, leading to a negative self-appraisal. The functional impairment and pain due to POP symptoms can cause the patient to withdraw from social activity, contributing to isolation and low self-esteem. This withdrawal may become a vicious cycle of avoidance behavior and subsequent chronic mental illness of anxiety and depressive disorders if left untreated. Since studies revealed emotional experience, relationships, and body image to correlate highly with treatment outcomes, psychological assessment and psychotherapy should be incorporated into POP management (N/A, 2019). Moreover, proper education and counseling of POP can enhance the self-esteem and mental health of women suffering from POP. The use of electronic patient-reported outcome measures such as ePAQ-PF can facilitate open communication regarding otherwise sensitive topics around POP, hence creating an enabling environment for articulation. Combined, these steps can empower patients to articulate their symptoms and treatment goals, which can have a beneficial effect on their mental health. Strategies aimed at relieving psychological distress and promoting improved self-esteem must be incorporated into clinical guidelines for the treatment of POP, recognizing that women's experiences range far beyond physical symptoms to incorporate overall well-being (N/A, 2019).

9.6.2. Social Stigma and Awareness

The stigma of POP is a significant feature of the condition in women with pelvic organ prolapse (POP). Stigma has a tendency to lead to avoidance of presentation to seek care, thereby maintaining the issue of pelvic floor dysfunction that remains untreated. Women will develop profound feelings of shame and embarrassment over physical alterations related to prolapse and find such alterations a failure or an inadequacy of theirs. Moreover, cultural beliefs and taboos around women's health add to the stigma, with sexually explicit subjects being discussed even less freely. Accordingly, most women choose to suffer in silence, as evidenced through a study that recognized 78.7% of women with POP as never having visited a doctor, indicating the need for increased awareness and education on the condition (Jokhio et al., 2020). Awareness of pelvic organ prolapse is crucial in demystifying social stigma and persuading women to seek appropriate care. Educational programs in the community that make discussions on women's health common are capable of giving a safe environment where people do not shy away from talking about delicate matters. Health experts have an overriding role to play whenever dealing with such issues; they must be trained on how to approach the talk on POP with empathy and knowledge. By promoting accurate information and dispelling myths regarding pelvic disorders, physicians can calm down women and make them understand that they are not alone and that help is available. Community engagement through workshops and classes can significantly lower misconceptions, destroying social stigma surrounding conditions like POP (Basappa et al., 2020). In addition, the cultural context within which the women live with pelvic organ prolapse can affect perception as well as stigma. Where reproductive health is traditionally an off-limits issue to talk about, the stigma of POP could be particularly pronounced. Where this is the case, the women could engage in coping methods that isolate them still further from potential support systems, whether social or medical. This points to the requirement for interventions to be specially crafted with consideration of local cultural beliefs and attitudes towards women's health. Facilitating the discussion of pelvic health, including the biological and emotional consequences, is needed to educate the population more. Empowering community dialogue can ultimately allow women to be active participants in their health, finally improving the quality of their lives and reducing the stigmatization of pelvic organ prolapse disorders (Jokhio et al., 2020).

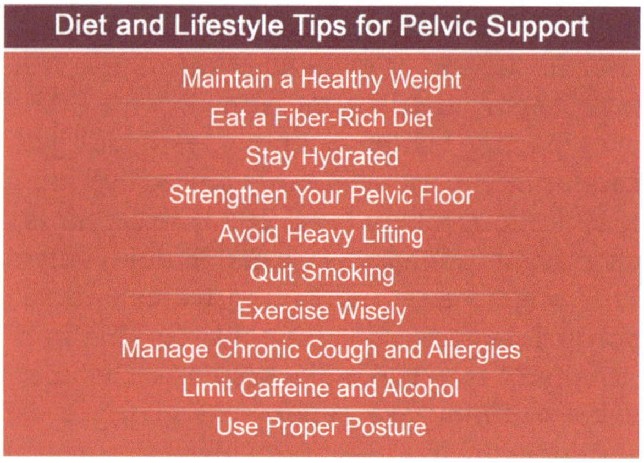

Source: https://www.herobgyn.com/wp-content/uploads/2025/03/pelvic-organ-prolapse-desktop.jpg

9.6.3. Importance of Support Systems

In prolapse of the pelvic organs, no part of the support systems can be overemphasized more. The systems involve both the formal support in the form of medical staff and informal support by friends and family. These networks provide enormous psychological and emotional support to patients afflicted with the pain and the shame of prolapse. Knowing that they are not the only victims of such a condition can motivate women to show up early for treatment and receive interventions that can relieve their symptoms. Besides emotional support, support systems can facilitate the sharing of information, enabling individuals to discuss treatment choices, experiences, and results, hence facilitating informed decision-making in the management of such a condition. The integration of support systems with pelvic organ well-being has the potential to promote recovery goals by supporting therapy adherence. For example, it has been found through research that pelvic floor muscle training can profoundly improve signs of prolapse, particularly when supplemented with provider and peer encouragement and counseling (Barry et al., 2013). Through providing concrete assistance and encouragement, support systems ensure that patients take recommended exercises or treatment regimens, leading to better health outcomes. In addition to facilitating mutual understanding between patients about successfully managing their condition, the systems also reduce the fear and stigma generally associated with conditions of the pelvis. Furthermore, the ultimate long-term care of prolapse of the pelvic organs always relates to the interaction between holistic support systems and care systems. Literature shows that mesh or graft surgery presents varying proportions of efficacy and safety, and patients are likely to render these choices more favorably under direction and support by information systems (Bain et al., 2008). Tight integration with medical professionals, with full involvement of family and friends, not only aids decision-making but also enables a comprehensive treatment and healing strategy. Ultimately, a solid support system can bridge gaps in care, providing consistent encouragement that maximizes the overall quality of life for patients with pelvic organ prolapse.

Test Your Knowledge

1. How can pelvic organ prolapse affect a patient's mental health and self-esteem?
2. What role does social stigma play in the diagnosis and treatment of pelvic organ prolapse?

SUMMARY

The synopsis of pelvic organ prolapse highlights the multi-factorial nature of the disease, recognizing intrinsic and extrinsic variables influencing its occurrence and severity. Various studies have shown that working and lifestyle factors have a significant impact on the incidence of pelvic organ prolapse, particularly in groups with distinct cultural practices. For instance, the occupational position of women appears to regulate their prolapse risk, as noted from research that found that women employed in sitting postures have a higher predisposition to uterine prolapse compared to women employed standing. In addition, the protective function of not wearing a patuka, usually employed for carrying loads, further contributes to the complexity of determining how one's day-to-day activities influence pelvic well-being (Bates et al., 2020). This multifactorial nature requires overall measures in prevention and awareness, ideally tailored to specific communities. Management of pelvic organ prolapse acutely includes consideration of surgery, particularly when conservative methods are ineffective. Use of mesh or graft material in repairs for anterior or posterior vaginal wall prolapse is controversial. Systematic reviews have shown that while mesh grafts will reduce short-term prolapse recurrence rates, mesh erosion complications necessitate a serious consideration of the type of surgery to be undertaken. In comparative studies reviewed for outcomes, it has been demonstrated that evidence shows that non-absorbable synthetic mesh significantly reduces recurrence but with a greater likelihood of erosion compared to biological grafts (Bain et al., 2008). These findings emphasize the importance of individualized patient education and informed consent, allowing women to make decisions that are rooted in their personal values and health goals during the navigation of treatment options. Overall, the resolution of prolapse of pelvic organs requires a holistic approach with modifications in lifestyle, surgery, and ongoing research seeking improved patient outcomes. With the multifactorial nature of risk factors such as occupational hazards and the body's inherent predispositions depending on the population, individualized preventive measures should be given priority. Additionally, the medical fraternity needs to promote greater awareness of pelvic health so that women are encouraged to seek intervention in advance of the deteriorating stage. As science continues to uncover the intricacies of pelvic organ prolapse, patients and providers must remain current with the existing evidence and available treatments, which have a direct influence on quality of life (Bates et al., 2020; Bain et al., 2008). This intricate approach ultimately results in enhancing women's health and sustaining their wellbeing.

In talking about the complexity of pelvic organ prolapse (POP), it is crucial to summarize the principal outcomes of more recent studies. The data refer to pelvic organ prolapse as a widespread condition, directly associated with such factors as childbirth and advanced age. One of the most interesting features of research is the emphasis on the effectiveness of pelvic floor muscle training (PFMT) as a conservative method of treatment. The evidence indicates that individualized PFMT can lead to a remarkable reduction in symptoms of prolapse over low-level lifestyle modifications (Abrams et al., 2008). This identifies the promise of non-surgical management for women who present with prolapse symptoms and indicates a move towards thinking in terms of understanding physical therapy in pelvic floor well-being. Greater scrutiny also recognizes that the quantification of the symptoms of prolapse of the pelvic organs through the utilization of standardized scoring scales, such as the Pelvic Organ Prolapse Symptom Score (POP-SS), is demonstrated to be highly internally consistent and responsive to change. In one study of the POP-SS, women who attended for operation had significantly elevated pre-operative symptom scores compared with women who were presented with conservative treatment (Abrams et al., 2008). Above all, this study also highlighted that post-operative scores showed major improvements, with the results of surgery delivering a greater reduction of symptoms in comparison with PFMT alone. This finding validates the notion that while surgery is beneficial, conservative measures must not be underestimated and should be part of a multidisciplinary approach to treatment. In addition, the cost-effectiveness of pelvic floor muscle training is an important factor that impacts clinical decision-making in treating pelvic organ prolapse. One comparison study on the cost-effectiveness of PFMT versus standard treatment determined that participants assigned to individualized PFMT reported fewer symptoms and higher satisfaction at 12-month follow-up compared to less intensive management group participants (Barry et al., 2013). Notably, the intervention group reported an impressive change in perceived condition, a key indicator of treatment success. As medical technology improves, being aware of these cost-benefit ratios will prove key to guiding patients and professionals along effective and knowledgeable treatment avenues for pelvic organ prolapse.

KEY TERMS FROM THIS CHAPTER

- Advanced imaging techniques
- Body mechanics
- Emotional support
- Intra-abdominal pressure
- Lifestyle interventions
- Medical interventions
- Nonoperative management
- Pathophysiological mechanisms
- Pelvic examination
- Pelvic floor muscle training (PFMT)
- Pelvic organ prolapse (POP)
- Biological xenografts
- Cystocele management
- Endocrine changes
- Labor process
- Manchester operation
- Mental health management
- Organ prolapse symptom scores (POP-SS)
- Patient experience
- Pelvic floor dysfunction
- Pelvic floor muscles
- Pelvic walls

CRITICAL THINKING QUESTIONS

1. **Which pelvic organ is most commonly involved in pelvic organ prolapse?**
   a. Bladder
   b. Small intestine
   c. Rectum
   d. Uterus
2. **What is the most common symptom of pelvic organ prolapse?**
   a. Vaginal bleeding
   b. Pelvic pain during menstruation
   c. Sensation of a vaginal bulge or pressure
   d. Sudden weight gain
3. **Which of the following is a risk factor for pelvic organ prolapse?**
   a. Nulliparity
   b. Obesity
   c. Early menopause
   d. Use of oral contraceptives
4. **The Pelvic Organ Prolapse Quantification (POP-Q) system is used to:**
   a. Diagnose urinary tract infections
   b. Stage endometriosis
   c. Classify the severity of pelvic organ prolapse
   d. Detect cervical cancer
5. **Which of the following is a non-surgical treatment option for pelvic organ prolapse?**
   a. Hysterectomy
   b. Vaginal mesh placement
   c. Pessary insertion
   d. Oophorectomy

Short Answer Questions

1. What are the main components of the pelvic floor anatomy?
2. Name three common types of pelvic organ prolapse.
3. What are the primary causes and risk factors for pelvic organ prolapse?
4. What symptoms might indicate the presence of pelvic organ prolapse?
5. What are common treatment options for pelvic organ prolapse?
6. How can pelvic organ prolapse affect a woman's psychological and social well-being?

Answer to Critical Thinking Questions

1. (a) 2. (c) 3. (b) 4. (c) 5. (c)

REFERENCES

1. Abdulaziz, M., Macnab, A., & Stothers, L. (2018). Effects of posture and gravity on pelvic organ prolapse. https://core.ac.uk/download/322437091.pdf (accessed on 15th June 2025).
2. Abramov, Y., Almeida, F. G., Berghmans, B., Bo, K., et al. (2016). An International Urogynecological Association (IUGA)/International Continence Society (ICS) joint report on the terminology for the conservative and nonpharmacological management of female pelvic floor dysfunction. https://core.ac.uk/download/293861075.pdf (accessed on 15th June 2025).
3. Abrams, P., Adams, E., Avery, K., Barber, M., Bugge, C., Bump, R., et al. (2008). Psychometric properties of the Pelvic Organ Prolapse Symptom Score. https://core.ac.uk/download/177138.pdf (accessed on 15th June 2025).
4. Adelowo, A., Coulter, A., Elders, A., Jordan, B., Shrestha, B., Haylen, B. T., Jaye, C., et al. (2019). Women's experiences of receiving care for pelvic organ prolapse: A qualitative study. https://core.ac.uk/download/293865525.pdf (accessed on 15th June 2025).
5. Allen, R. E., Anthony, S., Frudinger, A., Gilpin, S., Jackson, S., Johanson, R. B., et al. (2000). The effects of childbirth on the pelvic-floor. https://core.ac.uk/download/19418527.pdf (accessed on 15th June 2025).
6. Bain, C., Burr, J. M., Fraser, C. M., Glazener, C., et al. (2008). Efficacy and safety of using mesh or grafts in surgery for anterior and/or posterior vaginal wall prolapse: Systematic review and meta-analysis. https://core.ac.uk/download/177131.pdf (accessed on 15th June 2025).
7. Barry, S., Dickson, S., Elders, A., Frawley, H., et al. (2013). Individualized pelvic floor muscle training in women with pelvic organ prolapse: A multicenter randomized controlled trial. https://core.ac.uk/download/16462747.pdf (accessed on 15th June 2025).
8. Basappa, P. K., Gaddam, R., Gangadharan, K., Shivaraju, S., et al. (2020). Prevalence of pelvic floor dysfunction in women attending obstetrics and gynecology OPD at PES Institute of Medical Sciences and Research, Kuppa. https://core.ac.uk/download/539898299.pdf (accessed on 15th June 2025).
9. Bates, M. N., Devkota, H. R., Ghimire, D. J., Harris, M., et al. (2020). Bio-mechanical risk factors for uterine prolapse among women living in the hills of west Nepal: A case-control study. https://core.ac.uk/download/287623816.pdf (accessed on 15th June 2025).
10. Biskupski, M., Cygnarowicz, A., Hosseinnejad, N., Korotko, A., et al. (2024). Pelvic organ prolapse–General overview and latest therapy possibilities. https://core.ac.uk/download/636385615.pdf (accessed on 15th June 2025).
11. Bodean, O. M., Cirstoiu, M., Diaconu, C. C., Marcu, R., et al. (2018). Pelvic floor disorders in gynecological malignancies: An overlooked problem? https://core.ac.uk/download/216808110.pdf (accessed on 15th June 2025).
12. Braila, A. D., Braila, M., Deca, M., Lungulescu, C., et al. (2019). Conservative surgical treatment in cervical dysplastic lesions associated with cystorectocele. https://core.ac.uk/download/232440349.pdf (accessed on 15th June 2025).
13. Campbell, M., Rattray, C., Stewart, P., Stewart, K., Stewart, B., & Simms Stewart, D. (2022). Profile of women with pelvic organ prolapse at the University Hospital of the West Indies: Risk factors and presentation. *Journal of Obstetrics and Gynecology, 42*, 2220–2224. https://

www.semanticscholar.org/paper/7447ecb9dd45086e2766b865ea7db26ddba9c6fa (accessed on 15th June 2025).

14. Carpenter, J. S., Chen, C. X., Heit, M. H., Rand, C., et al. (2018). A scoping study of psychosocial factors in women diagnosed with and/or treated for pelvic organ prolapse. https://core.ac.uk/download/286682360.pdf (accessed on 15th June 2025).
15. Dave, A., Dave, A., Goel, V., Joshi, A., et al. (2017). MR imaging evaluation for the assessment of pelvic organ prolapses: A newer technique. https://core.ac.uk/download/544391465.pdf (accessed on 15th June 2025).
16. de Melo Andrade Coura, M. (2018). The role of three-dimensional endoanal ultrasound in preoperative evaluation of anorectal diseases. https://core.ac.uk/download/322436824.pdf (accessed on 15th June 2025).
17. Formosa, M. (2009). Le Fort colpocleisis: Re-visited and re-proposed. https://core.ac.uk/download/46602231.pdf (accessed on 15th June 2025).
18. Glazener, C. M. A., Hagen, S., Ramsay, I., Sinclair, L., et al. (2009). A randomized controlled trial of pelvic floor muscle training for stages I and II pelvic organ prolapses. https://core.ac.uk/download/177139.pdf (accessed on 15th June 2025).
19. Hamid, R., & Losco, G. (2014). Pelvic organ prolapse-associated cystitis. https://core.ac.uk/download/29410932.pdf (accessed on 15th June 2025).
20. Jokhio, A. H., MacArthur, C., & Rizvi, R. M. (2020). Prevalence of pelvic organ prolapse in women, associated factors and impact on quality of life in rural Pakistan: Population-based study. https://core.ac.uk/download/322820506.pdf (accessed on 15th June 2025).
21. Kalata, U., Jarkiewicz, M., Pomian, A., Zwierzchowska, A., Horosz, E., Majkusiak, W., Żelazowska-Rutkowska, B., et al. (2024). The influence of successful treatment of stress urinary incontinence and pelvic organ prolapse on depression, anxiety, and insomnia—A prospective intervention impact assessment study. *Journal of Clinical Medicine, 13*, 1528. https://doi.org/10.3390/jcm13061528 (accessed on 15th June 2025).
22. McKinlay, K. (2020). "I have no life and neither do the ones watching me suffer": Women's lived experiences of transvaginal mesh implant surgery. https://core.ac.uk/download/482252660.pdf (accessed on 15th June 2025).
23. Petros, P. (2021). Pelvic ligament repair with slings–A foundation stone for solution of the ageing crisis in female pelvic urology. *Central European Journal of Urology, 74*, 563–565. https://www.semanticscholar.org/paper/75189d8c3b11f2b4b23a23a9ba8eb2285cecae80 (accessed on 15th June 2025).
24. Razzak, L. (2018). Pathophysiology of pelvic organ prolapse. https://core.ac.uk/download/322436731.pdf (accessed on 15th June 2025).
25. Reid, F., Aucott, L., Glazener, C., Elders, A., Hemming, C., Cooper, K., Freeman, R., et al. (2022). PROSPECT: 4- and 6-year follow-up of a randomized trial of surgery for vaginal prolapse. *International Urogynecology Journal, 34*, 67–78. https://doi.org/10.1007/s00192-022-05308-0 (accessed on 15th June 2025).
26. Sinex, D. C. E. (2021). Shifting and shaping perceptions: Towards the characterization and literacy of female pelvic organ support. https://core.ac.uk/download/479151697.pdf (accessed on 15th June 2025).

27. Takano, C. C., Araujo, M. M., Joã, M., & Sartori, M. G. F. (2008). Learning with the Amerindians: The evaluation of pelvic floor disorders among indigenous women who live in the Xingu Indian Park, Brazil. https://core.ac.uk/download/pdf/287858.pdf (accessed on 15th June 2025).
28. Torgbenu, E. L., Aimakhu, C., & Morhe, E. (2020). Effect of Kegel exercises on pelvic floor muscle disorders in prenatal and postnatal women–A literature review. *Volume (16)*. https://www.semanticscholar.org/paper/8f2f4098ddfcf55f57ec10fb524c8fe19cd8bb61 (accessed on 15th June 2025).
29. Zhang, L., Lv, X., & Tang, J. (2021). Efficacy of pelvic floor magnetic stimulation combined with electrical stimulation on postpartum pelvic organ prolapse: A retrospective study. *Pelviperineology*. https://www.semanticscholar.org/paper/f4aa56d7c7899460e1416c52fad0b3a1c31f5f01 (accessed on 15th June 2025).

TUBERCULOSIS OF THE FEMALE GENITAL TRACT

10

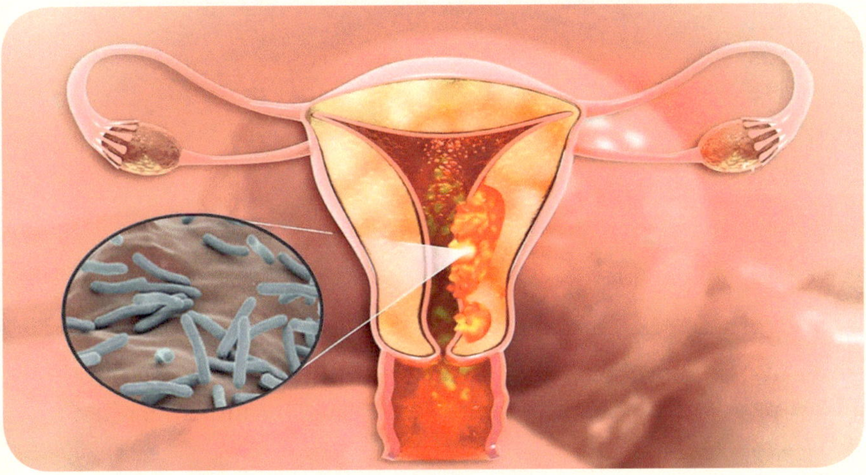

LEARNING OBJECTIVES

After studying this chapter, you will be able to:

1. Describe the epidemiology of tuberculosis (TB).
2. Explain the pathophysiology of tuberculosis.
3. Identify the clinical manifestations of tuberculosis.
4. Discuss the diagnostic methods used for tuberculosis.
5. Evaluate the treatment options available for tuberculosis (TB).

Introduction

Tuberculosis (TB), an illness traditionally associated with pulmonary infections, has also been found to be a significant problem in many extrapulmonary locations, the most prevalent being the female genital tract. The rarity of genital tuberculosis relative to other forms of the disease tends to result in underdiagnosis or misdiagnosis, which further leads to delayed or inadequate therapy. Physicians require knowledge of the pathophysiology, risk factors, and clinical presentation of genital TB for timely intervention. In addition, the overlap between systemic and localized manifestations presents diagnostic problems that are usually replicated by other gynecologic conditions. An emphasis on clinician and patient awareness of this condition may facilitate early diagnosis, which is key to good management and improved outcomes. The prevalence of genital TB has direct associations with socioeconomic status and geographical location, with endemic TB countries being developing nations. Contributing causes include inadequate access to medical care, malnutrition, and higher rates of HIV co-infection, which weaken immune systems. Symptoms can vary, with the patient presenting with dysmenorrhea, pelvic pain, or infertility; yet these are often subtle and lead to misattribution to benign gynecological disease. For instance, delayed diagnoses in certain cases reveal advanced disease states complicating treatment protocols. As emphasized in the literature highlighting the importance of awareness, such early detection protocols might have a promising potential to alter the disease's course among infected patients (Myrvang et al., 2009). Recent case reports have illustrated the tremendous impact of genital TB on women's reproductive health and thus emphasized the necessity for intensive gynecological examinations among high-risk populations. Patients may have atypical presentation, i.e., vulvovaginal mass or discharge, and can be interpreted wrongly as malignancy (Schneider et al., 2013). The integration of histopathological examination with microbiological investigation remains crucial in making the diagnosis and initiating appropriate anti-tuberculous treatment, which might significantly improve patient outcomes. As more and more doctors are brought to their notice about the nuances of genital tuberculosis, the chance of ideal treatment regimens increases. It may enhance diagnostic and therapeutic approaches by initiating interdisciplinary working relationships among medical disciplines, which remains imperative in addressing the burden of this disease among women globally.

Definition of Tuberculosis

Tuberculosis (TB) is a bacterial infectious disease caused primarily by Mycobacterium tuberculosis. The organism primarily infects the lungs; however, extrapulmonary types involving the female genital tract are of significant clinical significance. Tuberculosis is a pathogenic organism with a complex ability to infect numerous tissues, with the potential to cause severe health complications if not early diagnosed and treated. TB remains a worldwide issue with widespread prevalence in all parts of the world. In female reproductive health, it is crucial to be knowledgeable about the ability of TB to infect and colonize these locations since this can result in disabling complications like end-stage disease and infertility. Therefore, it is important for clinicians and public health practitioners who manage cases of extrapulmonary TB to understand the definition and extent of tuberculosis.

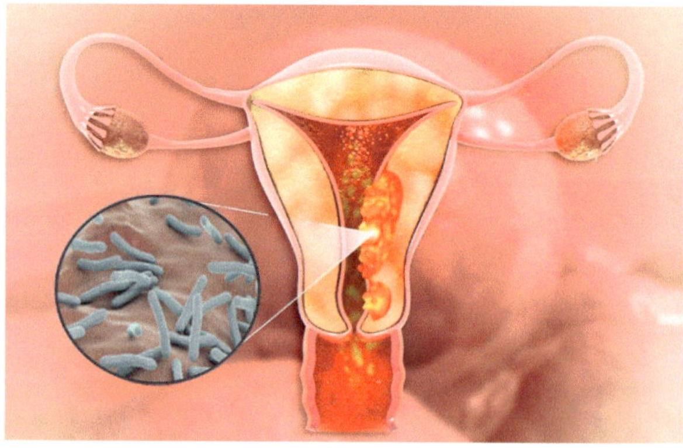

Source: https://www.medlineacademics.com/blog/female-genital-tuberculosis-and-infertility.php

Urogenital tuberculosis (UGTB) literally refers to the occurrence of TB in the urinary and genital tracts, including the kidneys, ureters, bladder, and genital organs. The presentation may be insidious, so diagnosis is delayed. All current evidence indicates that a high proportion of patients have an extremely protracted interval between symptom onset and starting treatment, and this underlines the need for greater awareness on the part of healthcare providers. With data from historical demographic figures revealing that a high proportion of UGTB cases are due to populations within endemic regions, strategic diagnostic and management approaches become imperative. The initial subtlety of the signs indicates that there is a risk of misdiagnosis, further emphasizing the imperative of understanding the idiosyncrasies of UGTB and their implications for female reproductive health (Chandran et al., 2021).

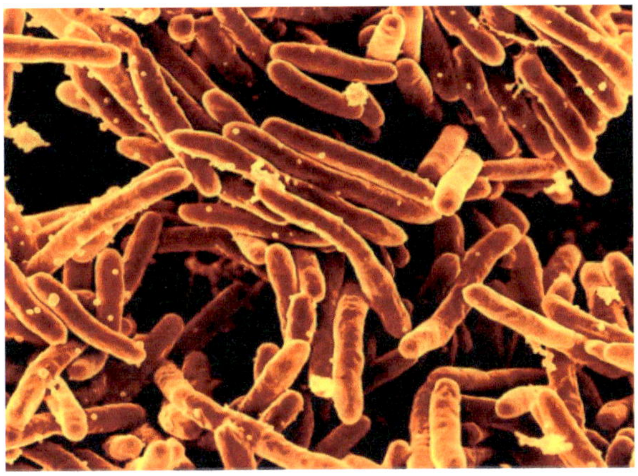

Figure 10.1. Urogenital tuberculosis (UGTB).

Source: https://en.wikipedia.org/wiki/Urogenital_tuberculosis#/media/File:Mycobacterium_tuberculosis_MEB_(1).jpg

Identification of UGTB as a differential diagnosis in women presenting with unexplained pelvic pain or menstrual abnormality is important. Radiologic imaging, including ultrasound and cross-sectional imaging, has been useful in defining the condition and distinguishing it from malignancies that may present similarly. Untreated UGTB has serious long-term effects that are typically severe, culminating in infertility or acute renal failure, which can considerably impact a woman's quality of life (Kearns et al., 2022). Clinicians must thus have a high index of suspicion for UGTB, especially in individuals with risk factors or histories consistent with exposure to tuberculosis. Early detection and appropriate treatment steps can significantly improve patient outcomes and avoid the risks of severe complications of this disorder.

Overview of Female Genital Tract Involvement

Involvement of the female genital tract in tuberculosis is often not accorded the respect it has in view of its serious impact on women's health. Tuberculosis may affect components of the female reproductive organs, such as the ovaries, fallopian tubes, and the uterus. The infection could present in the form of endometrial infection, which can lead to complications such as infertility, chronic pelvic pain, and ectopic pregnancy. Since the symptoms are likely to be similar to those of more common gynecological conditions, diagnosis can sometimes be challenging. Greater awareness within the medical community of this condition is necessary to avoid wrong diagnoses and delayed treatment, particularly since early treatment can dramatically enhance reproductive success. The practitioners must incorporate a full-scale response to the patient's history and differential diagnosis with tuberculosis in patients who present with unorthodox gynecologic symptoms, noting the need for robust educational programs within the medical profession. Studies have established that the pathogenesis of tuberculosis of the female genital tract is generally associated with hematogenous spread following post-primary pulmonary infection. Curiously, it is reported that women patients may present with solitary genital tuberculosis, modes of transmission differing from the common pulmonary dissemination (Balalau et al., 2017). Pelvic TB may result from more than one site of origin, including contiguous viscera or hematogenous infection, pointing towards its systemic nature. Depending upon the site of infection, the disease may result in extensive morbidity because of fibrosis, leading to blockade of reproductive organs, which consequently impairs fertility. Tuberculous salpingitis diagnoses are of particular interest as they can cause irreversible damage to fallopian tubes, precluding natural conception and necessitating advanced reproductive technologies for couples who want a child. Diagnosis and treatment of the infection are necessary for the resolution of greater public health issues in reproductive health. Treatment of active tuberculosis in the female genital tract greatly differs from standard gynecological procedures, necessitating integral, interdisciplinary care. The same routine treatment regimen of rifampicin, isoniazid, pyrazinamide, and ethambutol in pulmonary tuberculosis is likewise effective for genital tuberculosis cases. Aside from the pharmacologic management, the psychological and emotional aspects of the disease should now be dealt with in the context of the issues of fertility and chronic disease. Patient education is thus a key role of healthcare professionals in managing such complex cases. Emerging controversies during conferences, as presented by (Myrvang et al., 2009), revolve around the necessity of having collective healthcare strategies for increasing awareness and management of gynecological tuberculosis. Lastly, the integration of tuberculosis screening in routine gynecological examination among high-risk groups is capable of early diagnosis and intervention, improving reproductive health outcomes among infected women.

10.1. Epidemiology of Tuberculosis

Learning Outcome

1. Define global prevalence rates
2. Describe the risk factors for female genital tuberculosis
3. Understand the demographic variations in incidence

The epidemiology of tuberculosis (TB) is a critical public health concern due to its high prevalence and transmission patterns. TB is among the top infectious disease killers globally, particularly among low- and middle-income countries where healthcare access is limited. An estimated 10.6 million cases of TB were reported in 2021 alone, reflecting its widespread pervasiveness, as per the World Health Organization (WHO). In women's health, TB has likewise been directly associated with additional risks, such as the formation of extrapulmonary forms. These instances can complicate diagnosis and treatment because the symptoms may not be described in traditionally expected manners. Familiarizing ourselves with the epidemiological context that supports the development of TB in female populations is a recognition of the necessity of specialized interventions and health policies to contain the incidence as well as the morbidity in diverse groups. The relationship between psychiatric illnesses and infection rates, particularly that of tuberculosis, has emerged as a significant research focus. Psychological stressors such as adjustment disorder have been observed to increase the vulnerability towards infections such as TB significantly. A nationwide cohort study discovered that individuals who had adjustment disorder had higher rates of other infections, including sexually transmitted diseases, and may have implications for the spread of TB among women. The stress could lead to unhealthy lifestyles, suppress immune function, and increase susceptibility to infectious diseases like TB. By examining these root causes, it is clear that mental health plays a key role in the epidemiology of tuberculosis, and thus the public health response is further complicated and necessitates compounded efforts on psychological and physical health alike.

Further, gender-specific epidemiology offers evidence of a kind that implies that women may have unique difficulties in fighting tuberculosis. TB in women usually appears to be under-reported, particularly in populations where social stigma of female reproductive health is prevalent. Inter-action between TB and gynecological health requires an in-depth understanding of biological susceptibility to infection along with social determinants of health. Since one may see in studies on the interaction of infection and mental illness disorders, women might be overrepresented because of many cultural and systemic biases, such that there is increased susceptibility. With health systems evolving to combat TB, there remains an immediate call for integrated approaches based on both epidemiological data and the specific demands of women's health, ultimately resulting in better outcomes of female genital tract tuberculosis.

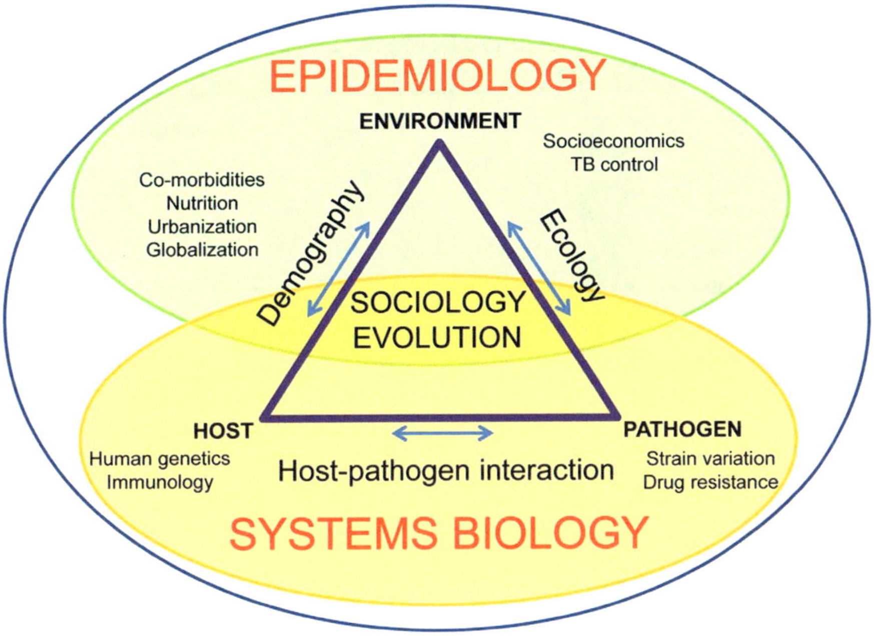

Figure 10.2. A systems epidemiology approach to TB research.

Source: https://www.researchgate.net/figure/A-systems-epidemiology-approach-to-TB-research-The-spread-of-TB-is-influenced-by-social_fig1_38035234

10.1.1. Global Prevalence Rates

The global burden of tuberculosis (TB), particularly of the female genital tract, is a serious public health problem. TB ranks as the second most common infectious cause of death globally, responsible for an enormous rate of morbidity and mortality among at-risk groups. In 2013, there were an estimated 9.0 million incident cases of TB, with about 1.5 million deaths from TB (predominantly among those with HIV infection). These statistics highlight a major need for awareness and targeted intervention in the field of women's health, addressing not only the immediate consequences of the disease but also the secondary conditions, such as infertility resulting from genital TB. The disparities in prevalence rates among different countries bring to the fore a wide need for targeted public health interventions to manage and mitigate the effects of this condition, particularly where the burden is highest, such as India, where 18% of women are estimated to be suffering from genital TB (Parks et al., 2017). Research has shown that TB is not only limited to pulmonary presentations but also significantly impacts the female reproductive system with catastrophic results if left untreated. Genital tuberculosis most commonly results from ascending infection pathways due to untreated sexually transmitted infections, causing pelvic inflammatory disease. These infections have the potential to cause structural damage to the reproductive tract, resulting in tubal ligation infertility, a serious concern for women of reproductive age. It must be observed that this disease often goes undetected since TB and reproductive health conditions are stigmatized. Furthermore, new findings suggest that infections such as *Chlamydia trachomatis* are a prime motive force of this condition, forecasting the necessity for additional clinical screening and early intervention methods (Parks et al., 2017).

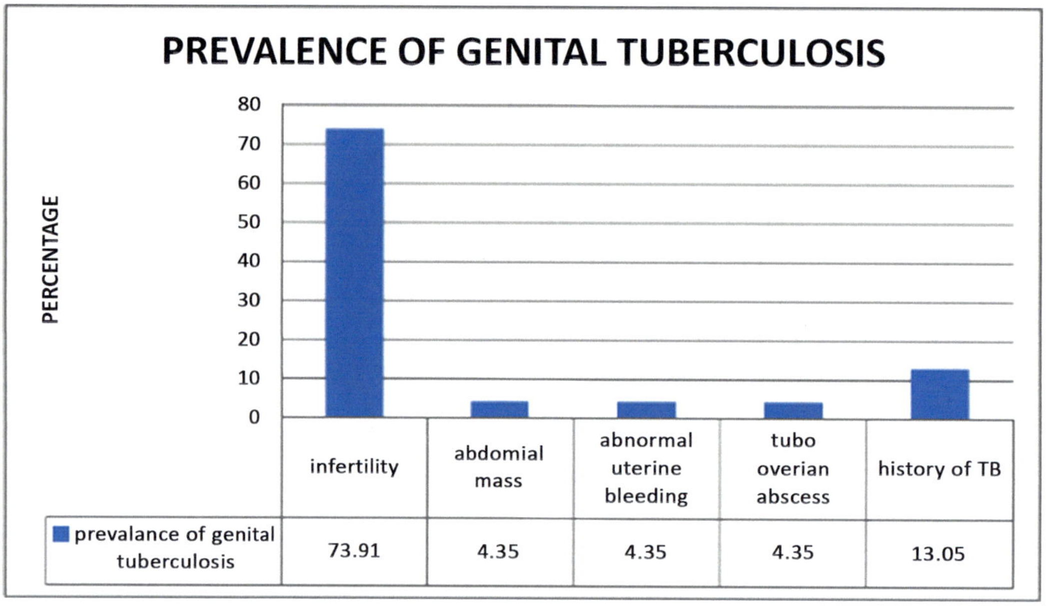

Figure 10.3. Prevalence of genital tuberculosis.

Source: https://www.researchgate.net/figure/Prevalence-of-genital-tuberculosis_fig1_276531833

The intricate interaction between infertility and TB necessitates multi-disciplinary intervention to address this urgent health crisis. The socio-economic implications of genital tuberculosis also extend to the issues of its emergence. Women suffering from the condition can face significant obstacles in pursuing fertility, causing psychological trauma and social stigmatization. This suffering is worse in low- and middle-income countries where the healthcare resources are limited, and diagnosis and treatment are delayed. Cultural beliefs on fertility also make the discussion of genital TB's impact on women's health more complicated. Handling the prevalence of tuberculosis among females calls for comprehensive health education interventions consisting of public symptom perception, rapid access to medical treatment, and the interconnection between STIs and TB. These interventions are paramount in diminishing the impact of genital tuberculosis alongside making women autonomous in their reproductive health process, ensuring that important resources are channeled towards solving the public health matter effectively (Kaur et al., 2019).

10.1.2. Risk Factors For Female Genital Tuberculosis

The pathophysiology of female genital tuberculosis (FGTB) involves a multifactorial interaction of causative risk factors, rendering it common and aggressive. In these, socioeconomic status emerges as the determining factor. Women with low socioeconomic status are deprived of access to health care, resulting in delayed treatment and diagnosis of tuberculosis (TB). Furthermore, these women are also more susceptible to TB due to improper nutrition and exposure to overcrowded places, where the transmission of the pathogen is more likely to occur. The convergence of poverty and health outcomes highlights the importance of focused interventions in which improving resources for health and education among marginalized populations is addressed. Adequate addressing of these socioeconomic disparities is critical in minimizing the risk of FGTB as well as in improving the health outcomes for the targeted women. Psychological distress has also been described as a prominent risk factor for FGTB. There has been an indication from previous research of a correlation between stress disorders, such as posttraumatic stress disorder (PTSD) and adjustment disorder, and increased vulnerability to infection, including TB. In general, research shows that people with high levels of stress can have compromised immune function, making them more susceptible to infection.

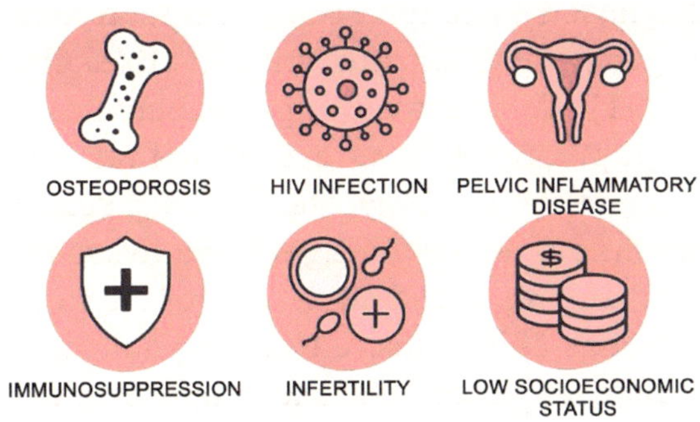

Figure 10.4. Risk Factors for Female Genital Tuberculosis.

Source: https://sdmntpreastus.oaiusercontent.com/files/00000000-9010-61f9-87d5-51fd424bf329/raw?se=2025-05-26T08%3A35%3A50Z&sp=r&sv=2024-08-04&sr=b&scid=e56a49c4-4deb-5b69-9ea9-f7d24cf12a3f&skoid=b0fd38cc-3d33-418f-920e-4798de4acdd1&sktid=a48cca56-e6da-484e-a814-9c849652bcb3&skt=2025-05-25T12%3A32%3A36Z&ske=2025-05-26T12%3A32%3A36Z&sks=b&skv=2024-08-04&sig=oPhad77I%2BVikVfhq1q/WZBXLQtHt8UQfEL9uWyGAad8%3D

The physical consequences of chronic stress can lead to inadequate nutrition and avoidance of medical care, adding to the risk of acquiring FGTB. Identification of psychological stressors in high-risk women is needed to provide proper prevention, ultimately leading to improvement in immune function and reduction in the prevalence of this disorder. A second critical risk area within the FGTB terrain is the intersection of sexually transmitted diseases (STIs) and reproductive health. Women are particularly vulnerable to STIs, and these can enhance the risk for the pathogenesis of FGTB by enhancing the inflammatory response to STIs. Cervical or pelvic inflammatory disease can create a terrain in which *Mycobacterium tuberculosis* can reside within the genital tract. Both sexual health and TB, furthermore, are stigmatized, discouraging women from seeking necessary medical interventions, resulting in cycles of unattended infections and arising complications. To effectively manage these interconnected issues, sexual health education and access to STI and TB testing must be part of a comprehensive response, ultimately aimed at dismantling obstacles that discourage effective healthcare delivery among at-risk women.

10.1.3. Demographic Variations in Incidence

Demographic variation in tuberculosis of the female genital tract is significant to comprehend in order to address the public health issue caused by the disease. Age, socio-economic status, and geographical site all have a vital role in shaping tuberculosis among women. Young women, particularly women of childbearing age, are more vulnerable due to biological and social factors like hormonal changes and increased exposure to sexually transmitted diseases. Evidence indicates that the prevalence of such tuberculosis is much higher in low-income communities and disadvantaged groups, as access to healthcare is limited. Therefore, being cognizant of these population conditions not only goes hand in hand with interpreting the rates of prevalence but also emphasizes the need for specially tailored interventions that respond to the specific vulnerabilities of the differing groups within the population.

Moreover, the intersection of socio-economic standing and patterns of health behavior further complicates the case of tuberculosis among women. Women of lesser socio-economic standing are disproportionately exposed to every possible health disparity, ranging from lower levels of access to preventive healthcare services to education regarding sexually transmitted diseases.

Research emphasizes that, if not treated, infection can potentially lead to severe complications, including tubal ligation infertility, which is a major problem linked with the presence of pathogens like *Chlamydia trachomatis* and *Neisseria gonorrhoeae* (Parks et al., 2017). The intricate relationship between socio-economic status, access to healthcare services, and the spread of infection necessitates an interdisciplinary approach towards the treatment and prevention of tuberculosis in the female genital tract.

Improvements in healthcare education and outreach in high-risk populations can erode these disparities and improve overall health outcomes. Beyond socio-economic determinants, cultural beliefs and practices also contribute to the spread of tuberculosis within different demographic groups. Cultural stigma regarding sexually transmitted diseases contributes to worsening delays in treatment and silence regarding reproductive health. In some societies, cultural values may discourage women from receiving effective healthcare, aggravating the health hazards of female genital tract tuberculosis.

For instance, lack of open communication and learning concerning infertility due to undiagnosed infections can perpetuate health emergency neglect and misuse (Uusküla et al., 2001). To effectively fight tuberculosis in such populations, it is essential that public health interventions involve culturally sensitive interventions, empowering women to seek care without stigma. The identification of the cultural dimensions of healthcare enables public health efforts to enhance awareness and eventually health improvement for at-risk women.

Test Your Knowledge

1. What are the estimated global prevalence rates of female genital tuberculosis?
2. Which key risk factors contribute to the development of female genital tuberculosis?

10.2. Pathophysiology of Tuberculosis

Learning Outcome

1. Define the mechanism of infection
2. Identify the immune response to Mycobacterium tuberculosis
3. Identify the impact on female reproductive health

The pathophysiology of tuberculosis (TB) is a complex interaction between *Mycobacterium tuberculosis* and the host immune system. After primary exposure, when the bacteria are inhaled into the lungs, they survive phagocytic evasion by macrophages and, at times, granuloma development in order to confine infection. Granulomas are made up of activated macrophages, T lymphocytes, and components of the extracellular matrix, which serve as a line of containment against the spread of the bacteria. Further, in some cases, M. tuberculosis can be transmitted from the primary site, leading to extrapulmonary expressions of TB, such as infection of the female genital tract. This spread is influenced by co-infection and immune status, such that impaired immune response, for instance, among HIV patients, tends to exacerbate the disease, leading to proliferation of the organism and severe manifestations requiring urgent clinical attention. In women, the importance of genital tuberculosis (GTB) lies particularly in its role in infertility and chronic pelvic pain. Histopathological features typically reveal endometrial and cervical involvement since the disease has the potential to result in chronic granulomatous inflammation and tuberculous lesions. A high-impact study noted that the prevalence of genital TB in women with idiopathic chronic pelvic pain was as much as 35.38%, indicating its value as a differential diagnosis in these patients. The study used both the AFB cultures and histological examinations to ascertain the existence of mycobacterial infection effectively. In addition, the frequency of nonspecific GTB manifestations that may overlap with other gynecological pathologies complicates timely diagnosis and delays effective treatment, thus pointing towards the importance of awareness and screening practice among health professionals (Bharadwaj et al., 2017). Cervical cancer-tuberculosis cross-talk is increasingly an area of interest, partly in light of M. tuberculosis involvement in tumors. Chronic inflammation induced by TB has been speculated to play a role somehow in carcinogenic processes in the cervix, particularly where there are co-infections with high-risk HPVs. The convergence of pathogens raises questions regarding the mechanisms allowing M. tuberculosis to coincide with neoplastic alterations. In rare instances, cervical cancer has been found together with cervical TB, which necessitates an integrated mode of therapy that addresses both diseases. The diagnostic challenges also persist, as histopathological examinations normally reveal granulomatous inflammation, covering up the malignancy underneath, thereby making management modalities more intricate. Along with diagnostic vigilance and cutting-edge imaging methods, early detection and patient outcomes for this outstanding convergence of disease would be enhanced (Degeratu et al., 2018).

10.2.1. Mechanism of Infection

Pathogenesis of tuberculosis (TB) infection of the female genital tract is complex and involves interaction between *Mycobacterium tuberculosis* and the host immune system. In the majority of instances, primary infection occurs through inhalation of airborne droplets, with subsequent hematogenous dissemination of the bacteria, spreading through the bloodstream. In women, the bacteria are localized in the reproductive organs, such as the ovary and uterus, and produce characteristic pathologic changes like granuloma formation. The localized infection, if untreated, leads to infertility or ectopic pregnancy. Since TB of the female genital tract is usually secondary to a pre-existing pulmonary infection, it is imperative to understand the interaction between the two sites for diagnosis as well as treatment. It is only through an elaboration of how TB maintains its peculiar mode of persistence that research can be further explored into its interaction with the immune response of its host in order to improve therapeutic responses and alleviate disease burden for women's reproductive health. *Mycobacterium tuberculosis*' intracellular survival tactic constitutes another crucial element of its infection mechanism, especially within the setting of the female genital tract.

When it infects host cells, M. tuberculosis can escape from immune responses through various mechanisms such as interference with phagosome-lysosome fusion and cytokine signaling pathways. This allows the bacteria to live in a latent form, also referred to as latency, which is chronic and hard to treat and eliminate. Secondly, the immune evasion processes facilitate chronic inflammation and tissue damage, culminating in scarring and dysfunction of the reproductive system. This chronic stage of inflammation portrays the complexity of TB pathogenesis, contributing to the risks of other co-infections such as *Chlamydia trachomatis*, whose role in reproductive morbidities and infertility has been highlighted in literature (Parks et al., 2017).

A clear understanding of these processes is imperative for the development of specific therapies and improved patient outcomes. Finally, the interplay between *Mycobacterium tuberculosis* and other sexually transmitted diseases (STIs) underscores the need for an interdisciplinary intervention in dealing with female genital tract tuberculosis. STIs such as *Chlamydia trachomatis* and *Neisseria gonorrhoeae* could cause inflammation and damage to the genitourinary system, which might facilitate the upward movement of the TB bacterium. The evidence suggests that ongoing infection will increase the risk of TB acquisition in the female genital tract, creating a morbidity pattern that is difficult to break (Parks et al., 2017). Furthermore, *Chlamydia trachomatis* has established mechanisms of chronic infection that make the host immune system more complex, such as the ability to downmodulate immunity via interferon gamma-induced mechanisms. This interaction between TB and other infections presents a rare challenge to public health strategies, and efficient screening, treatment at an early stage, and comprehensive sexual health education are required to avoid the risk of such interrelated infections..

10.2.2. Immune Response to Mycobacterium tuberculosis

The immune response to *Mycobacterium tuberculosis* (*M. tuberculosis*) is multifaceted and critical to the diagnosis of both pulmonary and extrapulmonary tuberculosis, including infections of the female genital tract. The activation of the innate immune system with infection causes an inflammatory response of macrophage and dendritic cell recruitment. These immune cells play a central role in the phagocytosis of the bacilli and also act as antigen-presenting cells, activating naive T cells and directing the immune response to a Th1 profile. The cytokine induction of cytokines such as interferon-gamma is also instrumental in driving macrophage activation to enable them to contain and control M. tuberculosis replication more effectively. But this very effective immune response can be seriously defective in immunocompromised states like severe HIV disease, conferring enhanced susceptibility to disseminated infection, making it more difficult to diagnose and treat further (Baez-Corujo et al., 2018).

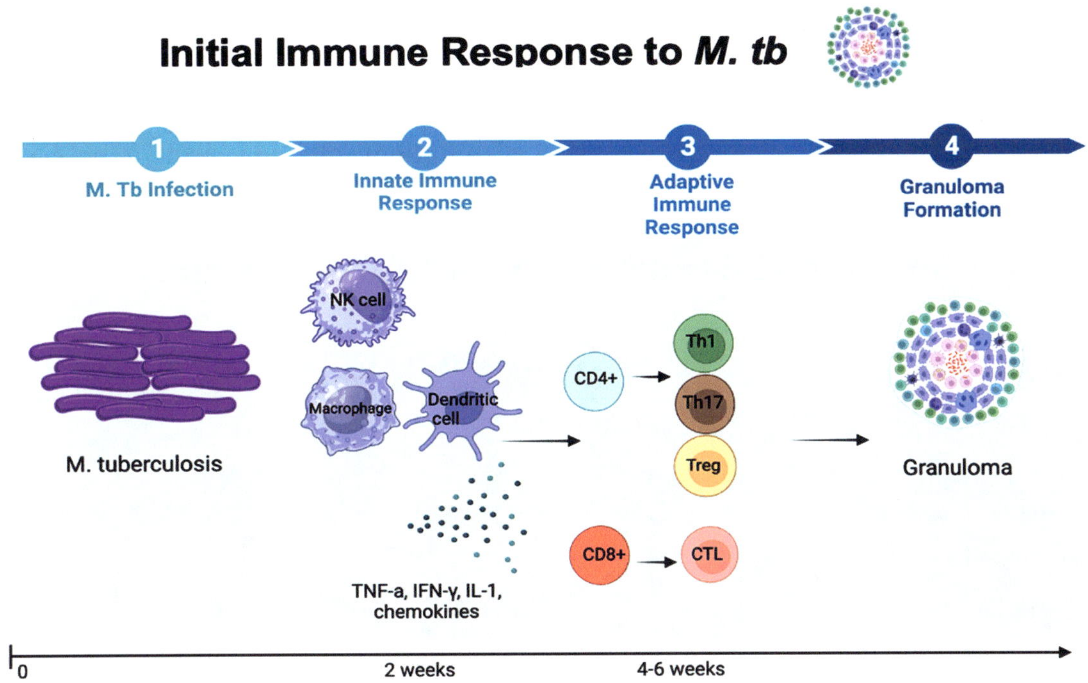

Figure 10.5. The introduction of *M. tb* into the host cell initiates the innate immune response, involving a coordinated effort of macrophages, natural killer cells, and dendritic cells. These immune cells release pivotal cytokines such as TNF-α, IFN-γ, IL-1, and other chemokines, subsequently activating CD4+ and CD8+ T cells to release their specific cytokines. This orchestrated immune cascade results in the formation of granulomas, representing the hallmark aspect of the host's strategy to confine and regulate the bacterial presence.

Source: https://www.mdpi.com/2076-393X/12/7/730

The role of cellular immunity is most crucial in the scenario of female genital tract tuberculosis, a site that can be infected with mycobacteria with varied clinical presentations. Activation of CD4+ T helper cells and CD8+ cytotoxic T lymphocytes plays a significant role in developing an effective immune response that can potentially limit the spread of the organism and enable healing of infected tissues. Though cellular immunity plays an important role in the control of infection, evidence shows that M. tuberculosis has evaded host defense through mechanisms such as inhibition of phagosome-lysosome fusion within macrophages. Immune system evasion could lead to chronic infection and the development of extrapulmonary forms of tuberculosis, commonly more challenging to diagnose and treat. The comprehension of such intricate interaction between the host immunity and pathogen is pivotal in devising effective therapeutic and preventative measures against tuberculosis (Hickey et al., 2008). Comprehension of how the immune response occurs against *Mycobacterium tuberculosis*, particularly in the context of the female reproductive tract, has significant public health implications. Despite ongoing efforts at control and eradication of tuberculosis globally, extrapulmonary tuberculosis continues to rise, highlighting the need for improved diagnostic tools and therapeutic regimens. The challenge of genital tuberculosis diagnosis stems from its often nonspecific clinical presentation, a fact that can mimic other conditions of the female reproductive system. Furthermore, coexistence with underlying immunosuppression tends to exacerbate disease presentation, further rendering the clinical picture challenging. Enhancing our understanding of immune mechanisms and providing focused interventions can ultimately enhance patient outcomes and reduce the burden of this silent infection in the female population (Baez-Corujo et al., 2018).

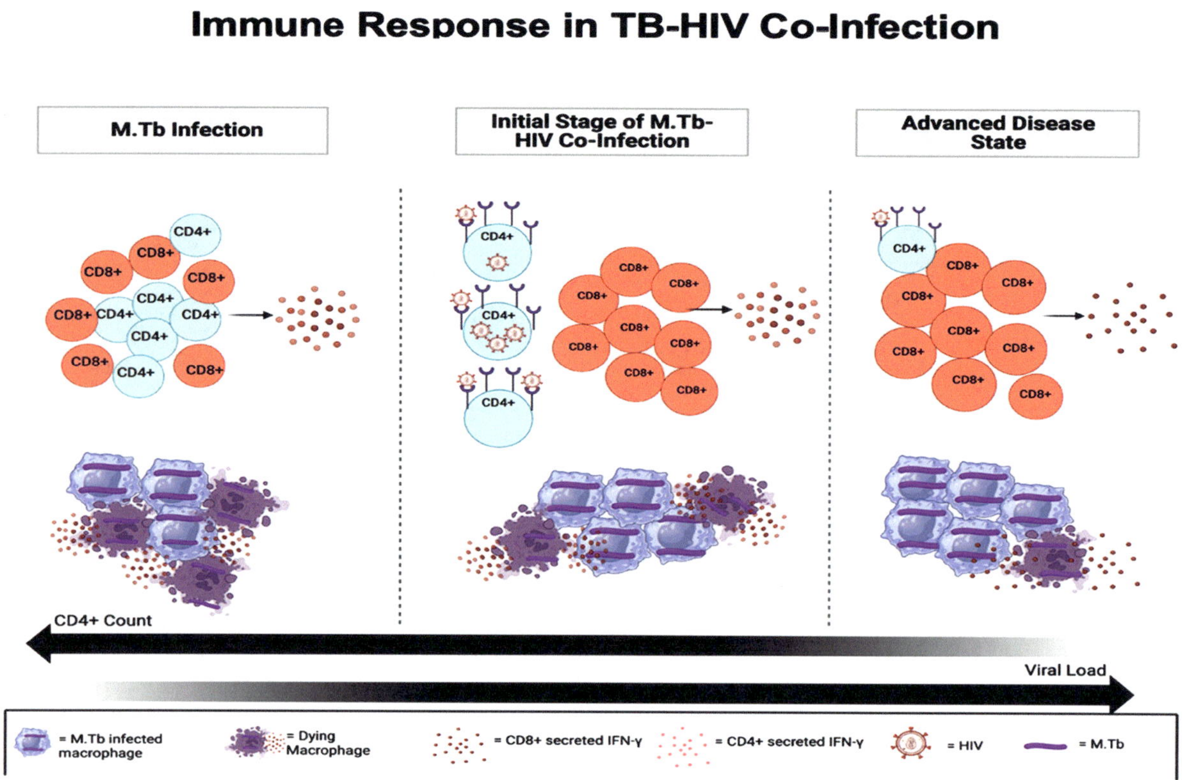

Figure 10.6. Both CD4+ and CD8+ T cells contribute to IFN-γ production in the body, with CD4+ T cells being the primary contributors. IFN-γ and other cytokines play a crucial role in macrophage activation and are responsible for cell-mediated immunity and phagocyte-dependent immune-protective responses in M. tb infection.

Source: https://www.mdpi.com/2076-393X/12/7/730

10.2.3. Impact on Female Reproductive Health

The impact of tuberculosis (TB) on the female reproductive system is increasingly emerging as a matter of concern, particularly with regard to fertility. Tuberculosis of the female genital tract can have serious reproductive consequences, such as infertility and fetal complications in pregnancy. Tuberculosis has a tendency to affect the fallopian tubes, with consequent scarring and occlusion that can severely impede fertility. It has been proven in research that tubal factor infertility, which accounts for much of infertility, is a consequence of occult infections ascending within the reproductive tract. In this regard, detection of such infections, particularly those due to *Chlamydia trachomatis* and *Neisseria gonorrhoeae*, is significant since they have been proven to be causative factors of reproductive morbidities like pelvic inflammatory disease and consequent tubal damage (Parks et al., 2017). Therefore, TB pathology demands a deep understanding of its implications on reproductive health in women, particularly where tuberculosis is endemic. Furthermore, the psychological implications of tuberculosis tend to complicate the physical health problems, hence further complicating the outcomes of reproductive health. Mental disorders, i.e., adjustment disorders, have been associated with increased risks of infection, which suggests the intersectional nature of psychological and physical health. Research has indicated that adjustment disorder patients have significantly higher rates of many types of infection, including sexually transmitted infections, which are essential to female reproductive health (Farkas et al., 2020).

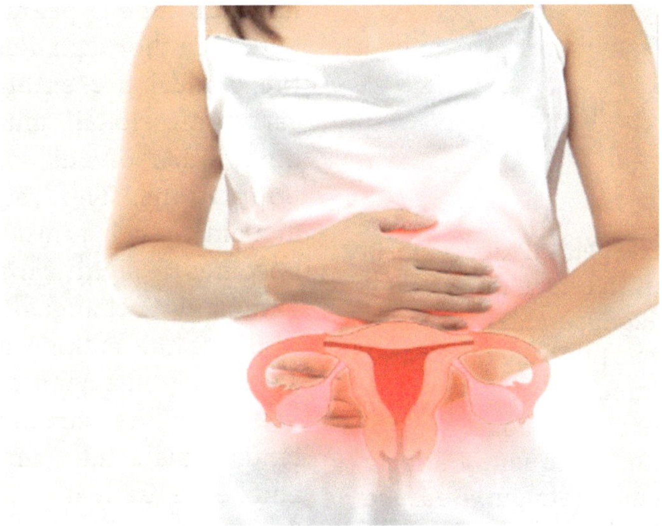

Source: https://external-content.duckduckgo.com/iu/?u=https%3A%2F%2Fh-leads.com%2Fwp-content%2Fuploads%2F2023%2F08%2Ftuberculosis.png&f=1&nofb=1&ipt=71f6f0e589ebac47d34c6261a58f0b3e9fe399aedb19e003e0d7412414145d29

Stress caused by the control of a long-term disease such as TB can lead to compromised immune function, thereby increasing susceptibility to infections that can hamper reproductive processes. This interaction emphasizes the need for addressing the mental factor in overcoming the broader consequences of TB on reproductive health with the same priority as both physical and psychological well-being. Lastly, the social stigma of tuberculosis may also lead to social isolation and defiance against medical intervention, further compromising the reproductive health of women. Women who have TB would be discriminated against, and this may deter them from seeking medical care or tests for reproductive health issues. Withholding access to such health resources raises the chances of an untreated infection that can lead to infertility or pregnancy complications. The intersection of social determinants of health, such as socioeconomic status, education, and access to health care, plays an important role in the reproductive health of women with tuberculosis. Therefore, awareness-raising, stigma reduction, and ensuring equitable access to reproductive health care interventions are important to address the multifaceted impact of tuberculosis on the reproductive health of women. This multi-disciplinary approach can eventually bring better health benefits to women afflicted with this debilitating disease.

Test Your Knowledge

1. How does Mycobacterium tuberculosis infect the female reproductive system?
2. What type of immune response is triggered by Mycobacterium tuberculosis infection?

10.3. Clinical Manifestations

Learning Outcome

1. Discuss the symptoms of female genital tuberculosis
2. Understand the diagnostic challenges and differential diagnosis

The clinical course of female genital tuberculosis (TB) is generally insidious in onset, making it a challenge to treat and diagnose early. Because the primary infectious focus typically originates from the lung or other extrapulmonary locations, the disease may spread hematogenously to the reproductive tract, but more frequently affects the fallopian tubes and endometrium. Because the majority of women with genital TB are of reproductive age, the subsequent infertility poses a significant issue. Presentations such as menstrual aberrations, pelvic pain, and abnormal vaginal discharge may initially be attributed to other female genital tract conditions, thereby further distorting the clinical presentation.

It is therefore critical that there is a subtle appreciation of these presentations by clinicians so that they can make an accurate diagnosis and apply therapeutic interventions accordingly, which will in turn find reflection in patient outcomes and quality of life. The variability of presentation of female genital tuberculosis underscores its complexity. Notably, the majority of patients have superficially similar presentations to those of common sexually transmitted diseases (STIs), hence leading to misdiagnosis. For instance, ulcerative masses or abnormal growths may superficially resemble conditions such as leishmaniasis or amoebiasis. In particular, endometrial lesions and occluded fallopian tube appearances may go undetected without a thorough diagnostic workup. Because the clinical presentation is so broad, health care professionals must possess an extremely high index of suspicion among susceptible populations. The requirement for imaging modalities such as hysterosalpingography (HSG) becomes a significant factor in illuminating pathological changes brought about by TB to facilitate the making of an accurate diagnosis and timely intervention (Akhbari et al., 2013). Moreover, the chronic nature of the disease tends to make the symptoms manifest gradually, and hence, early diagnosis is a challenging test. Over time, tuberculous lesion formation can lead to extensive scarring and dysfunction of the reproductive system, adding to infertility. Clinicians must remember that the majority of cases of genital tuberculosis are bilateral, that is, affecting both fallopian tubes, complicating reproductive outcomes in the process. Also, the presence of concomitant symptoms, such as abdominal pain, fever, or systemic evidence of active TB, can be red flags eliciting a prompt diagnostic response. Because differences in clinical presentation may hide the underlying pathology, healthcare providers must incorporate extensive diagnostic methods, including appropriate histories, physical examinations, and excellent imaging technology to ensure that female genital tract tuberculosis is adequately identified and managed (Richens et al., 2004).

10.3.1. Symptoms of Female Genital Tuberculosis

The clinical presentation of female genital tuberculosis (FGTB) is typically inconspicuous, primarily because the majority of the patients do not have a clear-cut symptom. In fact, the most common complaint is infertility, which occurs in an estimated 40 to 60 percent of women suffering from the disease and, thus, is a serious public health issue, particularly in the Indian subcontinent where its prevalence is predominantly high. Asymptomatic presentation of FGTB will most commonly be diagnosed during infertility investigations rather than by proactive screening.

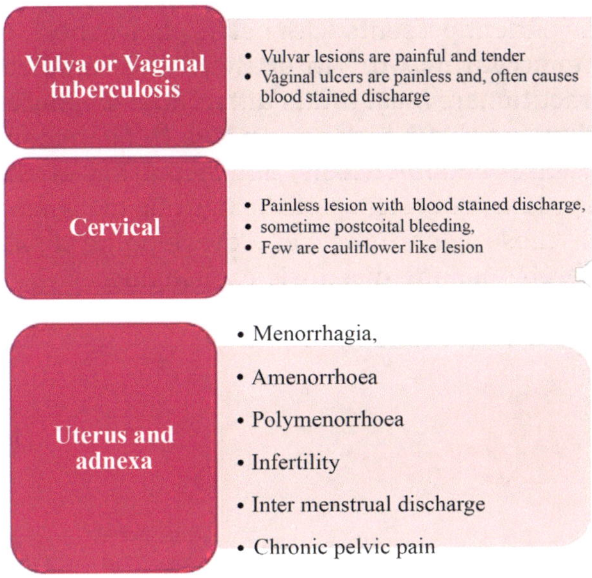

Figure 10.7. Symptoms of genital tuberculosis.

Source: https://www.slideshare.net/slideshow/genital-tuberculosis-234633741/234633741

Patients won't even become aware they have the condition until they have presented with complications related to infertility, thus emphasizing the insidious nature of the condition and the imperative need for increased awareness and targeted diagnostic activity among health care providers (Chate et al., 2016). Symptomatology of FGTB can also include abnormal menstrual cycles, dyspareunia, and pelvic pain, but they are not specific. Clinical presentation can even be subtle since FGTB will usually influence the endometrium and fallopian tubes by hematogenous dissemination from extra-genital sites like lymphatic tissues or the lungs (Akhbari et al., 2013).

With the advancement of the disease, the anatomical changes can lead to severe reproductive morbidity in the form of chronic pelvic inflammatory disease and ectopic pregnancy. Also, the involvement of the genitourinary tract makes the clinical situation problematic, leading to differential diagnosis issues with other gynecologic diseases. Hence, clinicians should be suspicious to a high degree while dealing with women of childbearing age, especially those experiencing difficulty in conceiving. Diagnostic challenge in the diagnosis of FGTB is also added to by the unpredictable clinical and radiological presentation of the condition. For instance, results from hysterosalpingography (HSG) may present classical patterns of tuberculosis, such as occluded fallopian tubes or irregular endometrial contours, to help in diagnosis. Normal results from HSG, however, do not rule out FGTB because there are cases where the endometrial biopsy will present unremarkable histopathology despite active disease. Accordingly, laparoscopic diagnosis emerges as an important diagnostic tool in diagnosing the existence of FGTB, with the advantage of direct visualization and biopsy of affected structures (Chate et al., 2016). This methodological approach enables good assessment of reproductive organs while opening the door for required therapeutic interventions, thus bridging the gap between diagnosis and patient management in the case of this debilitating disease (Akhbari et al., 2013).

10.3.2. Diagnostic Challenges

The diagnostic challenge arises from tuberculosis of the female genital tract because of the commonly indistinct presentation and the superimposition of signs and symptoms with other gynecological pathologies. The majority of patients present with nonspecific symptoms such as pelvic pain, irregular menstruation, or infertility that can easily be confused with more prevalent conditions, leading to misdiagnosis or delayed diagnosis. Moreover, the chronic nature of the disease can conceal its severity because symptoms may only manifest after extensive damage to reproductive organs, especially the fallopian tubes and endometrium, has already occurred. This diagnostic delay not only complicates the treatment but also puts the patients at critical risk, as without treatment, genital tuberculosis can lead to life-threatening complications, like infertility and ectopic pregnancy, contributing to the already growing public health concern due to tuberculosis in reproductive medicine. Imaging tests, endometrial biopsy, or laparoscopy are diagnostic tools that can provide critical information; however, they are not always diagnostic of genital tuberculosis. For instance, the sensitivity of imaging technologies like ultrasound or MRI is variable and fails to detect infection until late stages set in, which is often too late for conservative intervention. Moreover, sampling techniques can yield false negatives if the causative organism is present in minute quantities or if there's an atypical presentation, thereby complicating accurate diagnosis.

10.3.3. Differential Diagnosis

Differential diagnosis is a critical element in the diagnosis of female genital tract tuberculosis (TB), given its varied clinical presentation that can mimic other gynecological conditions. When the patient presents with pelvic pain, abnormal menstruation, or infertility, the medical practitioners must retain differential diagnoses in their minds, including pelvic inflammatory disease, endometriosis, and neoplasm of the reproductive system, both benign and malignant. All these conditions have overlapping signs, thereby making diagnosis challenging.

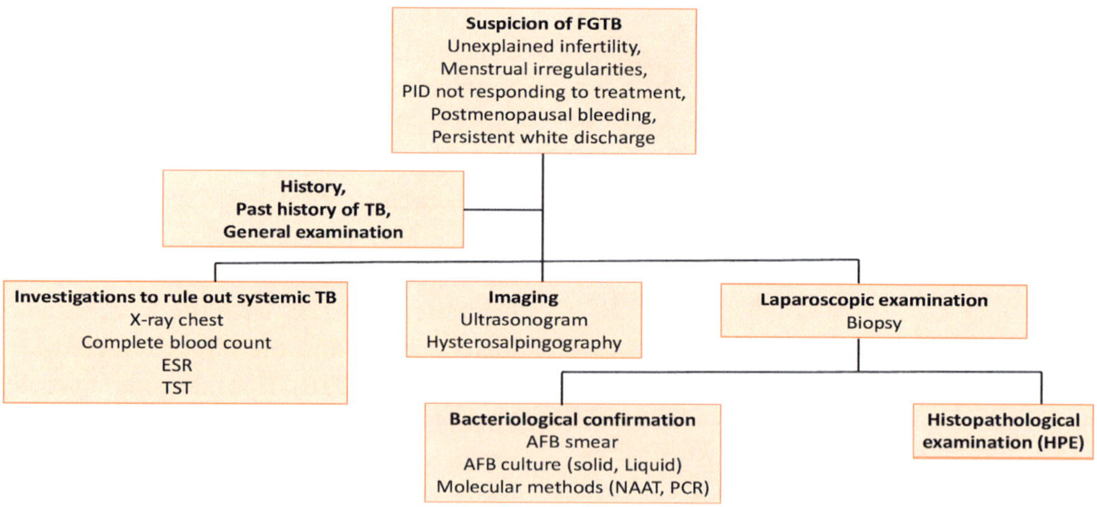

Figure 10.8. Diagnostic algorithm for female genital tuberculosis (FGTB).

Source: https://www.medlineacademics.com/blog/female-genital-tuberculosis-and-infertility.php

Effective differentiation largely hinges upon a combination of the clinical assessment, imaging investigations, laboratory testing, and medical history; thus, proper knowledge of less common presentations of these conditions and also TB is crucial so that one does not make any false diagnoses and can treat accordingly. The role of hysterosalpingography (HSG) cannot be overstated in the differential diagnosis of female genital tuberculosis. HSG is a radiologic procedure that provides significant information on the patency of the fallopian tubes and associated uterine disease. If there is genital tuberculosis, the appearance may be classic in the form of hydrosalpinx, ectopic endometrial outlines, or filling defects that would indicate the presence of disease. Because the fallopian tubes are typically bilaterally involved in TB, these imaging results can be extremely useful in distinguishing genital tuberculosis from other explanations for infertility, including chronic pelvic inflammatory disease or uterine fibroids. Precise interpretation of only these HSG findings is essential in establishing a certain diagnosis and determining appropriate management choices for the concerned patients, as highlighted in recent case reports of female genital tuberculosis (Akhbari et al., 2013).

Despite the promising progress in serological tests as well as nucleic acid amplification techniques, applicability and accessibility remain dominant issues in the use of such techniques in resource-poor settings that end up limiting early diagnosis and related therapeutic methods in affected populations. In terms of addressing such diagnostic issues, the implementation of a multidisciplinary approach is justified, including inputs from specialists in infectious diseases, gynecologists, and radiologists. Greater physician awareness of the characteristic presentation of tuberculosis in the female genital tract can equate with more astute clinical practice and a higher index of suspicion. Development of focused screening programs for the high-risk groups, such as women from high-burden countries, is crucial to ensure early detection and intervention. In addition, harmonization of diagnostic protocols and criteria between healthcare systems can result in better outcomes for patients. By the optimization of the diagnostic setting that shrouds genital tuberculosis, health workers can minimize the long-term effects of the disease, increasing reproductive health outcomes among infected women and minimizing the morbidity of this infectious chronic illness in populations (Myrvang et al., 2009; Sarkar et al., 2019).

Psychological factors, such as stress and anxiety, can further complicate the differential diagnosis of tuberculosis in the female genital tract. Emerging research has indicated that conditions like adjustment disorder may be associated with increased rates of infections, potentially masking or mimicking the symptoms of genital TB (Farkas et al., 2020). For example, the stress response may lead to changes in immune function that can affect the clinical presentation of infections. Therefore, healthcare providers must consider an integrated approach that not only addresses the physical symptoms but also evaluates the psychological well-being of the patient. This holistic view can contribute to more accurate diagnoses and improved patient outcomes, as psychological barriers may persist in delaying suitable medical intervention. Thus, a comprehensive assessment, incorporating both medical history and mental health considerations, is essential for effectively distinguishing tuberculosis from other overlapping gynecological disorders.

Test Your Knowledge

1. What are the common symptoms of female genital tuberculosis?
2. Why is diagnosing female genital tuberculosis often challenging?

10.4. Diagnostic Methods

Learning Outcome

1. Explain the role of laboratory tests and cultures in diagnosing tuberculosis
2. Describe the imaging techniques used in tuberculosis
3. Discuss the histopathological examination in tuberculosis diagnosis.

Precise diagnostic tests are vital for early detection of female genital tuberculosis (FGT) because, in most cases, the disease is characterized by mild and nonspecific symptoms. The approach proposed demands the use of multi-faceted diagnosis based on diversified methods such as the acid-fast bacilli (AFB) smear, culture, and molecular tests like Tuberculosis Polymerase Chain Reaction (TB-PCR) and CBNAAT. Experiences have confirmed that these methods have different sensitivities and specificities in the diagnosis of genital tuberculosis, a reflection of the necessity to screen the suspected cases in depth. Utilization of a combination of diagnostic techniques enhances the success of detection of the disease, which may be vital in the effective management and treatment of the subjects, particularly within groups with a higher level of risk, such as reproductive-aged women (Depan et al., 2019). The use of molecular diagnostics in FGT tuberculosis detection has become increasingly important with their rapid turnaround times and high sensitivity, particularly for paucibacillary presentations of the disease. As an example, studies have demonstrated that TB-PCR and CBNAAT are efficient at diagnosing genital tuberculosis with remarkable results reflected in P-values representing statistical significance. These procedures not only enable rapid diagnosis but also counteract the disadvantage of traditional procedures, which consume more turnaround time and depend on an adequate bacilli load. The use of such advanced diagnostic modalities is crucial in enhancing the overall diagnostic effectiveness, particularly under resource-poor settings where traditional culture methods might prove to be impractical (Depan et al., 2019). In addition, the diagnostic profile of FGT tuberculosis is also made complicated by the presence of numerous infectious agents that can produce overlapping clinical manifestations. As recent research has indicated, conditions such as schistosomiasis and amoebiasis have been discovered to produce overlapping clinical presentations of genital tuberculosis with the capacity to lead to misdiagnosis. The similarity further enhances the importance of in-depth clinical evaluation that is supported by certain laboratory tests in order to differentiate between the two conditions. Health care workers must have a high index of suspicion for tuberculosis, especially in endemic areas or among high-risk populations. Hence, a good understanding of some of the diagnostic methods, along with clinical acumen to put findings into perspective, is still of utmost importance to avoid misdiagnosis and proper treatment of tuberculosis in the female genital tract.

10.4.1. Laboratory Tests and Cultures

Laboratory examination and cultures are required in the diagnosis of female genital tract tuberculosis (TB) for accurate identification and management of the disease. The most common tests utilized include endometrial curettage and tissue histopathological examination, which provide direct visualization of the pathological lesion of TB. A Hyderabad study indicated that of 1102 presumptive genital TB cases, 23 were eventually diagnosed by these standard procedures, evidence of the role of lab examination in determining the causative pathology of the disease. Proper application of these tests is important, as a wrong diagnosis can lead to delay in treatment and increased morbidity, particularly in TB-endemic populations (Dass et al., 2017).

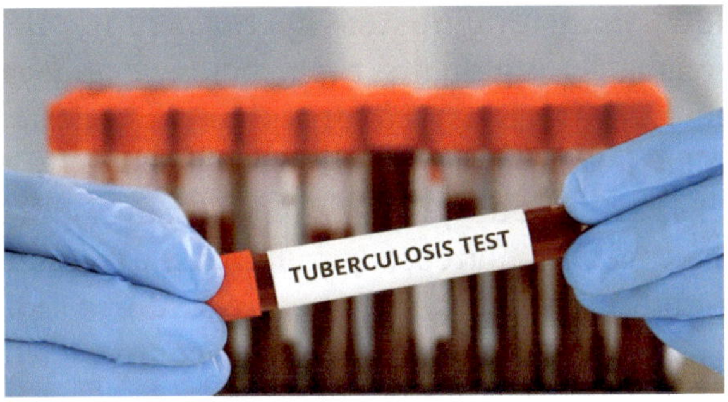

Source: https://external-content.duckduckgo.com/iu/?u=https%3A%2F%2Fimg.medscape.com%2Fthumbnail_library%2Fdt_200423_tuberculosis_blood_test_800x450.jpg&f=1&nofb=1&ipt=328e42daf8f8ea503a8c645323b7698137b86f1e2276d623907ad9105dbab381

Thus, knowledge and utilization of prolonged laboratory techniques have the potential to greatly impact clinical presentation in infected patients. Cultures remain a standard in the prolonged diagnostic approach to female genital tuberculosis, particularly in establishing *Mycobacterium tuberculosis*. While histopathological examination provides preliminary diagnostic data, cultures allow for species identification and drug susceptibility testing, which inform subsequent treatment protocols. Liquid culture systems have revolutionized TB diagnosis by delivering improved sensitivity and faster turnaround compared to traditional solid media. However, problems arise in resource-poor settings where laboratory infrastructures may not be satisfactory. It is crucial to ensure that doctors have access to robust laboratory facilities in bridging the gaps in diagnosis, treatment, and overall public health outcomes of TB (Ballard et al., 2012). Thus, the proper development of laboratory premises is a vital precaution against the spread of this disease and to improve prognosis in females suffering from genital TB. In addition to traditional forms of diagnosis, the application of new technologies is bound to enhance the detection of tuberculosis of the female genitalia. Recent advances in molecular diagnostics, such as polymerase chain reaction (PCR) techniques, facilitate rapid detection of *Mycobacterium tuberculosis* from tubercles. Not only do they improve diagnostic efficiency, but they also facilitate the timely initiation of appropriate therapy, which is critical in preventing complications such as infertility. However, despite the inherent benefits, the integration of such new technologies into already entrenched healthcare paradigms can be challenging. Factors such as health system constraints, socioeconomic determinants, and cultural perceptions of TB and diagnostic processes could inhibit the successful implementation of these innovations (Ballard et al., 2012). Ultimately, what is required is a combined approach that integrates high-tech diagnostic technology with an understanding of local healthcare dynamics in order to optimize care for tuberculosis of the female genital tract.

10.4.2. Imaging Techniques

Imaging modalities play a key role in the diagnosis of female genital tract tuberculosis (GTB), especially because the disease often presents subtly. Pelvic ultrasound is one of the first modalities to be used in the evaluation of reproductive health and can reveal suggestive findings like enlarged adnexal masses or hyperthickened endometrial lining. These can prompt further investigation, most significantly if symptoms like abnormal uterine bleeding (AUB) are noted. The flaws of ultrasounds, however, can force even more advanced imaging methods, especially in an endemic population for GTB. Magnetic resonance imaging (MRI), thus, has become increasingly valuable, with its capacity to show exquisite detail of soft tissue structures and to better ascertain any organ involvement, from the fallopian tubes to the uterus. This accuracy is critical, as accurate diagnosis prescribes direction for treatment and subsequent surgical interventions in the management of GTB. In GTB, computed tomography (CT) scans also have a significant diagnostic function, particularly in cases of suspected extragenital dissemination. CT scan is able to detect peritoneal disease, lymphadenopathy, and other disseminated tuberculosis complications. All of these are significant staging criteria for the disease and for treatment modality planning.

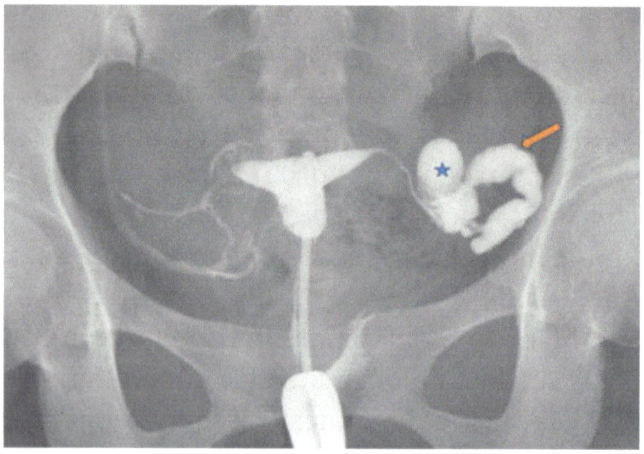

Figure 10.9. Imaging Spectrum of Female Genital Tuberculosis.

Source: https://ars.els-cdn.com/content/image/1-s2.0-S0363018821001122-gr4.jpg

Furthermore, integration of imaging findings with laboratory examinations, such as polymerase chain reaction (PCR) for *Mycobacterium tuberculosis*, validates increased diagnostic accuracy. As proposed by (Arpitha et al., 2016), laparoscopic visual assessment and endometrial TB-PCR positivity correlate positively with one another, validating the requirement for intensive diagnostic methods integrating imaging modalities with clinical evaluation. This combined strategy ensures that GTB is diagnosed promptly, which is critical in the prevention of irreversible damage to the reproductive system that may be caused by late treatment. The second appealing aspect of modern imaging in GTB is the use of new modalities, including hysterosalpingography (HSG) and diagnostic hysteroscopy. HSG particularly highlights tubal patency and can demonstrate scarring or tubal obstruction, which is prevalent in GTB patients. To find out more about postgraduate essays, go to www.postgraduateessays.com. As evidenced by multiple studies, such as the findings given in (et al., 2023), patients who come in with AUB not only undergo evidence of structural irregularities but also are diagnosed with unsuspected concomitant infections like GTB via routine screening procedures. This process is significant because it avoids mismanagement and unnecessary procedures that might be performed because of the misidentification of the cause of AUB. Lastly, application of a combination of these imaging modalities along with clinical examinations offers a thorough knowledge about GTB, therefore maximizing patient treatment and outcome results.

10.4.3. Histopathological Examination

Histopathological examination is a mainstay in the diagnosis and management of tuberculosis (TB) of the female genital tract, primarily with regard to the identification of *Mycobacterium tuberculosis*. Histopathological analysis of female genital TB can reveal typical granulomatous inflammation, one of the characteristic features of the disease, in tissue specimens. These findings are critical to the differentiation of TB from other infectious and non-infectious diseases that can affect the genital tract. Notably, histopathological examination is likely to miss cases based on sampling errors and therefore may necessitate even more utilization of complementary diagnostic tools. For 100 patients, histopathological examination diagnosed TB in only 2% of women, illustrating the potential limitations of this diagnostic tool when utilized alone (Chaudhary et al., 2022). Thus, histopathology has to be put into context with molecular techniques to enhance diagnostic yield in suspected cases of female genital tuberculosis. The introduction of newer diagnostic modalities, such as cartridge-based nucleic acid amplification tests (CBNAAT), has changed the TB detection scenario in the female genital tract. Use of CBNAAT was found to be more sensitive than histopathological methods, identifying TB in 5% of patients in the same cohort study (Chaudhary et al., 2022).

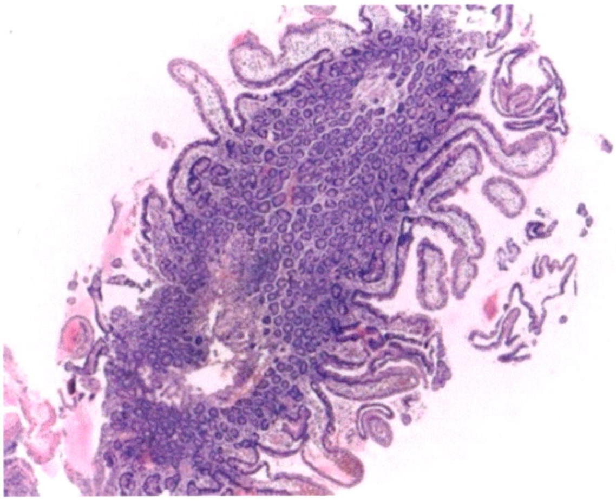

Figure 10.10. Histopathological examination.

Source: https://www.researchgate.net/figure/Histopathological-examination_fig3_302915945

Detection of the existence of *Mycobacterium tuberculosis* nucleic acids not only enables diagnosis at an earlier time than before but also facilitates various management practices in the clinic. These breakthroughs also work to highlight the significance of multi-faceted practice involving histopathology and molecular diagnostics for the optimal outcome of patients. With the devious nature of genital TB, often occult as a cause of unexplained infertility, it is the responsibility of healthcare providers to be equipped with diligent diagnostic tools to identify and treat this new public health indicator. Besides its application in diagnosis, histopathological analysis also plays a significant role in determining the extent of tissue disease in female genital tuberculosis. The presence of particular pathological features—e.g., caseating granulomas, lymphocytic infiltration, and necrosis—is important insofar as it can provide valuable information about the severity of the disease as well as potential impact on reproductive health. Awareness of these histopathological features is necessary for the guidance of treatment and prognosis. It also warns clinicians of potential sparing of reproductive function, an important consideration for affected women. Simple genital TB is not an innocent condition, and its sequelae may have long-standing effects on fertility, thus underlining the importance of detailed histological analysis in clinical situations. By clarifying our understanding of the histopathological landscape, we can enhance our capacity to design interventions to protect against the effects of this formidable disease on reproductive health in women.

Test Your Knowledge

1. What laboratory tests and cultures are used to diagnose tuberculosis?
2. How do imaging techniques assist in the diagnosis of tuberculosis?

10.5. Treatment Options

Learning Outcome

1. Discuss the antitubercular drug regimens
2. Define duration of tuberculosis treatment

Management of female genital tract tuberculosis is extensive and multi-disciplinary because it can create severe reproductive morbidity, i.e., infertility. The management is typically an association of surgery and anti-tubercular therapy (ATT), depending on the disease's severity. ATT is also needed to cure the causative infection and typically starts simultaneously with diagnostic investigations. In cases of tubal obstruction by TB, salpingostomy or salpingectomy might be necessary in order to achieve regular reproductive function. Because of the chronic course of genital TB, repeated follow-up and adjustment of treatment protocols are necessary to enhance the probabilities of a successful outcome, particularly in young women who desire future fertility (Sarkar et al., 2019).

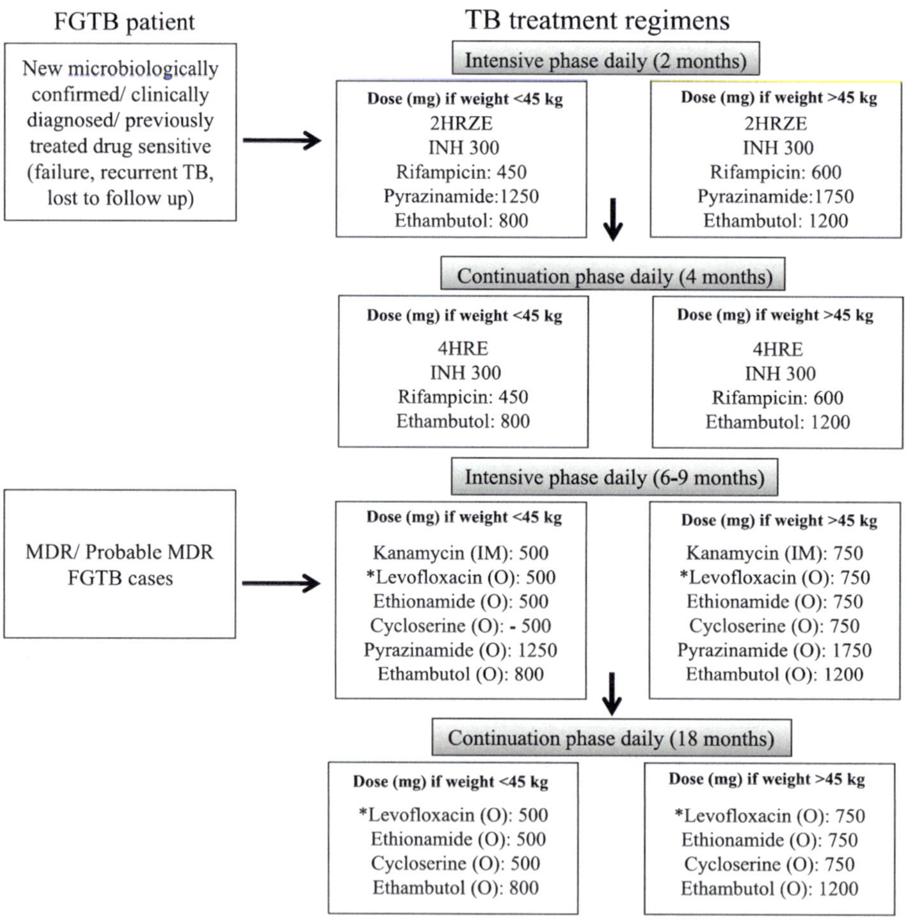

Figure 10.11. Treatment regimens for female genital tuberculosis (FGTB).

Source: https://www.researchgate.net/figure/Treatment-regimens-for-female-genital-tuberculosis-FGTB-Moxifloxacin-to-be-given-if_fig7_332572208

Moreover, imaging studies such as hysterosalpingography (HSG) play an important role in the diagnosis of infertility due to genital TB. HSG provides tubal patency and assessment of the uterine cavity, which provides important information regarding the severity of the disease. Bilateral patent fallopian tubes with a normal uterine cavity have been observed to be ideal, with this leading to increased reproductive opportunities. Following HSG, management may involve assisted reproductive technique (ART) like intrauterine insemination, which may be more advantageous for a few patients presenting with some conditions. Utilizing these interventions, clinicians can give hope to those afflicted with the reproductive pathologies of TB and emphasize the need for early diagnosis and appropriate treatment modalities (Mitra et al., 2022). In the management of genital TB, an integrated treatment plan would also include dealing with the psycho-social implications of infertility due to the disease. The psychological and emotional tension faced by the affected women can become extremely demanding, and supportive counseling along with medical therapy may become a necessity. Counseling of the patients about their condition and the possibilities available for the recovery of reproductive health is a key element for improving patient experience and outcomes. Besides, the awareness of potential postoperative and ongoing therapy complications can empower the patient, thereby improving decision-making. Thus, the interaction of medical, surgical, and psychological factors emphasizes the complexity of female genital tuberculosis, necessitating a collaborative multidisciplinary treatment regimen to optimize the care of infected patients (Sarkar et al., 2019).

10.5.1. Antitubercular Drug Regimens

Antitubercular therapy regimens are to blame for the management and treatment of tuberculosis, especially in the female genital tract, where the disease can have significant reproductive and overall health implications. A combination of first-line drugs, such as rifampicin, isoniazid, pyrazinamide, and ethambutol, also referred to as the RIPE regimen, forms the conventional treatment. The combination regimen is vital in preventing the development of drug resistance, a significant issue in the treatment of tuberculosis. In females, particularly reproductive-age women, the risk to pregnancy and fertility has prompted choosing these regimens cautiously to ensure maximal therapeutic effect while preventing risks. With increasing awareness about the implications of the disease, new drug delivery mechanisms are being explored to enhance the effectiveness of various treatments and minimize the side effects of traditional regimens. Recent advances in drug delivery systems have been promising in overcoming the obstacles of traditional antitubercular therapy using polyanhydride nanoparticles. Studies suggest that the encapsulation of first-line medications in biodegradable nanoparticles may increase their bioavailability and stability, as well as enhance treatment efficacy against *Mycobacterium tuberculosis*. An example depicted using a polyanhydride nanoparticle-based drug delivery platform co-delivering several antiparasitic and anti-tuberculous agents successfully to lower the amount of drugs needed to eliminate bacteria while reducing the time to therapeutic effect significantly. These technologies can potentially enhance compliance with treatment among women suffering from genital tract tuberculosis, particularly in resource-poor settings where conventional treatment may be compromised by such factors as drug resistance and side effects. Better delivery strategies can also minimize stigma and maximize health-seeking behavior among women entangled in the contradictions of the disease. The efficacy of antitubercular drug regimens, particularly among women, speaks to the imperative of effective therapeutic strategies tailored to the needs of this population. Guidelines set forth by the National

Institutes of Health and its cooperating agencies suggest that co-morbid conditions like HIV, which complicates enormously the tuberculosis complexities of women, should be considered in systemic approaches. The complexity of tuberculosis therapy in the female genital area also requires close monitoring of reactions and potential side effects on reproductive health. Furthermore, understanding the interface between tuberculosis treatment and appropriate hormonal treatments regarding women's health is important. As research continues to delve deeper into the efficiency of drug delivery via nanoparticles, the direction towards more tailored and effective antitubercular regimens would drastically enhance treatment success for women, thus addressing not only the disease itself but also its long-range repercussions on health and wellbeing as a whole.

10.5.2. Duration of Treatment

The duration of the treatment for female genital tuberculosis is an extremely important determinant of outcome in patients and public health. Antitubercular drugs are required to be administered chronically because *Mycobacterium tuberculosis* is a slow-growing bacillus, and the infection is intricately complex. Treatment with a standard schedule, in general, would take at least six months to ensure the complete elimination of the bacteria and prevent relapse. The World Health Organization suggests the implementation of a regimen involving a combination of first-line drugs, such as isoniazid and rifampicin, which are crucial for curing the disease in a sustained manner. Furthermore, sticking to the recommended duration can greatly promote the effectiveness of treatment, as lack of compliance directly involves drug resistance, making future treatment highly complicated and extending the disease process in case-positive individuals. In reality, the presence of such comorbidities as HIV, malnutrition, or drug resistance would necessitate extension of the treatment duration beyond the standard six months. Demands of women suffering from genital tuberculosis are also complicated by the peculiarity of social and health factors, particularly fertility. Those women suffering from genital tuberculosis also suffer a lot from the psychological and emotional pain, and this impacts whether or not they will adhere to long treatment regimens. Doctors must therefore provide candid talks with the patient on the need to complete treatment, as well as how long treatment will take to prevent these problems. Success of the treatment is also contingent upon individualized approaches that are able to treat specific patient conditions, thereby providing a reassuring setting for patients with protracted therapeutic regimens. Lastly, the success of treatment duration is often tracked not only in bacteriological terms but also in terms of reproductive health gains. The possibility of genital tuberculosis decreasing female fertility makes early and effective intervention imperative. It is discovered through studies that early treatment and diagnosis can significantly improve fertility outcomes in affected women, particularly if it is undertaken before irreversible harm. Recent studies have approximated that up to 13 percent of women visiting clinics for infertility are affected by genital tuberculosis, suggesting the need for sensitization and early treatment. As observed by previous research, histopathological characteristics vary extensively in women with genital tuberculosis, highlighting the need for individualized assessment to guide treatment duration and strategies, especially among women who present with concerns of infertility (Sankareswari et al., 2018; et al.).

10.5.3. Management of Complications

Complication management of female genital tract tuberculosis calls for a coordinated, timely, and multidisciplinary approach. Clinicians must first make the correct diagnosis, although this can be masked by asymptomatic presentation or mimicry of symptoms of another infectious process. The presence of vulvovaginal masses and abnormal discharge, for instance, may result in suspicion of malignancy, although granulomatous inflammation by *Mycobacterium tuberculosis* is in most cases the cause. The ultimate diagnosis is usually done on histopathological examination and culture techniques, which can clarify dubious cases. Early detection often matters because late intervention will lead to severe complications like the possibility of infertility and extensive pelvic damage, highlighting the need for early interventions in the management of tuberculosis sequelae (Richens et al., 2004). After diagnosis has been established, the management of female genital tuberculosis focuses on the administration of a standardized anti-tuberculous drug regimen. Treatment typically consists of a combination of isoniazid, rifampicin, ethambutol, and pyrazinamide for a long duration, typically six months or longer, depending on the severity of the disease and response of the patient. The management of complications, particularly the prevention of secondary infections and management of any obstructive uropathy, is critical in the process. The patients must also be monitored for drug side effects, which can hamper medication adherence. Failure to properly handle these complexities may result in treatment interruptions and subsequent complications, thus indicating the significance of an attentive follow-up regime in the clinical management of such patients (Richens et al., 2004). Patient psychosocial support and education are essential in the management of late complications of female genital tuberculosis. These patients can suffer tremendous emotional distress from stigma, fear of infertility, and the chronic nature of the disease. Mental health care can therefore enhance outcomes as well as compliance with treatment. Counseling for reproductive decisions and preservation of fertility should also be provided to the patients, especially when a future pregnancy is desired. Because fulfillment of such wishes varies, a multidisciplinary approach with the input of gynecologists, infectious disease experts, and psychiatrists or psychologists is required. Lastly, treatment of such complications over time of female genital tuberculosis is not only a cure for the infection but rather complete and compassionate care that addresses and considers the diverse implications for those who are infected (Schneider et al., 2013).

Test Your Knowledge

1. Describe the recommended duration of tuberculosis treatment.
2. Discuss strategies for the management of complications during tuberculosis therapy.

SUMMARY

The assessment of tuberculosis of the female genital tract is such that it is clear that this disease is a multifaceted interaction between the infectious process and host physiology. Clinical presentation tends to be imitative of other gynecologic diseases, thus potentially leading to delayed diagnosis and mismanagement. The ignorance of this entity on the part of healthcare professionals adds to the problem, so that by the time proper interventions are undertaken, the disease is well advanced. This writing has taken into account the intricacy of diagnosing and treating tuberculosis in this anatomical location, emphasizing the supreme necessity of heightened watchfulness in the case of women, particularly those in high-risk populations. As literature accounts, it is only by employing a multi-faceted approach that involves epidemiological sensitization, advanced diagnostic methods, and effective treatment regimens that the public health effects of this disease may be contained (Myrvang et al., 2009). Furthermore, the consequences of untreated genital tuberculosis extend beyond individual health to the broader public health concerns of reproductive health and maternal outcomes. The potential for infertility and pregnancy complications due to tuberculosis-induced structural changes in reproductive organs serves to underscore the need for early diagnosis and treatment. The lasting implications of this disease render continuing investigation of its pathogenesis and treatments imperative. A key area in managing tuberculosis of the female genital tract is through incorporating complete sexual health education, since greater awareness can allow for early symptom reporting. Encouragement of the practice of regular screenings for tuberculosis among high-risk individuals may also be a turning point toward stemming the tide of spread for this infectious disease (Dean et al., 2019). In essence, the treatment of female genital tract tuberculosis must be a concerted action through educational interventions, improved diagnosis, and multidisciplinary management strategies. Future research has to find out the complexities involved in co-infections and the immune response elicited by tuberculosis in the female reproductive tract. This research could enable the development of targeted therapeutic approaches that are directed towards minimizing sequelae and maximizing reproductive outcomes. In the end, addressing this issue in a holistic manner with prevention, education, and treatment will be essential to reversing the tide of this often-overlooked public health issue. Making current information available to healthcare providers will be paramount to ensuring enhanced health outcomes for women afflicted with this condition.

In the female genital tract, tuberculosis (TB) stands out in terms of the difficulties it presents that affect reproductive health in meaningful ways. The interdisciplinary character of TB as a disease resonates with the call for a broad-based understanding of how the infection operates across several systems of physiology. The function of cytokines, such as IL-36gamma, has emerged as an important area of study, specifically in describing immune responses at the mucosal level. This pro-inflammatory cytokine has an important role in early host defense mechanisms against sexually transmitted infections like HSV-2 and may be indicative of interactions between TB and other sexually transmitted infections. The interconnected and complex nature of these infections reflects the need for further research that integrates findings across disciplines of immunology and gynecology for effective treatment and to improve patient outcomes, especially in women at high-risk groups (N/A, 2019). The global burden of tuberculosis among women, particularly in low-resource settings, also reflects the need for focused research and intervention. Women suffering from reproductive health issues caused by TB are at a disadvantage since such conditions might disrupt their overall health and fertility. Current literature highlights the need to consider tuberculosis and

VAWG intersections, i.e., the ways in which these can exacerbate infection vulnerability, including the case of TB. Through solving these crosscutting issues, the scientists can develop targeted approaches to reduce the risk and burden of TB among women, ultimately aligning with global health initiatives that aim to enhance women's health and reduce gender-based violence (Heise et al., 2016).In a bid to effectively solve tuberculosis of the female genital tract, there should be an integrated approach that combines clinical research, public health practices, and community outreach. Collaborative practice must prioritize education on the complexities of TB in women's reproductive health for your healthcare providers so that early detection and treatment planning incorporate consideration of your individual physiological and social contexts. In addition, the construction of holistic models of care incorporating mental health provision will be key in combatting the psychological impacts of both TB and VAWG. By emphasizing the need for an integrative approach to women's health which unites the bodily and the social aspects, the struggle against tuberculosis can be made more effective, thereby leading to improved health outcomes among women worldwide and improved overall control of this pervasive disease (N/A, 2019; Heise et al., 2016).

KEY TERMS FROM THIS CHAPTER

- Abnormal menstruation
- Antitubercular therapy
- Extrapulmonary TB
- Genital tuberculosis
- Gynecological conditions
- Gynecological procedures
- Histopathological analysis
- Hydrosalpinx
- Abnormal uterine bleeding (AUB)
- Extra-genital sites
- Extrapulmonary tuberculosis,
- Granuloma formation
- Gynecological disorders
- Health care providers
- Histopathological examination
- Hysterosalpingography (HSG)

CRITICAL THINKING QUESTIONS

1. **The most common site of genital tuberculosis in females is:**
   a. Ovary
   b. Endometrium
   c. Fallopian tubes
   d. Cervix
2. **Which of the following is the primary route of infection in female genital tuberculosis?**
   a. Direct sexual transmission
   b. Hematogenous spread from a primary focus
   c. Lymphatic spread from pelvic lymph nodes
   d. Contamination from the urinary tract
3. **The typical clinical presentation of female genital tuberculosis includes:**
   a. Acute pelvic pain with fever
   b. Chronic pelvic pain, infertility, and menstrual irregularities
   c. Severe vaginal bleeding
   d. Painless vaginal mass
4. **Which diagnostic test is considered the gold standard for confirming genital tuberculosis?**
   a. Mantoux test
   b. Acid-fast bacilli (AFB) culture or PCR of endometrial biopsy
   c. Pelvic ultrasound
   d. ap smear
5. **The main treatment for genital tuberculosis is:**
   a. Surgical removal of the affected organs
   b. Broad-spectrum antibiotics
   c. Antitubercular therapy (ATT) for at least 6 months
   d. Corticosteroids

Short Answer Questions

1. What is the global epidemiology of tuberculosis?
2. Describe the pathophysiology of tuberculosis infection.
3. What are the common clinical manifestations of tuberculosis?
4. Which diagnostic methods are used to confirm tuberculosis?
5. What are the standard treatment options for tuberculosis?
6. How is drug-resistant tuberculosis managed differently from drug-sensitive TB?

Answer to Critical Thinking Questions

1. (c) 2. (b) 3. (b) 4. (b) 5. (c)

REFERENCES

1. Akhbari, F., Ahmadi, F., & Afzali, N. (2013). Various hysterosalpingography findings of female genital tuberculosis: A case series. https://core.ac.uk/download/pdf/26903495.pdf (accessed on 15th June 2025).
2. Arpitha, V., Jnanashree, V., Nagarathnamma, R., Rangaiah, S., Savitha, S., & Channaveeregowda, C. (2016). Diagnosis of genital tuberculosis: Correlation between polymerase chain reaction positivity and laparoscopic findings. https://core.ac.uk/download/539900297.pdf (accessed on 15th June 2025).
3. Baez-Corujo, S., Cantres-Fonseca, O. J., Del Olmo-Arroyo, F., Rodriguez-Cintrón, J., et al. (2018). *Extra Pulmonary Tuberculosis: An Overview*. https://core.ac.uk/download/322440357.pdf (accessed on 15th June 2025).
4. Balalau, C., Banu, P., Bratucu, M., Constantin, C., et al. (2017). Appendicular mass–A rare form of tuberculosis. https://core.ac.uk/download/144553186.pdf (accessed on 15th June 2025).
5. Ballard, R. C., Mabey, D., & Peeling, R. W. (2012). Introducing new diagnostics into STI control programmed: The importance of programmer science.
6. Bharadwaj, N., Lamba, I., Sharma, H., Sharma, R., et al. (2017). Role of AFB culture, histopathology and laparoscopy in female genital tuberculosis as a cause for chronic pelvic pain. https://core.ac.uk/download/539899292.pdf (accessed on 15th June 2025).
7. Binnebose, A. M. (2018). *Development of A Novel Anti-Infectivity Platform for The Treatment of Neglected Tropical and Infectious Diseases*. https://core.ac.uk/download/212819677.pdf (accessed on 15th June 2025).
8. Blanchfield, L., Margesson, R., Salaam-Blyther, T., Serafino, P., et al. (2011). *International Violence Against Women: U.S. Response and Policy Issues*. https://core.ac.uk/download/5131183.pdf (accessed on 15th June 2025).
9. Chandran, S., Kunst, H., Norris, J. M., Rahman, M., et al. (2021). Diagnostic pitfalls of urogenital tuberculosis. https://core.ac.uk/download/429942693.pdf (accessed on 15th June 2025).
10. Chate, P., & Khatri, M. (2016). A case of infertility with tuberculosis with multiple calcifications on both fallopian tubes. https://core.ac.uk/download/539898969.pdf (accessed on 15th June 2025).
11. Chaudhary, D., Gupta, S., Pandey, A., Tyagi, R., et al. (2022). Study of the frequency of female genital tract infection using cartridge-based nucleic acid amplification test. https://core.ac.uk/download/539902910.pdf (accessed on 15th June 2025).
12. Cools, P., Crucitti, T., Masha, S., Sanders, E., et al. (2017). High prevalence of curable sexually transmitted infections among pregnant women in a rural county hospital in Kilifi, Kenya. https://core.ac.uk/download/84044028.pdf (accessed on 15th June 2025).
13. Dass, M., Pavani, K., Kumari, K., Krishna, M., et al. (2017). To evaluate the prevalence of female genital tuberculosis in Hyderabad. https://core.ac.uk/download/543134794.pdf (accessed on 15th June 2025).
14. Dean, D., Ferrin, T. E., Hyuk Suh, J., Somboonna, N., et al. (2019). Clinical persistence of *Chlamydia trachomatis* sexually transmitted strains involves novel mutations in the functional αββα tetramer of the tryptophan synthase operon. https://core.ac.uk/download/323074473.pdf (accessed on 15th June 2025).

15. Degeratu, D., Nastasia, Ş., Russu, M. C., Stănculescu, R., et al. (2018). Breast and cervix uteri: Rare locations for *Mycobacterium tuberculosis* infections and complications—Cases report and literature review. https://core.ac.uk/download/322436007.pdf (accessed on 15th June 2025).
16. Depan, A., Narayan, S., Sharma, A., Sharma, R., et al. (2019). Prevalence of female genital tract tuberculosis in suspected cases attending gynecology OPD at tertiary center by various diagnostic methods and comparative analysis. https://core.ac.uk/download/539903002.pdf (accessed on 15th June 2025).
17. Farkas, D. K., Galea, S., Gradus, J. L., Jiang, T., et al. (2020). Associations between adjustment disorder and hospital-based infections in the Danish population. https://core.ac.uk/download/288432803.pdf (accessed on 15th June 2025).
18. Heise, L., & McGrory, E. (2016). *Greentree II: Violence Against Women and Girls, and HIV*. https://core.ac.uk/download/74229119.pdf (accessed on 15th June 2025).
19. Hickey, A. J., McMurray, D. N., & Padilla-Carlin, D. J. (2008). The guinea pig as a model of infectious diseases. https://core.ac.uk/download/345218068.pdf (accessed on 15th June 2025).
20. Induja, B. V., Dalvi, R. M., Potdar, M., Sawant, S., et al. (2023). A case report: Incidental diagnosis of endometrial tuberculosis in cases of abnormal uterine bleeding. https://core.ac.uk/download/588567929.pdf (accessed on 15th June 2025).
21. Kaur, S., Mor, S., & Santpur, U. (2019). The incidence detection of tuberculosis in patients with infertility and abnormal uterine bleed: A study in North Indian population. https://core.ac.uk/download/539902034.pdf (accessed on 15th June 2025).
22. Kearns, D., Kemp, B., Kundasamy, P., Lyon, R., et al. (2022). A rare case of disseminated genitourinary tract tuberculosis complicated by emphysematous prostatitis and seminal vesicle abscess. https://core.ac.uk/download/616662409.pdf (accessed on 15th June 2025).
23. Mitra, S., Patil, D., & Yazdani, S. (2022). Study of HSG findings in our clientele: A multicenter retrospective analytical study. https://core.ac.uk/download/544390457.pdf (accessed on 15th June 2025).
24. Myrvang, B., & Newport, M. J. (2009). *Proceedings of a Joint Meeting Held Between the Norwegian Society of Infectious Diseases and the Royal Society of Tropical Medicine and Hygiene, Oslo, 20th June 2008*. https://core.ac.uk/download/2709731.pdf (accessed on 15th June 2025).
25. Parks, C., Peipert, J. F., Tsevat, D. G., Wiesenfeld, H., et al. (2017). Sexually transmitted diseases and infertility. https://core.ac.uk/download/158967661.pdf (accessed on 15th June 2025).
26. Richens, J. (2004). Genital manifestations of tropical diseases. https://core.ac.uk/download/1669842.pdf (accessed on 15th June 2025).
27. Sankareswari, R., & Arthy, S. (2018). Histopathological features of endometrium in those with symptoms suggestive of female genital tuberculosis. https://core.ac.uk/download/544391466.pdf (accessed on 15th June 2025).
28. Sankareswari, R., & Sundharam, R. S. S. (2018). Histopathological features of endometrium in those with symptoms suggestive of female genital tuberculosis. https://core.ac.uk/download/543135603.pdf (accessed on 15th June 2025).
29. Sarkar, A. (2019). A case of endometrial tuberculosis leading to infertility in a young woman. https://core.ac.uk/download/480547362.pdf (accessed on 15th June 2025).

URINARY INCONTINENCE IN FEMALES

11

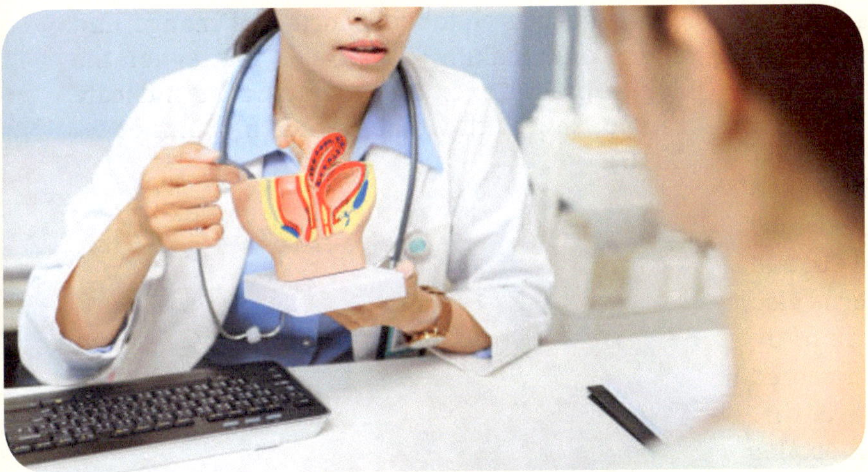

LEARNING OBJECTIVES

After studying this chapter, you will be able to:

1. Identify and differentiate the various types of urinary incontinence
2. Explain the underlying causes contributing to urinary incontinence
3. Recognize common risk factors associated with urinary incontinence
4. Describe the symptoms and diagnostic approaches used to assess urinary incontinence
5. Evaluate the available treatment options for managing urinary incontinence

Introduction

Urinary incontinence (UI) among women is an important public health problem, affecting millions of women worldwide. UI is a spontaneous loss of urine, a condition with extreme emotional and social impacts. UI can reach any woman independent of age, though its prevalence increases as the age advances, typically with compromised quality of life and increased healthcare costs. Causes of UI include a range of biological, environmental, and lifestyle factors. Pregnancy, childbirth, and menopause are specific physiological processes that can compromise pelvic floor support and make one susceptible to SUI and other forms of UI. Proper and timely intervention measures are essential in managing the condition and avoiding its effects on women's daily lives. Current advancements in medical procedures for urinary incontinence highlight the evolving nature of therapies available to women afflicted with the condition. A new approach involves the use of platelet-rich plasma (PRP), an autologous form of treatment that leverages high concentrations of platelets and growth factors for healing procedures. Emerging evidence is demonstrating the efficacy of PRP treatments to correct stress urinary incontinence in women, presenting evidence that regenerative medicine can be a real option for breakthrough therapy beyond accepted treatments. The research of such treatment is vital because it supplements existing management methods and addresses the various demands of women afflicted with UI. As medical researchers pursue this hopeful branch of research, understanding the mechanisms of UI and the various therapeutic options available is essential in advancing women's healthcare outcomes and overall healthcare advancement.

The relationship between sleep duration, obesity, and urinary incontinence is another key element in understanding this multifaceted condition. New evidence has illuminated how excess body weight is linked to increased SUI and UUI risks (Nan et al., 2024). Sleep patterns also play an enormous role in the prevalence of UI, with brief sleep duration accounting for increased incidence rates. This interaction suggests that obesity prevention and sleep hygiene lifestyles have potential impacts on the management of urinary incontinence. Encouraging women to be at a healthy weight and to enact behaviors that promote adequate sleep may be key prevention practices. Cumulatively, these results affirm the worth of interdisciplinary approaches to attaining increased insight and treatment of urinary incontinence and emphasizing holistic care practices that address both physiological and lifestyle conditions impacting women's health.

Definition of Urinary Incontinence

Urinary incontinence is only comprehensible through an in-depth examination of its definition, symptoms, and etiologic conditions. Urinary incontinence is defined as the involuntary loss of urine, and it contributes significantly to reducing the quality of women's lives. It occurs in various forms—stress incontinence, urge incontinence, overflow incontinence, and functional incontinence—and each has varied issues with corresponding treatment measures. Stress incontinence is most likely to occur with physical activity that stresses the bladder, whereas urge incontinence is a sudden and overwhelming urge to urinate. This multidimensionality of urinary incontinence is the reason why identifying the appropriate type is essential to designing effective management programs. Its existence can be traced back to causes such as childbirth, hormonal change, and aging, thus making it a serious matter for the health practitioner to understand its intricate relationship with women's health (Bunn et al., 2015).

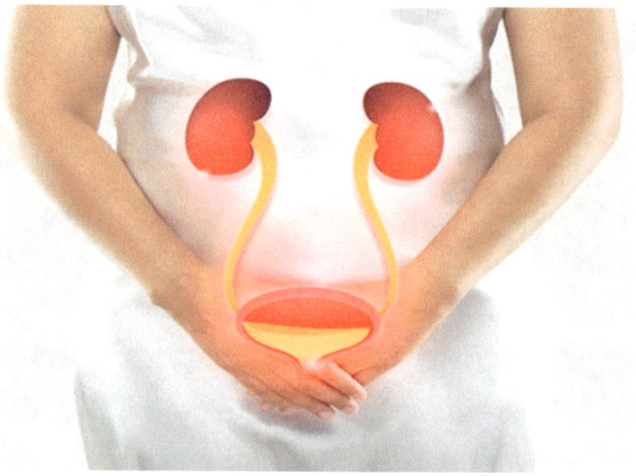

Source: https://www.rghospitals.com/assets/admin/images/blog/1721816407_197920316f6c9a0bdc83.jpg

Other than knowing the various types of urinary incontinence, it is important to recognize its relationship with other conditions, particularly in women. Research indicates that urinary incontinence can be associated with lower urinary tract symptoms and a complicated interaction between metabolic syndrome and overactive bladder, among others. Such relationships suggest an interdisciplinary approach to women's health, where urinary incontinence treatment requires a multi-dimensional approach. Studies report a greater occurrence of lower urinary tract symptoms in women patients with metabolic syndrome, thereby underscoring the importance of comprehensive assessment in clinical practice. The experts emphasize adopting this holistic perspective to administer more effective treatments, which further lead to an overall improvement in their patients' welfare with urinary incontinence (Ghoniem et al., 2012). Furthermore, the treatment of urinary incontinence involves both conservative and intervention therapy that is tailored to the patient. Non-surgical therapies typically involve pelvic floor exercises, lifestyle modifications, and bladder training maneuvers, which are sufficient to correct symptoms without embarking on invasive therapies. In women suffering from stress urinary incontinence, interventions like injection of polydimethylsiloxane—branded Macroplastique—are shown to have favorable results. A systematic review cited short-term improvement rates of 75% in women who undergo this minimally invasive therapy, noting that successful treatments can appreciably enhance quality of life. Both patient and healthcare provider must be aware of such treatment modalities since effective treatment of incontinence can engender better general health and social functioning in women afflicted with this condition (Ghoniem et al., 2012).

Prevalence Among Women

Prevalence of incontinence among women is a most significant public health issue, profoundly impacting their quality of life. Recent research shows that around 34.1% of women suffer from some kind of incontinence, showing a high health burden. The severity of the condition is not the same across all, with about 73.2% of affected individuals suffering from mild incontinence, while moderate and severe incontinence are seen in 19.6% and 7.2%, respectively. The effects extend beyond mere discomfort; women with urinary incontinence have evidenced considerable physical, emotional, and social complications. Indeed, such long-term conditions limit physical activities and social contacts, considerably reducing overall well-being. According to research, it becomes imperative to recognize the vast prevalence of the condition and the gravity of awareness and treatment availability for the afflicted population, which is supported by results of substantial health impacts among individuals with incontinence (et al., 2017). Moreover, age and menopause heighten the incidence of urinary incontinence in women. A prospective cohort study conducted on post-menopausal women illustrated the incidence of urinary incontinence to be 46.24%, indicating the enhanced risk caused by hormonal changes and age-related factors. Notably, women who have undergone surgical menopause show the same incidence as naturally menopausal women, leading to the conclusion that hysterectomy in itself is not an independent risk factor for the condition. Instead, other measures such as metabolic syndrome become playing factors; women who present with this syndrome have a significantly higher incidence of urinary incontinence, at 55.8%. Awareness of these relationships enables medical professionals to better counsel women about the risks of natural and surgical menopause and emphasize the importance of managing metabolic health to alleviate symptoms of urinary incontinence (Alexander et al., 2019). The intricate dynamic between urinary incontinence and other demographic and physiological factors underscores the need for worldwide public health initiatives to inform women about urinary health. Because urinary incontinence itself is stigmatized and underdiagnosed, many women quietly endure it, discounting those treatments available. Informal education campaigns must facilitate honest conversation about this ubiquitous condition, myths shattered, and encourage women so afflicted to seek assistance. Moreover, physicians must prioritize adding urinary incontinence screening to regular health checks, particularly in populations at greater risk, such as postpartum and post-menopausal women. By making it easier for women to discuss urinary incontinence, we can potentially improve early treatment and detection, as well as overall quality of life, in a broad segment of the female population suffering from this disease.

Importance of Addressing the Issue

It is necessary to address urinary incontinence in women because the severe impact of the condition on the physical and mental well-being of the subjects has a very adverse impact on their quality of life. The majority of women experience immense embarrassment and social stigma from urinary incontinence, and therefore, they avoid social activities, and their quality of life is reduced. Psychological impact results in depression and anxiety, and this further impairs treatment outcomes. An active intervention in this issue can help women to report and access help, thus facilitating early treatment and diagnosis, ultimately bringing improved outcomes in terms of their health. Health care providers play an integral part in creating a support network that facilitates open discussion of urinary incontinence, which is important in eradicating the stigma surrounding the condition and facilitating appropriate treatment according to the literature (Hegge et al., 2018). Furthermore, management of urinary incontinence can lead to better distribution of healthcare resources and policymaking. The prevalence of urinary incontinence among women suggests the importance of targeted interventions and health education in the healthcare system. Understanding the demographic and epidemiological characteristics of affected groups can guide policymakers to come up with overall programs for treatment and prevention. Specific focus should be given to educating healthcare professionals about best-practice interventions to enable them to effectively treat urinary incontinence and provide the necessary support to patients. Consequently, the use of focused training programs is capable of increasing practitioners' confidence in treating urinary incontinence, as research shows that this results in an improvement in the management of the condition, as well as higher patient satisfaction (Hegge et al., 2018). Finally, effective management of urinary incontinence permits research into new treatment options, improving outcomes for patients. Recent studies into treatment interventions, including percutaneous tibial nerve stimulation for related disorders, underscore the need for ongoing investigation into new therapies to effectively treat urinary incontinence. While initial findings are encouraging, research is required to establish efficacy and optimize treatment methods. This study can lead to the identification of some subgroups that can be responsive to individually tailored treatment techniques and thus enhance the overall care system in the case of women with urinary incontinence. Continuously evolving research and knowledge on this issue significantly assist in making measures reduce social as well as healthcare burdens caused by urinary incontinence.

11.1. Types of Urinary Incontinence

Learning Outcome

1. Define stress incontinence and urge incontinence
2. Explain the mixed incontinence

An appropriate understanding of urinary incontinence necessitates that the various types, which are indicative of the involved physiological mechanisms, are familiar. Its four broad categories are stress urinary incontinence, urge urinary incontinence, overflow incontinence, and functional incontinence. Stress urinary incontinence, prevalent in women, occurs when increased abdominal pressure during a physical activity such as exercise, coughing, or sneezing results in involuntary leakage of urine. This is usually due to weakened pelvic floor muscles and may be exacerbated by childbirth or hormonal changes during menopause. Alternatively, urge urinary incontinence is characterized by an urgent need to pass urine followed by involuntary leakage. This type is most often associated with overactive bladder syndrome and can significantly impact quality of life and daily function, hence the need for appropriate treatment modalities such as physical therapy (Wells et al., 1994). Overflow incontinence is also a frequent type, normally resulting from chronic urine retention due to bladder dysfunction or obstruction. This can lead to involuntary leakage in the course of an over-distended bladder, a setting commonly encountered in conditions such as urinary tract infection or neurological disease. Functional incontinence, alternatively, occurs as a consequence of physical or mental disorders, making toilet access delayed, but not from problems within the intrinsic urinary tract. This information is critical to clinicians with the aim of tailoring intervention strategies to the very type of urinary incontinence a patient presents with. Because of the multifaceted nature of the condition, dealing with an individual patient's case can lead to more effective treatment and improve the response to therapy as well as medication adherence (Alborz et al., 2009).

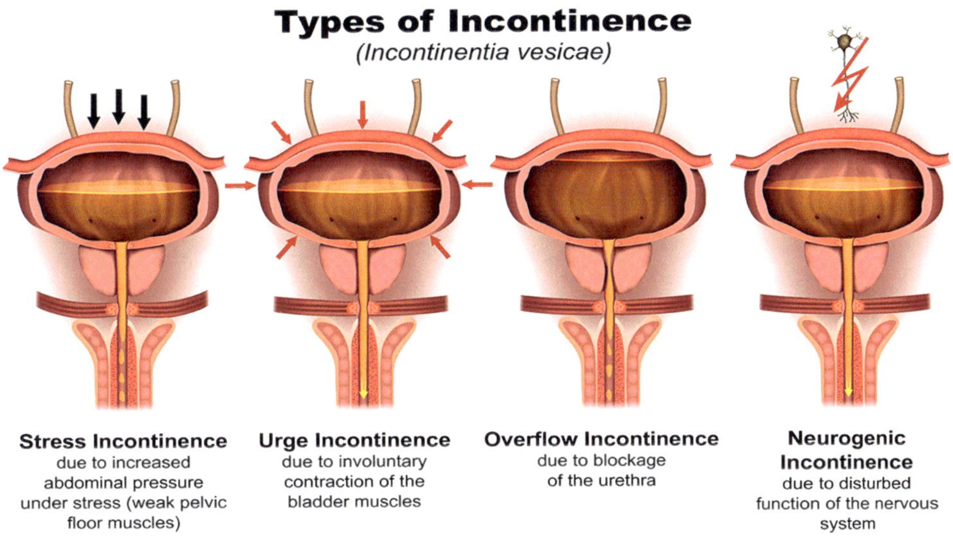

Figure 11.1. Types of Urinary Incontinence.

Source: https://www.nyp.org/womens/urogynecology/female-urinary-incontinence

The diversity of urinary incontinence types calls for an inclusive management strategy that is more than pharmacologic. Conservative management by pelvic floor muscle training and bladder training offers tremendous benefits without the urgency of surgery. These interventions have the potential to empower women by giving them control and reducing the frequency of leakage events. Furthermore, evidence suggests that an integrated strategy incorporating physical therapy can complement these conservative treatments. More frequently employed modes of treatment available to physical therapists will be addressed (Wells et al., 1994). These holistic interventions do not merely address the physiological signs of urinary incontinence but also consider the emotional and psychological impact most frequently linked to this disease. This multifaceted approach guarantees that women plagued by urinary incontinence are being treated with multifaceted and efficient mechanisms that ultimately improve the quality of their lives.

11.1.1. Stress Incontinence

In the examination of urinary incontinence in females, stress incontinence is a significant problem within this group, which is characterized by involuntary loss of urine with exertion, increasing abdominal pressure, and necessitating the activities of coughing, sneezing, or exercise. Weakened pelvic floor muscles and weakened connective tissue are generally the etiologies for this condition, making a person less capable of controlling urination. Notably, a study indicated the underreporting of stress urinary incontinence (SUI), with 26.1% of women reporting symptoms to doctors, thereby showing considerable underreporting of this uncomfortable condition. The association between the physiological variables and onset of SUI accentuates the role of women's health education and early intervention strategies, which work to maximize pelvic floor muscle strength in order to offset its adverse effect on quality of life and social functioning, deterring several women from taking part in physical exercises or sports for fear of urine leakage (Stoner et al., 2000).

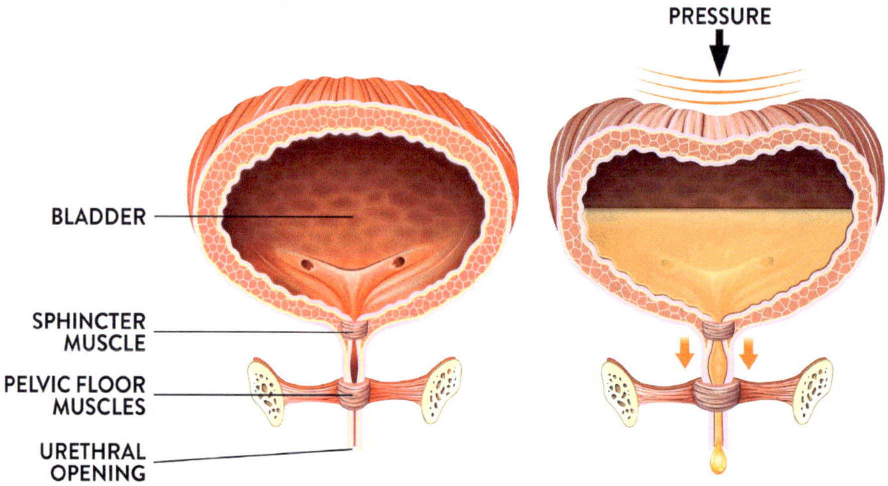

Figure 11.2. Stress urinary incontinence.

Source: https://nafc.org/female-stress-incontinence/

Other causative factors of stress incontinence include the nature of delivery experienced during childbirth, particularly vaginal delivery, since this has been found to be related to a greater incidence of pelvic floor dysfunction. The impact of childbirth on the support mechanisms of the pelvis cannot be overstressed, as vaginal delivery is likely to inflict tremendous trauma on the perineal muscles and the surrounding musculature. A pelvic floor dysfunction study noted that rising age, rising body mass index (BMI), and more childbirths contribute to SUI prevalence in women. Most notably, the study found that the majority of women who came in with symptoms had delivered vaginally, suggesting awareness and targeted treatment are most important to them. In the management of SUI, healthcare providers must go beyond medical treatment and ought to emphasize preventive measures and postpartum management for long-term pelvic improvement (Basappa et al., 2020). Finally, public stigma in urinary incontinence inspires fear to report symptoms, thus denying women access to proper care. The psychological effect of stress incontinence can be tremendous, leading to a loss of self-esteem and restricted lifestyle activities. Women may be withdrawn from social activities because they do not want to risk embarrassment or accidental leakage. In order to counteract these effects, education regarding the condition is crucial, to make conversation about urinary issues more acceptable and increase communication between patients and doctors. Also, effective management options like pelvic floor physical therapy, behavioral therapy, and, if needed, surgery should be readily accessible and clearly communicated to the victims of this condition. Promoting awareness and enhancing treatment accessibility can significantly improve the quality of life of women with stress incontinence (Stoner et al., 2000; Basappa et al., 2020).

11.1.2. Urge Incontinence

Urge incontinence, or involuntary urine loss with the abrupt, forceful sensation of the need to urinate, is a significant problem in most women in the United States. The symptom usually has causes such as an overactive bladder muscle, neurologic disease, or infection, which create a compulsive, immediate need to empty the bladder. The psychological impact of urge incontinence is very relevant, leading to feelings of embarrassment, anxiety, and social isolation in affected women. High numbers of patients delay treatment because of the stigmatization of urinary incontinence, leading to a lower quality of life. It is crucial for medical professionals to understand the multifactorial nature of this condition because it allows one to treat the condition in a more polydirectional way that can efficiently alleviate symptoms and enhance the daily functioning of patients. Treatment of urge incontinence is generally a combination of behavioral modification and pharmacology. The initial treatment may be bladder training to enable the patient to extend the time between voiding episodes, thus increasing bladder control.

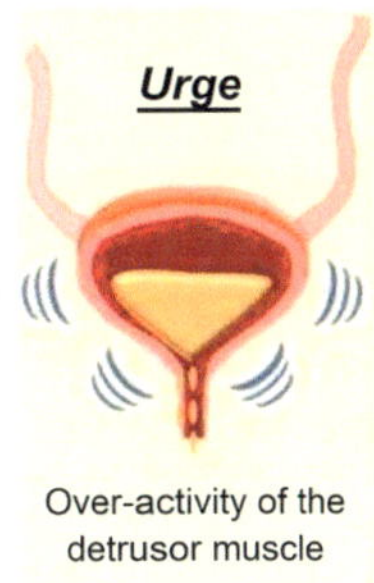

Figure 11.3. Urge incontinence.

Source: https://wecaregolp.com/wp-content/uploads/2023/03/Urinary-Incontinence-e1679984771105.jpg

Other techniques, such as pelvic floor exercises, are equally crucial since they make the muscles that support the bladder stronger and improve its function. Also, while patients may at first think that drugs are their only option, literature is increasingly directing us towards the significance of conservative management, and particularly physical therapy, in addressing this condition. While practitioners develop their awareness regarding the different treatment options that can be employed, they are in a position to instruct women to appreciate customized care programs which can incorporate lifestyle modifications, dietetic control, and exercise therapy interventions for improving the support mechanisms of the pelvis, thus addressing both the physical and psychologic aspects of urge incontinence (Wells et al., 1994).

Research has established that urge incontinence affects women disproportionately and frequently relates to age, menopause, and certain medical histories, including prior pregnancy. While examining the correlation between childbirth and frequency of urge incontinence, research has established an association, through which childbirth and vaginal deliveries cause pelvic floor dysfunction that ultimately increases the likelihood for urinary incontinence in old age (Stoner et al., 2000). Exploring this interaction educates the necessity of particular preventive treatments and early interventions in the healthcare apparatus. Through understanding these risk factors, healthcare providers can implement precautionary steps, such as education on pelvic floor maintenance, that might reduce the risk of urge incontinence among women, and educate the significance of a preventative model in urinary health administration.

11.1.3. Mixed Incontinence

Mixed incontinence, characterized by the coexistence of stress urinary incontinence (SUI) and urge urinary incontinence (UUI), presents a unique challenge to women with this condition. Compared to pure incontinence syndromes, mixed incontinence requires an advanced understanding of both mechanisms behind the symptoms. Stress incontinence typically manifests with activity that increases intra-abdominal pressure, such as coughing, sneezing, or exertion, while urge incontinence is characterized by a sudden, urgent need to void urine. The combination of the two complicates diagnosis and treatment, and healthcare providers must adjust therapy strategies in order to be able to restore the multidimensional condition. The prevalence of mixed incontinence is particularly noteworthy in older women, who accrue compounded risk factors over time, such as pelvic floor muscle weakness and neurologic changes. Studies have discovered that the presence of lower urinary tract symptoms (LUTS), such as mixed incontinence, has a strong correlation with other health domains, such as risk for falls. Specifically, the association of LUTS and falls is indicative of a broader issue of frailty in this group because both have overlapping etiological factors. Treatment of mixed incontinence thus needs an integrative approach that targets not just the urinary issue but also the overall physical well-being, including how to promote balance and mobility, which are critical determinants of reducing LUTS-related fall risk (Booth et al., 2017).

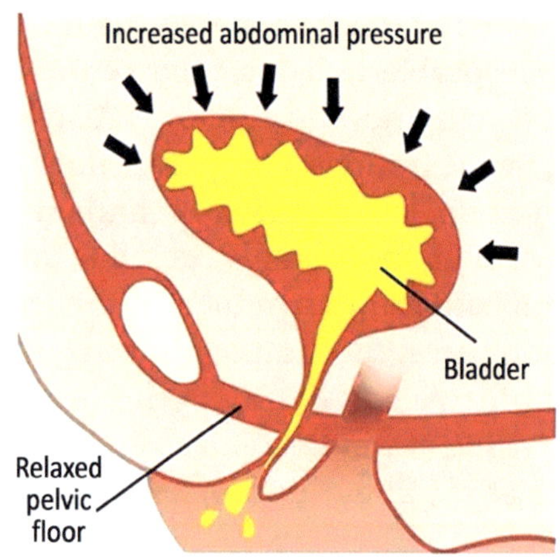

Figure 11.4. Mixed incontinence.

Source: https://alwaysdiscreet.com/en-us/incontinence-advice-support/what-is-mixed-incontinence

In understanding mixed incontinence, it is also important to remember the psychological impact and quality of life issues on women suffering from this condition. As per studies, urinary incontinence, particularly mixed, carries a significant adverse impact on sexual function and social relationships, causing a substantial amount of distress as well as lower self-esteem. As in studies, women with urinary incontinence are less satisfied with sexual relationships and perceive the tone of their vagina is weaker, particularly in vaginal delivery or non-exercising pelvic floor muscle exercises (PFMEs) women (Aung et al., 2008). Therefore, a good management plan not only treats the physiological symptoms but also includes counseling and education for pelvic floor health to enhance quality of life in women with mixed incontinence.

Test Your Knowledge

1. What is the primary cause of stress incontinence in women?
2. How does urge incontinence differ from stress incontinence in terms of symptoms?

11.2. Causes of Urinary Incontinence

Learning Outcome

1. Describe the anatomical factors contributing to urinary incontinence in females
2. Define hormonal changes
3. Explain the lifestyle and behavioral factors

The pathophysiology of female incontinence is multifactorial, with a series of physiological and lifestyle factors that can have a major impact on the function of the bladder. The most frequent cause is childbirth, particularly by the vaginal route, which causes weakening of the pelvic floor muscles and disruption of the support of the urethra.

This usually leads to SUI, an overactive type that is precipitated by physical maneuvers such as exercise or sneezing. Additionally, age is also a determining factor because elastin and collagen fibers also degenerate with age in pelvic tissues, and therefore, it becomes probable to be incontinent. Obesity also tends to make this issue more severe, placing additional pressure on the bladder and pelvic organs. All these factors together demonstrate a significant association between lifestyle choices and the prevalence of urinary incontinence in females, which establishes that preventive measures could well mitigate such threats. Sport participation, particularly in high-impact sports, is one of the strong etiological reasons for urinary incontinence. Sports such as weightlifting, gymnastics, and basketball, as recent studies have indicated, have been linked with a high incidence of SUI among sportswomen.

For instance, a 560 nulliparous Indian female sportswomen investigation concluded that weightlifters' sportswomen reported an unusually high prevalence of SUI, proving once again that undue physical stress could lead to pelvic floor dysfunction (Syeda et al., 2024). Again, the psychological and emotional impacts of urinary incontinence on athletes cannot be downplayed. Anxiety about leakage with practice or competition might prevent participation in sport, and thus, both adapted interventions and awareness campaigns that overcome the physical and psychological barriers to this group of women are indicated.

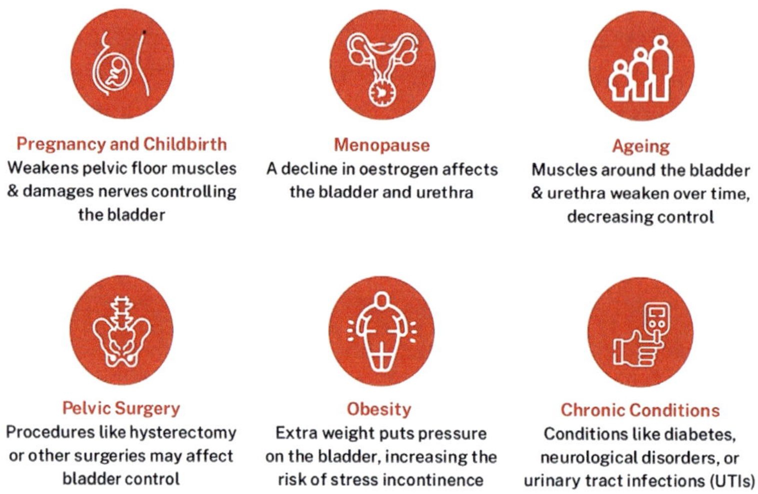

Figure 11.5. Causes of Urinary Incontinence in Women.

Source: https://ckbh.ckbirlahospitals.com/storage/cmri/uploadedfiles/gallery/article/causes-of-urinary-incontinence-03.webp

The social context of women experiencing urinary incontinence must also be taken into account, particularly where stigma and ignorance are dominant. In communities throughout sub-Saharan Africa, for instance, women will be reluctant to present themselves because of stigma around incontinence, resulting in underreporting of the condition (Whiting et al., 2022). This has significant implications, for quietly enduring women will not only affect their physical health but incur profound social and emotional expenditures in the form of relationship tension and depression. By putting a high value on properly designed education programs, this will be able to de-mystify urinary incontinence, will enable women to seek medical advice, and, in the end, sustain healthier lifestyles. Addressing social barriers to women's open discussion and management of this issue is vital for improving their quality of life and enabling timely treatment of urinary incontinence.

11.2.1. Anatomical Factors

The anatomical factors responsible for urinary incontinence among women are multifactorial and contribute to the prevalence and nature of incontinence that is present. Critical structures such as the pelvic floor muscles, bladder, and urethra play a key role in the maintenance of continence. The pelvic floor supports the base for the pelvic organs, and its integrity is critical in the prevention of inappropriate urine leakage. Weakness of such muscles, commonly seen in addition to conditions such as childbirth, obesity, or age, can lead to stress incontinence, wherein leakage takes place during activities of heightened abdominal pressure such as coughing or exercise. This compromise in structure points towards the importance of understanding physiological considerations in urinary incontinence, as this dictates successful treatments and preventive strategies for the betterment of pelvic health. Besides pelvic support, the role of the urethra is also critical in urinary continence. The anatomic position and length of the female urethra, being naturally shorter than that of men, render females more susceptible to involuntary leakage.

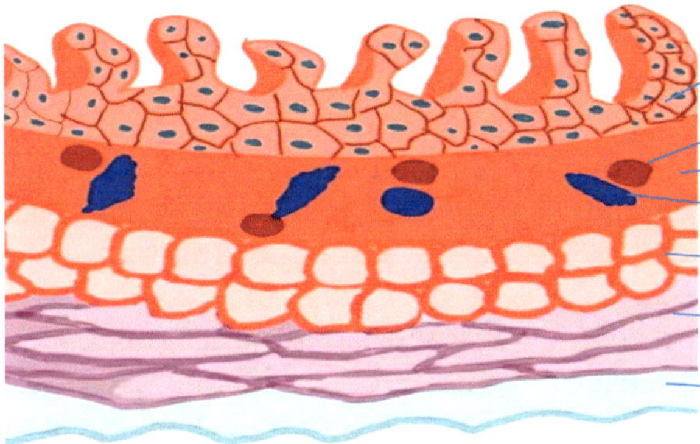

Figure 11.6. The normal transverse section of the urethral anatomy.

Source: https://www.mdpi.com/1648-9144/59/1/5

Coupling this anatomical susceptibility, hormonal changes during menopause also reduce urethral elasticity and muscle tone, thereby enhancing urinary incontinence among post-menopausal women. Urinary incontinence among post-menopausal women has been estimated at approximately 46.24% by research, thereby indicating a very high correlation between age and anatomical factors (Alexander et al., 2019). This information assists medical professionals in anticipating the issues faced by older women and highlights the necessity of certain interventions aimed at both anatomical reconstruction and symptomatic therapy through varied therapies. Moreover, surgical issues, particularly hysterectomy, demand extensive review due to their potential impact on urinary continence. Although hysterectomy remains a powerful therapy for many gynecological issues, its impact on urinary function is of greatest concern. There has been a proposal in some literature that there is a relationship between hysterectomy and the onset of urinary incontinence, though the evidence is not consistent. A recent study found that the prevalence of urinary incontinence is similar in women with natural menopause and surgical menopause, suggesting that hysterectomy per se is perhaps not an acute risk factor for its development (Alexander et al., 2019). These results highlight the importance of considering surgically induced anatomical changes, supporting the value of proper preoperative consultation regarding urinary health as a component of women's care.

11.2.2. Hormonal Changes

The interaction between hormonal shifts and urinary incontinence among women is most prominent during menopausal transition. With the decline in estrogen, the characteristic evidence of aging, several physiological changes occur within the female urogenital system. Hypoestrogenism, especially, results in pelvic floor muscle weakness and reduction of urethral support, aggravating stress urinary incontinence. The importance of these hormonal alterations is underscored by epidemiological data that show a striking relationship between hormonal change and the onset of urinary incontinence, both being major risk factors for this condition. Moreover, the psychological and emotional impact of urinary incontinence adds to the complexity in women during menopause, making a need for holistic management that considers both physiological and psychological factors of this chronic disorder. The link between urinary incontinence and obesity renders the hormonal profile of postmenopausal women more complex. Increased body mass index (BMI) has been identified as a strong, independent risk factor for urinary incontinence, with each 5-unit increase in BMI being associated with a 20%-70% increased risk of developing the disorder. The link necessitates an investigation of lifestyle factors affected by hormonal changes, such as fat distribution and metabolism, which can exacerbate the activities of incontinence. Consequently, the overlap of weight gain with hormonal alterations and risk of incontinence creates a complicated scenario that requires special treatment. Evidence has been provided through research that weight loss, either by surgical means or adjustment of lifestyle, can lead to major declines in urinary incontinence symptoms, precipitating an opening for treatment and improvement of quality of life for such women (Subak et al., 2011). Hormonal therapy is typically considered for menopausal urinary symptoms, but it may not always be suitable for all women. Since evidence on the Genitourinary Syndrome of Menopause shows that in around 70% of postmenopausal women, hypoestrogenism is the cause of multiple symptoms, including urinary incontinence. Traditional treatments like estrogen therapy alleviate symptoms; however, some women must use non-hormonal therapy because of contraindication or ineffectiveness with hormonal therapy. More modern treatments like topical prometriene or fractional CO_2 laser treatment have emerged and have demonstrated clinical benefit in the amelioration of urinary symptoms as well as in the reversal of the vaginal flora alteration and ecosystem (Aguiar et al., 2019). As the specialty expands, it remains important to pair treatments with patients based on their personal hormonal profiles and presentations, emphasizing the importance of an inclusive and individualized response to the treatment of urinary incontinence in women.

11.2.3. Lifestyle and Behavioral Factors

Lifestyle and behavioral factors occupy a central position in the etiology and management of urinary incontinence in women. One of the primary focuses has been obesity, which is a risk factor exacerbating the condition. Epidemiological studies have consistently demonstrated that there exists a very close correlation between body mass index (BMI) and urinary incontinence, demonstrating that for every rise of 5 units in BMI, exists risk of urinary incontinence ranging from 20% to 70% (Subak et al., 2011). This demonstrates how central weight management is to prevention and treatment planning as a most important aspect. Far too under-recognized, lifestyle issues like diet and exercise can be instrumental interventions that not only contribute to weight loss but also urinary well-being. In addition to obesity, physical activity level and behavioral factors are also instrumental in managing urinary incontinence symptoms. Physical exercise on a regular basis has been documented to enhance pelvic floor muscle strength and assist with bladder function management. Moreover, certain forms of exercise, for example, pelvic floor muscle training, are particularly effective in significantly decreasing the symptoms of urinary incontinence. The interplay between urinary health and lifestyle emphasizes the necessity for targeted educational interventions advocating exercise and its benefits. In particular, women would be recommended to engage in structured program exercise aimed at the strengthening of pelvic musculature as a non-surgical but effective method of management. Such interventions have been revealed to be evidence-supported, substantiating the connection between an active lifestyle and improved urinary continence outcomes. Further, behavioral habits, including smoking and alcohol, cannot be discounted in urinary incontinence. Smoking has been revealed to be linked with increased coughing, which can exacerbate stress incontinence, while excessive alcohol consumption will result in increased urgency and frequency of micturition. Intervention on such habits through counseling and lifestyle modification programs will go a long way in urinary well-being. Quitting smoking and restricted alcohol consumption, in fact, are at the heart of a comprehensive management of urinary incontinence. The better that women know the ill effects of such activities, the more likely they may be to make improved lifestyle choices, reducing the prevalence and severity of urinary incontinence even more. A comprehensive insight into the behavioral and lifestyle causes is significant for the formulation of effective interventions to improve the quality of life of women affected by this condition (Burgio et al., 2013).

Test Your Knowledge

1. How do anatomical factors such as pelvic floor weakness contribute to urinary incontinence?
2. In what ways can hormonal changes during menopause affect bladder control?

11.3. Risk Factors

Learning Outcome

1. Discuss the age and menopause
2. Explain the obesity
3. Define childbirth and pelvic floor damage

Knowledge of the risk factors for female urinary incontinence is critical to effective prevention and care. Various parameters dictate the risk for the condition, ranging from age to obesity to lifestyle. With advancing age, spontaneous changes in physiology during menopause, such as decreased levels of estrogen, may lead to pelvic floor muscle weakening, which is crucial for bladder control. Also, obesity significantly increases intra-abdominal pressure, which again loads the pelvic supportive apparatus. This synergy of obesity and age emphasizes the importance of exercise and a healthy weight to minimize the chance of urinary incontinence and general pelvic health. Besides age and obesity, other medical comorbidities and anatomic features also play a significant role in the etiology of urinary incontinence in women. Metabolic syndrome has also come into the limelight for its potential link with lower urinary tract symptoms (LUTS) and overactive bladder (OAB), both of which have a strong correlation with incontinence. The evidence suggests that there is a correlation between metabolic syndrome factors like blood pressure and diabetes and the prevalence of LUTS in women, i.e., metabolic health directly affects urinary function. These patients need to be evaluated for metabolic syndrome as part of their clinical evaluation, demonstrating the need for a complete approach in the management of urinary incontinence (Bunn et al., 2015).

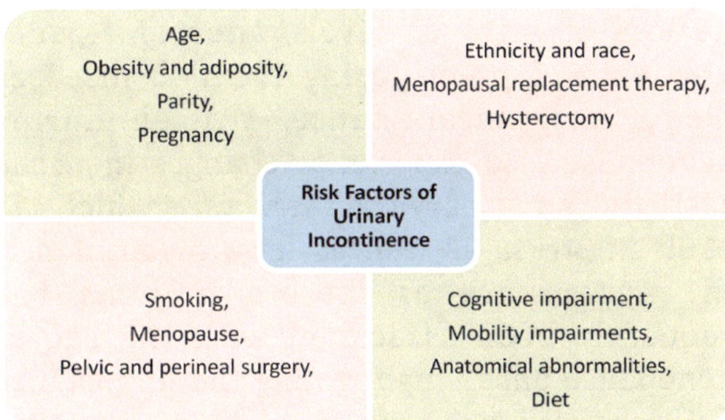

Figure 11.7. Risk Factors for Incontinence in Women.

Source: https://api.intechopen.com/media/chapter/53697/media/F2.png

Furthermore, habits of lifestyle, including diet, exercise, and the use of medication, can exacerbate or improve symptoms of urinary incontinence. For instance, consumption of some irritants, for example, alcohol and caffeine, may increase urinary frequency and urgency, and thus cause episodes of incontinence. Smoking is also a lifestyle habit linked to pelvic floor dysfunction in that it can induce chronic cough and bladder pressure. In some cases, the medications themselves can also be responsible for incontinence by affecting the control of the bladder directly or by exacerbating underlying medical conditions like urinary tract infections (UTIs). Older adults, particularly women, are at greater risk for UTI, which is further compounded by indwelling catheters, thus creating a vicious cycle that further deteriorates bladder health (Beveridge et al., 2011). Addressing these risk factors in an integrated manner is important to improving outcomes in women with urinary incontinence.

11.3.1. Age and Menopause

As women age, particularly as they reach menopause age, a complex combination of physiological processes occurs that has a direct influence on urinary health. Menopause significantly affects the urogenital system by the loss of estrogen levels, altering bladder function and predisposing them to diseases like urinary incontinence. Women during menopause also experience changes in tissue elasticity and urinary tract structure, which can result in stress as well as urge incontinence. The appearance of these symptoms has frequently been associated with the age at menopause onset, highlighting the importance of understanding this biological event. Moreover, urinary incontinence occurs in considerably higher numbers among postmenopausal women, and thus a better assessment of changes with age in hormones and how they impact urinary continence is significant. Recent studies highlight the interaction of menopausal status and age and the incidence of lower urinary tract symptoms (LUTS), a common complaint among older women. The interaction of LUTS and age exhibits an alarming pattern that not only affects quality of life but also serves as a marker for frailty, which itself is correlated with other health hazards such as falls and loss of mobility. The risk of falls in women with LUTS has odds ratios that suggest high correlation, between 1.5 and 2.3. The association assumes that as women age and reach menopause, their risk of incontinence may increase their risk of falls, necessitating integrated actions to address these concomitant conditions in practice (Booth et al., 2017). In order to counteract the undesirable effects associated with menopause, the use of individualized management approaches that consider patient profiles is required. The Treatment of Symptoms of the Menopause Task Force points out the necessity for individualized therapy, suggesting that menopausal hormone therapy (MHT) is highly effective in alleviating not only vasomotor symptoms but potentially also the genitourinary syndrome that typically occurs at the time of menopause. For those patients who are not candidates for MHT or refuse alternatives, low-dose vaginal estrogen and other non-hormonal treatment options can be used to adequately control urinary incontinence (Davis et al., 2015). Menopause's multifaceted nature and the attendant complications necessitate an integrative approach that encompasses lifestyle interventions, patient individualized healthcare approaches, and ongoing research directed at optimizing the health of aging women with urinary problems.

11.3.2. Obesity

It has also emerged as a significant public health problem, particularly in women, due to its severe correlation with other medical conditions, like urinary incontinence (UI). Moreover, epidemiological studies constantly reaffirm that obesity is an independent risk factor for both the incidence and prevalence of urinary incontinence. The connection between body mass index (BMI) and urinary incontinence is alarming; an increase in BMI by 5 units has been found to coincide with a 20% to 70% increased risk of acquiring urinary incontinence. The implications of this statistic are alarming, particularly considering the reality that women must often contend with extreme physiological challenges regarding weight dispersion and hormonal impacts that restrict urination function. Hence, obesity is a matter not just of significance for the betterment of overall health but even more so for the strategic management of urinary incontinence in women. The implications of weight management extend to therapeutic domains; successful weight loss can significantly suppress the signs of urinary incontinence. Surgical and non-surgical weight reduction procedures have been found to manage the frequency and occurrence of urinary incontinence in obese and overweight women. In several investigations, successful weight control resulted in considerable improvement not just in urinary symptoms but also in the quality of life of these patients. The linear dose-response relation shown in some investigations confirms the contention that modest weight loss can produce significant benefits, highlighting the significance of obesity management as a first-line treatment option.

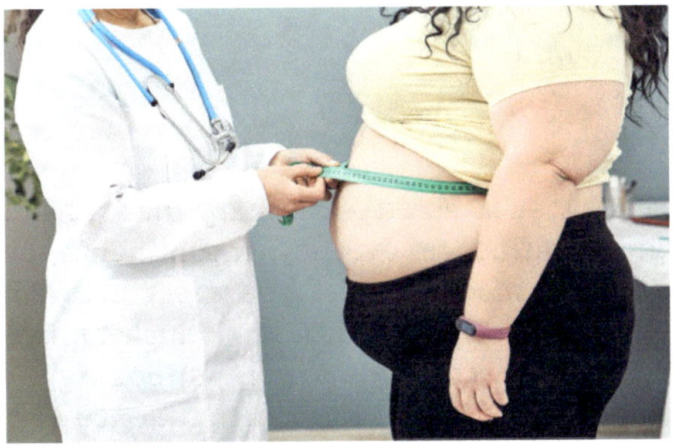

Source: https://media.istockphoto.com/id/1314797892/photo/obesity-unhealthy-weight-nutritionist-inspecting-a-womans-waist-using-a-meter-tape-to.jpg?s=612x612&w=0&k=20&c=1hsjTpScP_NJ-gYfMHStLV-fbyqi8iv1ORNJ2J06grE=

As a result, healthcare providers are increasingly being recommended to include weight loss management within treatment plans for urinary incontinence patients. In addition to direct effects on urinary incontinence, the connection between metabolic syndrome and lower urinary tract symptoms also makes it even more difficult to address obesity-associated urinary issues. Progressive research has indicated that components of metabolic syndrome, most commonly found to be present with obesity—such as hypertension, dyslipidemia, and insulin resistance—also contribute to the etiology of overactive bladder and directly related urinary dysfunction. Given the complex interrelationship of these diseases, medical experts must learn how obesity and secondary metabolic conditions interact to influence urinary health. Through such intricate examination, clinicians are more likely to create interventions that address both urinary incontinence and obesity at the same time in a comprehensive way, thereby improving patient outcomes while very low BMI potentially reducing the economic burden of these conditions among women (Subak et al., 2011; Bunn et al., 2015).

11.3.3. Childbirth and Pelvic Floor Damage

The intricate interaction of childbirth and pelvic floor trauma lies at the heart of the explanation of the high prevalence of urinary incontinence in women. Childbirth constitutes a severe stress event on the pelvic floor, particularly with vaginal delivery, which has been found to be connected with a number of complications, including urinary incontinence. As the pelvic floor consists of supporting structures such as muscles, fascia, and ligaments, all injuries incurred during childbirth can lead to weakened support systems. Alteration of these structures affects bladder control functions and leads to the development of urinary incontinence. This deficiency highlights that, in addition to being a physiological process, childbirth is also a strong determinant of women's long-term pelvic health, which calls for preventive interventions and postpartum rehabilitation. Research highlights that harm caused to the pelvic floor during childbirth is widespread and impacts urinary control, as well as conditions such as anal incontinence and pelvic organ prolapse. These secondary complications indicate the complexity of pelvic floor health and the multiple implications surrounding birth. As is underscored, the underlying pathophysiology of these complications lies with the normal trauma of delivery, which may include the stretching and tearing of the pelvic structures. Moreover, the integrity of the pelvic floor, having once been compromised, can predispose it to a cycle of constant complications, which necessitates that there be a critical examination of risk factors for childbirth. In efforts to keep such risks at a minimum, the mechanisms behind damage to the pelvic floor are important to understand, thereby enabling healthcare providers to design targeted prevention and management of such. Intensive interventions such as pelvic floor exercises, such as the mula bandha exercise, have become integral parts to condition the pelvic region and potentially prevent the development of urinary incontinence following childbirth. The exercises target the strengthening of the muscles supporting the bladder and urethra, addressing the causes of pelvic floor weakness. While pregnancy is a primary risk factor for pelvic floor dysfunction, the incorporation of regular pelvic floor exercises during pregnancy and postpartum is a proactive step toward optimal pelvic health. The efficacy of such exercises has been demonstrated in reducing symptoms of stress urinary incontinence, and there is a direct correlation between physical therapy and the return of pelvic floor function. By facilitating awareness and adoption of these exercises, healthcare workers have an effective tool to significantly enhance the quality of life for women experiencing the challenges of postpartum recovery, and reduce the risk of urinary incontinence (Awasthi et al., 2015).

Test Your Knowledge

1. How does menopause increase the risk of urinary incontinence in females?
2. What role does obesity play in the development or worsening of urinary incontinence?

11.4. Symptoms and Diagnosis

Learning Outcome

1. Identify the common symptoms experienced
2. Explain the diagnostic tests and assessments
3. Define the importance of medical history

Symptoms of female urinary incontinence can profoundly impact daily functioning as well as overall quality of life. Understanding the various forms in which incontinence may manifest is essential, such as stress urinary incontinence, urge incontinence, overflow incontinence, and functional incontinence. The most prevalent is stress urinary incontinence, which typically manifests with coughing, sneezing, or exercise. Conversely, urge incontinence is an overwhelming, sudden urge to urinate, resulting in involuntary leakage. It is critical to understand these distinctions in order to warrant immediate diagnosis and efficacious treatment intervention. Correct symptom recognition enables the medical team to create interventions tailor-made to each patient's needs, optimizing the recovery outcome and overall well-being. Urinary incontinence diagnosis begins with a complete medical history and physical examination, whereby health care professionals gather data on the patient's symptoms, their onset, and their precipitating factors. Additionally, a specific assessment may involve bladder diaries or questionnaires to quantify the frequency and severity of incontinence episodes. These tests not only help in the type of incontinence classification but also in identifying any hidden condition, such as urinary tract infections or prolapse of pelvic organs.

This type of systematic diagnosis is crucial because nearly 40-60% of patients admitted to hospitals after stroke have urinary incontinence, 25% have difficulty at the time of discharge, and 15% still have problems after one year. Hence, the appropriate assessments play a key role in deciding and managing the complexities in the case of urinary incontinence (Abrams et al., 2008). It is also important to assess the influence of general health complications, such as gynecological cancers, on the severity of urinary incontinence. Research indicates that pelvic tumors in women tend to produce pelvic floor dysfunction that, at times, leads to urinary complications. Despite the oncologic management of cancers like cervical, endometrial, and ovarian being a top priority, their effect on urinary function is substantial and largely underestimated.

Most women are likely to persist with urinary incontinence even after effective cancer treatment, and this highlights the requirement for post-treatment evaluations for the health of the pelvic floor. Ineffective reporting and description of pelvic floor disorders by the patients and clinicians can hinder future timely interventions, which are indispensable in enhancing the quality of life of cancer survivors (Bodean et al., 2018). As such, a holistic approach that incorporates post-cancer treatment evaluations is imperative to combat urinary incontinence holistically.

11.4.1. Common Symptoms Experienced

Female urinary incontinence produces a variety of symptoms that can have a profoundly detrimental impact on quality of life. The most common presentation may be leakage of urine inappropriately, and this may occur under a variety of circumstances, such as exercise, sneezing, or indeed with laughing. This involuntary loss of continence, generally characterized as stress incontinence, is particularly prevalent in women who have given birth or experienced hormonal alterations due to menopause. As the literature underlines, the severity of these symptoms significantly affects women's everyday life and mood, often leading to social isolation and low self-esteem. It is vital to understand these symptoms because they bring out the necessity of initial interventions and supportive management for the affected individuals. Another significant symptom of urinary incontinence is frequency or the need to urinate very often. Women can experience a strong and urgent feeling of having to void, leading to painful moments where they cannot make it to the bathroom in time. This is particularly common with overactive bladder (OAB), which may coexist with urinary incontinence. The impact of urgency is multiplied, encompassing physical, psychological, and social domains. Urgency can be related to an underlying health condition, such as metabolic syndrome, resulting in chronic lower urinary tract symptoms (Bunn et al., 2015).

This association indicates that healthcare professionals need to consider complete assessments to establish the primary causes of urgency among their patients in an effort to enhance the outcomes of treatment and client satisfaction. The other symptoms that are frequently reported alongside urinary incontinence include pain and pelvic pressure.

The majority of women feel fullness or heaviness in the pelvic region, a sign of pelvic organ prolapse. Evidence supports the existence of pelvic floor symptoms commonly occurring together with urinary incontinence, as supported by a study demonstrating effective treatment with pelvic floor muscle training (PFMT) for symptom improvement (Glazener et al., 2009). In addition, the symptoms can not only contribute to the physical burden of the condition but also become intertwined with emotional distress and anxiety. The interrelated nature of such symptoms demands a thoroughly integrated treatment strategy emphasizing the concurrent treatment of both the physical and emotional problems that beset patients with urinary incontinence.

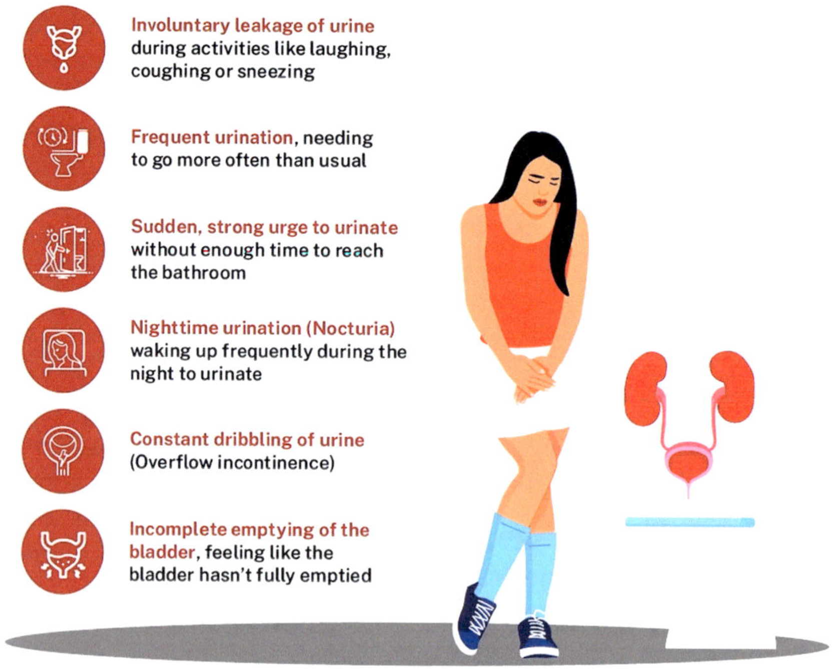

Figure 11.8. Common symptoms of urinary incontinence.

Source: https://ckbh.ckbirlahospitals.com/storage/cmri/uploadedfiles/gallery/article/symptoms-of-urinary-incontinence-02.webp

11.4.2. Diagnostic Tests and Assessments

In diagnosing incontinence of urine in women, a comprehensive diagnostic approach is the cornerstone for effective management and care. An extensive history of the patient is the first step, wherein clinicians take information regarding the timing, frequency, and nature of the symptoms along with the potential contributory factors such as comorbid conditions and lifestyle. This kind of assessment not only allows for the diagnosis of incontinence type—stress, urge, or mixed—but also of underlying conditions for which the need for further investigation can be established. As emphasized in studies investigating allied health conditions, an awareness of such factors is often necessary, as urinary incontinence could coexist with other disorders such as combative behavior in intellectually disabled adults and mental illness (Alborz et al., 2009).

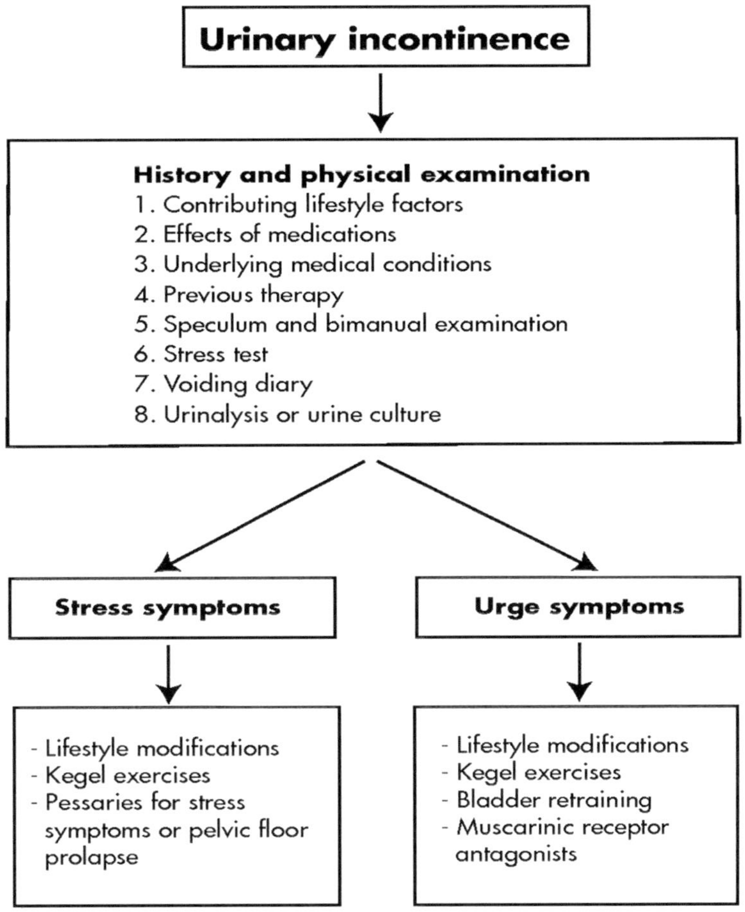

Figure 11.9. Management of urinary incontinence.

Source: https://external-content.duckduckgo.com/iu/?u=https%3A%2F%2Fd3i71xaburhd42.cloudfront.net%2F8705ee5f797a7721b4b144091651a41dc562d4d1%2F4-Figure1-1.png&f=1&nofb=1&ipt=68c7864d0ed53ce1b687f235f461ba327d28f2cf47e80cb87f8a3e89fcaf8a69

Thus, an adequate history forms the basis of an individualized plan of diagnosis that can lead to improved health for women with urinary incontinence. With the adequate history in place, clinical assessments and tests then fulfill a valuable role in defining the diagnosis and the best treatment. Physical exams, as well as attentive assessment of pelvic floor function, can reveal mechanical causes of incontinence. Also, urodynamic studies, which measure bladder pressure, capacity, and compliance, provide essential information to help distinguish between types of incontinence and define bladder function. Evaluation may include urinary diaries, in which patients record fluid intake, frequency of incontinence episodes, and related activities, again illustrating interference with daily activities. For the elderly, geriatric syndrome screening, such as urinary incontinence, is more critical due to the comorbid complications that characterize these conditions, as evidenced by diagnostic performance studies showing the necessity of early detection (Büla et al., 2018).

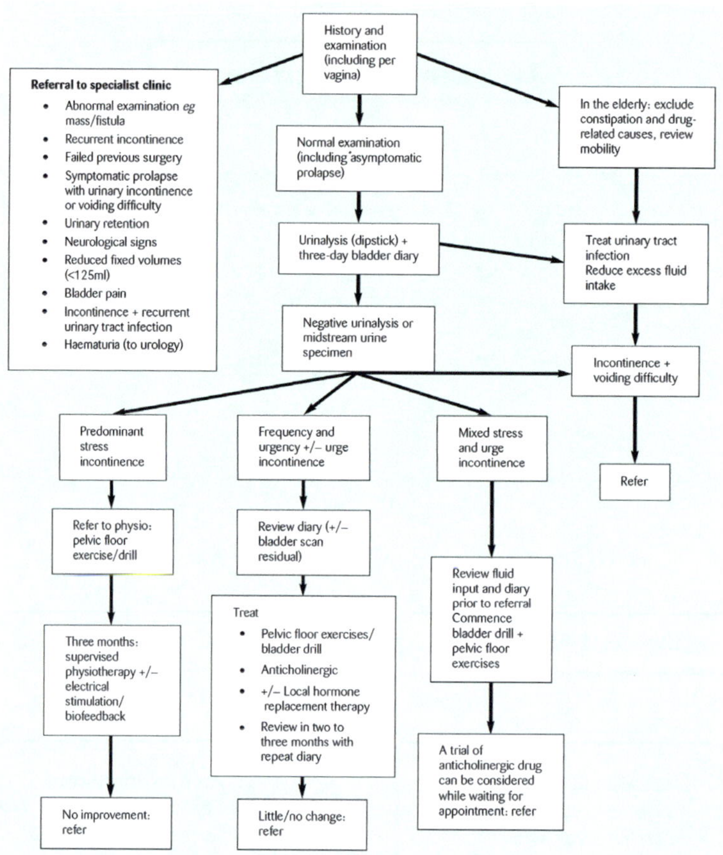

Figure 11.10. Flow chart for assessment of urinary incontinence in primary care.

Source: https://www.researchgate.net/profile/Swati-Jha-2/publication/264807601/figure/fig3/AS:296226105905181@1447637215762/Flow-chart-for-assessment-of-urinary-incontinence-in-primary-care14.png

Furthermore, symptoms need to be supplemented by quality-of-life questionnaires to measure the functional and psychological impact of urinary incontinence on affected patients. Including standardized questionnaires like the Incontinence Severity Index or the UDI-6 provides quantitative information on symptom severity as well as impact on society. These measurements not only allow clinicians to tailor individualized treatment plans but also elicit discussions about patient preference and concern. By focusing on the inclusive evaluation strategy with considerations of physiological as well as psychosocial implications, clinicians can overcome the multifaceted causes of urinary incontinence among women. As discussed above, the multifaceted nature of these aspects is not merely a matter of addressing a clinical sign but is necessarily at the core of improving total health outcomes and improvement among affected individuals.

11.4.3. Importance of Medical History

A patient's medical history is a precious guide to diagnosis and the treatment of urinary incontinence in females. An in-depth understanding of one's medical history can enlighten one regarding potential risk factors, causative conditions, and therapeutic response. For instance, previous instances of urinary tract infections (UTIs) or diseases such as pelvic organ prolapse, among others, can significantly impact the incidence of urinary incontinence.

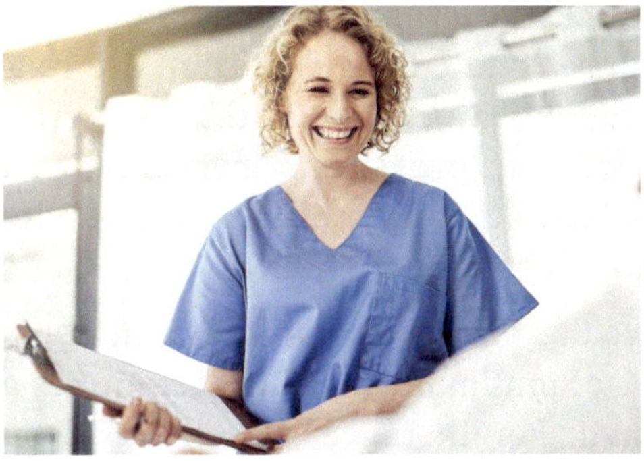

Source: https://cdn.prismcareerinstitute.edu/wp-content/uploads/2019/06/Assistant-Taking-Patient-History.jpg

The incontinence epidemiology determines the determinants applicable to age, parity, and hormonal status, and will only be fully understood through elicited medical histories in detail. In addition, the assessment of the patient's history enables clinicians to identify patterns of incontinence in relation to lifestyle factors and comorbid conditions and thus provide enhanced clinical practice and individualized treatment strategies. Furthermore, the medical history review aids in the discrimination between various types of urinary incontinence, for example, stress incontinence, urge incontinence, and overflow incontinence. Each of these subtypes can have specific diagnostic methods and treatment regimens. For example, if a patient has a history of frequent UTIs, this can lead to further workup to rule out complications like catheter-related urinary tract infection, which occurs frequently in specific populations. Incorporation of medical history into the diagnostic process can allow for the use of the naloxone antimicrobial drugs or modification of treatment modalities according to local resistance patterns, further improving patient outcomes. The implications of medical history are therefore profound, not only in directing clinical assessment but also in helping to develop evidence-based treatment modalities.

Talking about the role of medical history in urinary incontinence is particularly pertinent to issues of complications due to suboptimal exams. Inadequate documentation leads to misdiagnosis, which eventually compromises patient safety and therapeutic efficacy. For instance, inappropriate interpretation of symptoms without regard to history may lead to treatment in the form of excessive use of antibiotics for asymptomatic bacteriuria, which should not be treated as per guidelines. This emphasizes the need for educating medical professionals about the significance of taking adequate medical histories, particularly among culturally diverse patient populations with atypical symptomatology. Emphasis on this aspect of patient care is not only in accordance with best practice but further ensures a harmonized approach to the management of urinary incontinence that effectively addresses the concern while preserving quality of life in affected women and reducing public health concerns associated with this commonly identified problem.

Test Your Knowledge

1. What are common symptoms experienced by females with urinary incontinence?
2. Name two diagnostic tests commonly used to assess urinary incontinence in females.

11.5. Treatment Options

Learning Outcome

1. Discuss the behavioral therapies for urinary incontinence
2. Define surgical interventions

Treatment of urinary incontinence in women encompasses a broad range of measures, from conservative, nonoperative to more invasive surgical measures. Lifestyle modification and pelvic floor muscle training are starting points that tighten up the supportive tissues of the bladder and urethra. Behavioral therapies such as bladder training and fluid management can potentially alleviate the symptoms of urinary incontinence by a significant percentage, particularly in patients with stress urinary incontinence (SUI) (Petca et al., 2025). Nonsurgical treatment not only offers candidates a less aggressive alternative but also increases patient involvement, ultimately resulting in a better quality of life for patients.

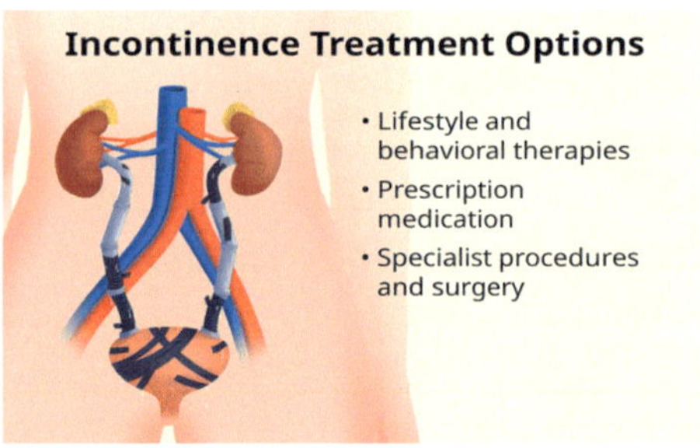

Figure 11.11. Urinary incontinence treatment options.

Source: https://www.verywellhealth.com/thmb/nDtKe35jHHi0K2ulBGpvDiDdoNY=/1500x0/filters:no_upscale():max_bytes(150000):strip_icc()/VerywellHealthNewCreate-ControllingIncontinence-WhatAreMyTreatmentOptions-final-e05089de43dd4c0587eacc6f66d79fcd.png

Educational efforts for these interventions are necessary, as the majority of the women are unaware of the alternatives, leading to underreporting and inappropriate management of the condition. If the nonsurgical measures do not succeed, more advanced treatments may be considered. Surgical therapies, particularly in moderate to severe SUI, have become a popular choice as good long-term options. Sling procedures and colposuspension are relatively well-studied interventions that are proven to be effective in preventing involuntary leakage during activities that create intra-abdominal pressure (Petca et al., 2025).

Besides this, new technologies incorporating the use of minimally invasive techniques are on the anvil. For instance, injections of bulking agents and platelet-rich plasma therapy are enhancing the treatment profile by targeting the cause of incontinence rather than just alleviating the symptoms. This indicates a direction towards customized treatment modalities, which are individualized to the unique patient's specific clinical profile and tendencies. Equally significant is that of education in the context of treatment decisions among young women, as emphasized by a recent study that identified vast awareness and information gaps.

The research conducted in Lahore found that a significant portion of young women were unaware of urinary incontinence and the treatment modalities available. The findings point to the urgent need for public awareness campaigns to educate women on urinary incontinence, its prevalence, and effective treatments. Raising awareness among this group is necessary, not only for early detection and treatment but also for de-stigmatizing the condition. With increased knowledge and access to treatment, women can make informed decisions that influence their health and wellbeing, thereby reducing the impact of urinary incontinence on the community.

11.5.1. Behavioral Therapies

Behavioral therapies are a standard technique in treating urinary incontinence, especially in women. They emphasize patient teaching, diet modification, and strengthening the pelvic floor muscles. One of the most popular methods is bladder training, where the time between urinations is slowly increased. The technique can help women regain control over the act of urination and frequently significantly reduce symptoms of involuntary leakage. Moreover, patients can be instructed to maintain a bladder diary, with frequency and amount of urination recorded, in order to familiarize them with their urinary patterns and identify their incontinence triggers. Utilizing these processes in combination, behavioral treatments not only support optimal physical outcomes but also allow women to actively participate in the management of their health and therefore improve their quality of life as a whole (Forcht et al., 2017).

In combination with bladder training, pelvic floor muscle training (PFMT) has proved to be a significant component of behavioral treatments. This technique focuses on exercising the muscles of the pelvic area that function to help support the bladder in a bid to strengthen them through systematic exercises such as Kegel exercises. Evidence has shown that women who regularly exercise their pelvic floor exhibit significant improvement in urinary function and in decreasing the severity of incontinence. Furthermore, biofeedback, which provides patients instant feedback regarding muscle activity, can further aid in the effectiveness of these exercises, allowing for more precise muscle control. The blending of these therapies not only permits symptom alleviation but also helps create an experience of controlling one's condition, with women able to utilize their body awareness (Davis et al., 2014).

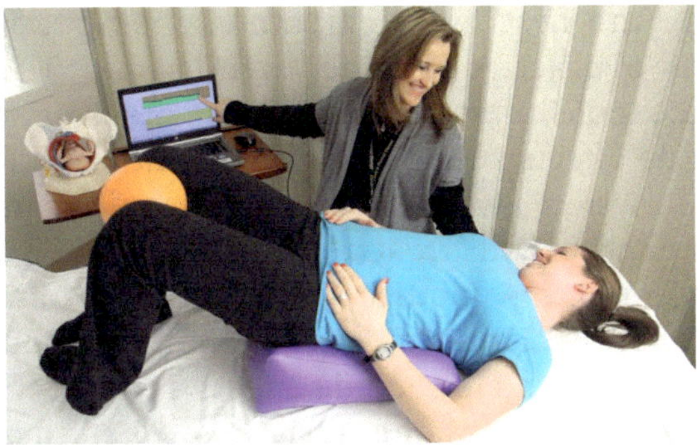

Figure 11.12. Pelvic floor muscle training.

Source: https://ptwfl.com/wp-content/uploads/2017/04/pelvic-floor-rehab.jpg

Besides the physical and behavioral therapies , psychological components of urinary incontinence, such as embarrassment and alienation, are also addressed. With guided sessions of therapy, women receive the necessary emotional support and can open up to others who face the same problems. Group therapy sessions or support groups can improve motivation and strength as women identify with each other and share coping strategies. In addition, cognitive-behavioral interventions aimed at modifying negative incontinence beliefs have the ability to empower women and modify body mindset as well as disease. As evidence continues to mount regarding the efficacy of these behavior therapies, it is certain that holistic treatment regarding the management of both physiological and psychological incontinence is very important in the management of urinary incontinence in women (Forcht et al., 2017).

11.5.2. Medications

Drugs are a focal aspect of managing urinary incontinence (UI) in women, providing therapeutic measures to reduce symptoms and improve quality of life. Anticholinergic drugs, being the class traditionally employed since they possess the ability to suppress bladder contractions in an involuntary manner, are often the first line of treatment for patients with overactive bladder symptoms. These medications, although beneficial to others, result in side effects such as dry mouth and cognitive dysfunction, which potentially undermine compliance with treatment. In addition, more contemporary medications, such as beta-3 adrenergic agonists, offer benefits through tolerability and fewer side effects and therefore increase the armamentarium for healthcare providers.

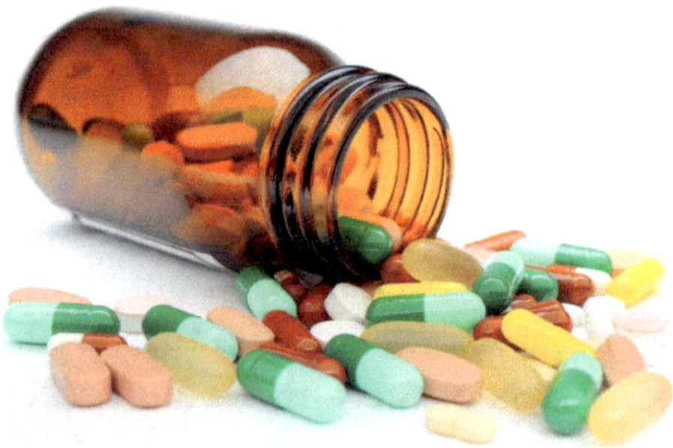

Source: https://firstaidforlife.org.uk/wp-content/uploads/2018/03/poisoning-pill-bottle.jpg

However, knowledge of the needs of the particular patient group and potential drug interactions remains relevant in light of the reality that certain women may have pre-existing conditions that make certain pharmacologic interventions contraindicated. In female urinary incontinence, an interdisciplinary medication plan necessitates a multidisciplinary approach that includes consideration of prior efficacy and history in the patient. While medications like anticholinergics decrease urgent urinary symptoms, efficacy often varies significantly between patients. For patients who are female and have incontinence that does not respond to pharmacologic therapy, the utilization of adjunctive treatments such as percutaneous tibial nerve stimulation is utilized as a complementary method of care to enhance results. In a study that assessed the influence of one treatment, it was stated that routine medications were not found to provide significant improvement in all patients, resulting in further research into electrical stimulation methods (Allescher et al., 2015).

This brings to the forefront the need for customized treatment protocols based on the symptomology, lifestyle, and personal options of each patient. In addition to traditional drugs, several alternative pharmacotherapeutics have been presented, giving rise to an extended discourse on their role in the management of UI. For example, topical estrogen therapy can increase urethral function and sustain pelvic floor health in postmenopausal women, indicating the hormonal etiology that most often leads to UI in older patients. In addition, research into norepinephrine and serotonin-targeting drugs has been promising for the treatment of both the physical and emotional aspects of UI, such as depression and anxiety associated with the disorder (Forcht et al., 2017). As medication evolves, continued education of healthcare providers on the latest evidence-based treatment is essential to maximize care practices in women suffering from urinary incontinence. Continuous testing and research are necessary to refine treatment advantages and ultimately decide on more effective treatment strategies.

11.5.3. Surgical Interventions

Surgical interventions have proven to be a valuable complement to the treatment of urinary incontinence in females, particularly if conservative management is ineffective. Of these interventions, mid-urethral sling procedures and colposuspension have gained more currency due to their minimal invasiveness and comparative efficacy. These interventions aim to provide physical support for the urethra and bladder neck to prevent involuntary leakage during maneuvers that increase abdominal pressure. The current literature sets high emphasis on selecting patients since conditions underlying and personal choice are partially the cause of the success or failure of the procedures. Females who wish to be rid of stress urinary incontinence (SUI) will be highly interested in the above-procedure options, particularly with the prospects of improved quality of life and less dependency on absorbent products. Nonetheless, determining the surgical method has to be undertaken in complete comprehension and mutual decision-making between the clinician and patient.

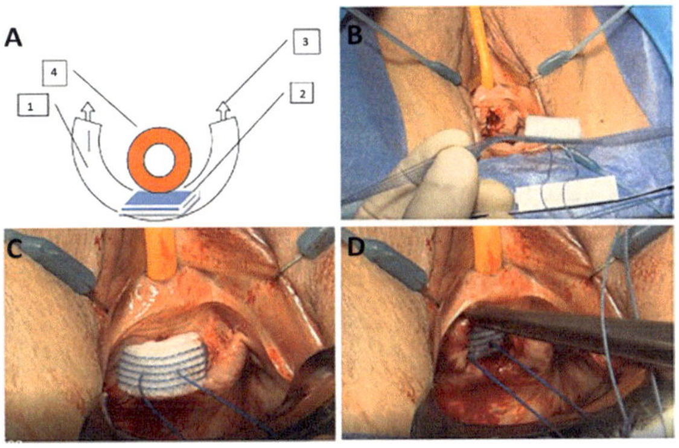

Figure 11.13. Suburethral synthetic adjustment-controlled tape compared with conventional treatment for female stress urinary incontinence.

Source: https://www.eu-focus.europeanurology.com/cms/10.1016/j.euf.2021.12.017/asset/bb8163aa-f112-472e-84d9-66d13c49d884/main.assets/gr1_lrg.jpg

Additional inspection of surgeries shows the intricacy of treating mixed urinary incontinence with both urgency and stress. Studies comparing traditional methods show that traditional methods may not always fully treat the multi-factorial component of mixed incontinence. For instance, a recent analysis compared the effectiveness of intradetrusor injections of onabotulinumtoxinA and mid-urethral slings in women who were not successful with conservative therapy. Results indicated significant benefits from both treatments, but also towards better relief for the stress incontinence component by mid-urethral slings. Such comparison not only contributes value to current clinical knowledge but also underscores the relevance of patient-specific treatment protocols. The necessity to address both facets of mixed urinary incontinence, that is stress and urgency, illustrates the intricacy faced by surgical interventions and emphasizes the worth of tailored interventions to achieve maximum outcomes in female patients (Petca et al., 2025; Harvie et al., 2025). Lastly, female urinary incontinence surgical treatment is to be seriously considered, but not without advisement and foresight. Risks of complications such as infection, pain, and urinary retention underscore the need for vigilant preoperative evaluation and informed consent processes. Moreover, ongoing patient education on what to expect following surgery can serve a crucial function in patient expectation management and achieving satisfactory outcomes. With evolving technology and technique refinement, it is increasingly necessary to incorporate patient-reported outcomes and quality-of-life measures into determining the true impact of surgical approaches. Additional studies must aim to improve techniques and identify subsets of women most likely to benefit from a given approach. This continued focus on individualized, evidence-based care will ultimately make surgical treatments for urinary incontinence more effective, with women receiving effective but individualized care that is also integrated into their own unique health goals (Harvie et al., 2025).

Test Your Knowledge

1. What are two common behavioral therapies used to manage urinary incontinence in females?
2. Under what circumstances is surgical intervention considered for urinary incontinence?

SUMMARY

Female urinary incontinence is, in general, an often-present health issue that interferes with the quality of life for the majority of women worldwide. The findings of the majority of studies, including large reviews of postpartum complications, ascertain that more than 50% of women have urinary incontinence, particularly after vaginal delivery. Pelvic floor muscle deterioration and other etiological factors, such as increasing age and body mass index (BMI), reflect the bidimensional nature of the condition. As highlighted in one of the studies, there was a strong correlation between urinary incontinence prevalence and age, which indicates that as people grow older, the likelihood of this condition also increases, particularly among those with high BMI (Aslam et al., 2023). This serves to underscore the need for expert intervention and education for the prevention and management of female urinary incontinence. Additionally, urinary incontinence management must be an integrated process that understands the diverse experiences and needs of women living with it. There is an implication from evidence that multidisciplinary assessment will optimize gains from treatment, especially for patients with chronic incontinence. Offer adequate resources—such as pelvic floor exercises education, lifestyle modification, and usage of continence aids—readily available. For instance, a study indicates outcomes after catheter removal among patients who were previously catheterized due to uncontrollable incontinence, indicating a significant percentage of patients regained continence after months following removal (Abela et al., 1995). This supports the concept that with the right support and management approaches, many women can achieve improved bladder health and quality of life. Finally, urinary incontinence entails breaking down social stigmas and misconceptions regarding the condition. Several women may be too embarrassed or ashamed to discuss their symptoms with health professionals. Public awareness campaigns to sensitize people about urinary incontinence and encourage open discussion will establish an enabling environment. In educating women further with better awareness, healthcare providers can encourage them to undergo evaluation and treatment, thereby leading to better outcomes. As evidence mounts, education of patients and healthcare providers about the issue and the solutions available will be critical in addressing urinary incontinence in females effectively. It is evident that through combined efforts in education, research, and clinical practice, it is possible to make some headway in effectively controlling this widespread condition.

The pathological complexity of female urinary incontinence encompasses many subtypes, including stress urinary incontinence (SUI) and urgency urinary incontinence (UUI), both of which have differing underlying mechanisms and treatment implications. Recent research emphasizes that urgency incontinence is the most prevalent form in elderly female patients, particularly among those after hip fracture fixation. Research has identified certain modifiable risk factors for certain incontinence patterns and demonstrated that their management is crucial to successful therapy. The combination of mixed urinary incontinence, a blend of elements of urgency and stress incontinence, complicates diagnosis and management even further, necessitating extensive application to geriatric assessment, which can sort out the subtypes and direct interventions appropriately (Hellman-Bronstein et al., 2024). In a revolutionary new approach, more recent scientific literature has directed focus towards the role played by the urethra in female urinary incontinence, challenging prevailing hypotheses that conceptualize incontinence overwhelmingly in terms of detrusor muscle function. The two-factor urethral theory, which attributes urgency urinary incontinence to overactive bladders and stress urinary incontinence to poor urethral support, fails to account for the nuanced dynamics of the urethra itself. Results of a recent overseas seminar emphasize the necessity for the integration of urethral function as a significant variable to account for both types of incontinence. This paradigm shift recognizes that urethral failure can have a significant impact on continence and emphasizes that there must be investigation into how urethral function will come into contact with existing mechanisms, thereby offering new avenues of research as well as potential treatment options (Hokanson et al., 2022). The evolving profile of urinary incontinence studies emphasizes the necessity of an appreciation for its multifactorial causation. As urinary incontinence becomes more prevalent, especially among older women, the implications for both clinical practice and public health are significant. Recognition of mixed urinary incontinence as a distinct entity highlights the importance of healthcare professionals adopting advanced diagnostic techniques that can accurately identify and treat the range of needs of this group. Further, identification of the urethral contribution to incontinence broadens the paradigm with which researchers view urinary incontinence and demands revision of treatment approaches that have heretofore been based on bladder function and support. With ongoing studies still entangling these intricacies, the necessity for interventions that are specifically tailored to take into account the entire range of urinary incontinence-contributing factors becomes more pronounced (Hellman-Bronstein et al., 2024; Hokanson et al., 2022).

KEY TERMS FROM THIS CHAPTER

- Behavioral therapies
- Bladder training
- Customized care programs
- Healthcare system
- Involuntary leakage
- Lifestyle modification
- Metabolic syndrome
- Onabotulinumtoxin
- Polydimethylsiloxane
- Bladder dysfunction
- Chronic lower urinary tract symptoms
- Gynecological issues
- In-depth examination
- Kegel exercises
- Lower urinary tract symptoms (LUTS)
- Mixed incontinence
- Overactive bladder (OAB)
- Postpartum rehabilitation

CRITICAL THINKING QUESTIONS

1. **The most common type of urinary incontinence in women is:**
   a. Overflow incontinence
   b. Urge incontinence
   c. Stress incontinence
   d. Functional incontinence
2. **Stress urinary incontinence is typically caused by:**
   a. Urinary tract infection
   b. Detrusor overactivity
   c. Increased intra-abdominal pressure and weakened pelvic floor muscles
   d. Neurological disorders
3. **Urge incontinence is most commonly associated with:**
   a. Urethral stricture
   b. Detrusor overactivity
   c. Vaginal prolapse
   d. Ureteric stones
4. **A key non-surgical management option for stress incontinence is:**
   a. Anticholinergic medication
   b. Kegel (pelvic floor) exercises
   c. Bladder catheterization
   d. Estrogen therapy
5. **Which of the following medications is commonly used to treat urge urinary incontinence?**
   a. Oxytocin
   b. Oxybutynin
   c. Omeprazole
   d. Ondansetron

Short Answer Questions

1. What are the main types of urinary incontinence?
2. List two common causes of urinary incontinence.
3. What are some key risk factors for developing urinary incontinence?
4. What symptoms are associated with urinary incontinence?
5. Which diagnostic methods are used to assess urinary incontinence?
6. What are common treatment options for managing urinary incontinence?

Answer to Critical Thinking Questions

1. (c) 2. (c) 3. (b) 4. (b) 5. (b)

REFERENCES

1. Abela, S., Dimech, J., Fiorini, A., Spiteri, M., et al. (1995). The outcome of elderly patients following removal of indwelling urinary catheter. https://core.ac.uk/download/46601752.pdf (accessed on 15th June 2025).
2. Abrams, A., Barer, B., Brittain, C., Brittain, D., Brittain, E., et al. (2008). Treatment of urinary incontinence after stroke in adults. https://core.ac.uk/download/339635.pdf (accessed on 15th June 2025).
3. Aguiar, L. B. (2019). Effects of fractional CO_2 laser in urinary symptoms of genitourinary syndrome of menopause and vaginal ecosystem: Randomized clinical trial. https://core.ac.uk/download/296900267.pdf (accessed on 15th June 2025).
4. Ahmed, W. A. R., Kamil, A. M., & Zeidan, M. A. K. (2024). An epidemiological study of urinary incontinence among a sample of adults in Baghdad City. https://core.ac.uk/download/618303051.pdf (accessed on 15th June 2025).
5. Alborz, A., Borthwick-Duffy, S., Cooper, C., Crocker, A., Deb, S., et al. (2009). Adults with intellectual disabilities: Prevalence, incidence and remission of aggressive behavior and related factors. https://core.ac.uk/download/1396177.pdf (accessed on 15th June 2025).
6. Alexander, M. C., Ebenezer, E. D., Jeyaseelan, V., Kekre, A., et al. (2019). Is hysterectomy a risk factor for urinary incontinence? https://core.ac.uk/download/539902137.pdf (accessed on 15th June 2025).
7. Allen, R. E., Anthony, S., Frudinger, A., Gilpin, S., Jackson, S., Johanson, R. B., et al. (2000). The effects of childbirth on the pelvic-floor. https://core.ac.uk/download/19418527.pdf (accessed on 15th June 2025).
8. Allescher, H., Allison, M. C., Arroyo, R., Asari, R., Bharucha, A. E., Boyle, D. J., et al. (2015). Double-blind randomized controlled trial of percutaneous tibial nerve stimulation versus sham electrical stimulation in the treatment of fecal incontinence: CONtrol of Faecal Incontinence using Distal NeuromodulaTion (the CONFIDeNT trial). https://core.ac.uk/download/30613726.pdf (accessed on 15th June 2025).
9. Ashton, L., Nataksuka, H., Johnson, C., Kenne, K., Kreder, K. J., Kruse, R., Eyck, P., et al. (2024). MP23-05: Platelet-rich plasma injection for the treatment of stress urinary incontinence in females: A randomized placebo-controlled trial. *The Journal of Urology, 211*, e383. https://www.semanticscholar.org/paper/04b58ca47250e7a9944979f6b445349d291f7cec (accessed on 15th June 2025).
10. Aslam, K., Jawale, A., Karim, A., Khursheed, M., et al. (2023). Prevalence and severity of urinary incontinence among females after normal vaginal delivery. https://core.ac.uk/download/568378581.pdf (accessed on 15th June 2025).
11. Ather, M. H., Ettinger, S., Hoffman, S., Martin, R. A., McLoughlin, M. A., Ross, L. A., Scott, R. C., et al. (2019). Endoscopic laser-ablation for the treatment of orthotopic and ectopic ureteroceles in dogs: 13 cases (2008–2017). https://core.ac.uk/download/213444929.pdf (accessed on 15th June 2025).
12. Aung, T., Dean, N., Glazener, C. M. A., Herbison, G. P., et al. (2008). Sexual function, delivery mode history, pelvic floor muscle exercises and incontinence: A cross-sectional study six years postpartum. https://core.ac.uk/download/177114.pdf (accessed on 15th June 2025).

13. Awasthi, H. H., & Maurya, P. (2015). Significance of Mula Bandha for urinary incontinence in women. https://core.ac.uk/download/354380663.pdf (accessed on 15th June 2025).
14. Basappa, P. K., Gaddam, R., Gangadharan, K., Shivaraju, P., et al. (2020). Prevalence of pelvic floor dysfunction in women attending obstetrics and gynecology OPD at PES Institute of Medical Sciences and Research, Kuppa. https://core.ac.uk/download/539898299.pdf (accessed on 15th June 2025).
15. Beveridge, L. A., Davey, P. G., McMurdo, M. E. T., Phillips, J., et al. (2011). Optimal management of urinary tract infections in older people. https://core.ac.uk/download/20450519.pdf (accessed on 15th June 2025).
16. Bodean, O. M., Cirstoiu, M., Diaconu, C. C., Marcu, E., et al. (2018). Pelvic floor disorders in gynecological malignancies: An overlooked problem? https://core.ac.uk/download/216808110.pdf (accessed on 15th June 2025).
17. Booth, J., Camicioli, R., Dumoulin, C., Gibson, W., et al. (2017). The association between lower urinary tract symptoms and falls: Forming a theoretical model for a research agenda. https://core.ac.uk/download/293883198.pdf (accessed on 15th June 2025).
18. Büla, C., Cornuz, J., Locatelli, I., Monod, S., et al. (2018). Performance of a brief geriatric evaluation compared to a comprehensive geriatric assessment for detection of geriatric syndromes in family medicine: A prospective diagnostic study. https://core.ac.uk/download/154364843.pdf (accessed on 15th June 2025).
19. Bunn, F., Cardozo, L., Chapple, C., Chester, K., et al. (2015). Is there a link between overactive bladder and the metabolic syndrome in women? A systematic review of observational studies. https://core.ac.uk/download/29849506.pdf (accessed on 15th June 2025).
20. Burgio, K. L., Newman, D. K., Rosenberg, M. T., Sampselle, C. M., et al. (2013). Impact of behavior and lifestyle on bladder health. https://deepblue.lib.umich.edu/bitstream/2027.42/98122/1/ijcp12143.pdf (accessed on 15th June 2025).
21. Davis, K. (2014). Clinical outcomes involving the use of extracorporeal magnetic innervation in the treatment of urinary incontinence. https://core.ac.uk/download/71425784.pdf (accessed on 15th June 2025).
22. Davis, S. R., Gompel, A., Lumsden, M. A., Murad, M. H., et al. (2015). Treatment of symptoms of the menopause: An endocrine society clinical practice guideline. https://core.ac.uk/download/42367511.pdf (accessed on 15th June 2025).
23. Forcht, D. J. (2017). Male urinary incontinence: A critical appraisal of the literature with practice recommendations. https://core.ac.uk/download/286607797.pdf (accessed on 15th June 2025).
24. Ghoniem, G. M., & Miller, C. J. (2012). A systematic review and meta-analysis of Macro plastique for treating female stress urinary incontinence. https://core.ac.uk/download/323075437.pdf (accessed on 15th June 2025).
25. Glazener, C. M. A., Hagen, S., Ramsay, I., Sinclair, L., et al. (2009). A randomized controlled trial of pelvic floor muscle training for stages I and II pelvic organ prolapses. https://core.ac.uk/download/177139.pdf (accessed on 15th June 2025).
26. Harvie, H., Menefee, S. A., Richter, H. E., Sung, V. W., Chermansky, C. J., Rahn, D., Amundsen, C. L., et al. (2025). Midurethral sling vs onabotulinumtoxinA in females with urinary

incontinence: The MUSA randomized clinical trial. *JAMA*. https://www.semanticscholar.org/paper/d5907a907a4f5e61237f0679cdd4e65b3b288a22 (accessed on 15th June 2025).

27. Hegge, J. B. (2018). A pilot professional development program for occupational therapy practitioners who work in home settings: Knowledge translation on urinary incontinence. https://core.ac.uk/download/200292811.pdf (accessed on 15th June 2025).
28. Hellman-Bronstein, A. T., Luukkaala, T., Ala-Nissilä, S., & Nuotio, M. (2024). Associated factors of stress, urgency, and mixed urinary incontinence in a geriatric outpatient assessment of older women with hip fracture. *European Geriatric Medicine, 15*, 861–869. https://www.semanticscholar.org/paper/73bf6477c97170d8b6d89aaf607943ba5cce0e8d (accessed on 15th June 2025).
29. Hokanson, J., & Delancey, J. (2022). Urethral failure is a critical factor in female urinary incontinence. Now what? *Neurourology and Urodynamics, 41*, 532–538. https://www.semanticscholar.org/paper/48af5e69285e569ca879ff4b03177766af50110e (accessed on 15th June 2025).
30. Masood, Z., Mushtaq, M., Javed, A., Shafi, M., & Majeed, R. (2024). Prevalence and knowledge of urinary incontinence and awareness about physical therapy treatment among young females of Lahore. *Journal of Health and Rehabilitation Research*. https://www.semanticscholar.org/paper/b3fbff45b2ad99981db872bba7f9dfc93a937d77 (accessed on 15th June 2025).
31. Nan, X., Dai, S., Zhao, S., Tian, T., & Gu, R. (2024). The interaction effect of obesity with sleep duration on urinary incontinence in adult females: A cross-sectional study of the NHANES database. *Urologic Internationalis, 108*, 525–538. https://www.semanticscholar.org/paper/513f55dbcd20337dd47df91a717094e1860b2b65 (accessed on 15th June 2025).
32. Petca, A., Fotă, A. E., Petca, R., & Rotar, I. (2025). Modern conservative management strategies for female stress urinary incontinence: A systematic review. *Journal of Clinical Medicine*. https://www.semanticscholar.org/paper/5b8c8681ef7019ecee976b5282dc865ecd8b93d6 (accessed on 15th June 2025).
33. Priyadharshini, M., & Poomalar, G. K. (2017). Prevalence of urinary incontinence in reproductive women and its impact on quality of life. https://core.ac.uk/download/543136749.pdf (accessed on 15th June 2025).
34. Stoner, L., & Way, M. (2000). Stress urinary incontinence: Parous versus nulliparous women ages 18–35. https://core.ac.uk/download/19980121.pdf (accessed on 15th June 2025).
35. Subak, L. L., & Whitcomb, E. L. (2011). Effect of weight loss on urinary incontinence in women. https://core.ac.uk/download/323079415.pdf (accessed on 15th June 2025).
36. Syeda, F., & Pandit, U. (2024). Prevalence of urinary incontinence in nulliparous Indian sportswomen. *Journal of Family Medicine and Primary Care, 13*, 3270–3274. https://www.semanticscholar.org/paper/1574ef79178e0999019b53d71bc2662381ec8d6b (accessed on 15th June 2025).
37. Wells, N. R. (1994). Treatment of urinary incontinence in females: A physical therapist's guide. https://core.ac.uk/download/235074006.pdf (accessed on 15th June 2025).
38. Whiting, D., Ian Shane, A., Pope, R., Payne, S., & Venn, S. (2022). Female urinary incontinence in sub-Saharan Africa. *BJU International, 130*. https://www.semanticscholar.org/paper/5cdc70981e813860c165f613841cc8a63d1a5178 (accessed on 15th June 2025).

RADIOTHERAPY, CHEMOTHERAPY, IMMUNOTHERAPY, AND GENE THERAPY IN GYNECOLOGY

12

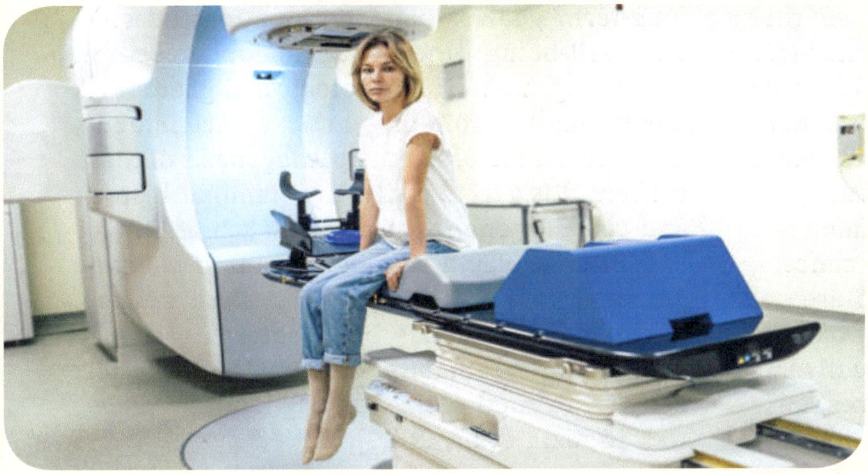

LEARNING OBJECTIVES

After studying this chapter, you will be able to:

1. Describe the overview and types of gynecological cancers.
2. Explain the role and principles of radiotherapy in gynecology
3. Discuss the use and mechanisms of chemotherapy in managing gynecology
4. Analyze the application and effectiveness of immunotherapy in gynecology
5. Evaluate the emerging role of gene therapy in the treatment of gynecology

Introduction

The gynecologic oncology scenario has undergone a dramatic shift in recent decades with the introduction of various therapeutic modalities like radiotherapy, chemotherapy, immunotherapy, and gene therapy. All these therapeutic modalities are developed to address the diversity of the gynecologic cancers with a plethora of malignancies having their own special biological behaviors and treatment responsiveness. The step-by-step unraveling of the molecular pathobiology of these cancers has provided an entry to more specific approaches. More specifically, the coming together of traditional modes like chemotherapy and radiotherapy with new modes like immunotherapy and gene therapy has been a milestone in therapeutic models. With continued study still cracking the code in tumor biology, the promise of enhancing treatment efficacy through combination therapy and targeted interventions remains a focus of investigation in the field. One of the significant advances in gynecological oncology is the application of immunotherapy to treat cancer, an approach that utilizes the patient's immune response to attack cancer. Early evidence indicates that immune checkpoint inhibitors have been promising in many cancers, but there are challenges in view of the establishment of an immunosuppressive tumor microenvironment that may limit therapeutic efficacy. This comprehension of mechanisms of immune evasion will help in maximizing the therapeutic efficacy of immunotherapy. For instance, the use of agents like Cucurbitacin B holds potential to reprogram myeloid-derived suppressor cells and tumor-associated macrophages so that immune responses against tumors become more potent (Anning et al., 2022). Further, research conducted today also illuminates which patient populations are most appropriate for these new treatments and conditions the strategy of treatment on the patient's profile. Treatment and prognosis of some of the gynecologic cancers, such as uterine sarcomas, are still an area of ongoing investigation. Uterine stromal sarcomas, for example, have been noted to assume diverse aggressive behaviors and unfavorable response to conventional therapy. Recent reports indicate that while conventional therapy in the form of chemotherapy and radiotherapy yields minimal survival benefit, newer agents of the immunotherapy type are emerging with potential for improved patient prognosis. Findings suggest that immunotherapy can uncover novel insights into tumor biology and prognosis, particularly in challenging cases such as undifferentiated uterine sarcomas (Hardell et al., 2020). These developments underscore the need for further research to identify useful biomarkers and targets for therapy, ultimately providing more tailored treatment regimens for women facing these daunting diagnoses.

Definition of Gynecological Cancers

Gynecologic cancers constitute a diverse group of tumors arising in the female reproductive system, including the ovaries, uterus, cervix, vagina, and vulva. Gynecologic cancers are largely classified based on their site of origin and share many histologic subtypes with other cancers, often with more characteristic clinical presentations. For example, ovarian cancer is more likely to be diagnosed later in life as it has no early symptoms, whereas cervical cancer is likely to be diagnosed earlier due to screening habits such as Pap smears. With growing knowledge about gynecologic malignancies, early diagnosis and proper classification are emerging as important factors in influencing treatment strategies in accordance with the long-term goal of enhancing patient survival and well-being. One of the major aspects in the management of gynecologic malignancies is identifying the role of genetic, environmental, and lifestyle factors in the pathogenesis of these cancers. Risk factors like age, familial history, and certain genetic mutations, such as BRCA1 and BRCA2, play a significant role in affecting personal susceptibility towards these cancers. Further evidence has been emerging on the role of lifestyle habits, i.e., diet and physical activity, in modulating or augmenting cancer risk (Bouzid et al., 2020).

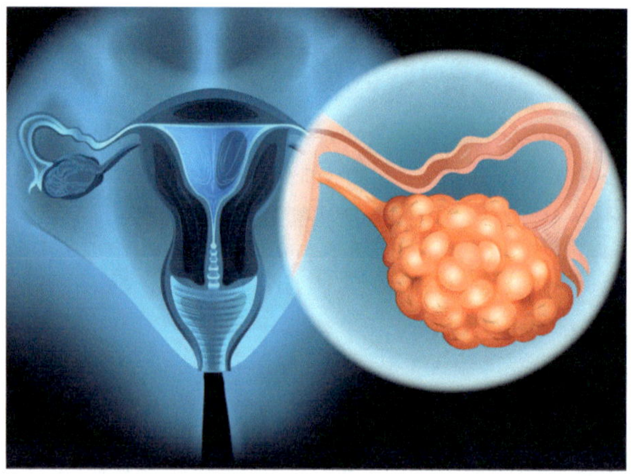

Source: https://www.openaccessgovernment.org/wp-content/uploads/2015/11/dreamstime_s_59495028.jpg

This multifactorial view of the gynecological cancers reemphasizes their complexity in prevention and therapy. The investigation of these factors gives an insight into creating specific interventions and personalized strategies, ultimately enhancing the efficacy of radiotherapy, chemotherapy, immunotherapy, and gene therapy. Improvements in the treatment of gynecologic cancer have been responsible for major advances in recent years, particularly with immunotherapy and gene therapy that have shown promise in addressing the specific needs of these patients. For instance, a variety of immunotherapeutic strategies, including checkpoint inhibitors, have been elicited to harness the body's immune system to recognize and kill cancer cells to improve outcomes in various subtypes of gynecologic cancer. In addition, gene therapy is a novel approach to treating genetic mutations that drive the development of tumors, with the possibility of curative interventions (Bouzid et al., 2020). Also, encounters such as the GYNOCARE COST Action have encouraged discussion of closure of clinical practice and research, focusing on the treatment of rare gynecological cancers and exploration of new treatment modalities that integrate the latest diagnostic techniques with the developing therapeutic avenues (Calleja-Agius et al., 2023). These innovations speak to a trend toward personalized gynecologic oncology, which is essential to optimizing patient outcomes and addressing the unique challenges posed by these neoplasms.

Importance of Treatment Modalities

Successful treatment modalities of gynecologic oncology are very important in improving patient outcomes, particularly against challenging diagnoses such as cancer of the ovary. The disease is often treated with a multi-faceted approach, which involves radiotherapy and chemotherapy as the central components. This traditional modality is employed to systematically eradicate tumor burdens, something that is also very vital in view of the extremely aggressive nature of gynecologic cancers. The latest development has also considered the addition of immunotherapy, which tries to exploit the immune response of the body to better combat cancer. The concurrent use of these treatments not only enhances treatment efficacy but also promises the potential to boost overall survival rates, as shown with trials involving new agents that provide benefit in improving the tumor microenvironment and triggering immune activation in addition to classic treatments (Hamade et al., 2024). New therapeutic modalities such as gene therapy and the use of smart nanoparticles are opening new horizons in oncological therapeutic modalities. Gene therapy can potentially treat genetic abnormalities at the molecular level by treating the etiologic factors of gynecologic cancers. Similarly, smart nanoparticles capable of delivering therapeutic agents with extreme specificity have the capability to make treatment more efficient with fewer side effects. The ability of these nanoparticles to be sensitized to particular biological signals enables personalized medicine approaches that enable individualized therapeutic treatment dependent on an individual's tumor characteristics. The use of these new technologies not only enables increased treatment specificity but also overcomes significant challenges, such as treatment resistance and systemic toxicity, inevitably leading to improved patient quality of life and better prognoses (Sun et al., 2023). The incorporation of multiple modalities of treatment underlines the utility of an integrated therapy for gynecologic oncology. Multimodal treatment takes advantage of synergistic effects of combined therapy, with the best possible outcome, with the least possible side effects of therapy. As an example, the combination of radiotherapy and immunotherapy has been noted to enhance tumor control and induce long-term immune memory, with a sustained response in selected patients with ovarian cancer. Moreover, the early finding supporting the application of precision therapies like targeted immunotherapy and gene intervention also indicates more personalized treatment planning. With ongoing development in the area, investigation and trials will continue to be important in identifying the best combinatory approaches to improve survival and quality of life among gynecologic cancer patients, abetting the critical importance of various treatment modalities (Hamade et al., 2024; Sun et al., 2023).

12.1. Overview of Gynecological Cancers

Learning Outcome

1. Explain the types of gynecological cancers
2. Define prevalence and statistics of gynecological cancers
3. Identify risk factors and prevention of gynecological cancers

Gynecologic cancers are a group of neoplasms that affect the female reproductive system, and they primarily include malignancies of the ovary, uterus, cervix, and vulva. Epithelial ovarian cancer (EOC) is the most malignant among them and is responsible for the highest proportion of gynecologic cancer-related deaths. The heterogeneity of these cancers is due to their various histological types, distinct molecular characteristics, and distinct metastatic behaviors, and hence, diagnosis and treatment become difficult. Early diagnosis remains a significant challenge due to the typically asymptomatic presentation of gynecological tumors until advanced disease. Health systems thus emphasize prevention and education in order to encourage increased rates of early diagnosis as well as survival for affected groups. As research progresses, understanding the molecular and genetic pathogenesis of such diseases becomes increasingly critical to the development of targeted therapies and individualized treatment regimens employing both traditional and new modalities. The therapeutic scenario for gynecologic malignancies has, in the past, been multimodal and incorporates surgical therapy, radiation, and chemotherapy. Surgery continues to be the mainstay for localized disease, but systemic regimens are important in advanced stages. Of particular interest, chemotherapeutic modalities have proved to be effective or ineffective based on tumor type; platinum-based therapy, for instance, is extremely effective in ovarian malignancy, but other cancers have limited response to conventional agents. The recent years have witnessed the introduction of a more advanced perspective of the biological behavior of these tumors, thus paving the way for novel therapeutic modalities such as immunotherapy. The advent of immune checkpoint inhibitors is a beaming spot in the therapy of several gynecological cancers. However, while they are very promising, research has revealed that the same treatments currently yield inadequate outcomes in some forms, and hence there is a need for ongoing clinical trials to maximize treatment techniques and enhance outcomes for patients (Benedetto et al., 2020). Further, the study of newer forms of treatment, such as gene therapy, suggests where gynecologic cancer treatment is headed. Gene therapy aims to correct genetic defects or increase therapeutic benefits and holds the potential to alter gynecologic cancer refractory treatment. As there is a greater understanding of the molecular basis of cancers, individualized medicine approaches are increasingly being integrated into models of therapy. For instance, the development of chimeric antigen receptor (CAR)-T cell therapy has caused a buzz around using this novel method on solid tumors as well as exploring its use in gynecologic cancer. This is a paradigm shift where traditional treatment methods marry new techniques in focusing on the distinctive biology of the patient-specific tumor. With further research shedding light on the intricate biology of such cancers, the incorporation of target therapies into clinical practice emerges as a top avenue forward in improving patient prognosis and quality of life (Altavilla et al., 2021).

12.1.1. Types of Gynecological Cancers

Gynecologic cancers comprise a group of neoplasms of the female reproductive system with the most frequent being cervical, ovarian, and endometrial cancer. Cervical cancer, which is primarily caused by human papillomavirus (HPV), constitutes a significant public health problem, particularly among developing nations where screening tests may not be easily accessible. Ovarian cancer is known for its nonspecific presentation and late diagnosis, hence an unfavorable prognosis. The endometrial carcinoma, which arises from the uterine lining, is commonly associated with hormonal imbalance and is marked by variable histological forms. These various forms play a critical role, for the physiologic and pathologic distinctions not only impact treatment methods such as radiotherapy and chemotherapy but also underscore the importance of early detection and prevention measures to improve survival in the afflicted. Also, vulvar and vaginal cancers, while less common, are crucial components of gynecologic oncology. Vulvar cancer is most commonly diagnosed in elderly women and might be manifested as lesions on the external genitalia and needs careful study and treatment. Similarly, vaginal cancer, which might arise from adjacent tissues or metastasize from other sites, raises certain diagnostic difficulties due to the unsolvability of early diagnosis. Both malignancies are HPV-associated and typically require a multidisciplinary treatment for their successful management, in combination with various surgical techniques, radiotherapeutic modalities, and adjuvant therapy such as chemotherapy. Advances in the pathophysiology of these malignancies have brought to the forefront the importance of targeted therapies, particularly in relation to their unique biological behaviors and response to conventional therapies. Advances in treatment modalities such as immunotherapy have revolutionized the management of advanced gynecologic malignancies. With widespread tumor heterogeneity, particularly in endometrial and ovarian cancer, immune-based therapies have emerged quite recently as valuable tools, with the potential to both enhance patient responses and reduce the side effects generally associated with conventional therapies. The emerging clinical data indicate that immune checkpoint inhibitors have promising avenues of treatment, with sustained responses even in previously refractory diseases. The application of biomarkers to guide immunotherapy has the potential to lead to more personalized and effective therapies for a patient's tumor profile, enhancing clinical outcomes. As ongoing research moves forward with these new treatments, the promise lies in the combination treatment approaches that can potentially overcome resistance and enhance efficacy against many gynecologic malignancies, as noted in recent reports (Sharma et al., 2020; Heinzelmann-Schwarz et al., 2017).

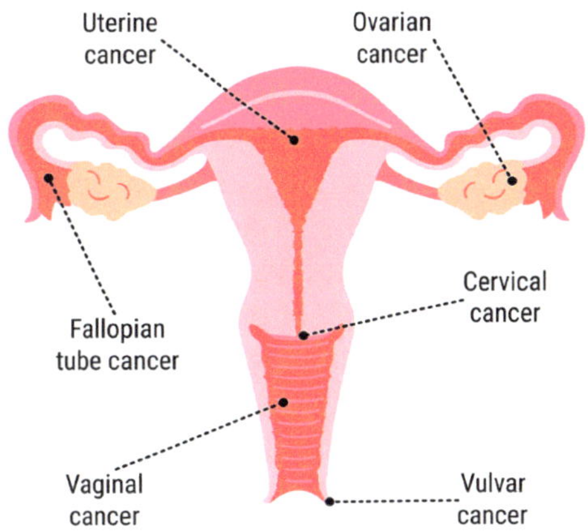

Figure 12.1. Gynecological cancers.

Source: https://www.aurorahealthcare.org/-/media/Project/Health-System-Enterprise/AuroraHealthCareOrg/aurorahealthcare/images/images/services/gynecological-cancers.webp?h=1200&iar=0&w=1200&rev=3b255cde29e0467e9b9d91245c111160&hash=3FC676C030645E9A2C717C893E6E17A4

12.1.2. Prevalence and Statistics

The prevalence of gynecologic cancers strongly emphasizes the necessity of ongoing research and therapeutic interventions such as radiotherapy, chemotherapy, immunotherapy, and gene therapy. Cervical cancer remains one of the leading causes of cancer morbidity and mortality among women globally, particularly in resource-limited countries where screening and vaccination are not readily available. The need to create novel therapeutic strategies has been fueled by the poor prognosis in stage IV cervical cancer, prompting clinicians to achieve a greater understanding of the disease's etiology, specifically its modulation of the immune response. In this context, new immunotherapeutic interventions have surfaced into the spotlight, with encouraging results in pipeline clinical trials to improve the prognosis for advanced disease patients. The incorporation of newer therapies with traditional treatment modalities is a paradigm shift in gynecologic oncology to precision medicine and individualized paradigms in patient care, underscoring the need for rigorous statistical analysis of disease prevalence. Endometrial carcinoma, the leading gynecologic malignancy, has demonstrated a staggering rise in incidence rates, partly fueled by lifestyle factors such as obesity and physical inactivity. According to The Cancer Genome Atlas research network, endometrial carcinomas can be divided into four molecular subgroups with varying prognostic significance. This classification is clinically significant; it not only helps in the refinement of treatment regimens but also in the interpretation of disease progression and potential therapeutic responses. Notably, although molecular profiling helps individualize patient care, prevalence within specific subgroups can also be representative of population patterns and thus impact public health policy. The advances in molecular diagnostics enable a more accurate determination of risks due to traditional factors and enhancement of the prediction of treatment responses, which supports evidence-based management of endometrial carcinoma as a discrete disease process (Bützow et al., 2022). Integration of statistical data into the identification of prevalence rates and treatment responses in gynecological cancers offers important information regarding patient outcomes and efficacy of treatment. As shown through the advances in immunotherapy, the quantifiable success rates of early-phase trials have provoked research into other treatment procedures, specifically those with immune checkpoint inhibitors and tumor-infiltrating lymphocytes. Such treatments have emerged as a result of a higher rate of advanced cervical cancers, where traditional treatments often proved to be insufficient. The positive trends observed in ongoing trials reflect the promise of immunotherapy, and greater investigation of the best therapeutic algorithms is warranted. Based on the insights obtained from large clinical trials and molecular subgroup investigations, clinicians are increasingly able to create interventions that are informed by today's prevalence data and evolving treatment environments. The constant stream of robust data needs to inform clinical decision-making, thereby improving patient outcomes (Valsecchi et al., 2022).

12.1.3. Risk Factors and Prevention

Risk factors for gynecologic cancers are important to know in order to create successful prevention programs. They are advanced age, family history of cancer, and genetic susceptibility, such as BRCA1 and BRCA2 mutations, which significantly increase ovarian and endometrial cancer risks. Lifestyle and socioeconomic status, such as dietary intake and physical activity level, also impact cancer risk. A sedentary life has been correlated with increased instances of obesity, a known risk factor for many gynecological cancers. These factors can serve to inform screening programs for early diagnosis, which goes a long way in guiding treatment outcomes. Furthermore, educational programs for high-risk groups can promote active health habits, emphasizing the necessity of frequent screenings and genetic counseling, ultimately aimed at preventing the development of gynecological cancers while enhancing patient outcomes through early intervention. Preventative interventions have, of late, moved beyond traditional risk factor awareness to novel methods such as immunotherapy.

The developments in immunotherapy in recent years have been towards the use of immune checkpoint inhibitors to treat gynecologic cancers, particularly endometrial and cervical cancers. Such therapies work through the enhancement of the body's immune reaction to cancer cells, and their success points to the importance of identifying the individual patient risk factors to select appropriate candidates for such therapy. Notably, a combined strategy employing genetic profiling can identify patients whose disease can be anticipated to be responsive to immunotherapies, thereby instilling personalized prevention strategies. With continued research, responsiveness and resistance to immunotherapies are anticipated to be made more accurate by biomarker-guided randomized trials, opening up opportunities for more targeted and effective prevention interventions in gynecological oncology (Heinzelmann-Schwarz et al., 2017). The relationship between older modalities, such as chemotherapy and radiotherapy, and newer modalities, such as gene therapy and targeted therapies, also plays a critical role in solving risk factors as well. Gene therapy holds promise in modifying the genetic predisposition to cancer by directly targeting specific gene mutations and repairing them to prevent cancer development.

Moreover, its combination with existing therapies like immunotherapy may result in additive effects, increasing effectiveness and minimizing resistance. Current studies examining the application of immunotherapy to neoadjuvant settings demonstrate the shift towards preemptive options, aiming to prevent cancer from becoming advanced (de Vries et al., 2022). These broader strategies for dealing with cancer not only address treatment after diagnosis but also emphasize prevention, shifting the focal point toward the optimization of health benefits through the combination of complete knowledge of individualized risk factors with the latest available therapy options.

Test Your Knowledge

1. What are the main types of gynecological cancers?
2. Which gynecological cancer is the most prevalent worldwide?

12.2. Radiotherapy in Gynecology

Learning Outcome

1. Define the mechanism of action of treatments used in gynecological oncology
2. Explain the types of radiotherapy used in gynecological cancer treatment
3. Identify side effects and management of radiotherapy

Radiotherapy is a key modality in the management of the majority of gynecologic cancers, to which it is applicable both as a single modality and adjuvant therapy with other modalities such as mastectomy and chemotherapy. The precision of modern radiotherapy techniques, especially IMRT and IGRT, has been crucial in maximizing the treatment outcome with decreased damage to the normal tissues surrounding the target. This is especially so in gynecologic malignancies, where patients have tumors in fragile anatomical locations. The addition of more advanced radiotherapy techniques has been documented by the European Society for Radiotherapy and Oncology to enhance rates of local control and survival in locally advanced cervical cancer patients, validating the use of these technologies in cancer care as a whole (Amaral et al., 2021). Radiotherapy is particularly valuable in the management of uterine cancers such as uterine sarcomas, where surgery may be extremely limited. Uterine stromal sarcomas actually display a variety of biological behavior and response to treatment. Experience indicates that traditional radiotherapy and chemotherapy have been of small impact on survival rates in the past, but that technical advances in imaging and radiotherapeutic approaches are needed to improve therapeutic effort. Investigation into molecular subgroups and how they respond to radiotherapy can render treatments more specifically tailored. Low-grade endometrial stromal sarcomas, for instance, can respond differently from their undifferentiated forms, which suggests differential responsiveness in the design of treatment (Hardell et al., 2020). Being aware of these nuances can guide more individualized radiotherapeutic strategies that are aligned with the unique tumor biology of each patient. In addition, ongoing research is needed to more precisely delineate the role of radiotherapy within the multimodal treatment protocol of gynecological cancers. With evolving treatment protocols that move toward more integral approaches, the association of radiotherapy with immunotherapy or targeted therapy is very promising. Early evidence indicates the potential for radiotherapy to enhance the efficacy of immunotherapeutic agents by causing an immune response against tumor cells, particularly in endometrial cancer patients harboring specific immune markers. Investigations on biomarkers and radiotherapy's ability to alter the tumor microenvironment would be extremely valuable towards improving treatment protocols. These advances point towards the urgent need for the continuous expansion of radiotherapy uses to ensure its position as a pillar of therapy in the multi-faceted treatment of gynecological malignancies, ultimately translating to improved patient outcomes (Amaral et al., 2021; Hardell et al., 2020).

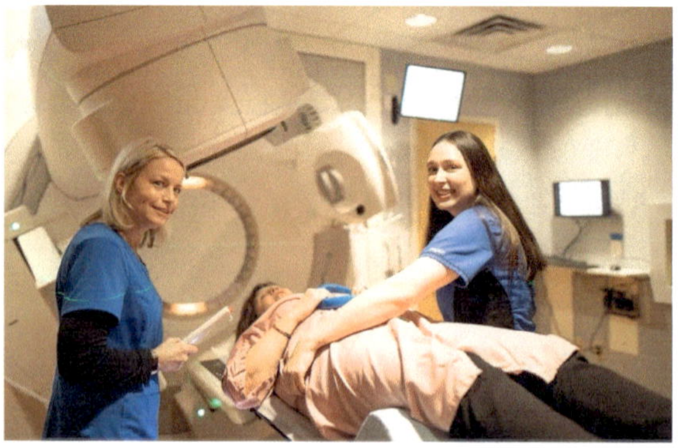

Figure 12.2. Radiation therapy used for gynecologic cancers.

Source: https://georgiaradiationtherapy.com/hubfs/radiation%20for%20gynecologic%20cancers.jpg

12.2.1. Mechanism of Action

In gynecologic oncology, it is crucial to have a complete understanding of the mechanisms of action of various treatment modalities. Radiotherapy acts primarily by the mechanism of ionizing radiation, which damages the DNA of neoplastic cells and kills them. This modality is particularly advantageous in treating localized neoplasms because the radiation acts preferentially on cells that proliferate rapidly, as in neoplastic tissues. Besides, radiotherapy can induce secondary effects such as the release of tumor antigens, which can enhance immune response.

By understanding the precise mechanisms, clinicians may optimize dosages and schedules to achieve maximum efficacy with minimum harm to adjacent healthy tissue, thus supporting treatment schedules for most gynecologic malignancies. Chemotherapy employs cytotoxic agents that disrupt the proliferation of cancer cells by inhibiting some cellular processes. Most of the chemotherapeutic agents target a particular phase of the cell cycle—synthesis phase (phase) or mitotic phase (phase)—inhibiting the replication or division of DNA. Drug action most often leads to cancer cell apoptosis induction. Combination regimens enhance overall treatment efficacy by using drugs with multiple mechanisms of action and resistance patterns.

However, the intricacy of tumor microenvironments could make these interactions complicated, and more research on how to optimize chemotherapy to allow it to reach the tumor tissues and minimize normal cell damage is necessary. Immunotherapy has also emerged as a game-changer in the management of most malignancies, particularly through immune checkpoint blockade mechanisms with the inhibition of programmed death-1 (PD-1) and cytotoxic T-lymphocyte-associated protein 4 (CTLA-4) pathways. These routes are of vital importance to immunomodulation of immune responses and, if blocked, can enhance anti-tumor immune responses. In some gynecologic cancers, TME can be immunosuppressive, with devastating consequences on the effectiveness of such treatments.

For instance, T-helper 17 and tumor-associated macrophages have the ability to create an unfavorable TME, as proposed in uterine cervical cancer (Cicinelli et al., 2020). Agents such as the small molecule Cucurbitacin B have been promising to reprogram the immune microenvironment by inhibiting myeloid-derived suppressor cells and tumor-associated macrophages, showing the potential of combining agents that modulate the TME with immunotherapeutic approaches (Anning et al., 2022).

12.2.2. Types of Radiotherapy Used

Radiotherapy is one of the important modalities in the treatment of gynecologic cancers, with multiple techniques for specific malignancies. External beam radiotherapy (EBRT) is used frequently to irradiate tumors in cervical, endometrial, and vulvar cancers. The method involves the delivery of high-energy photons or electrons from external sources directed to the tumor, which allows precise and effective shrinking of the tumor. Because it is non-invasive, EBRT is especially applicable to those patients who may not be good candidates for surgery. Moreover, the newer generation of radiotherapy machines enables oncologists to restrict treatment exposure to normal tissues surrounding the target as much as possible, which can reduce potential side effects and enhance the patient's quality of life during treatment.

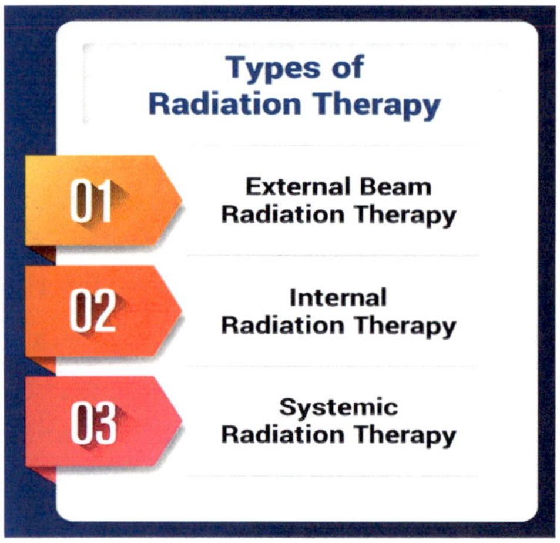

Figure 12.3. Types of radiotherapy.

Source: https://actchealth.com/images/the-power-of-radiation-therapy-for-cancer-treatment/02.webp

In contrast, brachytherapy is a localized form of radiotherapy involving the placement of radioactive sources directly into or close to tumor tissues. It is ideally suited to the treatment of cervical and endometrial cancer because it allows the administration of high doses of radiation over the shortest duration possible without causing ionizing radiation damage to adjacent organs. Brachytherapy has also evolved with advances in technology, as image-guided brachytherapy further enhances the precision and outcomes of treatment. It has been proposed that synergy occurs in combining brachytherapy with external beam radiotherapy, which is synergistic and increases the local control rates and overall survival benefit in locally advanced gynecologic cancers. These modalities of radiotherapy collectively point the direction towards personalized oncology in the management of gynecologic cancers. With the progress in the area of medicine, research is carried out on newer radiotherapy methods that are constantly on the rise, particularly when used for recurrent and metastatic diseases. More recent methods like SBRT are coming into the limelight for their accuracy in providing high doses of radiation with minimal side effects, reducing the duration of treatment, and improving patient comfort. This method is promising for the treatment of isolated metastatic lesions, for example, in the brain, an issue area commonly faced in endometrial cancer cases (Bonasera et al., 2025). Collectively, these different modalities of radiotherapy enhance the arsenal available to the oncologists to deal more effectively with the gynecological cancers' challenges (Mackay et al., 2015). This complex approach results in improved clinical results and emphasizes the need for ongoing research for the refinement of therapeutic options in this field.

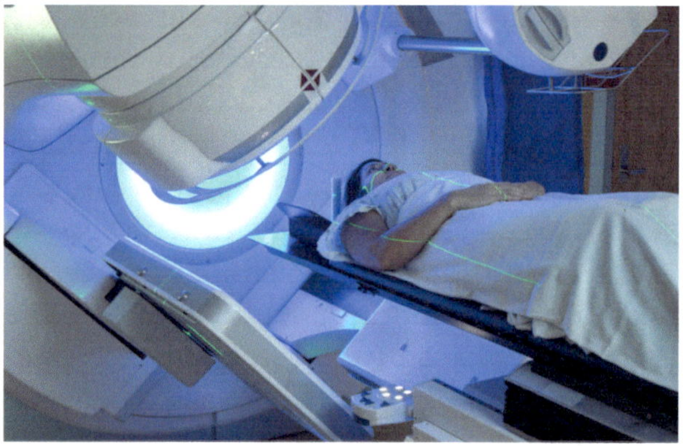

Figure 12.4. Stereotactic body radiotherapy (SBRT).

Source: https://external-content.duckduckgo.com/iu/?u=https%3A%2F%2Fchblob.icloud-hospital.com%2Fthumbnailcontainer%2F10-134578c0-56ae-414f-b6e5-5318e07db4e0.jpg%3Fw%3D1536%26q%3D75%26format%3Dwebp&f=1&nofb=1&ipt=5d738c6a28f780a30adcd91d3b4b41dda8fc7e0cbf807e33f3a9df5ec819b4b7

12.2.3. Side Effects and Management

Application of radiotherapy, chemotherapy, immunotherapy, and gene therapy in gynecology is known to induce a range of side effects, of concern to both patients and healthcare providers. Side effects induced by radiotherapy include fatigue, skin reaction, and pain during and at the site of treatment, which impact a patient's quality of life to a great extent. Chemotherapy, while successful in destroying cancerous cells, may cause nausea and vomiting, hair loss, and various hematologic side effects such as anemia and neutropenia. These side effects call for integrated management processes to help ensure patient comfort and adherence to treatment protocols. Care teams must closely monitor symptoms, providing supportive therapy that may include antiemetics for nausea or growth factors to stimulate white blood cell production, thereby minimizing some of the adverse effects that can accompany such treatment. If immunotherapy is contemplated, side effects come about differently with the different mechanisms of action involved.

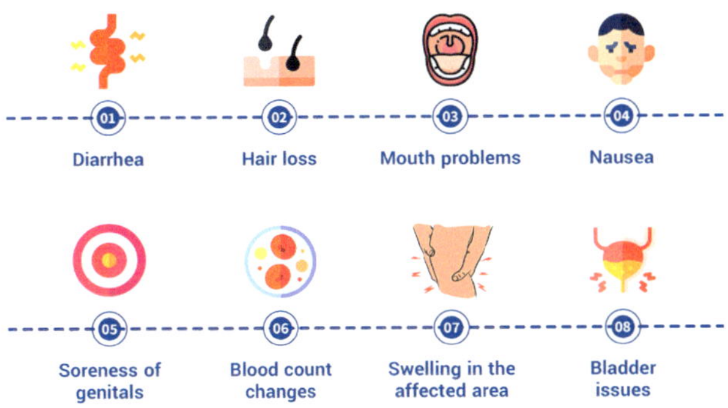

Figure 12.5. Common side effects of radiation therapy.

Source: https://actchealth.com/blogs/four-ways-to-cope-with-side-effects-of-radiation-therapy

Immune-related adverse events (irAEs) may present as a response of the immune system to cancer cells, but can also initiate autoimmunity. Common presentations of irAEs are dermatitis, colitis, pneumonitis, and endocrinopathies, which make the entire treatment course for patients with cancer more complicated. Treatment of these irAEs typically involves corticosteroids and immunosuppressants to counteract severe effects and achieve immune homeostasis. Moreover, recent research is exploring how certain therapies, such as Cucurbitacin B, can induce tumor immunity along with simultaneously reprogramming the immunosuppressive cells in the tumor microenvironment, possibly decreasing the severity of side effects and increasing patient benefit in the area of immunotherapy in gynecologic malignancies (Anning et al., 2022).

Gene therapy, although still an emerging field, also comes with its own set of side effects for clinicians to manage. Gene therapy patients may experience local reactions where the injection was administered, as well as systemic reactions depending on the route of delivery. The challenge is to optimize the therapeutic index with minimal reaction. Remarkably, with the gene-targeted approaches still being evaluated via clinical trials, there is a need to understand the long-term impacts of these therapies on organ function as well as overall well-being. According to research, treatments based on immunotherapy are being formulated as safer options for gynecological cancer that can have significant results (Sharma et al., 2020). Therefore, active monitoring, management, and planning of treatment regimens are most important in the total care of patients receiving these new treatments.

Test Your Knowledge

1. What is the general mechanism of action of treatments used in gynecological oncology?
3. Name two types of radiotherapy commonly used in gynecological cancer treatment.

12.3. Chemotherapy in Gynecology

Learning Outcome

1. Discuss the common chemotherapeutic agents of various gynecological cancers
2. Define treatment protocols and regimens of chemotherapy in gynecology
3. Understand the challenges and side effects of chemotherapy in gynecology

In gynecologic oncology, chemotherapy takes center stage in managing most malignancies such as ovarian, cervical, and endometrial cancer. As a systemic modality of treatment, this modality employs chemotherapeutic drugs to kill rapidly growing malignant cells, most often with tumor regression and an improved survival rate. The effectiveness of chemotherapy relies on numerous factors, including the extent and type of cancer, the overall health of the patient, and the sensitivity of the tumor to specific cytotoxic agents. It is used either as adjuvant therapy to eliminate microscopic residual disease after surgery or as neoadjuvant therapy to decrease tumor size prior to surgery.

While helpful, chemotherapy's toxicity, including nausea, fatigue, and immunosuppression, makes its impact on patients' quality of life questionable. Thus, the balance between therapeutic effect and toxicity continues to be a key issue in gynecological oncology. The evolving situation of treatment for gynecological cancers continues to highlight a combination of chemotherapy with other modes of treatment, including radiotherapy and immunotherapy. For instance, concurrent chemoradiation has proved beneficial in the management of cervical cancer through the augmentation of radiotherapy effectiveness with overall better outcomes. Moreover, ongoing investigations into the integration of chemotherapy with immunotherapy agents like immune checkpoint inhibitors may be able to leverage synergism advantages for further enhancement of tumor response. Chemotherapy has been demonstrated to be able to induce immunogenic cell death and condition the immune system to subsequent immune checkpoint blockade, but resistance mechanisms more often present significant hurdles to tumor growth. Therefore, current research attempts to elucidate optimal combinations and timing of treatment, attempting to improve therapeutic results while minimizing adverse effects associated with extended chemotherapy courses.

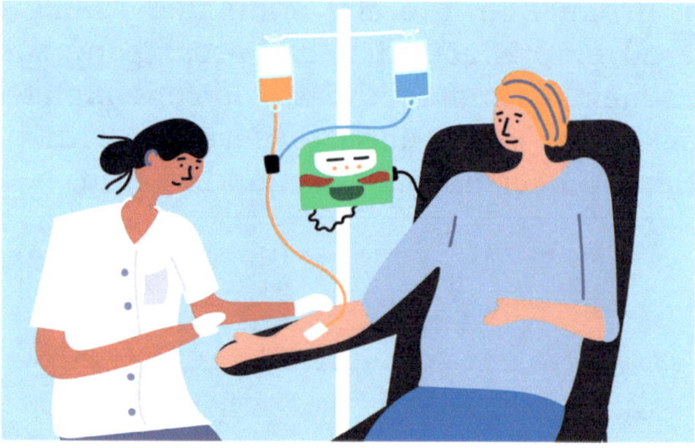

Figure 12.6. Chemotherapy.

Source: https://www.oncoplus.co.in/wp-content/uploads/2021/03/chemo.jpg

There has been a recent advancement in the identification of novel therapeutic agents to enhance chemotherapy effectiveness in gynecologic malignancies. Cucurbitacin B stands out for its ability to inhibit immune-suppressive cancer microenvironments and enhance chemotherapy efficiency. As detailed in the current literature, Cuc. B inhibits key signaling pathways in tumor progression and immune evasion through reprogramming tumor-associated macrophages and myeloid-derived suppressor cells. By addressing these challenges, Cuc. B not only maximizes the efficacy of standard chemotherapy protocols but also paves the way for improved immunotherapeutic treatments in cancers of the gynecological tract. With the development of the field, the combination of chemotherapy with new agents and therapies, such as those against tumor microenvironments, promises to deliver improved clinical results and patient survival rates in gynecological oncology (Anning et al., 2022; Sharma et al., 2020).

12.3.1. Common Chemotherapeutic Agents

Chemotherapy remains the cornerstone in the treatment of most gynecologic cancers, with some of the traditional drugs being essential to practice. The most famous of these is cisplatin, which is particularly valuable in ovarian and cervical cancer. Cisplatin, by the mechanism of DNA cross-links, disrupts cell replication, ultimately inducing apoptosis in rapidly dividing cells. Its infusion, however, is typically followed by cytotoxic toxicities, including nephrotoxicity and hematologic toxicities. This highlights the key need for personalized treatment regimens based on patient profiles and tumor characteristics, particularly when combined with other modalities such as radiotherapy (Giannios et al., 2012). With new chemotherapy regimens on the horizon, optimizing efficacy with the least amount of adverse effects is the goal, a process that is particularly challenging in the case of gynecologic cancers. Another widely used chemotherapeutic drug is paclitaxel, which also plays a crucial role in the treatment of ovarian and endometrial cancers. Paclitaxel acts by causing microtubule stabilization, preventing normal mitotic spindle formation, and thereby cell division. This action is particularly helpful for the treatment of very mitotic tumors. However, paclitaxel administration is also linked with side effects such as peripheral neuropathy and hypersensitivity reactions, necessitating continual monitoring and regulation of the therapeutic approaches (Giannios et al., 2012).

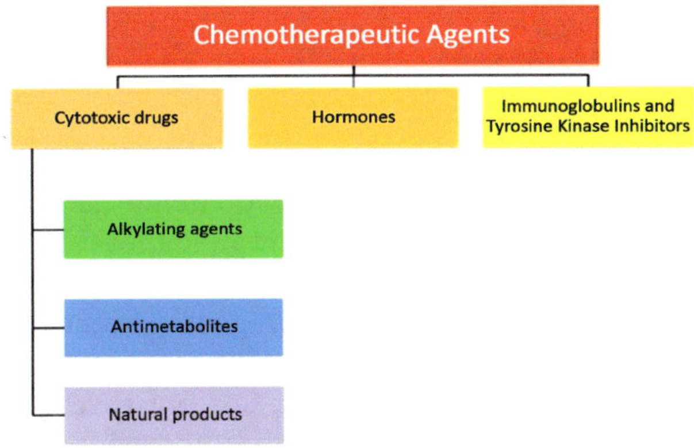

Figure 12.7. Chemotherapeutic agents.

Source: https://www.pharmacologyeducation.org/sites/default/files/Chemotherapeutics.jpg

Furthermore, the activity of paclitaxel may be altered by tumors' molecular and genetic makeup, resulting in increased interest in the application of personalized medicine strategies aimed at maximizing patient responses through genomic profiling and customized treatment regimens. The overlap between chemotherapy and newer modalities of therapy is transforming gynecologic cancer therapy. For instance, combinations of targeted therapy and immunotherapy are now becoming more common, which may be promising to give greater efficacy of conventional chemotherapeutic agents like doxorubicin. This drug, which can intercalate DNA and inhibit topoisomerase II, has established itself as a therapeutic agent against many gynecologic cancers. Despite its effectiveness, administration of doxorubicin needs careful attention due to its cardiotoxicity and cumulative toxicity. The continually evolving universe of gynecologic oncology highlights the importance of multidisciplinary regimens extending not only to chemotherapeutic agents but also immunologically derived therapies, toward an expanding trend toward more personalized regimens emphasizing optimization of efficacy coupled with prevention of harm.

12.3.2. Treatment Protocols and Regimens

Treatment modalities in gynecologic oncology embrace a broad, multidisciplinary intervention with radiotherapy, chemotherapy, immunotherapy, and gene therapy. Radiotherapy has been criticized for a long time due to its side effects, particularly gastrointestinal toxicity, which limits its application in ovarian cancer and other conditions. Current research uncovers the importance of new strategies that minimize radiotherapeutic side effects while enhancing its efficacy. For instance, the inclusion of agents like *Limosilactobacillus reuteri* has emerged as a thrilling adjunct to radiotherapy regimens. As demonstrated in model systems in the laboratory, the agent was able to induce immune responses that could alter the tumor microenvironment, eventually leading to improved overall survival rates when combined with standard treatment regimens. Integration of these advances in standard treatment protocols is a paradigm-shifting step in the treatment modalities of gynecologic cancers, in accordance with the goal of improving patient outcomes and doing away with the toxicity inherently associated with cancer treatments (Hamade et al., 2024). Chemotherapy remains the leading treatment protocol in gynecologic cancers, particularly advanced ovarian cancer. Traditional chemotherapy regimens involve the combination of platinum drugs and taxanes, yet resistance has been a key challenge, and hence, unabated exploration for new agents and combination regimens continues. The major toxicities of the regimens necessitate the institution of supportive care treatments, including immunotherapy, that can enhance treatment effectiveness without maximizing patient toxic load. Tumor-infiltrating lymphocytes (TILs) are also being explored for their potential to improve the treatment outcomes in this situation. By augmenting the body's immune response against neoplastic cells, TIL therapy has the capacity to make existing chemotherapy regimens more effective. The evolving understanding of the tumor microenvironment and immune checkpoints is central to tailoring these combined regimens to deliver the greatest curative benefit while maintaining patient safety and quality of life (Kazemi et al., 2022).

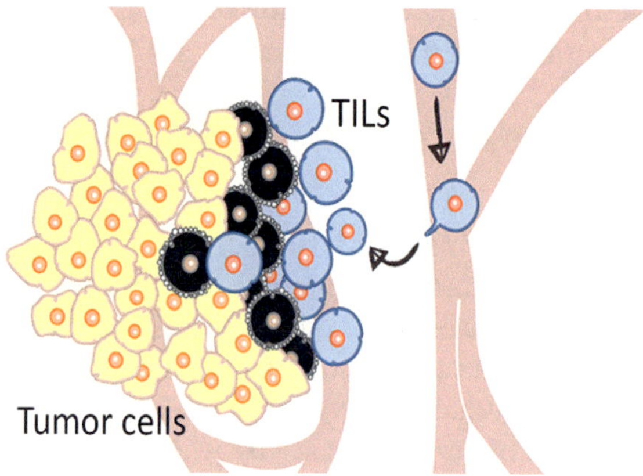

Figure 12.8. Tumor-infiltrating lymphocytes (TILs).

Source: https://www.arigobio.com/files/editor/images/TILs%281%29.jpg

Gene therapy also becomes increasingly prominent in the treatment regimens for gynecologic cancers, particularly as an instrument in treating the genealogy of such cancers. By utilizing techniques such as CRISPR-Cas9 and viral vector systems, gene therapy attempts to mend mutations or introduce therapeutic genes to repress tumor development. This new approach has an unprecedented potential to tailor cancer therapy to the individualized molecular profile of each patient's tumor. Gene therapy combined with conventional modalities such as chemotherapy and immunotherapy has the potential to utilize a synergistic interaction, possibly to improve clinical outcomes. In addition, current clinical trials are assessing the therapeutic efficacy and toxicity of these multimodal treatments, which could pave the way for their use in clinical practice guidelines. As research continues to unveil the complexities of gynecologic cancers, an interdepartmental approach encompassing gene therapy can redefine the treatment landscape for oncologists and their patients.

12.3.3. Challenges and Side Effects

Use of radiotherapy in gynecologic tumors is associated with several challenges and severe side effects that have to be tolerated by the patient. Though radiotherapy is a valuable tool for cancer cell destruction using ionizing radiation, it tends to cause injury to surrounding normal tissues. This is experienced as acute side effects like erythema, asthenia, and gastrointestinal symptoms in pelvic cancers. Chronic side effects include potential long-term damage to reproductive organs, leading to infertility and menstrual function disruption. Psychosocial challenges could also be faced by patients when coping with the physical and emotional impacts of these side effects. The need for effective management modalities to overcome these adverse effects is a clinical practice priority, emphasizing the need for continuous advancements in radiotherapy technology to enhance accuracy and reduce damage to non-target tissues. Chemotherapy treatment of gynecologic oncology is also hindered by critical barriers, particularly regarding its systemic toxicity and development of resistance. The traditional chemotherapy employs cytotoxic drugs that target proliferating cells indiscriminately, but this strategy of generic targeting often leads to severe side effects. Patients tend to experience gastrointestinal distress, fatigue, and myelosuppression that leaves them vulnerable to infection and anemia. More sinister is the risk of persistent complications such as chemobrain, or cognitive impairment induced by chemotherapy, which affects memory and mental capacity. Furthermore, the emergence of resistant tumor subtypes complicates the treatment; tumors can become resistant to chemotherapy through adaptive mechanisms, including enhanced DNA repair mechanisms and genomic and epigenomic changes (Giannios et al., 2012). All these factors bring about a shift in paradigm towards personalized treatment strategies based on individual patients' molecular profiles to maximize benefits with minimized side effects. Immunotherapy, while being touted as a game-changer in cancer treatment, has its own set of challenges, including those that are related to its efficiency and immune-related toxicities. Some types of gynecologic cancers are inherently resistant to immunotherapy drugs due to the presence of an immunosuppressive tumor environment that may limit the body's ability to deploy therapies that should activate the immune system against cancer (Anning et al., 2022). The infiltration of inhibitory cells like TAMs and MDSCs further prevents treatment by downregulating anti-tumor immune responses. Additionally, the immunologically mediated side effects can be severe, ranging from dermatitis and colitis to more systemic organ involvement, such as pneumonitis and endocrinopathies. Therefore, ongoing research into ways of maximizing the effectiveness of immunotherapy and minimizing its side effects remains crucial in the quest for optimal treatment options in gynecologic cancers.

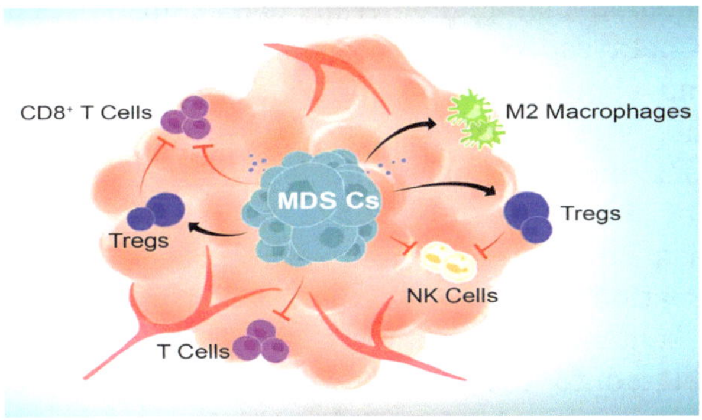

Figure 12.9. Myeloid-derived suppressor cells (MDSCs).

Source: https://resources.rndsystems.com/images/blog/blog-mdsc-header.jpg?v=1

Test Your Knowledge

1. What factors influence the choice of treatment protocols and regimens in gynecologic oncology?
2. What are two major challenges or side effects associated with chemotherapy, and how are they managed?

12.4. Immunotherapy in Gynecology

Learning Outcome

1. Describe the principles of immunotherapy
2. Explain the current immunotherapeutic agents
3. Define clinical trials and outcomes

The combination of immunotherapy with oncology in gynecology has emerged as a revolutionary approach to the treatment of various cancers, particularly in cases where traditional therapies have yielded low results. This innovative type of treatment exploits the body's own immune response to recognize and eliminate cancer cells, making it a good option for advanced or chemotherapy-resistant tumor patients. Current investigations indicate the potential of immunotherapy to maximize patient benefit, especially in neoplasms such as cervical and endometrial cancer, where the choice of therapies is currently limited. It is demonstrated that manipulation of the immune system can not only increase response to therapy but may also induce lasting remissions, reshaping the treatment paradigm in gynecologic oncology essentially. Of specific interest are the findings related to the human microbiota in cancer treatment, which report a symbiotic relationship between microbial communities and the host immune response to treatments. Research indicates that some bacterial signatures correlate with patient responses to immune checkpoint inhibitors, suggesting the microbiome as an "assistant" to achieving optimal therapeutic response. For instance, the role of gut bacteria has been explored extensively in melanoma and cervical cancer, and it has been demonstrated that microbiome profiling can be employed to potentially personalize immunotherapy strategies. This line of study hinges on the complex relationship between microbiome and immunotherapy, with the implication that successful integration of microbiome interventions would boost the effectiveness of immunotherapeutic drugs against gynecological cancers, and more particularly against those which have been the most difficult to treat, as highlighted in Tsakmaklis et al. (2024). Further, growing interest in immunomodulation has been accompanied by interest in novel strategies for the therapy of endometrial cancer. Because this neoplasm is often associated with limited treatment choices for recurrent and metastatic disease, the use of immunotherapy brings new hope. Current updates highlight the significance of active and passive immunotherapies as a means to alter the tumor microenvironment with therapeutic potential in such challenging cases. Evidence shows that these immunotherapeutic approaches are not only more effective but can also possess an improved side effect profile compared to conventional treatments. Extending the armamentarium of endometrial cancer using immunotherapy could lead to new, customized regimens of therapy that address the pressing clinical need for efficacious treatments, as explained in Bobirca et al. (2023).

12.4.1. Principles of Immunotherapy

Immunotherapy has been a revolutionary technique in treating gynecological cancer by utilizing the body's own immune response to fight and destroy cancer cells. Unlike traditional therapies such as chemotherapy or radiotherapy, which target rapidly growing cells directly, immunotherapy enhances the immune system activity against cancer cells by making use of various mechanisms, including monoclonal antibodies and immune checkpoint inhibitors. These medications can harness the strength of T cells and other immune cells to recognize and kill cancer, boosting the survival of patients where conventional treatments have failed. More recent studies indicate the efficacy of immunotherapy for conditions like undifferentiated uterine sarcomas, where previous treatments have been of little help, and researchers have started to study the intricate interaction between tumor biology and immunity (Hardell et al., 2020).

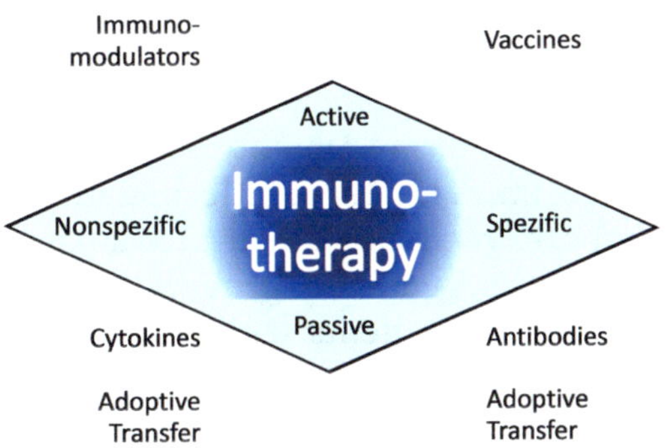

Figure 12.10. The four principles of an immunotherapy intervention: active or passive, and specific or nonspecific.

Source: https://www.researchgate.net/figure/The-four-principles-of-an-immunotherapy-intervention-active-or-passive-and-specific-or_fig6_223136709

A key element of immunotherapy is the detection and application of specific biomarkers to direct decision-making around treatment and predict response. Research has shown that tumors exhibit a heterogeneous phenotype of immune markers, which can influence prognosis in addition to therapeutic strategy. For instance, in low-grade endometrial stromal sarcomas, a favorable prognosis correlated with a low ratio of CD8+/FOXP3+ cells, indicating an improved cytotoxic T cell response. With continuous improvement in the comprehension of immune profiles associated with various gynecologic cancers, personalized immunotherapeutic interventions are now being designed that are specific to a patient's individuality.

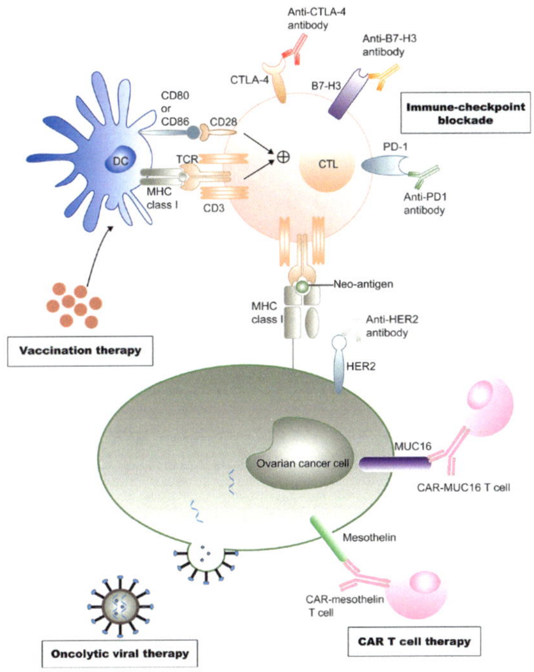

Figure 12.11. Current immunotherapy treatments of ovarian cancer. Ovarian cancer vaccine therapy is based on dendritic cell (DC)-mediated presentation of neo-antigens derived from malignant ovarian cancer cells to T cells through MHC class I–T cell receptors (TCRs) and a co-stimulation signal of CD80 and/or CD86-CD28 interactions.

Source: https://www.frontiersin.org/journals/immunology/articles/10.3389/fimmu.2020.577869/full

These advancements reflect a paradigm shift towards more and more personalized treatment that is attuned to both safety and efficacy in oncology, away from the traditionally dominant one-size-fits-all approach (Giannios et al., 2012). Further, the synergistic effect of immunotherapy with other treatments poses interesting possibilities of enhanced treatment outcomes. The combinatorial treatment is found to increase the overall effectiveness of treatments, particularly for advanced or refractory diseases. For instance, a combination of immunotherapy with chemotherapy or radiotherapy has shown enhanced results in some tumor types by reducing the resistance mechanisms and enhancing immune infiltration. As emerging evidence reveals the complex relationship between cancer and the immune system, it is more and more clear that the manipulation of such interactions can lead to more effective treatment regimens. The exploration of novel immunotherapeutic targets, in association with standard therapies, represents a new era for the fight against gynecologic neoplasias, bringing new hope for doctors and patients (Hardell et al., 2020).

12.4.2. Current Immunotherapeutic Agents

The evolving situation of gynecological cancer therapy puts more emphasis on the potential of immunotherapeutic agents. The novel strategy revolves around the unique challenge of malignancies such as endometrial and ovarian cancers, for which traditional therapies are less effective, particularly in stages of progression. Immunotherapeutic agents attempt to enlist the body's immune system to recognize and attack cancer cells, addressing important deficiencies pertaining to chemotherapy and radiotherapy. Active and passive immunotherapy in endometrial cancer is increasingly promising, emphasizing the importance of new treatment modalities that induce enhanced antitumor reactions. This shift toward tumor microenvironment immunomodulation expresses significant progress, suggesting that current immunotherapeutic agents can greatly improve the outcomes for patients with recurrent or metastatic disease, as evidenced by recent research (Bobirca et al., 2023). Key immunotherapeutic approaches in the context of gynecologic cancer are immune checkpoint inhibitors, monoclonal antibodies, and cancer vaccines. Immune checkpoint inhibitors like pembrolizumab and nivolumab are drugs that block proteins utilized by cancer cells to evade immune-mediated destruction and hence allow intense mechanisms of tumor rejection. In gynecologic contexts, these agents have had promising outcomes in the context of endometrial carcinomas, especially those with microsatellite instability. Monoclonal antibodies, on the other hand, specifically target specific markers of cancer cells to enhance identification and targeting by the immune system. In addition, therapeutic vaccines are designed to trigger an immune response to tumor-associated antigens, promoting long-term immunity. The adoption of these novel immunotherapeutic modalities into standard care regimens constitutes a paradigm shift in the management of gynecologic cancers, offering hope to patients with limited options (Pockley et al., 2013). Although considerable hope is vested in these immunotherapeutic modalities, challenges lie in optimizing their use in the clinic. Tumor microenvironment heterogeneity, immune evasion mechanisms employed by cancer cells, and the presence of immunosuppressive cell populations can all contribute towards the effectiveness of immunotherapy. Notably, tumors can also create immunoregulatory milieus that suppress the growth and activity of protective immune cell populations like T cells and natural killer cells. Overcoming these mechanisms is crucial to further optimizing current therapies as well as activating the maximal potential of immunotherapy in gynecological oncology. Recent research aims to explain how tumor-derived factors influence immune cell migration and function, providing valuable information on the development of more targeted and effective therapeutic interventions. With advances in knowledge, the potential of immunotherapeutic medicines in combination with existing treatment modalities in gynecology continues to be active (Bobirca et al., 2023; Pockley et al., 2013).

12.4.3. Clinical Trials and Outcomes

The therapeutic scenario of gynecologic malignancies, especially epithelial ovarian cancer (EOC), has come a long way with various clinical trials. Besides the application of standard therapies such as cytoreductive surgery along with platinum-based chemotherapy, the survival in most patients is not satisfactory, with 80% recurrence and a median progression-free survival of merely 12 to 18 months. Clinical trials increasingly have focused on novel treatments, including immune checkpoint inhibitors (CPIs), that aim to exploit the body's immune system against cancer. Previous trials have produced disappointing results for CPIs, though, which serve to highlight both the difficulty tumors present for immune evasion and the necessity of continued innovation in treatment design. The study emphasizes the need for research activities to enhance outcomes in patients through complementary treatments to routine treatments (Benedetto et al., 2020).

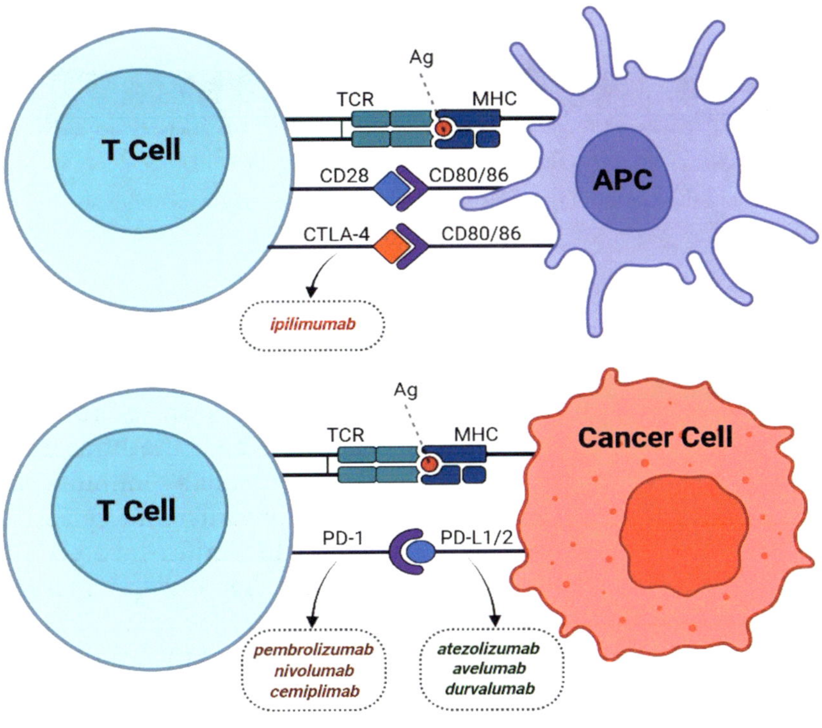

Figure 12.12. FDA-approved classes of immune checkpoint inhibitors (CPIs).

Source: https://www.mdpi.com/2039-7283/13/1/3

New treatment strategies also realize the promise of precision medicine in the future of gynecologic oncology. The most exciting research likely targets Poly (ADP-ribose) polymerase (PARP) inhibitors, which take advantage of the malignant cell's dependence on certain cellular processes for DNA repair. Since 10-15% of EOC patients are hereditary for BRCA mutations, current research has illustrated that these inhibitors have been extremely effective at enhancing the efficacy of treatment in not just BRCA-mutated cells but in a broader category designated as BRCAness. Information regarding tumor genetic profiles is instrumental in tailoring therapy to accommodate patient-specific characteristics. The clinical relevance is robust, with current trials looking at combination therapies that pair PARP inhibitors with other therapies, supporting further continuing these studies to establish the optimal treatment architectures (Caruso et al., 2016). Overall, the exploration of clinical trials in gynecologic cancers underscores the collaboration between researchers, clinicians, and patients in refining treatment paradigms. Clinical outcomes are linked to the evolution of treatment modalities, and these become increasingly individualized. The integration of new treatments into traditional schemas is a turning point in oncology, particularly for malignancies such as ovarian cancer with notoriously unfavorable prognoses. With functional barriers being overcome and new therapies being advanced through trials, the future promises much for improved survival and quality of life for patients with gynecologic malignancies. Continued investment in research plays a key role in opening up not just to an understanding of the complex nature of these cancers but also to the provision of more effective and targeted treatment (Benedetto et al., 2020; Caruso et al., 2016).

Test Your Knowledge

1. What are the basic principles behind immunotherapy in cancer treatment?
2. Name one current immunotherapeutic agent used in the treatment of gynecological cancers.

12.5. Gene Therapy in Gynecology

Learning Outcome

1. Discuss the basics of gene therapy
2. Explain the applications in gynecological cancers
3. Define ethical considerations and challenges

The gynecologic community has now recognized the potential of gene therapy as a therapeutic modality of the future, especially for gynecologic cancers such as cervical cancer. Gene therapy relies on the alteration of genes in an effort to prevent or treat disease, a process that is uniquely advantageous in the instance of malignancies that are resistant to conventional forms of treatment. For cervical cancer, which is still one of the most common gynecologic malignancies and a leading cause of female cancer deaths, there is active research in developing new gene delivery approaches. These involve methods of correcting altered genes, enhancing immune responses, and using oncolytic viruses to selectively destroy cancer cells. This multi-faceted approach holds the promise not only to increase response rates, but to decrease some of the noxious side effects that come with traditional treatments, and thereby enhance the quality of life in those being treated for this disabling illness. And yet, even with encouraging results in preclinical testing with various different targeted systems of gene delivery, translating these developments into effective clinical applications is a formidable challenge. One of the most significant challenges has been the ineffectiveness of current gene delivery vectors, which limit the potential for obtaining sufficient gene expression in target tissues without causing toxicity in normal cells. Further, the heterogeneity of patient responses to gene therapy puts emphasis on personalized approaches based on individual tumor profiles and genetic backgrounds. Advances in nanotechnology, for instance, offer the prospect of improving the specificity and efficiency of gene delivery systems. As more is learned, these obstacles must be addressed to establish gene therapy as a common treatment approach in gynecology (Tsakmaklis et al., 2024). Current research has also demonstrated the vitally important relationship between the human microbiome and the efficacy of cancer treatments, including gene therapy treatments. For example, immune checkpoint inhibitor response has been demonstrated to correlate with gut microbiota differences, indicating personalized therapy could be further refined by considering the effect of microbiomes. Cervical cancer, as an example, in one instance where cervical microbiota composition and bacterial load were analyzed before and after undergoing chemoradiation treatment, exhibited significant variation in composition and bacterial load, making it imperative to discover these interactions in the context of gene therapy. Investigating the microbiome function could bring about synergistic therapies that enhance not only the outcomes of gene therapy but also the treatment regimen of gynecologic cancers. Therefore, integrating microbiome research with the paradigms of gene therapy could provide novel means of augmenting the effectiveness of treatment and the survival of patients (Tsakmaklis et al., 2024).

12.5.1. Basics of Gene Therapy

Gene therapy is a revolutionary approach in the field of oncology, particularly in gynecological oncology, where traditional treatments like radiotherapy and chemotherapy have been found to have numerous limitations. Basically, gene therapy involves changing the genetic composition of a patient's cells to combat disease and consequently treat the root cause of cancers rather than managing symptoms. This new approach includes the insertion of therapeutic genes into a patient's cells using various vectors, for example, virus-engineered vectors, to ensure safety and efficiency. These therapies aim to replace damaged genes, repair aberrant genetic expressions, or even induce apoptosis of cancer cells to enhance outcomes. Since gynecologic malignancies such as cervical and ovarian cancers typically present with significant challenges in treatment, gene therapy is a very promising option or adjuvant to standard therapy, hopefully improving patients' survival and quality of life. Increasing evidence has been gathered in recent years, implying the promise of gene therapy as an effective treatment strategy in gynecologic cancers. Notably, adenoviral vectors have shown promise in delivering therapeutic genes to target cells, demonstrating efficacy in preclinical models and early-phase clinical trials. For instance, investigations into the use of gene therapy for cervical cancer have reported favorable outcomes when combined with existing treatments, such as chemoradiation. These findings suggest that gene therapy could enhance the antitumor efficacy of conventional approaches while potentially mitigating their adverse effects. Besides, as researchers probe further into the molecular origins of gynecological malignancies, the combination of advances in proteomics and genomics can make more precise gene therapy interventions possible, where therapy is customized to individual patient profiles for maximum efficacy (N/A, 2022). Despite the promising progress of gene therapy, barriers are present for the implementation of this novel approach to widespread clinical use for gynecologic cancers. Issues such as the need for target-delivery systems, minimization of off-target effects, and sustained expression of therapeutic genes must be addressed in order to maximize the safety and efficacy of such treatments. In addition, incorporation of gene therapy into established treatment regimens, including immunotherapy and chemotherapy, will necessitate careful understanding and collaborative efforts among oncologists, geneticists, and scientists. As indicated in current literature, the incorporation of gene therapy into gynecologic oncology may prove to be the remedy for breaching the bounds of current conventional treatment strategies (Roche et al., 2019). Increased research and refinement of gene therapy techniques will be key in increasing the clinical efficacy of treatments for cancer patients with gynecologic malignancies, making research in this new subject a necessity.

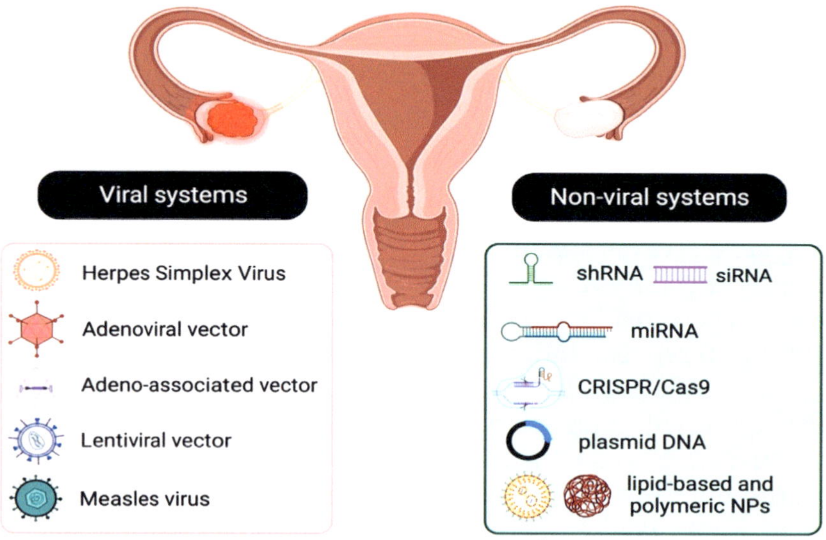

Figure 12.13. Gene therapy strategies for ovarian cancer. These employ viral vectors, such as Herpes Simplex Virus, adenoviral and adeno-associated viral vectors, lentiviral vectors and Measles virus, and non-viral systems, such as shRNA/siRNA/miRNA, DNA plasmids, lipid-based and polymeric NPs and CRISPR/Cas9 approaches. Of note, some of the above approaches, e.g., shRNA, were also delivered via lentiviral vectors.

Source: https://www.mdpi.com/2072-6694/14/13/3238

12.5.2. Applications in Gynecological Cancers

The treatment paradigm for gynecologic cancers has been revolutionized, particularly with the introduction of targeted drugs and immunomodulators that enhance prognoses in patients. Traditionally, surgery combined with adjuvant radiotherapy has been the cornerstone of therapy for locoregional endometrial cancer. However, with the occurrence of metastatic or recurrent disease, conventional chemotherapy is often accompanied by modest results and worry regarding toxicity. Research into immunomodulation within the tumor environment has been a fruitful area of investigation. Present studies show that both active and passive immunotherapy hold the potential to treat endometrial cancer, offering hope for patients with advanced disease whose conventional treatment options have been exhausted (Bobirca et al., 2023). New modalities of treatment, such as personalized medicine, are increasingly being used in gynecologic oncology. Personalized medicine capitalizes on pharmacogenomics to tailor treatment protocols to the molecular signature of every patient's tumor. This is intended to decrease the harmful side effects of conventional chemotherapy, which inadvertently stimulate drug resistance and induce severe side effects like immunosuppression and organ toxicity (Giannios et al., 2012). With a comprehension of the unique genetic and epigenetic alterations within a tumor, clinicians can more effectively personalize therapeutic interventions, reducing systemic toxicity while increasing effective response. Not only does this personalized approach maximize the potential for successful treatment, but it also helps contribute to optimizing the patient's quality of life as they navigate the gynecologic cancers. Beyond that, the integration of gene therapy in the treatment of gynecologic cancers provides yet another field of possible innovation. This method involves the direct manipulation of cancer cell genetic material to alter its function. By targeting specific tumorigenic mutations, gene therapy can potentially halt or even reverse disease progression. Emerging evidence indicates that the combination of gene therapy with immunotherapeutic drugs can enhance antitumor response and thus overall therapeutic efficacy. As the gynecologic oncology science evolves, it is important to adopt these newer therapeutic modalities, since they not only bypass the limitations of the conventional modalities but also hold promise for patients with challenging gynecologic cancers.

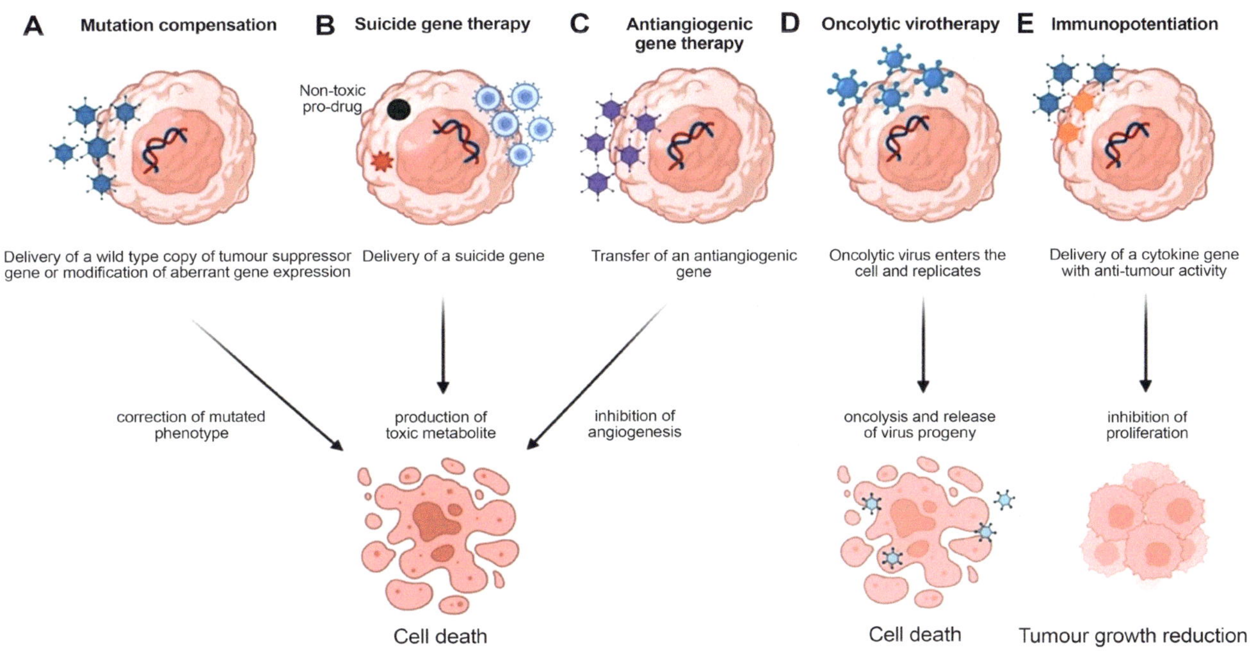

Figure 12.14. Main targeted gene therapy approaches for gynecological benign and malignant disorders. Strategies include (A) mutation compensation using adenoviral vectors to correct gene expression; (B) suicide gene therapy, such as HSV-TK, inducing cell death via toxic metabolites; (C) antiangiogenic gene therapy to inhibit tumor angiogenesis; (D) oncolytic virotherapy, where viruses replicate within and destroy cancer cells; and (E) immunopotentiation through delivery of cytokine genes to stimulate anti-tumor immunity.

Source: https://www.mdpi.com/2072-6694/14/13/3238

12.5.3. Ethical Considerations and Challenges

In the management of gynecologic cancer—such as with radiotherapy, chemotherapy, immunotherapy, and gene therapy—the ethical conflict is rather usual due to the complexity of patient care and variability of conceivable benefits and risks for each modality. One of the larger ethical concerns is informed consent, since patients must navigate complicated treatment choices that are often full of jargon and technicalities. It is required that healthcare professionals give patients full knowledge of their treatment choices, such as the chances of unwanted side effects and the rates of success. This requirement points towards the requirement of effective communication strategies in clinical practice, where healthcare professionals are tasked with de-mystifying treatment choices and establishing a relationship of trust. With changing treatment modalities, primarily immunotherapy and gene therapy, the need for broad-based ethical guidelines becomes increasingly pertinent to allow patients to make decisions based on well-informed choices that reflect their values and beliefs. The second important ethical concern is inclusive access to novel therapies because healthcare disparities can have a significant impact on the outcomes of treatment. They may be deprived of access to new drugs such as immunotherapy and gene therapy, which are very costly. This inequality raises traditional ethical dilemmas of fairness and justice in the distribution of healthcare. Furthermore, the evolving landscape in personalized medicine, in which the treatment plan is tailored to a patient's unique genetic patterns, necessitates that all patients, regardless of socioeconomic status, have access to the necessary testing and therapies. Correcting these disparities is critical to making advancements in gynecologic oncology accessible to a diverse patient population, thereby maintaining the ethical ideal of justice in medical ethics, which fosters equal opportunities of treatment for all members, irrespective of their background. Lastly, the unpredictability of the long-term outcomes of novel therapies adds another ethical twist to their integration into practice. For instance, while gene therapy is theoretically able to transform the treatment of gynecological cancers, its long-term patient and intergenerational implications are as yet largely unexplored. Clinicians and patients are therefore forced to weigh up short-term therapeutic advantage against untold long-term implications as gene therapy evolves. Additionally, there are bioethics concerns about monitoring and handling potential complications, and the clinician's responsibility to monitor patients for long periods after treatment. Moreover, as explained by Awada et al. (2016), the need for specialist training and adherence to ethical guidelines becomes imperative in delivering the safety and efficacy of these evolving therapies. By addressing these ethical concerns, the health profession can play an important role in enhancing patient outcomes while upholding ethical concepts in gynecologic oncology.

Test Your Knowledge

1. What is the basic concept of gene therapy and how does it work?
2. How can gene therapy be applied in the treatment of gynecological cancers?

SUMMARY

With the evolution of the specialty of gynecologic oncology, the combination of radiotherapy, chemotherapy, immunotherapy, and gene therapy is a significant advance in maximizing patient outcomes. All modalities of treatment have their role to play in the killing of gynecological cancers and constitute an arsenal that can be tailored to patient profiles. Radiotherapy and chemotherapy are established stalwarts in the management of malignancies, with different mechanisms operating to kill cancer cells. Conversely, immunotherapy is grabbing the limelight in the use of the body's immune system and giving hope to patients since traditional therapies are not doing much. The entire system facilitates the notion that there is no one treatment modality that can fit every patient, thereby stressing the use of a personalized medicine paradigm in gynecologic oncology. The recent findings in the investigation of tumor microenvironments indicate that therapies, particularly immunotherapies, can face many barriers. As noted, immune checkpoint blockade therapies are hindered by immunosuppressive cells, including tumor-associated macrophages and myeloid-derived suppressor cells that create resistance to treatment (Anning et al., 2022). Innovative solutions, for instance, Cucurbitacin B, have emerged, targeting such cells with the hope of enhancing the effectiveness of immunotherapy. This highlights a key focus area of future research where bridging the gap between basic research and therapeutic application has the ability to yield paradigm shifts in the management of refractory forms of gynecological malignancies. Extensive discussion at conventions, such as that conducted by GYNOCARE, is the arena where these findings get disseminated and encourages interaction among researchers, clinicians, and biotechnologists (Calleja-Agius et al., 2023). The outcome of these processes is one aspect of a broader trend towards better patient care. Ongoing clinical trials and innovative treatment approaches are holding out the promise of more efficient ways of treating rare gynecologic malignancies. The emphasis on individualized treatment indicates the necessity of knowing individual patient characteristics, such as genetic profile and tumor biology. Greater collaboration among the pharmaceutical industry, biotech firms, and universities will assist in finding new answers in gynecological oncology. Cooperation is central to bringing research discoveries into clinical practice, ultimately aiming not only to improve survival rates but also patients' quality of life with a gynecologic cancer diagnosis. Thus, ongoing refinement of therapeutic modalities, coupled with an emphasis on innovative research, will be required to advance the discipline further.

The therapeutic context for gynecologic cancers provides a variety of treatment modalities, such as radiotherapy, chemotherapy, immunotherapy, and gene therapy, all of which play significant roles in improving patient outcomes. Radiotherapy, typically used as a localized modality, impacts the cancer cells with minimal damage to surrounding tissues. It is most beneficial in the treatment of cervical cancer and is often employed in combination with other treatments to generate synergistic effects. Chemotherapy, on the other hand, is a systemic therapy that eliminates proliferating cancer cells, but may cause damage to normal tissues and lead to severe side effects. The use of these treatments combined is generally patient-specific, emphasizing the role of personalized medicine in gynecologic oncology for a more successful treatment. Immunotherapy has emerged as a novel approach in recent years through which the body's immune system is used to combat gynecologic cancers. This treatment has a number of agents, such as monoclonal antibodies and immune checkpoint inhibitors, that enhance the immune response to cancer cells. The efficacy of immunotherapy in diseases like ovarian cancer has sparked significant interest in ongoing clinical trials on the understanding of its long-term impact and co-administration with existing therapies. In addition, the exploration of newer technologies such as CAR-T cell therapy holds a promising future for immunotherapeutic interventions in improving survival and quality of life among women with these cancers. Gene therapy is a groundbreaking technique in the management of gynecologic cancers by enabling the direct manipulation of the genetic material of cancer cells. This new strategy aims to correct damaged genes or introduce new genes with the potential to initiate a healing response, thereby inhibiting tumor growth or enhancing existing therapy. Genetic alteration studies are also aided by breakthroughs in areas such as genomics and epigenomics, extensively discussed in articles such as those in the special issue of Biomedicines (N/A, 2022). With continued study, it will be necessary to understand the molecular landscape of gynecologic cancers in order to create targeted therapies with better prognoses against this increasingly prevalent class of diseases, underlining continued funding for both basic and clinical research initiatives (Institute A of Health and Welfare).

KEY TERMS FROM THIS CHAPTER

- Cervical cancers
- Chemotherap
- Gastrointestinal toxicity
- Gene therapy
- Genetic pathogenesis
- Gynecologic cancers
- Gynecological tumors
- Immune microenvironment
- Individualized therapeutic treatment
- Radiotherapy technology
- Checkpoint inhibitors (CPIs)
- External beam radiotherapy (EBRT)
- Gene delivery
- Genetic mutations
- Gynecologic cancer treatment
- Gynecologic oncology
- Immune infiltration
- Immunomodulators
- Radiotherapy
- Systemic toxicity

CRITICAL THINKING QUESTIONS

1. **Which of the following is the primary goal of radiotherapy in gynecologic cancers?**
   a. To stimulate the immune system to attack cancer cells
   b. To kill or damage cancer cells using high-energy radiation
   c. To deliver genetic material into cancer cells
   d. To block hormone receptors in cancer cells
2. **Which chemotherapy drug is commonly used in the treatment of cervical cancer?**
   a. Paclitaxel
   b. Imatinib
   c. Rituximab
   d. Trastuzumab
3. **Immunotherapy in gynecologic oncology often involves:**
   a. Using radiation to shrink tumors
   b. Using antibodies or checkpoint inhibitors to enhance the immune response
   c. Delivering genes that code for tumor suppressors
   d. Directly killing cancer cells with cytotoxic drugs
4. **Gene therapy in gynecological cancers aims to:**
   a. Replace mutated or defective genes to restore normal cell function
   b. Increase the dosage of chemotherapy drugs
   c. Enhance radiotherapy effects by increasing radiation dose
   d. Stimulate hormone production in cancer cells
5. **Which of the following is a common side effect of chemotherapy in gynecologic cancer patients?**
   a. Hair loss (alopecia)
   b. Increased bone density
   c. Improved fertility
   d. Hyperpigmentation of the skin

Short Answer Questions

1. What are the common types of gynecological cancers?
2. What are the basic principles of radiotherapy in treating gynecological cancers?
3. How does chemotherapy work in managing gynecological cancers?
4. What are the advantages and limitations of immunotherapy in gynecologic oncology?
5. How effective is immunotherapy in treating advanced-stage gynecological cancers?
6. What is the role of gene therapy in the treatment of gynecological cancers?

Answer to Critical Thinking Questions

1. (b) 2. (a) 3. (b) 4. (a) 5. (a)

REFERENCES

1. Ahmad, M. F., Chang, S. J., Chen, X., Chung, Y., et al. (2019). Asian Society of Gynecologic Oncology International Workshop 2018. https://core.ac.uk/download/628899334.pdf (accessed on 15th June 2025).
2. Altavilla, A., Brighi, N., Casadei, C., Conteduca, V., De Giorgi, U., Farolfi, A., Iaia, M. L., et al. (2021). Immunotherapy and its development for gynecological (ovarian, endometrial and cervical) tumors: From immune checkpoint inhibitors to chimeric antigen receptor (CAR)-T cell therapy. https://core.ac.uk/download/490668382.pdf (accessed on 15th June 2025).
3. Amaral, T., Audisio, R., Dopazo Taboada, C., Sandrucci, S., et al. (2021). The ESSO core curriculum committee update on surgical oncology. https://core.ac.uk/download/534957948.pdf (accessed on 15th June 2025).
4. Anning, E. (2022). Cucurbitacin B: A potential natural agent for targeting tumor immune cell population. https://core.ac.uk/download/578747814.pdf (accessed on 15th June 2025).
5. Australian Institute of Health and Welfare. (2025). *National Health Data Dictionary: Version 16.2*. https://core.ac.uk/download/pdf/30672426.pdf (accessed on 15th June 2025).
6. Awada, A., Eniu, A., Grothey, A., Kiss, A., Palumbo, A., Glaudemans, A. W. J. M., Coiffier, B., et al. (2016). ESMO/ASCO recommendations for a global curriculum in medical oncology edition 2016. https://core.ac.uk/download/187972852.pdf (accessed on 15th June 2025).
7. Benedetto, C., Borella, F., Cosma, S., Ghisoni, M., et al. (2020). Immune checkpoint inhibitors in epithelial ovarian cancer: An overview on efficacy and future perspectives. https://core.ac.uk/download/326909114.pdf (accessed on 15th June 2025).
8. Bobirca, A., Bobirca, F., Gaube, A., Georgescu, M., et al. (2023). The evolving landscape of immunotherapy in uterine cancer: A comprehensive review. https://core.ac.uk/download/581039138.pdf (accessed on 15th June 2025).
9. Bonasera, A., Caputo, G., Centonze, D., Di Mattia, A., et al. (2025). Brain metastasis in endometrial cancer: A systematic review. https://core.ac.uk/download/639005159.pdf (accessed on 15th June 2025).
10. Boulaiz Tassi, H., Jiménez Martínez, Y., & Áyen, Á. (2020). Targeted gene delivery therapies for cervical cancer. https://core.ac.uk/download/328867906.pdf (accessed on 15th June 2025).
11. Bouzid, R., Buschow, S. I., & Peppelenbosch, M. P. (2020). Opportunities for conventional and *in situ* cancer vaccine strategies and combination with immunotherapy for gastrointestinal cancers: A review. https://core.ac.uk/download/322667979.pdf (accessed on 15th June 2025).
12. Bützow, R., Loukovaara, M., & Pasanen, A. (2022). Molecular classification of endometrial carcinoma: A clinically oriented review. https://core.ac.uk/download/558722577.pdf (accessed on 15th June 2025).
13. Calleja-Agius, J. (2023). Bridging the gap between research and cure in rare gynecological cancers: Where do we stand? Report from the GYNOCARE Conference in Naples (17th–18th February 2023). https://core.ac.uk/download/566460289.pdf (accessed on 15th June 2025).
14. Caruso, D., Papa, A., Strudel, M., Tomao, S., et al. (2016). Update on poly-ADP-ribose polymerase inhibition for ovarian cancer treatment. https://core.ac.uk/download/98332573.pdf (accessed on 15th June 2025).

15. Cicinelli, E., Cormio, G., De Nola, R., & Loizzi, V. (2020). Dynamic crosstalk within the tumor microenvironment of uterine cervical carcinoma: Baseline network, iatrogenic alterations, and translational implications. https://core.ac.uk/download/589941771.pdf (accessed on 15th June 2025).

16. Copeland, L. I. B. T., James, D., Duinkerken, M. S. I., Kelsey, G., et al. (2019). Jefferson Digital Commons quarterly report: October–December 2019. https://core.ac.uk/download/286097805.pdf (accessed on 15th June 2025).

17. de Vries, E. G. E., Eggen, A. C., Hooiveld-Noeken, J. S., Jalving, M., et al. (2022). Towards less mutilating treatments in patients with advanced non-melanoma skin cancers by earlier use of immune checkpoint inhibitors. https://core.ac.uk/download/548540705.pdf (accessed on 15th June 2025).

18. Giannios, J. (2012). From cancer researcher to opinion leadership and advocacy in translational medicine. https://core.ac.uk/download/573860047.pdf (accessed on 15th June 2025).

19. Hamade, D. F., Epperly, M. W., Fisher, R., Hou, W. C., Shields, D., van Pijkeren, J. P., Leibowitz, B. J., et al. (2024). Genetically engineered probiotic *Limosilactobacillus reuteri* releasing IL-22 (LR-IL-22) modifies the tumor microenvironment, enabling irradiation in ovarian cancer. *Cancers, 16*, 474–474. https://doi.org/10.3390/cancers16030474 (accessed on 15th June 2025).

20. Hardell, E. (2020). Prognosis based classification and tumor biology of uterine sarcomas. https://core.ac.uk/download/323274871.pdf (accessed on 15th June 2025).

21. Heinzelmann-Schwarz, V., & Vetter, M. (2017). Immunotherapy in gynecologic cancers. https://core.ac.uk/download/322430184.pdf (accessed on 15th June 2025).

22. Kazemi, M., Sadri, M., Najafi, A., Rahimi, A., Baghernejadan, Z., Khorramdelazad, H., & Falak, R. (2022). Tumor-infiltrating lymphocytes for treatment of solid tumors: It takes two to tango? *Frontiers in Immunology, 13*. https://doi.org/10.3389/fimmu.2022.1018962 (accessed on 15th June 2025).

23. Mackay, H. J., Mileshkin, L., & Wenzel, L. (2015). Nonsurgical management of cervical cancer: Locally advanced, recurrent, and metastatic disease, survivorship, and beyond. https://core.ac.uk/download/591731101.pdf (accessed on 15th June 2025).

24. Pockley, A. G., Multhoff, G., Foulds, G. A., Radons, J., & Kreuzer, M. (2013). Influence of tumors on protective anti-tumor immunity and the effects of irradiation. https://core.ac.uk/download/30630615.pdf (accessed on 15th June 2025).

25. Sharma, D., & Sharma, N. (2020). Immunotherapy in gynecological malignancies. https://core.ac.uk/download/322446073.pdf (accessed on 15th June 2025).

26. Sun, L., Liu, H., Ye, Y., Yang, L., Islam, R., Tan, S., Tong, R., et al. (2023). Smart nanoparticles for cancer therapy. *Signal Transduction and Targeted Therapy, 8*. https://doi.org/10.1038/s41392-023-01642-x (accessed on 15th June 2025).

27. Torres de la Roche, L. A. (2019). Clinical outcomes of therapies for early-stage invasive uterine cervical cancer: A single-institution retrospective study. https://core.ac.uk/download/622925094.pdf (accessed on 15th June 2025).

INDEX

D

E

F

W

Z